Hepatitis: Clinical Research

Hepatitis: Clinical Research

Edited by Sophie Harrison

hayle
medical

New York

Hayle Medical,
750 Third Avenue, 9th Floor,
New York, NY 10017, USA

Visit us on the World Wide Web at:
www.haylemedical.com

ISBN: 978-1-63241-909-5

Cataloging-in-Publication Data

Hepatitis : clinical research / edited by Sophie Harrison.
p. cm.
Includes bibliographical references and index.
ISBN 978-1-63241-909-5
1. Hepatitis. 2. Hepatitis--Treatment. 3. Hepatology. I. Harrison, Sophie.
RC848.H42 H47 2020
616.362 3--dc23

Table of Contents

Preface

Hepatitis is a clinical condition in which the tissues of the liver become inflamed. It can be a temporary manifestation or a chronic condition lasting for six months or more. The former may resolve by itself, or may progress to chronic disease and even to acute liver failure. The chronic state may potentially lead to liver scarring, liver failure and even cancer. Viruses are primary cause of hepatitis. Other factors such as excessive alcohol consumption, certain toxins and medications, non-alcoholic steatohepatitis and autoimmune diseases may also contribute to this condition. Hepatitis A, B, C, D and E are the main types of viral hepatitis. Symptoms such as yellowing of the skin or the whites of the eyes, vomiting, abdominal pain, poor appetite or diarrhea may occur in this condition. Its diagnosis is generally possible through an evaluation of presenting signs and symptoms, substance use history, sexual history, blood tests and liver biopsy. Once diagnosed, hepatitis is treated depending on the type and severity of the disease and its underlying cause. Hepatitis is largely preventable through immunization, in particular the A, B and D types. Medication, healthy lifestyle, proper diet and weight loss are important for its management. This book brings forth some of the most innovative concepts and elucidates the unexplored aspects of hepatology. Different approaches, evaluations, methodologies and advanced studies on hepatitis diagnosis and management have been included in this book. It will prove to be immensely beneficial to students and researchers in hepatology.

This book is a result of research of several months to collate the most relevant data in the field.

When I was approached with the idea of this book and the proposal to edit it, I was overwhelmed. It gave me an opportunity to reach out to all those who share a common interest with me in this field. I had 3 main parameters for editing this text:

1. Accuracy – The data and information provided in this book should be up-to-date and valuable to the readers.

2. Structure – The data must be presented in a structured format for easy understanding and better grasping of the readers.

3. Universal Approach – This book not only targets students but also experts and innovators in the field, thus my aim was to present topics which are of use to all.

Thus, it took me a couple of months to finish the editing of this book.

I would like to make a special mention of my publisher who considered me worthy of this opportunity and also supported me throughout the editing process. I would also like to thank the editing team at the back-end who extended their help whenever required.

Editor

Hepatitis C Virus Induces the Cannabinoid Receptor 1

David van der Poorten[1], Mahsa Shahidi[1], Enoch Tay[1], Jayshree Sesha[1], Kayla Tran[2], Duncan McLeod[2], Jane S. Milliken[2], Vikki Ho[1], Lionel W. Hebbard[1], Mark W. Douglas[1,3], Jacob George[1]*

1 Storr Liver Unit, Westmead Millennium Institute, University of Sydney at Westmead Hospital, Sydney, Australia, **2** Department of Anatomical Pathology, Institute of Clinical Pathology and Medical Research (ICPMR), Westmead Hospital, Sydney, Australia, **3** Centre for Infectious Diseases and Microbiology, Westmead Hospital, Sydney, Australia

Abstract

Background: Activation of hepatic CB_1 receptors (CB_1) is associated with steatosis and fibrosis in experimental forms of liver disease. However, CB_1 expression has not been assessed in patients with chronic hepatitis C (CHC), a disease associated with insulin resistance, steatosis and metabolic disturbance. We aimed to determine the importance and explore the associations of CB_1 expression in CHC.

Methods: CB_1 receptor mRNA was measured by real time quantitative PCR on extracted liver tissue from 88 patients with CHC (genotypes 1 and 3), 12 controls and 10 patients with chronic hepatitis B (CHB). The Huh7/JFH1 Hepatitis C virus (HCV) cell culture model was used to validate results.

Principal Findings: CB_1 was expressed in all patients with CHC and levels were 6-fold higher than in controls ($P<0.001$). CB_1 expression increased with fibrosis stage, with cirrhotics having up to a 2 fold up-regulation compared to those with low fibrosis stage ($p<0.05$). Even in mild CHC with no steatosis (F0-1), CB_1 levels remained substantially greater than in controls ($p<0.001$) and in those with mild CHB (F0-1; $p<0.001$). Huh7 cells infected with JFH-1 HCV showed an 8-fold upregulation of CB_1, and CB_1 expression directly correlated with the percentage of cells infected over time, suggesting that CB_1 is an HCV inducible gene. While HCV structural proteins appear essential for CB_1 induction, there was no core genotype specific difference in CB_1 expression. CB_1 significantly increased with steatosis grade, primarily driven by patients with genotype 3 CHC. In genotype 3 patients, CB_1 correlated with SREBP-1c and its downstream target FASN (SREBP-1c; R=0.37, FASN; R=0.39, p<0.05 for both).

Conclusions/Significance: CB_1 is up-regulated in CHC and is associated with increased steatosis in genotype 3. It is induced by the hepatitis C virus.

Editor: Jean-Pierre Vartanian, Institut Pasteur, France

Funding: This work was funded by the Gastroenterological Society of Australia (GESA) Postgraduate Medical Scholarship (DVDP), Australian National Health and Medical Research Council #402577, #219282 (JG), CJ Martin Fellowship (MD) and the Robert W. Storr Bequest to the University of Sydney (JG). The funders had no role in study design, data collection and analysis, decision to publish, or preparation of the manuscript.

Competing Interests: Dr. David van der Poorten, Mark Douglas and Jacob George have filed a provisional patent on their findings of the relationship between CB_1 and the hepatitis C virus.

* E-mail: jacob.george@sydney.edu.au

Introduction

Chronic Hepatitis C (CHC) is one of the most common causes of hepatic fibrosis and cirrhosis with the World Health Organization (WHO) estimating that up to 3% (180 million people) of the world's population are affected [1]. The pathogenic processes by which hepatitis C virus (HCV) causes liver fibrosis are incompletely understood, but include immune activation, direct cytopathic effects, activation of hepatic stellate cells, induction of insulin resistance and hepatic steatosis [2]. A number of clinical factors are associated with fibrosis progression in CHC including male gender, duration of infection, age at infection, excessive alcohol use [3] and most recently, daily cannabis smoking [4]. There are genotype-specific associations with steatosis: HCV genotype 1 induces steatosis in association with insulin resistance [5]; HCV genotype 3 directly induces steatosis [6] independent of other metabolic risk factors, which resolves following successful

anti-viral therapy [7]. Steatosis in CHC is associated with liver fibrosis [8], an increased risk of liver cancer [9], and higher levels of viral replication [10].

Cannabis (*Cannabis Sativa*, marijuana) has been used for medicinal and ritual purposes for over 3 millennia, and remains the most commonly used recreational drug in the western world [11]. The identification of the cannabinoid receptor 1 (CB_1) in human brain some twenty years ago [12] and the subsequent discovery of endogenous cannabinoids, has led to an understanding of the importance of the endocannabinoid system in health and disease. There are two G protein-coupled cannabinoid receptors; CB_1 and CB_2 [13]. CB_1 is found in high concentrations in the brain, but is also present in many peripheral tissues such as the liver, adipose tissue and gut. CB_2 is found primarily in the immune system, but is also expressed in peripheral tissues including the liver [14]. The two best characterised endocannabinoids (ECBs) are arachidonoylethanolamide (anandamide) and

2-arachidonoyl-glycerol (2-AG). ECBs acting through CB_1 have a strong anabolic effect and play an important role in appetite stimulation and normal energy homeostasis [14,15]. CB_1 blockade confers resistance to the development of diet-induced obesity [16], increases adiponectin levels, reduces triglyceride levels and causes weight loss independent of food intake [17,18]. CB_1 activation therefore is associated with obesity, insulin resistance and dyslipidaemia.

Data detailing the importance of the endocannabinoid system to hepatic disease remains limited. CB_1 and CB_2 receptors are weakly expressed in normal liver, but are strongly up-regulated in experimental liver injury and cirrhosis due to alcohol, hepatitis B, and primary biliary cirrhosis [19]. CB_1 inactivation has been shown to inhibit the progression of fibrosis in three models of liver injury [19]; conversely, CB_2 blockade enhances experimental liver fibrosis [20] and CB_2 activation causes partial fibrotic reversal in cirrhotic rats [21]. CB_1 receptors have been shown to mediate both alcohol [22] and diet [18] induced hepatic steatosis by up regulating the lipogenic transcription factor SREBP-1c and increasing *de novo* fatty acid synthesis [18]. In the obese Zucker rat model, treatment with a CB_1 antagonist abolished hepato-megaly and steatosis, and caused normalisation of liver enzymes [23]. Furthermore, in well characterised cohorts with CHC, daily cannabis use, which was reported in 32% of patients, was significantly associated with the progression of fibrosis and the development of severe steatosis and fibrosis [4,24].

Thus, there is good reason to believe that the endocannabinoid system is of importance in hepatitis C and may be involved in the metabolic dysregulation, hepatic steatosis, hepatic fibrogenesis and insulin resistance of CHC. To date however, the cannabinoid receptors have not been definitively identified in association with hepatitis C, nor has their significance been directly examined. In this study we demonstrate for the first time that the CB_1 receptor is present in all patients with hepatitis C and is significantly up-regulated when compared with controls. We show that CB_1 receptor expression increases with fibrosis stage and is associated with increased steatosis. Moreover, through the use of the Huh7/JFH1 HCV cell culture model, we demonstrate that CB_1 up-regulation is also a viral effect, independent of hepatic inflammation and fibrosis.

Methods

Ethics statement

The study protocol was approved by the Human Ethics Committee of the Western Sydney Area Health Service and written informed consent was obtained from all participants.

Patient selection

Study subjects were selected from a prospectively collected database of over 400 patients with chronic HCV infection who underwent liver biopsy at Westmead Hospital. All subjects had antibodies against HCV (Monolisa anti-HCV; Sanofi Diagnostics Pasteur, Marnes-la-Coquette, France) and detectable HCV RNA by PCR (Amplicor HCV; Roche Diagnostics, Branchburg, NJ, USA). Hepatitis C virus genotyping was performed with a second generation reverse hybridization line probe assay (Inno-Lipa HCV II; Innogenetics, Zwijndrecht, Belgium). Of 446 patients in total, only the 372 with genotype 1 or 3 disease were included. Of these, 193 patients with additional risk factors for liver steatosis or fibrosis other than HCV; ie those with diabetes, obesity (BMI>30 kg/m^2), significant alcohol intake (>20 g/day) or dyslipidaemia (Total cholesterol >5.5 mmol/L, LDL >4 mmol/L, HDL <1 mmol/L or TG >2 mmol/L) were excluded. 87 were excluded due to lack

of stored liver tissue or serum, or poor quality RNA. 11% of the cohort had smoked cannabis within the last year. Four patients who used cannabis daily were excluded in line with recent data showing that only regular daily use is a risk factor for the progression of fibrosis and steatosis [4,24]. This left 88 study participants. No patient had clinical evidence of hepatic decompensation at the time of biopsy.

Clinical and Laboratory Evaluation

A complete physical examination was performed on each subject. On the morning of the liver biopsy, venous blood was drawn after a 12 hour overnight fast to determine the serum levels of alanine aminotransferase (ALT), albumin, bilirubin, platelet count, international normalized ratio, glucose and insulin. Hepatitis C viral load was measured by PCR (Amplicor HCV; Roche Diagnostics, Branchburg, NJ, USA) with a dynamic range of 100–850,000 IU/mL. Serum insulin was determined by radio-immunoassay (Phadaseph insulin RIA; Pharmacia and Upjohn Diagnostics AB, Uppsala, Sweden). Insulin resistance was calculated by the homeostasis model (HOMA-IR) using the following formula: HOMA-IR = fasting insulin (mU/L) × plasma glucose (mmol/L)/22.5. All other biochemical tests were performed using a conventional automated analyzer within the Department of Clinical Chemistry at Westmead Hospital.

Histopathology

All liver biopsy specimens were scored semi-quantitatively using the Scheuer score [25] by an experienced hepatopathologist blinded to clinical data. Portal/periportal inflammatory grade and fibrosis stage was scored from 0 to 4. Steatosis was graded 0 to 3 as follows; 0: <2% fat, 1: 2–10% fat, 2: 10–30% fat, 3: >30% fat. Patients with steatosis grades 2–3 were grouped together for statistical purposes.

Control and Hepatitis B subjects

Twelve healthy controls had a core liver biopsy at the time of cholecystectomy or benign tumor resection. All had normal liver tests, negative serology for chronic viral hepatitis and no history of liver disease or T2DM and normal liver histology. Ten patients with chronic hepatitis B, low fibrosis and no steatosis on biopsy (F0-1) were selected from a prospectively collected database. These patients had a positive HBsAg, and raised ALT at the time of biopsy.

Huh7/JFH-1 (Japanese fulminant hepatitis) cell line

Huh7 cells were transfected with JFH-1 strain of hepatitis C by electroporation and passaged in culture for 3 weeks until over 90% of cells were infected, as previously described [26]. HCV infection was confirmed by immunofluorescence, using antibodies against HCV NS5A protein (provided by Prof Mark Harris, University of Leeds). For the time course studies, Huh7 cells were infected by incubating overnight with supernatant from JFH-1 infected Huh7 cells. Cells were then monitored for 26 days, with HCV infection confirmed by immunofluorescence microscopy as above.

Subgenomic replicon and Genotype 1 and 3 Chimeric virus

Huh7 cells were transfected with a subgenomic replicon based on the JFH-1 HCV strain, expressing nonstructural proteins NS3 to NS5B and containing a neomycin (G418) resistance gene [27]. Cells were passaged for 3 weeks in G418 (250 μg/mL) until only transfected cells survived. Immunofluorescence confirmed that over 90% of cells were infected. Chimeric viruses containing core protein from genotype 1b (N strain) or genotype 3a (HCV3a-GLa)

[28] were used to transfect Huh7 cells as described above. Cells were passaged in culture until over 90% were infected.

RNA extraction and cDNA synthesis

Total RNA was isolated from liver and cell culture samples using the RNeasy Mini Kit (Qiagen, Hilden, Germany) according to the manufacturer's protocol. RNA quality analysis was then performed using an Agilent 2100 Bioanalyser (Agilent Technologies, Palo Alto, CA, USA) as per the manufacturer's instructions. Total RNA with an integrity number >7 was considered acceptable. 200 ng and 1 ug of liver and cell RNA respectively was then reverse transcribed to first strand complementary DNA (cDNA) using Superscript III RT kit (Invitrogen, Carlsbad, CA, USA) and random primers.

Gene expression by Real-time PCR

Real-time quantitative PCR (qPCR) was performed using a Corbett Rotor-gene 6000 (Corbett life sciences, Mortlake, Australia). Amplifications were performed in a 10 uL reaction containing 4 uL of cDNA, 5 uL of Platinum qPCR Super-mix (Invitrogen, Carlsbad, CA, USA) and 0.25 uL of either CB_1, SREBP-1c or FASN Taqman primer probe (Applied Biosystems, Foster City, CA, USA). Amplification conditions were according to the manufacturer's protocol. The housekeeper gene 18S was used as an internal control. CB_1 mRNA was quantitated using Corbett Rotor-gene series software v1.7 (Corbett life sciences, Mortlake, Australia) and values were expressed relative to 18S. For all cell culture experiments, 3 replicates of control and infected cells were assayed and the mean values reported.

Western Blot and Immunohistochemistry

The relative tissue content of CB_1 protein was assessed by western blot analysis using CB_1 receptor antibody (Sigma, product no. C1233). Cells or liver biopsy tissue was processed using the Proteo-extract ^{TM} sub cellular proteome extraction kit (Calbiochem, San Diego, USA) to purify membrane fraction associated protein. Protein (100 µg) was run on a 10% PAGE gel and blotted onto nitrocellulose membranes. Membranes were blocked with 5% skim milk powder in TBST (0.1% Tween) for 1 hour and incubated overnight at 4°C with anti-CB_1 antibody at a dilution of 1:1000 (diluted in 5% skim milk powder/TBST). Membrane were then washed 3X in TBST and incubated with appropriate horse-radish peroxidase conjugated secondary antibody and the resulting signal detected using the Supersignal luminescent detection system (Thermo Scientific, Rockford IL, USA). CB_1 bands were further quantitated by densitometry using ImageJ software (ImageJ, NIH, Bethesda USA [29]), with values normalised to the loading control dye (Amido Black). For immunohistochemistry, formalin fixed, paraffin embedded 4 µsections were stained using a Ventana Benchmark Immunostainer (Ventana Medical Systems, Inc, Arizona, USA). Detection was performed using Ventana's Ultra View DAB kit (Roche/Ventana 05269806001) using the following protocol: The sections were dewaxed with Ventana EZ Prep. Endogenous peroxidase activity was blocked using the Ventana inhibitor in the kit. Anti cannabinoid receptor 1 antibody (Cayman, product no. 10006590; Cayman Chemical, Ann Arbor, MI, USA) was diluted in Biocare's DaVinci Green diluent (Biocare Medical-Concord, CA 94520) for 32 mins at 42°C. The site of the antigen was visualised with Ventana's Ultra View DAB kit. The sections were counterstained with Ventana Haematoxylin and blued with Ventana Blueing Solution. On completion of staining the sections were dehydrated in alcohol, cleared in Xylene and mounted in Permount. Negative controls where the primary antibody was excluded confirmed the specificity of immunostaining.

Statistical Analysis

Statistical analysis was carried out using SPSS version 16.0 (SPSS Inc., Chicago, IL). Results are reported as mean ± standard deviation (SD). Univariate analysis of variance (ANOVA) was used to examine factors associated with increasing histology grades/stages as these were categorical variables with multiple end-points. Student t-tests were used to compare means of continuous variables. The strength of association between continuous variables was reported using Spearman rank correlations due to the non-parametric nature of certain variables. Multiple ordinal regression analysis was performed to determine the independent associations of viral load, steatosis grade and fibrosis stage. For the steatosis and fibrosis models all variables significant on univariate analysis were entered, and backward stepwise removal of variables to create a best-fitting model was performed. An interaction term (genotype multiplied by CB_1) was used in the steatosis model to determine if the association between CB_1 and steatosis was genotype dependent. P-values of <0.05 were considered significant.

Results

The baseline characteristics of the 88 patients with chronic hepatitis C is presented in table 1. The mean age for these patients was 42, with the majority male (64.8%) and of normal body mass. 56% had genotype 1 disease and 44% had genotype 3 infection. Over a third had advanced fibrosis (F3–4; 37.5%) and steatosis was present in 54.5%. Control patients are compared to the 31 hepatitis C patients with low fibrosis (F0-1) and no steatosis, and to 10 patients with chronic hepatitis B in table 2. Controls had a

Table 1. Baseline characteristics of patients with Chronic hepatitis C.

	Hepatitis C
	(n = 88)
Age	42.6 (9.7)
Sex (male)	57 (64.8%)
BMI	24.9 (2.9)
Genotype 1	49 (56%)
Genotype 3	39 (44%)
Fibrosis Stage	
0	12 (13.6%)
1	39 (44.3%)
2	4 (4.5%)
3	20 (22.7%)
4	13 (14.8%)
Steatosis Grade	
0	40 (45.5%)
1	22 (25%)
2	22 (25%)
3	4 (4.5%)
Portal Inflammation Grade	
1	11 (12.5%)
2	39 (44.3%)
3	22 (25%)

Variables are reported as mean (SD) or frequency (percentage) as appropriate.

Table 2. Baseline characteristics of patients with Chronic Hepatitis C (F0-1), Chronic hepatitis B (F0-1) and controls.

	Hepatitis C (F0-1)	Hepatitis B (F0-1)	P-value*	Control	P-value**
	(n=31)	(n=10)		(n=12)	
Age	39.7 (11.1)	37 (11.8)	0.44	42.2 (9.4)	0.5
Sex (male)	16 (51.%)	8 (80%)	0.3	3 (25%)	<0.01
BMI	24.1 (2.6)	22.7 (2.9)	0.1	29.6 (9.8)	<0.01
HOMA-IR	1.7 (0.9)	1.4 (1.3)	0.5	2.4 (1.1)	0.04
Fibrosis Stage					
0–1	31 (100%)	10 (100%)	-	12 (100%)	-
2–4	0	0		0	
Steatosis Grade					
0	31 (100%)	10 (100%)	-	12 (100%)	-
1–3	0	0		0	
Portal Inflammation Grade					
1	7 (22.6%)	4 (40%)	0.4	0	-
2–3	24 (77.4%)	6 (60%)		0	

Variables are reported as mean (SD) or frequency (percentage) as appropriate.
*p-values for Hepatitis C (F0-1) and Hepatitis B (F0-1), **p-values for Hepatitis C (F0-1) and control.

similar mean age to those with hepatitis C, but were more insulin resistant, obese and contained a lower percentage of males. Control liver biopsies were histologically normal. The 10 hepatitis B patients studied all had low fibrosis (F0-1), but comparable hepatic inflammation to those with hepatitis C.

CB_1 expression in hepatitis C, controls and hepatitis B

CB_1 was expressed in all patients with hepatitis C, and there was a 6-fold up-regulation when compared to controls ($P<0.001$, figure 1A and 1F). Within the hepatitis C cohort, CB_1 expression significantly correlated with increasing viral load (figure 1B). Patients with a high viral load (>800,000 IU/ml) had significantly higher CB_1 than those with intermediate (400,000–800,000 IU/mL), or low viral load (<400,000 IU/mL, $p=0.03$), even when controlled for fibrosis stage ($p=0.05$). There was no difference in CB_1 expression between those who had smoked cannabis in the last year (n = 10) and those who had not.

CB_1 expression increased with increasing fibrosis stage, with cirrhotics having up to a 2 fold up-regulation compared to those with low fibrosis stage (F0/1- figure 1C) and results were confirmed on tissue lysates by western blot (figure 1G). Despite this relationship to fibrosis, CB_1 levels in hepatitis C patients with low fibrosis and no steatosis were still substantially greater than those in controls ($p<0.05$, figure 1D).

To determine if CB_1 gene expression was a non-specific response to virus-mediated liver injury, we next compared CB_1 expression in 10 patients with hepatitis B and low fibrosis to the controls and to hepatitis C patients with low fibrosis and no steatosis. In the hepatitis B patients, CB_1 expression was increased when compared with controls, but was almost three-fold lower than that seen in a similar cohort with hepatitis C (figure 1E).

JFH-1/Huh7 HCV cell culture model and genotype 1 and 3 chimeric virus

To exclude any potential changes that could be due to fibrosis or the injury milieu in the liver and to determine if CB_1 up-regulation is in part a HCV-specific effect, we assessed receptor expression in the JFH-1/Huh7 model of replicating virus *in vitro*.

Huh7 cells infected with the JFH1 strain of HCV showed a 4-fold upregulation of CB_1 mRNA compared to control Huh7 cells (figure 2A, $p<0.05$). Immunoblotting confirmed an 8-fold induction of CB_1 protein as measured by densitometry (figure 2B). We next examined the expression of CB_1 over time following *de novo* infection of Huh7 cells with JFH-1. CB_1 expression increased slowly between day 5-22 and then rapidly between day 22–26 (p <0.001 for change in CB_1, figure 2C) Importantly, the changes in CB_1 expression paralleled increasing HCV infection, in particular when over 50% of cells were infected (R = 0.73, figure 2C and D).

To determine if CB_1 induction was due to structural or non-structural viral proteins, we next transfected Huh7 cells with a subgenomic replicon expressing only the non-structural proteins NS3 to NS5B. Compared with control, there was a 60% reduction in CB_1 expression in the HCV replicon containing cells (figure 3A), suggesting that HCV structural proteins are essential for promoting CB_1 expression in HCV infection.

We therefore went on to investigate the genotype-specific effect of HCV structural proteins on CB_1 expression using chimeric viruses containing core protein from genotype 1b and genotype 3a. CB_1 expression in Huh7 cells infected with chimeric HCV increased as the proportion of infected cells increased. This was similar to the results obtained using wild type JFH-1 (data not shown). When over 90% of the cells were infected, there was a corresponding 4.7 and 6.3 fold up-regulation of CB_1 from genotype 1b and 3a chimera's respectively, as compared to control Huh7 cells (p<0.01, figure 3B). However, there was no difference in the up-regulation of CB_1 between genotypes 1b and 3a ($p = 0.19$), suggesting that although the HCV structural proteins are essential for CB_1 induction, there is no genotype-specific effect of core protein.

Immunohistochemistry in Hepatitis C

CB_1 receptor protein expression by immunohistochemistry correlated with RNA expression by qPCR. Patients with high CB_1 expression exhibited diffuse cytoplasmic and nuclear staining of hepatocytes in addition to strong staining of hepatic stellate cells

n = number of patients

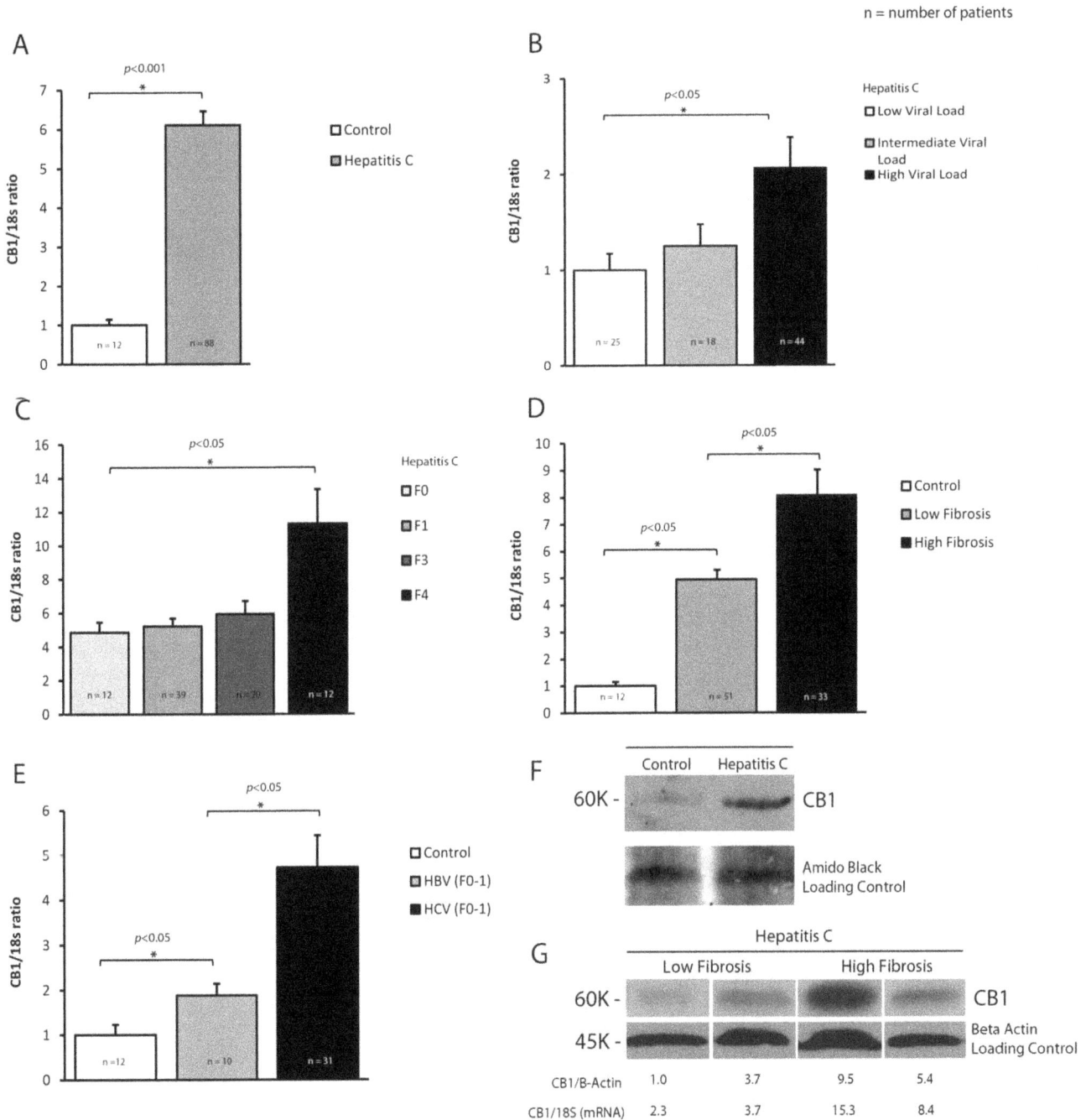

Figure 1. CB$_1$ is up-regulated in chronic hepatitis C and associated with viral load and fibrosis. Relative hepatic CB$_1$ mRNA expression in 88 patients with Chronic Hepatitis C, 12 controls and 10 patients with chronic hepatitis B normalised to 18s;, A) 6-fold up-regulation of CB$_1$ in hepatitis C patients compared to control, B) Viral load: Significant association between CB$_1$ expression and increasing viral load. C) Fibrosis stage: Increasing expression of CB$_1$ with increasing fibrosis stage in hepatitis C, D) Significant up-regulation in CB$_1$ even in those with low fibrosis stage and no steatosis (F0-1) compared to control, E) Hepatitis B patients with low fibrosis had increased CB$_1$ expression when compared to control, but at significantly lower levels than hepatitis C patients with low fibrosis, F) Western blot from representative control and hepatitis C patients demonstrating significant CB$_1$ up-regulation and G) Western blot from representative patients with hepatitis C and differing levels of fibrosis, showing increased CB$_1$ expression in patients with high fibrosis. The relative protein expression (CB$_1$/B-Actin) and mRNA expression (CB$_1$/18S) are presented for validation.

and cholangiocytes (figure 4A and B). Immunostaining in patients with low CB$_1$ expression and low fibrosis was less intense, patchy and confined to hepatocytes (figure 4D). A negative control image where the primary antibody was excluded is provided (figure 4C) to demonstrate the specificity of immunostaining. Low power

images in patients with high and low fibrosis respectively are presented as supplementary material (Figure S1). The nuclear localisation of CB$_1$ receptors is in keeping with recent evidence that trans-membrane G-protein coupled receptors can internalise on the cell nucleus [30,31].

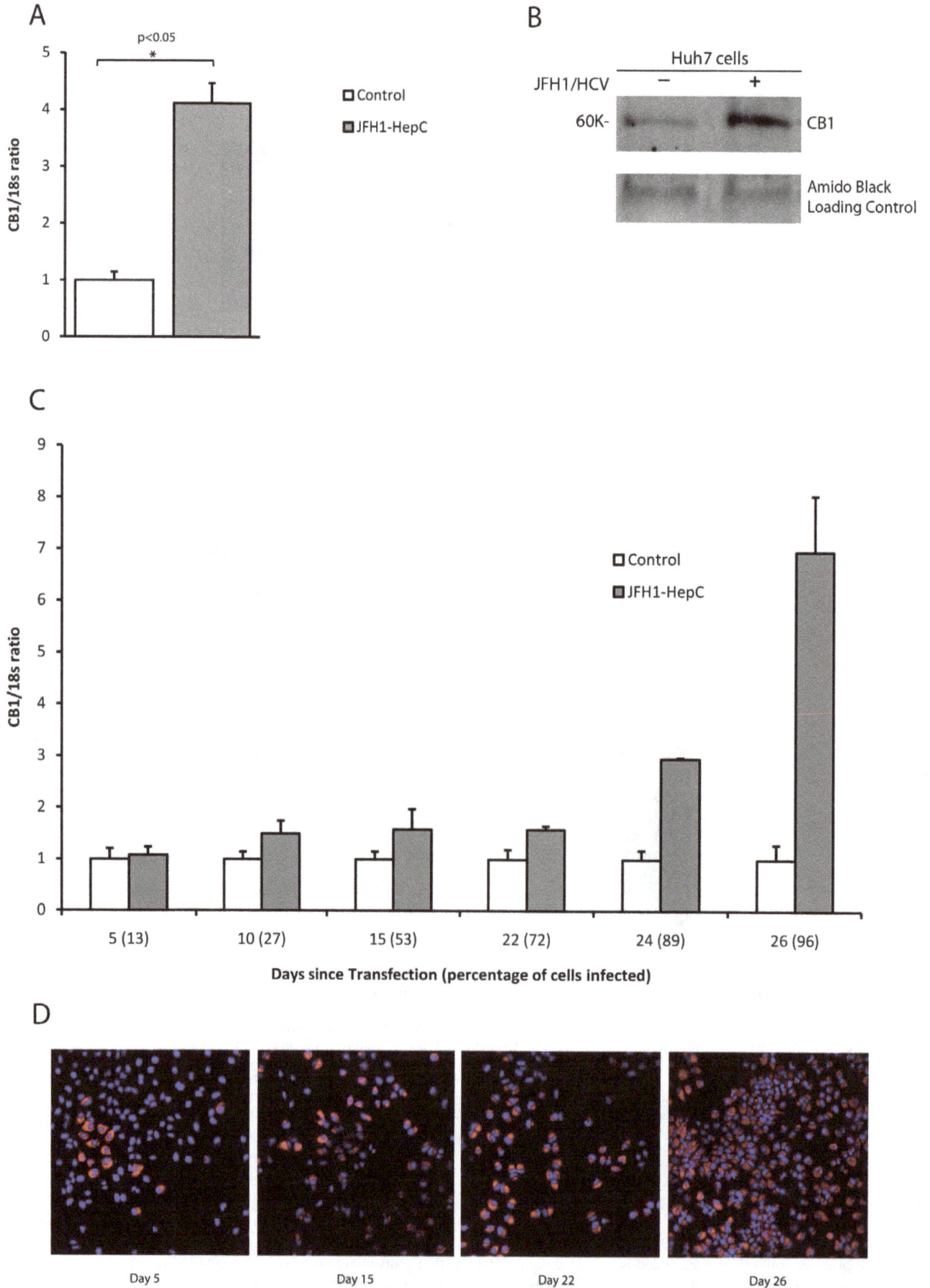

A

B

C

D

Day 5   Day 15   Day 22   Day 26

Figure 2. CB$_1$ is directly up-regulated by hepatitis C virus in a cell culture system. Relative hepatic CB$_1$ mRNA expression in Huh7 cells infected with the JFH$_1$ strain hepatitis C virus as compared to mock infected control cells normalised to 18s; A) 4-fold up-regulation of CB$_1$ mRNA in JFH-1 infected cells compared to control and B) Western blotting confirmed CB$_1$ protein up-regulation by at least >8-fold as measured by densitometry. C) Time course of CB$_1$ expression following de novo infection with JFH-1 hepatitis C virus. CB$_1$ expression increases with time ($p<0.01$), in parallel to the percentage of Huh7 cells infected (see horizontal axis) D) representative immunostaining for NS5a showing increasing infection of Huh7 cells at day 5, 15, 22 and 26.

The relationship of CB$_1$ expression to hepatic inflammation and steatosis

There was no difference in CB$_1$ expression between genotypes 1 and 3, nor was there any association between CB$_1$ and portal inflammatory activity. The presence of steatosis was associated with significantly increased CB$_1$ expression in the hepatitis C cohort (figure 5A, $p<0.05$) and CB$_1$ expression increased with steatosis grade (figure 5B, p<0.01). Genotype was significantly associated with steatosis grade, so an interaction term was used to test if the association between CB$_1$ and steatosis grade was genotype dependent. This demonstrated that CB$_1$ expression was highly associated with steatosis grade for genotype 3, but not genotype 1 (p-value for interaction term = 0.006).

We next examined genes that have been shown to be up-regulated by CB$_1$ receptor activation and are associated with lipogenesis (table 3). Overall, CB$_1$ had a modest correlation with sterol regulatory element binding protein (SREBP-1c; R = 0.21, $p<0.05$) and its downstream target fatty acid synthase (FASN; R = 0.25, $p<0.05$), but this was significantly stronger in genotype 3 patients (SREBP-1c; R = 0.37, FASN; R = 0.39, p<0.05 for both) and not present in those with genotype 1 disease. CB$_1$ had a modest correlation with insulin resistance as measured by the HOMA-IR (R = 0.23, $p<0.05$), but had no association with other steatogenic factors such as measures of adiposity, BMI, lipids, or increasing age.

Independent association between CB$_1$, steatosis and fibrosis

Multivariate analysis was performed to determine if CB$_1$ was independently associated with steatosis and fibrosis in CHC and controls. Input variables included CB$_1$, BMI, HOMA-IR, ALT, age, viral load, gender, steatosis grade and fibrosis stage. For fibrosis, input variables identified on univariate analysis were CB$_1$, HOMA-IR, BMI, age and steatosis grade. CB$_1$ remained a significant independent predictor of increasing fibrosis stage ($p=0.04$), as did HOMA-R ($p=0.008$), BMI ($p=0.04$) and steatosis grade ($p=0.001$). For steatosis, input variables were CB$_1$, HOMA-IR, viral load, genotype and fibrosis stage. CB$_1$ remained an independent predictor of increasing steatosis ($p=0.03$) along with viral load ($p=0.007$) and genotype (p<0.001).

Discussion

In this study we demonstrate the presence of cannabinoid receptor 1 (CB$_1$) in the livers of patients with chronic hepatitis C, a finding that has not been previously reported. We found CB$_1$ receptor to be expressed in all patients with CHC, with a significant up-regulation compared to control patients. While CB$_1$ expression was highest in those with advanced fibrosis, the levels in patients with early hepatitis C (Fibrosis 0-1 and no steatosis) were still 4-fold greater than that of controls. Moreover, there was a strong positive association between CB$_1$ expression and HCV viral load. This suggested a direct viral effect, and led us to examine CB$_1$ receptor expression in an *in vitro* system in which infectious virus is produced.

The Huh7/JFH-1 system, first described by Wakita *et al* in 2005 [26], uses full genomic RNA from the JFH1 genotype 2a strain of HCV, isolated from a patient with fulminant hepatitis. Once transfected into the human hepatoma cell line Huh7, JFH-1 virus replicates efficiently and virus particles are produced that are infectious in both tissue culture and chimpanzees [26]. In Huh7

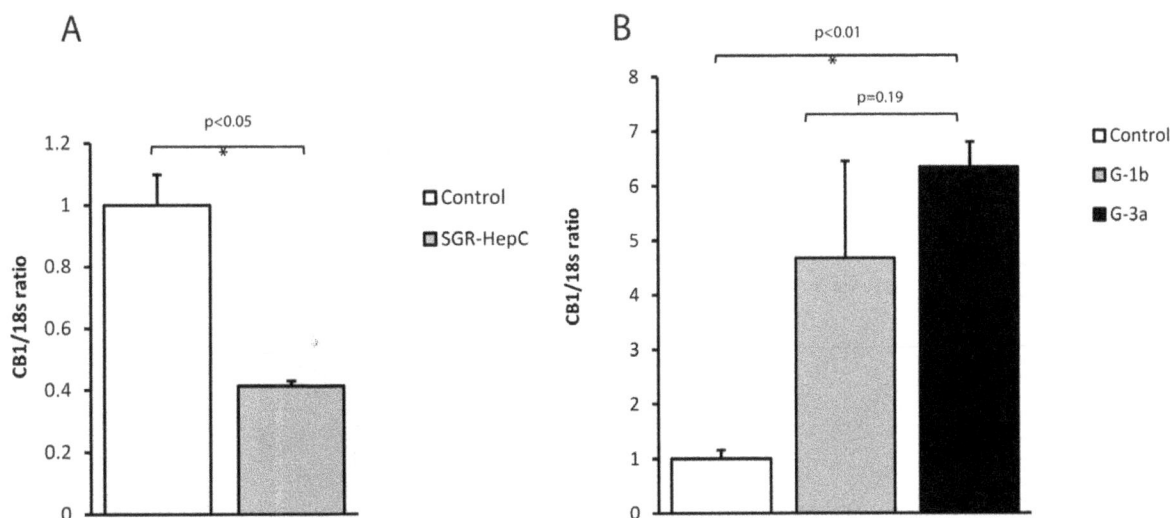

Figure 3. CB$_1$ expression in a subgenomic HCV replicon and genotype specific chimeric virus. Relative hepatic CB$_1$ mRNA expression in Huh7 cells infected either with a subgenomic HCV replicon (expressing JFH-1 NS3-NS5B) or genotype specific chimeric virus as compared to control. A) There was a 60% reduction in CB$_1$ expression in the HCV replicon containing cells compared to control and B) There was a 4.7 and 6.3 fold up-regulation in CB$_1$ expression in the genotype 1b and 3a chimera viruses when compared to control. There was no difference, however, in CB$_1$ expression between the two different genotype chimeras.

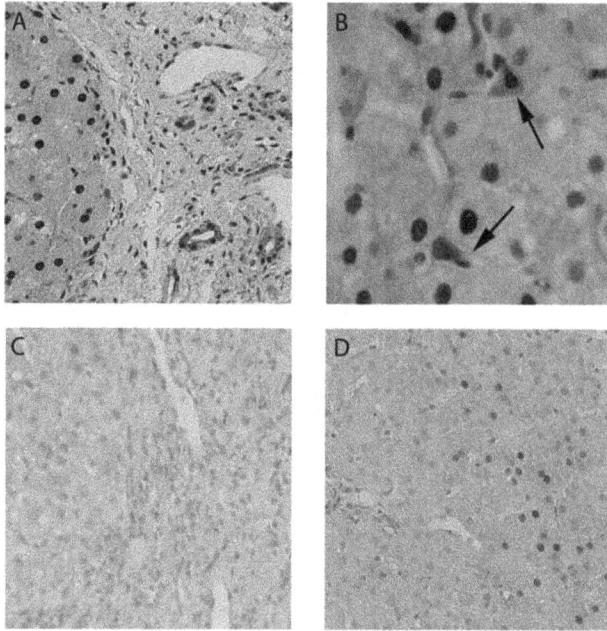

Figure 4. Representative immunostaining for CB$_1$ receptor protein in hepatitis C patients with high and low CB$_1$ expression. High CB$_1$ expression and advanced fibrosis: A) strong, diffuse cytoplasmic and nuclear immunostaining of hepatocytes is evident in addition to cholangiocyte and B) hepatic stellate cell immunostaining (arrows). Negative control: C) No immunostaining apparent in negative control where the primary antibody was excluded. Low CB$_1$ expression and low fibrosis: D) low intensity and patchy cytoplasmic and nuclear immunostaining of hepatocytes is evident.

cells infected with HCV (JFH-1) we showed that CB$_1$ expression was increased over 8-fold compared to control cells. The enrichment of CB$_1$ expression in JFH1-infected cells suggests for the first time that CB$_1$ receptor is an HCV-inducible gene. Our results using the JFH-1 subgenomic replicon suggest that HCV structural proteins are essential for induction of CB$_1$, as there was no increase seen with nonstructural proteins alone. We were unable to demonstrate an effect of core protein genotype on CB$_1$

expression using chimeric viruses, which supports our clinical data showing no difference in CB$_1$ expression between patients infected with HCV genotypes 1 and 3.

One limitation of this and other liver biopsy-based human studies relates to the cross-sectional nature of the data. Reports of this type can demonstrate significant associations, but inference of cause and effect are always difficult. We used a number of methods to strengthen our finding that CB$_1$ was directly induced by hepatitis C. Firstly, we demonstrated an up-regulation of CB$_1$ in those with very mild hepatitis C (F0-1 and no steatosis) compared with controls, and an association with viral load, which would not be expected if this was a non-specific effect of fibrosis or inflammation. We then went on to show that CB$_1$ expression in comparable patients with mild hepatitis B (F0-1) was significantly lower (almost 3-fold) than those with mild hepatitis C. Finally, we used a cell culture system to demonstrate a direct relationship between CB$_1$ expression and hepatitis C viral infection, both in time course and static experiments. Cannabis smoking did not appear to be a confounder as no difference in expression was seen in the small number of cannabis smokers compared to the remaining cohort. While the numbers were too small to determine if cannabis smoking regulates CB$_1$ expression, published reports indicate that this is the case only in daily smokers [4,24] and these patients were excluded from the study. It should be noted that control subjects had significantly higher BMI and HOMA-IR scores than those with hepatitis C. However, since CB$_1$ expression has been associated with insulin resistance and obesity, this would if anything lead to an underestimate of the difference in expression. Further work however clearly needs to be done to define the mechanisms by which HCV up-regulates CB$_1$ and the specific viral proteins involved.

The pathophysiology of steatosis in CHC is complex. In HCV genotype 1, steatosis is associated with metabolic disturbance, obesity and insulin resistance [5], while steatosis in genotype 3 appears principally to be virally mediated [32]. HCV is known to directly induce steatosis via interactions between core protein [33,34] and lipogenic regulators such as SREBP-1c [35] and microsomal triglyceride transfer protein (MTP) [36]. In our cohort, hepatic CB$_1$ expression correlated with the extent of steatosis and was significantly up-regulated in those with increased steatosis grade, suggesting CB$_1$ receptor activation and signalling. This association was highly significant for genotype 3, but not 1.

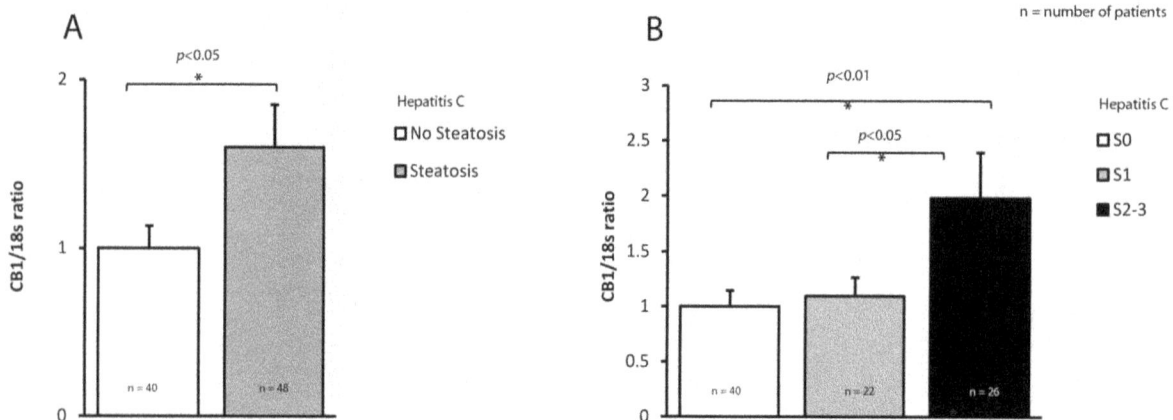

Figure 5. CB$_1$ expression is associated with increasing steatosis in chronic hepatitis C. Relative CB$_1$ mRNA expression in 88 patients with Chronic Hepatitis C normalised to 18s; A) Steatosis: Significantly increased CB$_1$ expression in hepatitis C patients with steatosis, B) Steatosis grades: Significantly increased CB$_1$ expression with increasing steatosis grade.

Table 3. Rank correlations between CB_1 and factors associated with steatosis in HCV by genotype.

	SREBP-1c	FASN	HOMA-IR	BMI	HDL	TG	Age
CB_1 - HCV all	0.21*	0.25*	0.23*	0.10	0.03	0.01	0.15
CB_1 - HCV G1	0.08	0.19	0.19	0.11	0.11	−0.04	0.21
CB_1 - HCV G3	0.37*	0.39*	0.24	0.20	0.01	0.02	0.14

*p-value <0.05.
SREBP-1c; Sterol regulatory element binding protein, FASN; fatty acid synthase, HOMA-IR; homeostasis model assessment of insulin resistance, BMI; body mass index, HDL; high density lipoprotein, TG; triglyceride.

Moreover, in genotype 3 patients, CB_1 expression correlated strongly with the lipogenic transcription factor SREBP-1c and its downstream target FASN, but in genotype 1 patients there was no correlation. Clinical studies in CHC have hinted at the importance of CB_1 stimulation to steatosis, with daily cannabis use a risk factor for steatosis severity in over 300 patients with CHC [24]. In experimental work, endocannabinoid stimulation of CB_1 mediates diet-induced steatosis, since CB_1 knockout mice fed a high fat diet are resistant to steatosis [18]. Likewise, treatment of wild type mice with a CB_1 agonist induces de novo fatty acid synthesis via increased hepatic expression of SREBP-1c and its downstream targets FASN and acetyl coenzyme-A carboxylase-1 (ACC1) [18]. Finally, the selective deletion of hepatocyte CB_1 receptors alone is sufficient to prevent diet [37] and alcohol-induced [22] hepatic steatosis [22,37].

The endocannabinoid system plays an important role in liver fibrosis. In three murine models of chronic liver injury, CB_1 receptor antagonism by pharmacological or genetic means reduced fibrosis area, TGF-β1 expression and the accumulation of fibrogenic cells. It has also been shown that CB_1 can mediate liver fibrosis through effects on apoptosis and the growth of hepatic myofibroblasts [19]. Clinical studies first demonstrated the likely importance of this system in patients with CHC, showing daily cannabis smoking to be independently associated with the progression and severity of fibrosis [4]. In our study, CB_1 was expressed in all patients with CHC and increased with advancing fibrosis, with the highest levels present in those with cirrhosis. We were unable to show any relationship between CB_1 receptor expression and inflammatory grade, although this does not exclude that the endocannabinoid system via CB_1 may mediate fibrosis in this way. Rather, it has been suggested that HCV can directly activate and stimulate hepatic stellate cells through its core and non-structural proteins, or via secretions from infected hepatocytes [38,39]. In this context, activated HSCs not only secrete collagens and cytokines, but also the endocannabinoid 2-AG, which in turn up-regulates and activates hepatocyte CB_1 [22]. Stimulation of hepatocyte CB_1 through this pathway or directly by HCV as we demonstrate will serve to amplify the pathways by which liver fibrosis develops in CHC [2,32]. It is interesting to note from our immunohistochemistry that CB_1 receptors were up-regulated on hepatic stellate cells in CHC. One could therefore speculate that the direct pro-fibrogenic interactions between HCV and stellate cells demonstrated by Battaler and colleagues [38] may in part, be mediated through and exaggerated by the induction of CB_1.

There has been much recent interest in the use of CB_1 antagonists to treat both hepatic and metabolic disease and our findings emphasize the likely usefulness of these compounds in patients with hepatitis C. In addition to the amelioration of steatosis and fibrosis, CB_1 blockade reduces portal pressure and can reverse mesenteric arterial dilation [40], making them useful in end stage liver disease as well. We speculate that CB_1 antagonism may also have an inhibitory effect on HCV replication. This is prompted both by the significant, genotype independent association we found between CB_1 expression and viral load, and by reports that blockade of the SREBP and FASN signalling in hepatitis C cell culture models reduces HCV replication [41,42]. Clearly this needs further study before any conclusions can be drawn. Unfortunately, several CB_1 receptor antagonists were recently withdrawn from clinical development including Rimonabant (SR141716A) and Taranabant (MK-0364). These withdrawals followed an EU medicines safety edict that Rimonabant be suspended due to excessive psychiatric side effects including depression, anxiety and suicide [43]. Nonetheless, our findings and those of others, showing the importance of hepatic CB_1 receptors in CHC, suggest that the development of a peripherally selective CB_1 antagonist with minimal neurotoxicity remains a promising future option.

In conclusion, we have demonstrated that CB_1 receptor is widely expressed in the livers of patients with CHC and is associated with advanced fibrosis and steatosis. Importantly, CB_1 is also highly enriched in those with low fibrosis and is induced by HCV in a cell culture system, findings that underscore the unique susceptibility of patients with CHC to cannabis-induced liver damage. CB_1 has already been implicated in the genesis of fibrosis and steatosis in experimental and metabolic liver disease. We have now shown that it is important in CHC and may be a future target for pharmacotherapy in this disease.

Acknowledgments

The authors wish to thank Keshni Sharma and Lee Russell for assistance with Data and sample collection, David Warton for assistance with statistical methods and Dr John McLauchlan, MRC Virology Unit, Glasgow for providing the Huh7 clone.

Author Contributions

Conceived and designed the experiments: DvdP LWH MWD JG. Performed the experiments: DvdP MS ESET JS KT DM JSM VH. Analyzed the data: DvdP KT LWH MWD. Contributed reagents/materials/analysis tools: MWD. Wrote the paper: DvdP LWH MWD JG.

References

1. World Health Organisation Initiative for vaccine research (IVR); Hepatitis C page. Available at: http://www.who.int/vaccine_research/diseases/viral_cancers/en/index2.html Accessed January 15, 2008.
2. van der Poorten D, George J (2008) Disease-specific mechanisms of fibrosis: hepatitis C virus and nonalcoholic steatohepatitis. Clin Liver Dis 12: 805–824, ix.

3. McCaughan GW, George J (2004) Fibrosis progression in chronic hepatitis C virus infection. Gut 53: 318–321.

4. Hezode C, Roudot-Thoraval F, Nguyen S, Grenard P, Julien B, et al. (2005) Daily cannabis smoking as a risk factor for progression of fibrosis in chronic hepatitis C. Hepatology 42: 63–71.

5. Hui JM, Sud A, Farrell GC, Bandara P, Byth K, et al. (2003) Insulin resistance is associated with chronic hepatitis C virus infection and fibrosis progression [corrected]. Gastroenterology 125: 1695–1704.

6. Hui JM, Kench J, Farrell GC, Lin R, Samarasinghe D, et al. (2002) Genotype-specific mechanisms for hepatic steatosis in chronic hepatitis C infection. J Gastroenterol Hepatol 17: 873–881.

7. Kumar D, Farrell GC, Fung C, George J (2002) Hepatitis C virus genotype 3 is cytopathic to hepatocytes: Reversal of hepatic steatosis after sustained therapeutic response. Hepatology 36: 1266–1272.

8. Asselah T, Rubbia-Brandt L, Marcellin P, Negro F (2006) Steatosis in Chronic Hepatitis C: Why does it really matter? Gut 55: 123–130.

9. Ohata K, Hamasaki K, Toriyama K, Matsumoto K, Saeki A, et al. (2003) Hepatic steatosis is a risk factor for hepatocellular carcinoma in patients with chronic hepatitis C virus infection.[see comment]. Cancer 97: 3036–3043.

10. Su AI, Pezacki JP, Wodicka L, Brideau AD, Supekova L, et al. (2002) Genomic analysis of the host response to hepatitis C virus infection. PNAS 99: 15669–15674.

11. Smart RG, Ogborne AC (2000) Drug use and drinking among students in 36 countries. Addict Behav 25: 455–460.

12. Devane WA, Hanus L, Breuer A, Pertwee RG, Stevenson LA, et al. (1992) Isolation and structure of a brain constituent that binds to the cannabinoid receptor. Science 258: 1946–1949.

13. Pacher P, Batkai S, Kunos G (2006) The endocannabinoid system as an emerging target of pharmacotherapy. Pharmacol Rev 58: 389–462.

14. Kunos G, Osei-Hyiaman D, Liu J, Godlewski G, Batkai S (2008) Endocannabinoids and the control of energy homeostasis. J Biol Chem 283: 33021–33025.

15. Di Marzo V, Goparaju SK, Wang L, Liu J, Batkai S, et al. (2001) Leptin-regulated endocannabinoids are involved in maintaining food intake. Nature 410: 822–825.

16. Ravinet Trillou C, Delgorge C, Menet C, Arnone M, Soubrie P (2004) CB1 cannabinoid receptor knockout in mice leads to leanness, resistance to diet-induced obesity and enhanced leptin sensitivity. Int J Obes Relat Metab Disord 28: 640–648.

17. Despres JP, Golay A, Sjostrom L, Rimonabant in Obesity-Lipids Study G (2005) Effects of rimonabant on metabolic risk factors in overweight patients with dyslipidemia.[see comment]. New England Journal of Medicine 353: 2121–2134.

18. Osei-Hyiaman D, DePetrillo M, Pacher P, Liu J, Radaeva S, et al. (2005) Endocannabinoid activation at hepatic CB1 receptors stimulates fatty acid synthesis and contributes to diet-induced obesity.[see comment]. Journal of Clinical Investigation 115: 1298–1305.

19. Teixeira-Clerc F, Julien B, Grenard P, Tran Van Nhieu J, Deveaux V, et al. (2006) CB1 cannabinoid receptor antagonism: a new strategy for the treatment of hepatic fibrosis. Nat Med 12: 671–676.

20. Julien, Grenard, Teixeira C, Van N, Li, et al. (2005) Antifibrogenic role of the cannabinoid receptor CB2 in the liver. Gastroenterology 128: 742–755.

21. Munoz-Luque J, Ros J, Fernandez-Varo G, Tugues S, Morales-Ruiz M, et al. (2008) Regression of fibrosis after chronic stimulation of cannabinoid CB2 receptor in cirrhotic rats. J Pharmacol Exp Ther 324: 475–483.

22. Jeong WI, Osei-Hyiaman D, Park O, Liu J, Batkai S, et al. (2008) Paracrine activation of hepatic CB1 receptors by stellate cell-derived endocannabinoids mediates alcoholic fatty liver. Cell Metab 7: 227–235.

23. Gary-Bobo M, Elachouri G, Gallas JF, Janiak P, Marini P, et al. (2007) Rimonabant reduces obesity-associated hepatic steatosis and features of metabolic syndrome in obese Zucker fa/fa rats. Hepatology 46: 122–129.

24. Hezode C, Zafrani ES, Roudot-Thoraval F, Costentin C, Hessami A, et al. (2008) Daily cannabis use: a novel risk factor of steatosis severity in patients with chronic hepatitis C. Gastroenterology 134: 432–439.

25. Scheuer PJ (1991) Classification of chronic viral hepatitis: a need for reassessment. J Hepatol 13: 372–374.

26. Wakita T, Pietschmann T, Kato T, Date T, Miyamoto M, et al. (2005) Production of infectious hepatitis C virus in tissue culture from a cloned viral genome. Nat Med 11: 791–796.

27. Kato T, Date T, Miyamoto M, Furusaka A, Tokushige K, et al. (2003) Efficient replication of the genotype 2a hepatitis C virus subgenomic replicon. Gastroenterology 125: 1808–1817.

28. Shaw ML, McLauchlan J, Mills PR, Patel AH, McCruden EA (2003) Characterisation of the differences between hepatitis C virus genotype 3 and 1 glycoproteins. J Med Virol 70: 361–372.

29. Rasband W ImageJ. U.S. National Institutes of Health, Bethesda, Maryland, USA, 1997-2007.

30. Boivin B, Vaniotis G, Allen BG, Hebert TE (2008) G protein-coupled receptors in and on the cell nucleus: a new signaling paradigm? J Recept Signal Transduct Res 28: 15–28.

31. Ellis J, Pediani JD, Canals M, Milasta S, Milligan G (2006) Orexin-1 receptor-cannabinoid CB1 receptor heterodimerization results in both ligand-dependent and -independent coordinated alterations of receptor localization and function. J Biol Chem 281: 38812–38824.

32. Negro F (2006) Mechanisms and significance of liver steatosis in hepatitis C virus infection. World J Gastroenterol 12: 6756–6765.

33. Shi ST, Polyak SJ, Tu H, Taylor DR, Gretch DR, et al. (2002) Hepatitis C virus NS5A colocalizes with the core protein on lipid droplets and interacts with apolipoproteins. Virology 292: 198–210.

34. Barba G, Harper F, Harada T, Kohara M, Goulinet S, et al. (1997) Hepatitis C virus core protein shows a cytoplasmic localization and associates to cellular lipid storage droplets. PNAS 94: 1200–1205.

35. Kim KH, Hong SP, Kim K, Park MJ, Kim KJ, et al. (2007) HCV core protein induces hepatic lipid accumulation by activating SREBP1 and PPARgamma. Biochem Biophys Res Commun 355: 883–888.

36. Perlemuter G, Sabile A, Letteron P, Vona G, Topilco A, et al. (2002) Hepatitis C virus core protein inhibits microsomal triglyceride transfer protein activity and very low density lipoprotein secretion: a model of viral-related steatosis. FASEB Journal 16: 185–194.

37. Osei-Hyiaman D, Liu J, Zhou L, Godlewski G, Harvey-White J, et al. (2008) Hepatic CB1 receptor is required for development of diet-induced steatosis, dyslipidemia, and insulin and leptin resistance in mice. J Clin Invest 118: 3160–3169.

38. Bataller R, Paik YH, Lindquist JN, Lemasters JJ, Brenner DA (2004) Hepatitis C virus and nonstructural proteins induce fibrogenic effects in hepatic stellate cells. Gastroenterology 126: 529–540.

39. Schulze-Krebs A, Preimel D, Popov Y, Bartenschlager R, Lohmann V, et al. (2005) Hepatitis C virus-replicating hepatocytes induce fibrogenic activation of hepatic stellate cells. Gastroenterology 129: 246–258.

40. Parfieniuk A, Flisiak R (2008) Role of cannabinoids in chronic liver diseases. World J Gastroenterol 14: 6109–6114.

41. Su AI, Pezacki JP, Wodicka L, Brideau AD, Supekova L, et al. (2002) Genomic analysis of the host response to hepatitis C virus infection. Proc Natl Acad Sci U S A 99: 15669–15674.

42. Yang W, Hood BL, Chadwick SL, Liu S, Watkins SC, et al. (2008) Fatty acid synthase is up-regulated during hepatitis C virus infection and regulates hepatitis C virus entry and production. Hepatology 48: 1396–1403.

43. European Medicines Agency (2008) The European Medicines Agency recommends suspension of the marketing authorisation of Acomplia. pp. London, 23 October, Doc. Ref. EMEA/CHMP/537777/532008.

2

IP-10 can be Measured in Dried Plasma Spots in Patients with Chronic Hepatitis C Infection

Morten Ruhwald[1]*, Ellen Sloth Andersen[2,3], Peer Brehm Christensen[4], Belinda Klemmensen Moessner[4], Nina Weis[2,5]

1 Clinical Research Centre, Copenhagen University Hospital, Hvidovre, Copenhagen, Denmark, 2 Department of Infectious Diseases, Copenhagen University Hospital, Hvidovre, Copenhagen, Denmark, 3 Department of Infectious Diseases, Copenhagen University Hospital, Rigshospitalet, Copenhagen, Denmark, 4 Department of Infectious Diseases, Odense University Hospital, Odense, Denmark, 5 Faculty of Health Sciences, Copenhagen University, Copenhagen, Denmark

Abstract

The chemokine IP-10 (CXCL10) is a candidate marker for hepatitis C virus (HCV) fibrosis monitoring. The aim of this proof-of-concept study is to assess if IP-10 measurements from dried plasma spots (DPS) are accurate in HCV-infected patients with either minimal or significant fibrosis. We measured IP-10 levels in plasma and DPS of 21 HCV-infected patients with cirrhosis and 19 patients with no/little fibrosis (determined with FibroScan). Cirrhotic patients had significantly higher levels of IP-10 compared to patients with minimal fibrosis. DPS and plasma measurements of IP-10 are comparable and the correlation was excellent ($r^2 = 0.97$, $p < 0.0001$). The DPS based method for IP-10 detection performs well in HCV-infected patients with either minimal or significant fibrosis.

Editor: Matthew L. Albert, Institut Pasteur, France

Funding: The work was supported by the Danish National Advanced Technology Foundation. The funders had no role in study design, data collection and analysis, decision to publish, or preparation of the manuscript.

Competing Interests: Nina Weis and Morten Ruhwald are employed at Copenhagen University Hospitals, Hvidovre, which is the proprietor of a pending patent disclosing the use of IP-10 and filter paper for the monitoring of liver fibrosis (PCT/DK/11162289.0). Morten Ruhwald is registered as inventor. Ellen Sloth Andersen, Peer Brehm Christensen, and Belinda Klemmensen Moessner have no conflicts of interest to disclose.

* E-mail: mruhwald@gmail.com

Introduction

Globally, 170 million individuals are chronically infected with Hepatitis C virus (HCV). The hallmark of HCV infection is the progressive development of liver fibrosis, leading to liver cirrhosis and potentially hepatocellular carcinoma. The level of liver fibrosis predicts liver related complications and therefore the assessment of liver fibrosis is a cornerstone in the management of patients chronically infected with HCV. Each year 0.5 million people die of HCV-related diseases.

For the last fifty years, liver biopsy has been considered the gold standard for fibrosis and cirrhosis assessment, but recent reports indicate that biopsy does not fulfill the requirements of a surrogate marker; mainly because of its high complication and sampling error rate, high inter- and intra observer variability, cost and patient reluctance to undergo serial monitoring [1,2]. In the last decade, several promising non-invasive alternatives have emerged. Liver stiffness measurement using FibroScan (Echosens, Paris, France) is a rapid method with high accuracy for the monitoring of HCV induced fibrosis and cirrhosis [1]. Also blood sample tests, such as the FibroTest (Biopredictive, Paris, France), have been shown to have a good correlation with advanced liver fibrosis.

There are limitations to the novel non-invasive tools. The FibroScan is expensive to acquire and the blood tests rely on accurate measurement using multiple assays. These tests are therefore only offered in a few, validated laboratories. As these promising novel modalities will most likely not reach the large majority of HCV infected patients in the developing world, simpler and cheaper alternatives are needed.

A series of reports have demonstrated that chemokine Interferon-γ Inducible protein 10 (IP-10, CXCL10) is a promising single marker correlate for liver fibrosis, and an IL-28b independent negative predictor of treatment outcome in HCV infected patients[3–7]. IP-10 is a key driver in both innate and antigen specific immune responses by directing Th1 cells to the site of inflammation [8,9]. IP-10 is secreted by HCV infected hepatocytes into the blood and can therefore be seen as a direct proxy of ongoing inflammation in the liver [10,11]. Recently, it was shown that in patients with chronic HCV infection the majority of plasma IP-10 exists in a 2 amino-acid truncated antagonist form, which inhibits the desired antiviral effects of IP-10 and could play an important role in pathology [12]. Compared to most of the key pro-inflammatory T cell cytokines (e.g. IFN-γ), IP-10 is expressed in 100 fold higher levels making it easy to measure also with simple technology [13].

Drying of plasma and blood on filter paper is a reliable method for conserving proteins. The method is state-of-art in national screening programs of neonates and it enables very simple sample acquisition (e.g. a finger or heel prick), and safe and cheap long distance transport using normal mail service [14]. Recent publications have demonstrated that dried blood spots (DBS) are a reliable alternative to serum specimens for detecting anti-HCV, quantifying HCV RNA and genotyping HCV [15]. We have recently developed an ELISA based assay for IP-10 detection in DBS and dried plasma spots (DPS) [16]. Using this assay we have demonstrated a very high correlation between DPS, DBS and plasma IP-10 levels in sample from healthy donors and patients with *M.tuberculosis* infection, and that this method renders comparable diagnostic accuracy as the current state-of-art diagnostic assay for infection with *M.tuberculosis*, the Quantiferon test (Aabye et al unpublished). It is unknown how the filter paper based method for IP-10 detection performs in samples from patients with chronic HCV infection. The aim of this study was to assess if the filter paper based method for IP-10 detection compares to IP-10 detected in plasma from HCV infected patients with either minimal or significant liver fibrosis.

Materials and Methods

Ethics Statement

The study has been approved by the Danish National Committee on Biomedical Research Ethics (H-D-2007-0087) in accordance with the Helsinki Declaration. All patients had given written and oral consent to participate in the study.

Patient Material

A detailed description of the patients included has previously been published [17]. In brief, we included 40 patients with HCV genotype 1 infection. Twenty-one had cirrhosis and 19 had no/mild fibrosis. Transient elastography (FibroScan®, medium probe, software version 1.30) was used for diagnosing the stage of fibrosis. Liver stiffness measurements were considered to be successful if ten valid measurements were obtained (valid measurements >60% and interquartile range <25%). Patients were diagnosed as having no/mild fibrosis when the liver stiffness was below 7.7 kPa, and as having cirrhosis when the values were equal to or above 13.0 kPa. Patients with hepatocellular carcinoma, previous liver transplantation or co-infection with other HCV genotypes than 1, hepatitis B virus or HIV were excluded. Compared to patients with no/mild fibrosis, the patients in the cirrhotic group were older (median age was 57 vs. 46 years, p<0.0001), predominately male (15/21 (71%) vs. 8/19 (42%), p = 0.117) and had a higher body mass index (median 26.5 kg/m^2 (inter quartile range (IQR) 23.9–29.9 kg/m^2) vs. 22.6 kg/m^2 (IQR 20.4–26.1 kg/m^2), p = 0.019).

Sample Preparation

Blood was drawn on the day of FibroScan and EDTA plasma was stored at -80°C until analysis. Plasma samples were thawed and IP-10 concentration was determined with ELISA. DPS samples were prepared as described in detail elsewhere [16], in brief 25 μl plasma was added to filter paper (903 Protein Saver™ cards,Whatman) in duplicates. After 4 hours drying on the lab bench, DPS samples were stored in gas-impermeable plastic bags with a desiccator at room temperature for 7 days before analysis.

IP-10 Measurement in Plasma and DPS with ELISA

IP-10 levels in plasma and DPS samples were determined with an ELISA based assay, developed and optimized for the monitoring of IP-10 in plasma and filter paper samples [16]. In brief, we made rat and murine hybridoma cell lines producing monoclonal antibodies (mAbs) specific for IP-10. Maxisorb plates (Nunc, Denmark) were coated with murine mAb in carbonate buffer, washed, blocked and dried for later use. On day of assay 20 μl of each plasma sample was diluted 5 times in assay buffer with HRP-conjugated detection mAb. When used for DPSs, 2 discs of 5.5 mm were punched from the centre of the DPS using a standard office paper puncher (Impega, UK) and incubated with 100 μL assay buffer. Plasma samples and DPS discs were incubated for 2 hours at room temperature (23°C) and washed x

3. HRP-substrate (TMB One, Trichem) was added, plates were revealed for 30 minutes before colour reaction was stopped with 100 μL H$_2$SO$_4$ and absorbance was read. Concentrations were calculated using a standard curve with a linear range from 2.5–600 pg/ml (Peprotec, USA). Plasma concentrations were corrected for the dilution factor (multiplied x5), DPS samples are presented as pg/2 discs.

Statistics

IP-10 concentrations were compared with non-parametric methods (Mann Whitney U test and Spearman correlation). Data were plotted and analysed using GraphPad Prizm 5.0 for Mac OS X (GraphPad, USA).

Ethical

The study has been approved by the Danish National Committee on Biomedical Research Ethics (H-D-2007-0087) in accordance to the Helsinki Declaration. All patients gave written and oral consent to participate in the study.

Results

Plasma samples from patients with cirrhosis had significantly higher levels of IP-10 median 385 pg/ml (IQR 282–595 pg/ml)) compared to patients with no/mild fibrosis 174 pg/ml (IQR 120–335 pg/ml, p<0.0001, Figure 1). Similar differences were found in the DPS samples median 34 pg/2 DPS discs (IQR 25–49 pg/2 DPS discs)) compared to 9pg/2 DPS discs (IQR 4–20 pg/2 DPS discs, p<0.0001). There was an excellent correlation between plasma and DPS samples (r^2 = 0.97, p<0.0001, Figure 2). ROC curve analysis revealed a comparable discriminatory capability between the two methods AUC 0.82 and 0.85 for IP-10 determined in plasma and DPS samples, respectively (Figure 3).

Discussion

In this proof-of-concept study we assess whether IP-10 can be measured in HCV-infected patients by the DPS method. We show that IP-10 determined in plasma and DPS samples have excellent correlation and comparable discriminatory capability between patients with no/mild fibrosis and patients with cirrhosis.

Plasma levels of IP-10 have proven to be a valid correlate for HCV fibrosis [18], a measure of chronic HCV disease activity [19], and an IL-28b independent negative predictor of treatment effect[4–7,11,19]. We have previously developed and validated the filter paper method for IP-10 detection in DBS and DPS samples, and we have shown that the recovery and stability of IP-10 in filter paper samples is very high and comparable to IP-10 detected in plasma (r^2>0.97). The range of the assay allows for accurate detection of both the levels of IP-10 found in the blood, and the high levels seen after in-vitro stimulation of whole blood with disease specific antigens and mitogens ([16] and Aabye et al. unpublished). This report supports our previous work in terms of technical performance of the filter paper IP-10 method and extends the usefulness IP-10 detection in un-stimulated patient samples.

Liver biopsy, and to some extend FibroScan and FibroTest, are surrogate markers for fibrosis in liver disease. In contrast, the plasma level of IP-10 appears a more dynamic and functional marker, directly linked to interplay of virus and immune response [10,11]. IP-10 appears to reflect both the extent of liver fibrosis as well as the immune activity (e.g. IP-10 increase during a flare-up and after interferon treatment in responsive patients [11,12,18]).

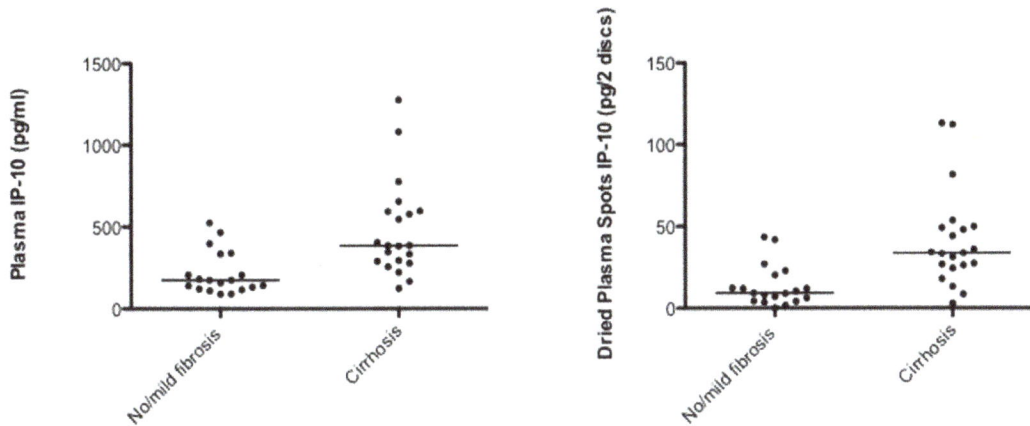

Figure 1. IP-10 measurements. IP-10 measured in plasma (left) and dried plasma spots (right) from 19 patients with chronic hepatitis C infection and no/mild liver fibrosis and 21 patients with liver cirrhosis. Line denote median. There was a significant difference between the groups in both plasma and dried plasma spots, $p < 0.0004$.

Further prospective studies, with sequential measurements of IP-10, are needed to assess the contribution of these two potential components in the total plasma IP-10 level, and to explore if this can be used to guide patient management.

Limitations: In this study we use plasma and not whole blood. Whole blood from a finger prick would be the optimal and simplest source of material for the filter paper application if this method should prove valid for clinical use. We have previously demonstrated that IP-10 levels detected in DPS discs are comparable to DBS discs in terms of signal intensity ($r^2 = 0.99$; regression slope = 1.01, $p < 0.0001$) and IP-10 stability [16], wherefore we think that our DPS results can be transferred to DBS analysis. We use FibroScan as a proxy for biopsy and histological classification of fibrosis, FibroScan readings can differ from biopsy results and the data should be interpreted in this light [20]. However, of the 40 patients included, ten had within 5 years of inclusion undergone a percutaneous liver biopsy of which, 9 (90%) had a fibrosis stage determined by liver biopsy in agreement with the fibrosis stage determined by FibroScan [17]. Another limitation is the comparison of the two highly selected groups of HCV genotype 1 infected patients and that the two groups were not matched with respect to age, gender or body mass index. This comparison of the least and the most affected within a strictly defined disease entity is artificial, and can lead to over interpretation of the associations observed. Nevertheless, a clear case-control design is essential, in the early stages of validating a new biomarker or a new method such as the DPS/DBS method; if no association is found, then the biomarker or method should probably not be explored further [21]. Future studies including patients representing intermediate degrees of fibrosis are needed to define cut offs and establish correlates between plasma levels of IP-10 and other surrogate markers of fibrosis. In addition the investigations of IP-10 as marker of fibrosis must be extended to patients infected with other genotypes than 1. Finally the median levels in the no/mild fibrosis detected with the DPS method were only 4 fold higher than the lower limit of detection for the assay [16]. This could compromise the ability to accurately compare uninfected controls to patients with no/low fibrosis, but not when comparing patients infected with HCV with varying degree of fibrosis.

Regardless of the limitations in this study, it appears from this and other recent studies that the filter paper method is as reliable as a plasma sample for detection of chemokines such as IP-10 [16,22]. Given that IP-10 can be demonstrated to be a valid fibrosis monitoring- and clinical decision tool in well-powered prospective studies, the filter paper based method opens new possibilities for HCV screening and monitoring, especially in combination with filter paper based HCV RNA quantification and genotyping [15]. IP-10 is readily detectable in DBS as in DPS, which makes sampling as simple as a home blood glucose monitoring [14], and could enable a new approach to HCV disease monitoring, based on frequent at-home testing. Automated high-throughput filter paper punching and analysis equipment is already standard for neonatal screening and can be adapted for IP-10 measurement to centralize analysis and reduce analytical imprecision.

In conclusion, this study we establish that IP-10 levels in plasma can be detected after the plasma has been dried on filter paper, but more studies are needed to substantiate IP-10 as a valid biomarker for liver fibrosis.

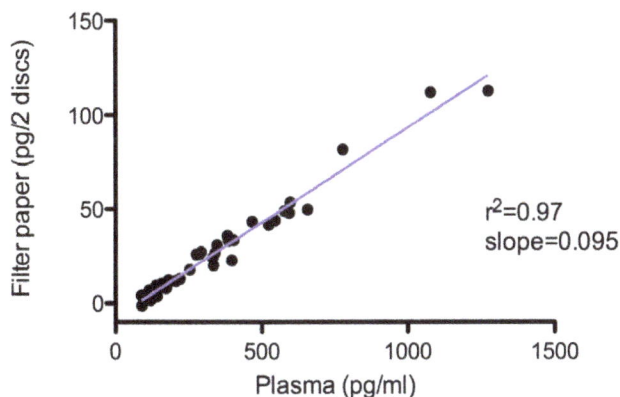

Figure 2. Correlation between IP-10 detected in plasma and dried plasma spots. Samples from 19 patients with chronic hepatitis C infection and no/mild liver fibrosis and 21 patients with liver cirrhosis were compared. There was a highly significant correlation between IP-10 detected with the two methods ($r^2 = 0.97$, $p < 0.0001$).

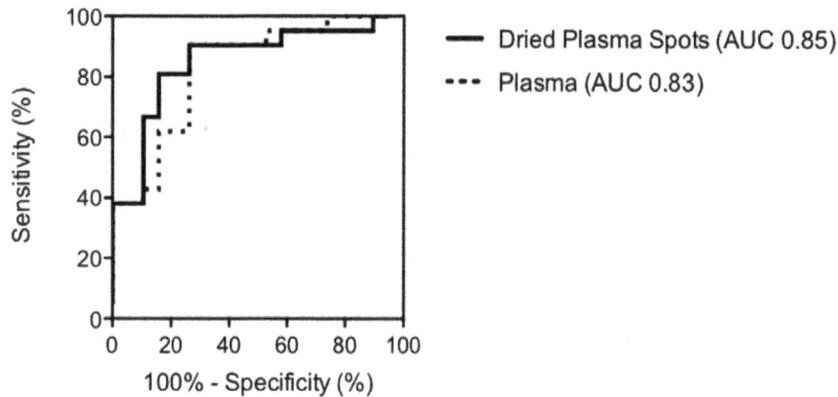

Figure 3. A comparison of Receiver Operation Characteristic Curves of IP-10 determined in dried plasma spots and plasma. Analysis included samples from 21 patients with cirrhosis (regarded as cases) and 19 patients with no/mild fibrosis (regarded controls in the analysis). The Area Under the Curve reflects the markers' ability to differentiate between the two groups of patients. There was no significant difference between the two methods.

Author Contributions

Conceived and designed the experiments: MR ESA NW BKM PBC.

Performed the experiments: MR ESA BKM. Analyzed the data: MR. Contributed reagents/materials/analysis tools: MR. Wrote the paper: MR.

References

1. Vergniol J, Foucher J, Terrebonne E, Bernard P-H, le Bail B, et al. (2011) Noninvasive tests for fibrosis and liver stiffness predict 5-year outcomes of patients with chronic hepatitis C. Gastroenterology 140: 1970–1979, 1979.e1–3. doi:10.1053/j.gastro.2011.02.058.

2. Bedossa P, Dargère D, Paradis V (2003) Sampling variability of liver fibrosis in chronic hepatitis C. Hepatology 38: 1449–1457. doi:53/jhep.2003.09022.

3. Darling JM, Aerssens J, Fanning G, McHutchison JG, Goldstein DB, et al. (2011) Quantitation of pretreatment serum interferon-γ-inducible protein-10 improves the predictive value of an IL28B gene polymorphism for hepatitis C treatment response. Hepatology 53: 14–22. doi:10.1002/hep.24056.

4. Beinhardt S, Aberle JH, Strasser M, Dulic-Lakovic E, Maieron A, et al. (2012) Serum level of IP-10 increases predictive value of IL28B polymorphisms for spontaneous clearance of acute HCV infection. Gastroenterology 142: 78–85.e2. doi:10.1053/j.gastro.2011.09.039.

5. You CR, Park S-H, Jeong SW, Woo HY, Bae SH, et al. (2011) Serum IP-10 Levels Correlate with the Severity of Liver Histopathology in Patients Infected with Genotype-1 HCV. Gut Liver 5: 506–512. doi:10.5009/gnl.2011.5.4.506.

6. Zeremski M, Dimova R, Brown Q, Jacobson IM, Markatou M, et al. (2009) Peripheral CXCR3-associated chemokines as biomarkers of fibrosis in chronic hepatitis C virus infection. J. Infect. Dis 200: 1774–1780. doi:10.1086/646614.

7. Askarieh G, Alsiö A, Pugnale P, Negro F, Ferrari C, et al. (2010) Systemic and intrahepatic interferon-gamma-inducible protein 10 kDa predicts the first-phase decline in hepatitis C virus RNA and overall viral response to therapy in chronic hepatitis C. Hepatology 51: 1523–1530. doi:10.1002/hep.23509.

8. Groom JR, Luster AD (2011) CXCR3 ligands: redundant, collaborative and antagonistic functions. Immunol Cell Biol 89: 207–215. Available: http://dx.doi.org.ep.fjernadgang.kb.dk/10.1038/icb.2010.158. Accessed 12 Jan 2011.

9. Liu M, Guo S, Hibbert JM, Jain V, Singh N, et al. (2011) CXCL10/IP-10 in infectious diseases pathogenesis and potential therapeutic implications. Cytokine Growth Factor Rev. 22: 121–130. doi:10.1016/j.cytogfr.2011.06.001.

10. Li K, Li NL, Wei D, Pfeffer SR, Fan M, et al. (2012) Activation of chemokine and inflammatory cytokine response in hepatitis C virus–infected hepatocytes depends on toll-like receptor 3 sensing of hepatitis C virus double-stranded RNA intermediates. Hepatology 55: 666–675. doi:10.1002/hep.24763.

11. Zeremski M, Petrovic LM, Chiriboga L, Brown QB, Yee HT, et al. (2008) Intrahepatic levels of CXCR3-associated chemokines correlate with liver inflammation and fibrosis in chronic hepatitis C. Hepatology 48: 1440–1450. doi:10.1002/hep.22500.

12. Casrouge A, Decalf J, Ahloulay M, Lababidi C, Mansour H, et al. (2011) Evidence for an antagonist form of the chemokine CXCL10 in patients chronically infected with HCV. J. Clin. Invest 121: 308–317. doi:10.1172/JCI40594.

13. Ruhwald M, Aabye MG, Ravn P (2012) IP-10 release assays in the diagnosis of tuberculosis infection: current status and future directions. Expert Rev. Mol. Diagn. 12: 175–187. doi:10.1586/erm.11.97.

14. Mei JV, Alexander JR, Adam BW, Hannon WH (2001) Use of filter paper for the collection and analysis of human whole blood specimens. J. Nutr 131: 1631S–6S.

15. Santos C, Reis A, Dos Santos CV, Damas C, Silva MH, et al. (2012) The use of real-time PCR to detect hepatitis C virus RNA in dried blood spots from Brazilian patients infected chronically. J. Virol. Methods 179: 17–20. doi:10.1016/j.jviromet.2011.06.012.

16. Aabye MG, Eugen-Olsen J, Werlinrud AM, Holm LL, Tuuminen T, et al. (2012) A Simple Method to Quantitate IP-10 in Dried Blood and Plasma Spots. PLoS ONE 7: e39228. doi:10.1371/journal.pone.0039228#s5.

17. Andersen ES, Ruhwald M, Moessner B, Christensen PB, Andersen O, et al. (2011) Twelve potential fibrosis markers to differentiate mild liver fibrosis from cirrhosis in patients infected with chronic hepatitis C genotype 1. Eur J Clin Microbiol Infect Dis 30: 761–766. Available: http://www.ncbi.nlm.nih.gov/pubmed/21229279. Accessed 1 Mar 2011.

18. Zeremski M, Hooker G, Shu MA, Winkelstein E, Brown Q, et al. (2011) Induction of CXCR3- and CCR5-associated chemokines during acute hepatitis C virus infection. J Hepatol 55: 545–553. Available: http://www.ncbi.nlm.nih.gov/pubmed/21256906. Accessed 5 Aug 2011.

19. Reiberger T, Aberle JH, Kundi M, Kohrgruber N, Rieger A, et al. (2008) IP-10 correlates with hepatitis C viral load, hepatic inflammation and fibrosis and predicts hepatitis C virus relapse or non-response in HIV-HCV coinfection. Antivir. Ther 13: 969–976.

20. Lai M, Afdhal NH (2011) Editorial: Staging Liver Fibrosis in Hepatitis C: A Challenge for This Decade. The American Journal of Gastroenterology 106: 2121–2122. doi:10.1038/ajg.2011.343.

21. Zhou X-H, McClish DK, Obuchowski NA (2002) Statistical Methods in Diagnostic Medicine. 1st ed. Wiley-Interscience.

22. Skogstrand K (2005) Simultaneous Measurement of 25 Inflammatory Markers and Neurotrophins in Neonatal Dried Blood Spots by Immunoassay with xMAP Technology. Clinical Chemistry 51: 1854–1866. doi:10.1373/clinchem.2005.052241.

3

The Role of Serum Biomarkers in Predicting Fibrosis Progression in Pediatric and Adult Hepatitis C Virus Chronic Infection

Pamela Valva[1]*, **Paola Casciato**[2], **Juan M. Diaz Carrasco**[1], **Adrian Gadano**[2], **Omar Galdame**[2], **María Cristina Galoppo**[3], **Eduardo Mullen**[4], **Elena De Matteo**[1], **María Victoria Preciado**[1]

1 Laboratory of Molecular Biology, Pathology Division, Ricardo Gutiérrez Children's Hospital, Buenos Aires, Argentina, **2** Liver Unit, Hospital Italiano de Buenos Aires, Buenos Aires, Argentina, **3** Liver Unit of University of Buenos Aires at Ricardo Gutiérrez Children's Hospital, Buenos Aires, Argentina, **4** Pathology Division, Hospital Italiano de Buenos Aires, Buenos Aires, Argentina

Abstract

Background/Aims: Liver biopsy represents the gold standard for damage evaluation, but noninvasive serum markers that mirror liver fibrosis progression are actual goals both in adults and especially in children. The aim was to determine specific serum markers that correlate with liver fibrosis progression during chronic HCV infection.

Methods: Liver biopsies and concomitant serum samples from 22 pediatric and 22 adult HCV patients were analyzed. Histological parameters were evaluated. On serum TGF-ß1, tissue inhibitor of matrix metalloprotein inhibitor-1 (TIMP-1), hyaluronic acid (HA) and aminoterminal peptide of procollagen type III (PIIINP) were tested.

Results: Significant fibrosis (F≥2) and advanced fibrosis (F≥3) represented 64% and 20%, respectively in children; while 54% F≥2 and 23% F≥3 in adults. Hyaluronic acid ($p = 0.011$) and PIIINP ($p = 0.016$) were related to worse fibrosis stages only in adults, along with TIMP-1 ($p = 0.039$) just in children; but TGF-ß1 was associated with mild fibrosis ($p = 0.022$) in adults. The AUROC of TIMP-1 in children to discriminate advanced fibrosis was 0.800 (95%IC 0.598–0.932). In adults, the best AUROCs were that of HA, PIIINP and TGF-ß1 [0.929 (IC95% 0.736–0.994), 0.894 (IC95% 0.689–0.984) and 0.835 (IC95% 0.617–0.957)], respectively. In children, according to the cut off (165.7 ng/mL) value for TIMP-1, biopsies could have been avoided in 72% (18/25). Considering the cut off for HA (109.7 ng/mL), PIIINP (9.1 µg/L), and TGF-ß1 (10,848.3 pg/mL), biopsies could have been avoided in 87% (19/22) of adult patients by using HA and 73% (16/22) using PIIINP or TGF-ß1.

Conclusions: In adults given the diagnostic accuracy of HA, PIIINP, TGF-ß1, their combination may provide a potential useful tool to assess liver fibrosis. This first pediatric study suggests that TIMP-1 is clinically useful for predicting liver fibrosis in HCV patients.

Editor: Ravi Jhaveri, Duke University, United States of America

Funding: This study was funded by grants from the International Society for Infectious Diseases (2009). No additional external funding received for this study. PV and JMDC are supported by a fellowship from National Research Council (CONICET), MVP is a member of the CONICET Research Career Program, and EDM is a member of the Research Career of Buenos Aires City Government. The funders had no role in study design, data collection and analysis, decision to publish, or preparation of the manuscript.

Competing Interests: The authors have declared that no competing interests exist.

* E-mail: valvapamela@yahoo.com

Introduction

Hepatitis related to HCV is a progressive disease that may result in chronic active hepatitis, cirrhosis, and hepatocellular carcinoma [1,2,3]. It represents a global health problem since there is no vaccine currently available and furthermore, liver failure due to chronic hepatitis C (CHC) is one of the most common reasons for liver transplants. Liver disease seems to be milder in children than in adults; however, the natural history of chronic HCV infection acquired in infancy and childhood remains poorly characterized and the long-term outcome of the disease is still a matter of debate [4,5]. The mechanisms leading to liver cell injury, inflammation, steatosis and fibrosis are still under study. Staging liver fibrosis is considered to be an essential part in the management of patients with CHC, because it provides prognostic information and, in many cases, assists in therapeutic decisions [6]. Although liver biopsy represents the gold standard for evaluating presence, type and stage of liver fibrosis and for characterizing necroinflammation; it remains a costly and invasive procedure with inherent risks. Thus, it cannot be performed frequently to monitor therapeutic outcomes [7,8]. Moreover, in children, biopsy is still perceived to carry a higher risk of complications, so it is less accepted than in adults. Therefore, developing noninvasive tests that can accurately predict initial disease stage and progression over time represents a high priority and growing medical need [9,10].

Currently, there are several noninvasive diagnostic methods for determining liver fibrosis that are being validated such as blood markers and imaging methods, but little progress has been achieved in clinical practice [11].

In recent years, many studies have been dedicated to the evaluation of noninvasive indirect serum markers of fibrosis such as serum aminotransferases, aspartate aminotranferase (AST)-to-platelet ratio (APRI) and AST-to-alanine aminotranferase (ALT) ratio (AAR), but they reflect alterations in hepatic function rather than in extracellular matrix metabolism. Since, several HCV reports have described normal aminotransferase levels in about 25%–30% CHC patients, there may be a potential advantage in assessing serum direct fibrosis markers that do not involve transaminases [4,12,13,14]. The extracellular matrix remodelling markers represent attractive candidates because they measure directly the fibrogenic process that leads to clinical complications [15]. These markers include several glycoproteins (hyaluronan, laminin etc), the collagen family (procollagen III, type IV collagen and type IV collagen 7s domain), collagenases and their inhibitors (metalloproteinases and tissue inhibitors of metalloproteinases) and a number of cytokines involved in the fibrogenic process (in particular TGF-ß1). These have been analysed individually as well as combined, in order to assess severity and progression of hepatic fibrosis and to follow up changes related to viral treatment [16,17,18,19,20,21,22,23].

On the other hand, many authors have combined several biochemical and clinical data (i.e. Fib-4, Forns, Fibrotest) to predict fibrosis stages, but others have brought these together with serum fibrosis markers (i.e. Hepascore, SHASTA, Fibrometer) to do so. [24,25,26]. However, this calculation system is tough and complicated to perform routinely in every case.

Finally, considering that most noninvasive approaches for evaluating liver fibrosis have been performed in adults and taking into account the above mentioned considerations about biopsies, there is a clear need to assess these markers in children. Hence, the purpose of our study was to evaluate the presence of a pro-fibrogenic cytokine (TGF-ß1) and matrix deposition markers [hyaluronic acid (HA), type III procollagen amino-terminal peptide (PIIINP) and tissue inhibitor of matrix metalloprotein inhibitor-1 (TIMP-1)] that correlate with liver injury during chronic hepatitis C virus infection, in a cohort of pediatric and adult patients.

Methods

Patients and samples

Twenty two pediatric patients with chronic HCV infection (8 male, 14 female; range of age at biopsy: 1–17 years, median: 8 years) who attended the Ricardo Gutierrez Children's Hospital; and 22 adult patients (13 male, 9 female; range of age at biopsy: 38–74 years, median: 51 years) from Hospital Italiano de Buenos Aires were enrolled in the present study.

Diagnosis was based on the presence of anti-HCV antibodies in serum at or after 18 months of age and HCV RNA in plasma at one or more separate occasions. Patients had no other causes of liver disease, autoimmune or metabolic disorders, hepatocellular carcinoma and coinfection with hepatitis B virus and/or human immunodeficiency virus. In adult cases, patients with a history of habitual alcohol consumption were excluded (>80 g/day for men and >60 g/day for women). Patients were naïve of treatment. This study has the approval of the Institutional Review Board and the Ethics Board of both Ricardo Gutierrez Children Hospital and Hospital Italiano de Buenos Aires and is also in accordance with the Helsinki Declaration of 1975, as revised in 1983. A written informed consent was obtained from all the included adult patients

and from parents of pediatric patients after the nature of the procedure had been fully explained.

Formalin-fixed paraffin-embedded liver biopsies and serum samples at time of biopsy were used for histological and serological analysis, respectively. Histological sections were evaluated by two independent pathologists in a blind manner. Fibrosis staging were semiquantitatively assessed according to the METAVIR system [27]. Serum samples were stored frozen at −80°C. Serum AST and ALT levels, HCV viral load and genotype, smoking status and alcohol consumption were obtained from clinical records. In pediatric patients, normal ALT and AST levels were ≤32 and ≤48 IU/L, respectively. In adult patients, normal ALT and AST levels were ≤40 and ≤42 IU/L, respectively. In two pediatric cases, more than one sample was analyzed. As controls, serum samples from pediatric (n = 9) and adult (n = 9) healthy subjects without known systemic or liver disease and with normal biological liver test as well as absence of anti-HCV antibodies, were included.

In adult cases, liver samples were not obtained from patients diagnosed as having liver cirrhosis based on clinical, biochemical and imaging findings. Although, there are no pediatric specific guidelines about the need for and timing of a liver biopsy in children, the probability of a child undergoing liver biopsy in this study reflected the current practice at our centre, which is based mostly on the national experts consensus [28].

Quantitative measurement of human TGF-ß1, TIMP-1, HA and PIIINP

Serum TGF-ß1 and TIMP-1 were determined by commercial quantitative sandwich enzyme immunoassay technique (Quanti-kine, R&D System Inc) according to the manufacturer's instructions. Serum concentration for each marker was determined from the constructed standard curves. Serum TGF-ß1 was expressed as pg/mL and TIMP-1 as ng/mL.

Serum HA levels were assessed by ELISA (Corgenix) according to the manufacturer's instructions. The HA test kit is an enzyme-linked binding protein assay that uses a capture molecule known as hyaluronic acid binding protein (HABP) and an enzyme-conjugated version of HABP. Hyaluronic acid levels in patient and control samples were determined from the constructed reference curve and expressed as ng/mL.

The levels of PIIINP were measured using a commercial competitive radioimmunoassay technique (UNniQ, Orion Diagnostica) according to manufacture's instructions. Concentrations of PIIINP (µg/L) were obtained from a calibration curve.

Each serum marker concentration was assessed in duplicate.

Operators who perform the laboratory tests were blinded for patient's clinical and histological data.

Statistical analysis

Statistical analysis was performed using GraphPad InStat software, version 3.05. To compare the means between groups, ANOVA or Student's t test were performed. To determine differences between groups not normally distributed, medians were compared using the Mann-Whitney U test or Kruskal Wallis test. Pearson's correlation coefficient was used to measure the degree of association between continuous, normally distributed variables. The degree of association between non-normally distributed variables was assessed using Spearman's nonparametric correlation. To compare categorical variables Fisher's exact Test was applied. P values<0.05 were considered statistically significant. Results of serum fibrosis markers were expressed as box plots.

To assess the ability of the four serum fibrosis markers for differentiating significant (F≥2) and advanced fibrosis (F≥3), we calculated the sensitivity and the specificity for each value of each fibrosis marker and then constructed receiver operating characteristic (ROC) curves by plotting the sensitivity against the reverse specificity at each value. The diagnostic value of each serum marker was assessed by the area under the ROC (AUROC). AUROC of 1.0 is characteristic of an ideal test, whereas 0.5 indicates a test of no diagnostic value. We determined the cut-off value for the diagnosis, as the maximal value at the sum of the sensitivity (Se) and specificity (Sp). The diagnostic accuracy was calculated by sensitivity, specificity and positive and negative predictive values, considering significant and advanced fibrosis of the disease. Area under the ROC, cut off values, positive predictive values (PPV) and negative predictive values (NPV) were determined using the MedCalc demo statistical software (Mariakerke, Belgium).

Due to the heterogeneous distribution of fibrosis stages on liver biopsies, we applied the DANA method described by Poynard et al [29]. The DANA is an index for standardizing comparisons in order to transform any different fibrosis prevalence profile into a homogeneous distribution of fibrosis stages from F0 to F4, as defined by a prevalence of 0.20 for each of the five METAVIR stages (standard prevalence). The DANA method was applied for each biological non-invasive test. The formula to calculate the adjusted AUROC (AdAUROC) according to a uniform DANA of 2.5 was ObservedAUROC+(0.1056) (2.5-ObservedDANA). Observed AUROC represents the AUROC of the studied group [29].

Finally, we calculated the percentage of patients in whom the results of each serum marker could have avoided the biopsy. Patients correctly classified [true positive (TP)+true negatives (TN)] by a certain test would not have needed the biopsy procedure.

Results

1. Clinical and liver biopsy findings

Clinical, virological, and histological features of patients are described in Table 1 (pediatric patients) and Table 2 (adult patients).

In both groups genotype 1 was predominant. It was present in 86% of pediatric cases and 77% of adult cases. Only one pediatric patient displayed genotype 4, two adults genotype 2 and three adults genotype 3. The risk factors for HCV infection in pediatric cases were maternal HCV infection in 46% of patients (10/22), transfusion in 36% (8/22) and unknown in 18% (4/22). In adults, seven cases (32%) had a history of injecting drug abuse, one case (5%) described an occupational exposure to infected blood, four (18%) a transfusion as a risk factor and 10 (45%) an unknown source for transmission. The AST and ALT levels at time of biopsy (considering multiple biopsies from the same patient in 2 pediatric cases) were elevated in 52% (13/25) and 76% (19/25) serum samples of pediatric patients, respectively and in 59% (13/22) and 77% (17/22) serum samples of adult patients as well.

Concerning fibrosis, bridging fibrosis was predominant among studied pediatric biopsies (44%). However, one case harbouring thalassemia displayed complete cirrhosis and one case, with an actual progression of liver disease during follow up, incomplete cirrhosis. In adult cases, the fibrosis profile displayed 32% stage 1, 32% stage 2 and 23% stage 3. Finally, three adult patients showed absence of fibrosis. The prevalence of significant fibrosis (F≥2) and advanced fibrosis (F≥3) in the pediatric cohort were 64% and 20%, respectively; meanwhile it was 54% F≥2 and 23% F≥3 in adults.

The comparative statistical analysis of all histological parameters between adult and pediatric patients studied did not show any significant difference. However, it should be taken into account that adult cases with liver cirrhosis based on clinical, biochemical and imaging findings were not biopsied.

Aminotransferase values showed no statistical correlation with fibrosis stages (AST r = 0.04, p = 0.85 and ALT r = 0.08, p = 0.70 in pediatrics; AST r = 0.14, p = 0.50 and ALT r = 0.05, p = 0.81 in adults), as well as viral load did not correlate with it either (r = 0.55, p = 0.12 in pediatric patient, r = 0.26, p = 0.31 in adults). Concerning gender, it has no statistically significant difference related neither to advanced nor significant fibrosis in any of the studied series (p = 1.0 for F≥3, p = 0.23 for F≥2 in pediatric patients; p = 0.11 for F≥3, p = 0.41 23 for F≥2 in adults. With regards to the smoking status, none of the pediatric patients is a smoker and in the adult cohort, 12 were no smokers, 7 were smokers and there were no available data in the medical records for the other 3. Smoking status showed no statistically significant difference related either to advanced or significant fibrosis in the studied adult series [Adults F≥2 (p = 1), Adults F≥3 (p = 0.60)].

2. Quantitative measurement of TGF-ß1, TIMP-1, HA and PIIINP

Serum concentrations of studied markers were compared between HCV patients and control healthy subjects. In chronic HCV patients TGF-ß1, TIMP-1, HA and PIIINP levels were higher than in controls (Table 3).

Serum TGF-ß1 showed no statistically significant differences among fibrosis stages in pediatric patients; however it was associated with mild fibrosis (p = 0.022) in adults (Figure 1). Higher values of TIMP-1 and HA were observed in both pediatric and adult patients with worse fibrosis stages. The same pattern was observed with PIIINP in adults, but not in children (Figure 1). However, the differences among fibrosis stages were significant for HA (p = 0.011) and PIIINP (p = 0.016) only in adults, along with TIMP-1 (p = 0.039) just in children.

Interestingly, the uppermost values for HA (228.2 ng/mL) and TIMP-1 (845.2 ng/mL) in children correspond to a patient with complete cirrhosis. In adults, the extremely elevated HA value (2,225 ng/mL; result confirmed in three independent assay) and the TIMP-1 (977.5 ng/mL) and PIIINP (39.42 µg/L) uppermost values correspond to the case with stage 4 fibrosis according to modified Knodell scoring system.

3. Diagnostic performance of serum markers for significant and advanced fibrosis

The efficiency of these markers to differentiate significant (F≥2) and advanced fibrosis (F≥3) were evaluated using ROC (Figure 2). Table 4 showed the best AUROC for the four serum fibrosis markers. These AUROCs had low but similar diagnostic accuracies for significant fibrosis. In the pediatrics cohort, the best AUROC was that of TIMP-1, which discriminates advanced fibrosis from other stages, with an AUROC of 0.800. On the other hand, in adults, the best AUROCs were that of HA, PIIINP and TGF-ß1 (0.929, 0.894 and 0.835, respectively). For most markers, the accuracy for discriminating significant fibrosis was lower than that for discriminating advanced fibrosis.

Standardization of AUROC by DANA method was carried out for each marker. The analysis showed that AdAUROC were always higher than the corresponding AUROC, but these increments were not significant (Table 4)

Cut off values for each marker in both cohorts for significant and advanced fibrosis stages were shown in Table 5. Many fibrosis experts would consider noninvasive tests for fibrosis with an AUROC value of 0.850–0.900 to be as good as liver biopsies for

Table 1. Clinical, virological and histological features of HCV pediatric patients.

Pediatric Patients		Sex	Ages (ys)	Risk factor for HCV infection	Genotype	Transaminases		Knodell	Lymphoid Follicle	Bile duct damage	Steatosis
						AST (U/L)	ALT (U/L)				
1		M	13	T	1a	47	43	8(5+3)	no	no	absent
2		F	14	T	1b	55	86	11(9+2)	no	no	minimal
3		F	4	V	1a/c	46	34	10(7+3)	yes	yes	absent
4		F	17	T	1a/c	39	43	8(4+4)	no	yes	moderate
5		M	4	V	1a/c	84	97	10(9+1)	yes	yes	severe
6	BxI	F	6	V	1a/c	13	11	7(3+4)	no	no	absent
	BxII		13			23	21	8(5+3)	no	yes	minimal
7		F	16	Unknown	1a/c	30	41	12(10+2)	yes	yes	minimal
8	BxI	M	3	V	1a/c	71	91	6(5+1)	yes	yes	minimal
	BxII		6			314	364	11(8+3)	no	yes	severe
	BxIII		13			225	260	21(16+5)	no	yes	moderate
9		F	6	V	1a/c	35	50	8(7+1)	yes	yes	minimal
10		F	8	Unknown	1a	41	38	9(7+2)	yes	yes	absent
11		M	13	Unknown	ND	56	71	10(7+3)	no	yes	absent
12		F	17	V	1a/c	21	11	6(3+3)	no	yes	minimal
13		F	3	V	1a/c	84	137	6(5+1)	no	yes	moderate
14		F	3	V	1b	65	75	9(6+3)	yes	yes	moderate
15		F	1	V	4	57	33	11(7+4)	yes	yes	absent
16		F	17	T	1a/c	22	16	10(7+3)	no	yes	minimal
17		M	1	T	1b	159	213	14(11+3)	yes	yes	minimal
18		F	8	T	1b	10	12	6(5+1)	no	no	absent
19		M	15	T	ND	58	76	16(10+6)	no	yes	absent
20		F	6	V	1a/c	56	55	6(5+1)	no	yes	severe
21		M	15	T	1b	20	24	13(10+3)	yes	yes	absent
22		M	12	Unknown	1a/c	83	113	11 (8+3)	no	yes	minimal

F: female, M: male. ND: not determined Bx I, Bx II, Bx III denote: multiple liver biopsies. Risk factor for HCV infection: T: transfusion, V: maternal HCV infection. ALT: alanine aminotransferase; AST: aspartate aminotransferase. Normal ALT and AST levels were ≤32 and ≤48 IU/L, respectively when test was done at 37°C.

staging fibrosis [9]; however others consider lower AUROC values to be predictors of fibrosis. In this analysis, those markers with AUROCs higher than 0.800 were only considered. The cut off value for pediatric TIMP-1 in advanced fibrosis was 165.7 ng/mL (80% sensibility, 70% specificity). In adults, the cut-off values of HA, PIIINP and TGF-ß1 were 109.7 ng/mL, 9.1 μg/L and 10,848.3 pg/mL respectively. The sensitivity and specificity for these cut off values were 100% and 82.3% for HA, 100% and 64.7% for PIIINP and 100% and 64.7% for TGF-ß1, respectively.

Although PIIINP for F≥2 and HA for F≥3 in pediatric patients had an excellent 100% PPV (Table 5), the diagnostic values were quite low (PIIINP AUROC: 0.648 and HA AUROC: 0.562) (Table 4). The same was observed in adults' TIMP-1 for F≥3 (AUROC: 0.553) (Table 4). The NPV was quite low for all the non-invasive markers of F≥2 in children (always <67%), so that significant fibrosis could not be reliably excluded by any of these markers. The noninvasive methods with best AUROCs (TIMP-1 in the pediatric cohort and HA, PIIINP and TGF-ß1 in adults) showed high NPV (>90%) for advanced fibrosis.

In children, according to the cut off values for advanced fibrosis (F≥3), using TIMP-1 as a serum marker, 14 of 20 (70%) patients with F<3 were correctly categorized, while only 1 of 5 (20%)

patients with F≥3 were misclassified (40% PPV and 93.3% NPV). Considering the above, biopsies could have been avoided in 72% (18/25) of pediatric patients. In adults, when the cut-off value for HA was applied, 19 patients were correctly classified (5 patients were TP and 14 patients were TN), and 3 patients were misclassified [False Positive (FP)]. Taking into consideration the cut off for PIIINP, 16 patients were correctly identified (5 patients were TP and 11 patients were TN), and 6 patients were misclassified (6 FP). According to the cut off value for TGF-ß1, 16 patients were correctly identified (5 patients were TP and 11 patients were TN), and 6 patients were misclassified (6 FP). Consequently, biopsies could have been avoided in 87% (19/22) of adult patients by using HA and 73% (16/22) using PIIINP or TGF-ß1.

Discussion

A major clinical challenge is finding the best means for evaluating liver impairment and managing the increasing number of HCV infected patients. Prognosis and treatment of CHC are partly dependent on the assessment of histological activity, namely cell necrosis and inflammation, and on the

Table 2. Clinical, virological and histological features of HCV adult patients.

Adult Patients	Sex	Ages (ys)	Risk factor for HCV infection	Genotype	Transaminases AST (U/L)	Transaminases ALT (U/L)	Knodell	Lymphoid Follicle	Bile duct damage	Steatosis
							Histological characteristics*			
1	M	38	Unknown	1b	82	89	6(5+1)	yes	yes	absent
2	F	52	T	1b	45	52	8(6+2)	yes	yes	minimal
3	M	42	Unknown	1a	44	56	9(8+1)	yes	yes	absent
4	F	62	T	1a	42	32	11(7+4)	no	yes	moderate
5	M	48	DA	1b	40	63	10(7+3)	no	yes	severe
6	M	40	DA	1a	34	45	10(6+4)	yes	yes	moderate
7	M	47	Unknown	1a	29	54	8(6+2)	yes	yes	minimal
8	M	40	DA	2a	63	79	4(4+0)	yes	no	absent
9	M	41	DA	3a	79	86	7(4+3)	no	yes	absent
10	F	61	Unknown	1a	31	28	17(12+5)	yes	yes	absent
11	F	72	Unknown	1a/c	52	71	9(6+3)	yes	yes	minimal
12	F	74	T	1*	106	85	15(12+3)	yes	yes	absent
13	M	62	Unknown	1b	22	32	10(7+3)	no	yes	absent
14	F	55	Unknown	3b	49	60	8(6+2)	yes	yes	severe
15	F	67	Unknown	2a	28	26	6(6+0)	yes	yes	minimal
16	F	41	Unknown	1a	192	105	6(2+4)	yes	yes	absent
17	M	51	OE	1b	65	74	5(4+0)	yes	yes	absent
18	M	51	DA	1a	73	109	10(7+3)	yes	yes	minimal
19	F	67	T	1b	106	103	13(9+4)	yes	yes	absent
20	M	73	Unknown	1b	31	42	8(6+2)	yes	yes	absent
21	M	41	DA	1a	32	50	10(7+3)	yes	yes	severe
22	M	47	DA	3	38	59	3(2+1)	yes	yes	minimal

F: female, M: male.
*Subtype not determined Risk factor for HCV infection: T: transfusion, DA: drug abuse, OE: occupational exposure.
ALT: alanine aminotransferase; AST: aspartate aminotransferase. Normal ALT and AST levels were ≤40 and ≤42 IU/L, respectively when test was done at 37°C.

degree of liver fibrosis. These parameters have so far been provided by liver biopsy, because conventional laboratory tests are unable to precisely evaluate liver lesions. Biopsy, because of its limitations and risks, is no longer considered mandatory as the 1st-line indicator of liver injury in HCV patients [30,31,32,33]. In addition to the risks related to an invasive procedure, liver biopsy has been associated with sampling error mostly due to suboptimal biopsy size [34,35,36]. To avoid these pitfalls, several markers have been proposed as noninvasive alternatives for predicting fibrosis; but few, particularly those which combine clinical and biochemical parameters, have been applied to pediatric patients [37,38].

Table 3. TGF-ß1, TIMP-1, HA and PIIINP levels in chronic HCV patients vs healthy subjects.

	Pediatrics Healthy*	Pediatrics HCV+*	Pediatrics P value	Adults Healthy*	Adults HCV+*	Adults P value
TGF-ß1 (pg/ml)	2,866	12,178	<0.0001	5,257	12,384	<0.0001
	(770.3–7,125)	(1,400–24,407)		(1,566–7,898)	(2,151–25,679)	
TIMP-1 (ng/ml)	79.75	142.9	0.0029	114.9	302.6	<0.0001
	(53.98–120.2)	(71.66–845.2)		(92.58–181.1)	(113.5–977.5)	
HA (ng/ml)	6.36	10.22	0.03	10.22	80.12	<0.0001
	(0–11.03)	(2.67–228.2)		(4.51–48.41)	(7.90–2,225)	
PIIINP (µg/L)	11.43	12.37	0.04	5.54	9.58	0.0004
	(8.64–13.65)	(6.91–27.77)		(3.30–6.61)	(3.41–39.42)	

*Results are expressed as median (min-max).

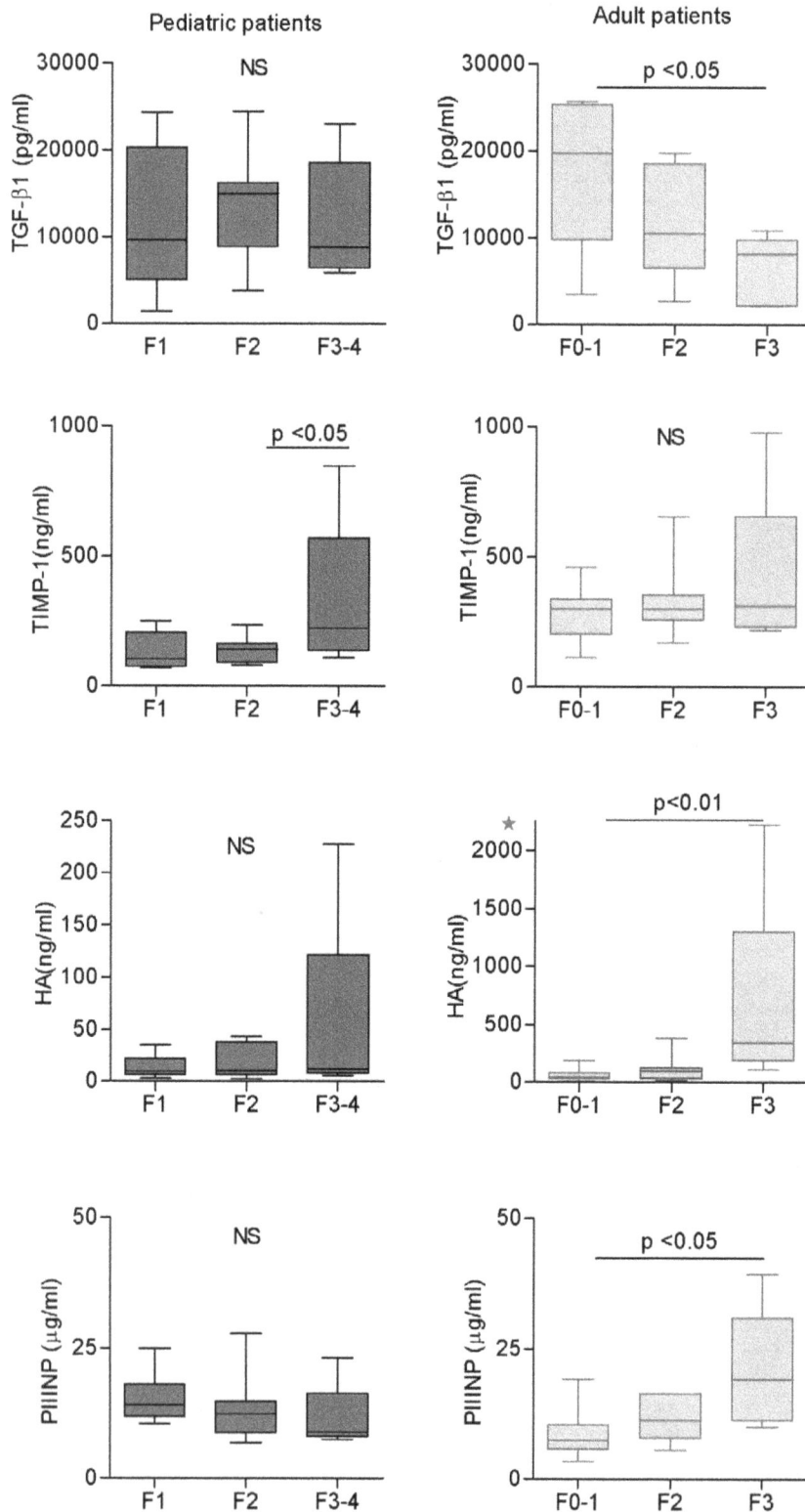

Figure 1. Serum markers related to fibrosis stages in chronic hepatitis C patients. A) TGF-ß1, B) TIMP-1, C) HA, D) PIIINP. Horizontal lines inside each box represent the median, and the lower and upper borders of the box encompass the interquartile range. The vertical lines from the ends of each box encompass the extreme data points. Fibrosis stages according to METAVIR. *NS*: no significant. * Note: different scale compared with pediatric values.

A Significant Fibrosis

B Advanced Fibrosis

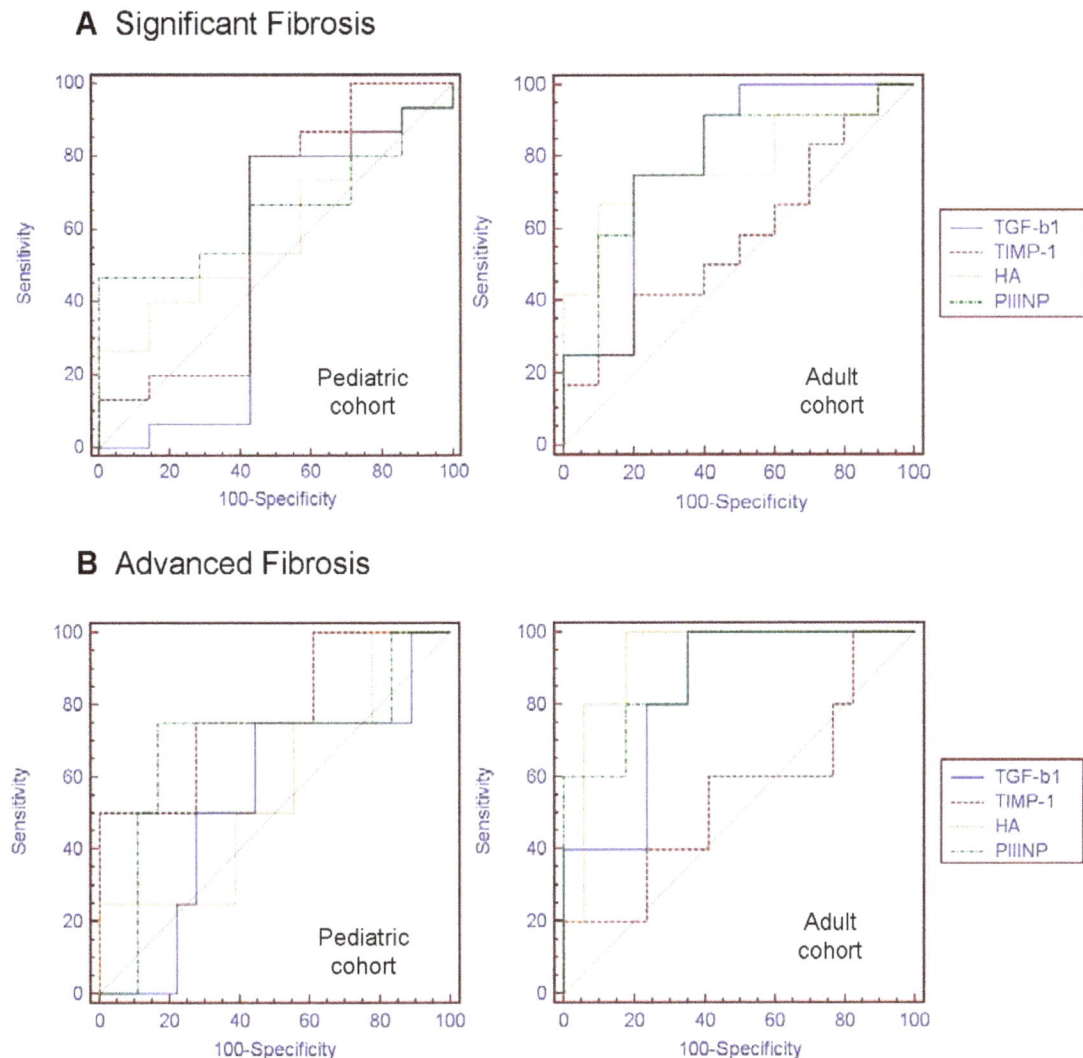

Figure 2. AUROC of TGF-ß1, TIMP-1, HA and PIIINP in pediatric and adult cohorts A) for significant and B) for advanced fibrosis.

Table 4. AUROC for significant and advance fibrosis.

	Significant fibrosis (F≥2)			Advanced fibrosis (F≥3)	
	AUROC	95% CI	AdAUROC	AUROC	95% CI
PEDIATRICS					
TGF-ß1	0.549	0.339–0.746	0.661	0.570	0.359–0.764
TIMP-1	0.625	0.411–0.809	0.737	0.800	0.593–0.932
HA	0.585	0.368–0.780	0.697	0.562	0.347–0.762
PIIINP	0.648	0.417–0.836	0.760	0.694	0.464–0.870
ADULTS					
TGF-ß1	0.792	0.567–0.933	0.875	0.835	0.617–0.957
TIMP-1	0.575	0.349–0.780	0.658	0.553	0.329–0.762
HA	0.783	0.558–0.928	0.866	0.929	0.736–0.994
PIIINP	0.792	0.567–0.933	0.875	0.894	0.689–0.984

The key step in the pathophysiology of liver fibrogenesis is the balance between extracellular matrix (ECM) deposition and removal [39]. It is characterized by the activation and proliferation of hepatic stellate cells (HSCs) which undergo a phenotypic switch when exposed to soluble factors including transforming growth factor beta-1 (TGF-ß1) [40,41,42]. Hepatic stellate cells secret excess matrix proteins such as collagens, elastin, glycoproteins, and proteoglycans, then matrix degradation, initiated by a family of enzymes called the matrix metalloproteins (MMPs), occurs. MMP are in turn inhibited by tissue inhibitors of metalloproteins (TIMPs) [17,43,44].

Hepatitis C virus Core protein is thought to be involved in the disruption of lipid metabolism leading to the production of the pro-inflammatory cytokine TGF-ß1 [45,46,47]. Hyaluronic acid (HA) is synthesized and distributed throughout the extracellular space by HSC, therefore its serum levels reflect the activity state of these cells [48]. Tissue inhibitor of matrix metalloprotein inhibitor-1 (TIMP-1) protects collagen from MMP fibrolysis and also inhibits the apoptosis of HSC [49]. On the other hand, initiating events in HSC activation are occurring on a background of progressive disease changes in the surrounding ECM. Over the time, the subendothelial matrix composition changes from one

Table 5. Diagnostic accuracy of the serum markers measurement for significant and advance fibrosis.

	Significant fibrosis (F≥2)					Advanced fibrosis (F≥3)				
	Cut off	Se%	Sp%	PPV	NPV	Cut off	Se	Sp	PPV	NPV
PEDIATRICS										
TGF-ß1 (pg/ml)	6,950.6	87.5	44.4	73.7	66.7	8,755.7	60	70	33.3	87.5
TIMP-1 (ng/ml)	105.4	81.2	55.6	76.5	62.5	**165.7**	**80**	**70**	**40**	**93.3**
HA (ng/ml)	23.9	40	88.9	85.7	47.1	43.4	25	100	100	87
PIIINP (µg/L)	10.1	46.7	100	100	46.7	9.62	75	83.3	50	93.7
ADULTS										
TGF-ß1 (pg/ml)	10,848.3	75	80	81.8	72.7	**10,848.3**	**100**	**64.7**	**45.5**	**100**
TIMP-1 (ng/ml)	336.2	41.7	80	71.4	53.3	654.8	20	100	100	81
HA (ng/ml)	103.1	66.7	90	89	62.2	**109.7**	**100**	**82.3**	**62.5**	**100**
PIIINP (µg/L)	9.1	75	80	81.8	72.7	**9.1**	**100**	**64.7**	**45.5**	**100**

Se: sensitivity Sp: specificity PPV: positive predictive value. NPV: negative predictive value.
In bold are shown the parameters for those markers with best AUROC.

comprised of type IV collagen, heparan sulfate proteoglycan, and laminin to one rich in fibril-forming collagen, like collagen type III [44].

Concerning our results, there are different points to be emphasized. First, the circulating concentration of TGF-ß1, HA, TIMP-1, PIIINP were higher in CHC patients than in healthy control subjects. Second, many markers seemed to be related to liver fibrosis progression, but with different association patterns in the two cohorts: TIMP-1 levels were associated with fibrosis progression in the pediatric cohort and HA, PIIINP and TGF-ß1 in adults.

Many authors have explored these markers as a potential noninvasive tool to predict fibrosis changes. Most of them evaluated HA in adult HCV patients, and many applied a combined panel of TIMP-1, PIIINP and HA named ELF test [16,17,21,23,50]. This test which has shown good performance in predicting advanced fibrosis, it is not commercially available worldwide [10]. In our analysis, these above mentioned markers seemed to be also related to liver fibrosis progression, but probably not to be applied altogether as a panel. In accordance with the results published by Patel et al [21], Sanvisens et al [18] and Resino et al [50] our adult studied cohort displayed levels of HA strongly associated with advanced stages of liver fibrosis. Furthermore, our findings also go along with Saitou et al [16] and Leroy et al [17] who described that both HA and PIIINP were related to worse fibrosis stages. However, concerning TIMP-1 conflicting results were reported. Leroy et al [17] found association between TIMP-1 levels and fibrosis stage in adults, while Macias et al [24] did not. Interestingly our results were also discordant, since no association was evidenced in adults but it was presented in children. Although there are few data related to TIMP-1 in children as a single marker of liver injury in different hepatic diseases, our results suggested that TIMP-1 would be suitable as a fibrosis marker in HCV children. This observation is in agreement with data reported by Lebensztejn et al on pediatric HBV patients [51], It is worthwhile to note that the highest TIMP-1 values were those of the cirrhosis case, so it would be interesting to analyze more cases from this condition to assess the actual diagnostic accuracy for cirrhosis.

Diagnostic accuracy is evaluated using the area under the ROC curve [30,31,32]. In the studied cohort most markers displayed an AUROC increment between significant and advanced fibrosis.

According to Leroy et al [17] in our adult cohort HA and PIIINP were also the markers with the best diagnostic accuracy for advanced fibrosis. Moreover, HA showed moderate accuracy for diagnosis of significant fibrosis (AUROC: 0.783), while it seemed to be a very useful method for detection of advanced fibrosis (AUROC: 0.929). This observation is in agreement with the data published by many reports including adult monoinfected as well as HIV/HCV coinfected patients [16,17,18,50]. Many authors have described the reliability of this marker in series of pediatric HBV infected patient as well as non-alcoholic fatty liver disease [51,52,53,54,55,56]. Although in our HCV pediatric cohort HA showed 100% specificity in advanced fibrosis, a remarkable point for a diagnostic tool, it usefulness seemed to be limited. Finally, a novel finding was the TIMP-1 diagnostic accuracy for advanced fibrosis which was described for the first time in HCV pediatric series.

Poynard et al had proposed that for a disease defined as a combination of stages vs. a combination of other stages, the AUROCs for the diagnosis of it must be expressed in a standardized fashion according to the prevalence of a given stage [57]. They suggested to use a uniform distribution with the same prevalence for each stage (corresponding to a difference in DANA of 2.5 fibrosis METAVIR units between F≥2 and F<2). This finding is clinically significant, because it is easier to discuss the apparently discordant results of a given biomarker observed in the literature [29].Through the literature different AUROCs for significant fibrosis concerning several markers were described. Resino et al [50] reported an AUROC for HA of 0.676, while Levoy et al [17] showed a HA AUROC of 0.75 and a PIIINP AUROC of 0.77 and finally, Saitou et al [16] described an AUROC of 0.805 for HA and of 0.747 for PIIINP. Based on their population distribution published data we could assess DANA values and estimate the AdAUROC for HA and PIIINP. When comparing the HA and PIIINP AdAUROC results of our adult series with the above mentioned estimated AdAUROCs; no significant differences were observed. This confirms that although our series is small, the conclusions drawn concerning the usefulness of HA and PIIINP as fibrosis markers, are in accordance to the data published in larger studies.

The facts that both HA and TGF-ß1 have close relationship with stellate cells and that the activation of stellate cells is crucial for developing hepatic fibrosis led to the hypothesis that serum levels of both HA and TGF-ß1 could be significantly associated with fibrosis [18]. However, the relationship between TGF-ß1, a pro-fibrogenic cytokine, and the hepatic fibrosis is not well established. Nelson et al [58] stated that fibrogenesis is a long process and that the level of fibrosis was the summation of all the effects in the past; therefore, active TGF-ß1 at a certain time point might not correlate with the fibrosis score. In this study adult TGF-ß1 levels displayed an inverse relationship with fibrosis stages, where the lower TGF-ß1 values correspond to the worse stages. Moreover, lower levels of TGF-ß1 were detected when serum samples from 4 adult cirrhotic patients were included (data no shown). In accordance with other authors, lower levels of TGF-ß1 might indicate advanced liver fibrosis suggesting that this marker may reflect fibrogenesis rather than fibrosis [59,60].

The final aim of a serum marker is to find molecules that mirror liver fibrosis progression as an alternative of the biopsy when it is contraindicated. In our cohort, all adult patients with advanced fibrosis were correctly classified according to each cut off by HA, PIIINP and TGF-ß1 markers. A better sorting of the cases should be achieved if these markers were applied sequentially taking into account their NPV and PPV. Given the diagnostic accuracy of HA it would be chosen as the first line assay, then HA values over cut off could be re-evaluated according either PIIINP or TGF-ß1 cut off. Finally, only those cases with values over each marker cut off should not avoid liver biopsy since it is the gold standard method to assess actual damage of liver.

Finally, there are several reports that analyze APRI and AAR as surrogate indirect serum markers of liver fibrosis. When assessed in our cohorts, these approaches did not improve the diagnostic accuracy performance of the proposed selected markers for each group. In adults APRI showed a low performance which not reach the 0.800 AUROC value proposed to be enough for staging fibrosis, while AAR displayed a limited diagnostic value since it only slightly improved the AUROC of TGF-ß1 to predict only advanced fibrosis. (Table S1 and Figure S1). However, in the pediatric series neither APRI nor AAR reached the 0.800 AUROC value, thus TIMP-1 remained to be the best option.

The present study does have several limitations. First, this was in fact a retrospective study, with a quite limited number of cases, so the small sample size makes it difficult to validate the utility of serum markers. However, the results obtained from our adult patients were similar to the ones reported in other larger adult cohorts. Second, due to medical management protocols from our institutions, pediatric patients without liver fibrosis (F0) and adults with cirrhosis or hepatic decompensation were not available for this study. Third, since we did not take into account biopsy length and fragmentation, the potential for sampling error and under-staging of fibrosis remains possible.

This study represents the first analysis performed on pediatric chronic HCV patients and the first comparative study between pediatric and adult cohorts related to a pro-fibrogenic cytokine and matrix deposition markers. Our proposal represents a significant step forward because we suggested that these markers of fibrosis could be easily measured by a single assay without need of special equipment and could be simply interpreted. The solely evaluation of TIMP-1 may be enough to predict fibrosis in children. The availability of a single marker test as TIMP-1, avoids the need of not yet accessible complex tests, such as ELF, that require the evaluation of predictive algorithms. Then, pediatric patient with lower levels of TIMP-1 should avoid liver biopsy. Continued monitoring of markers of liver fibrosis in pediatric patients will help to establish their role in predicting clinical outcomes. Serum TIMP-1 levels below the cut off values could act as a surrogate marker of non-advanced liver fibrosis, thus facilitating the clinical management of patients with HCV disease when liver biopsy is unavailable or contraindicated. It would be useful to study larger pediatric cohorts, perhaps in a multicentre study, to validate and confirm our findings. Perhaps if these parameters are validated in the near future, they would be so easy to assess and interpret as are AST and ALT nowadays. In consequence, this approach would be potentially translatable to the bedside.

Acknowledgments

The authors thank Galoppo M, Pedreira A, Giacove G, Lezama C (Medical Staff of the Liver Unit at Ricardo Gutiérrez Children's Hospital) for providing assistance in reviewing clinical records, Pellizzari E (CEDIE-CONICET, Ricardo Gutiérrez Children's Hospital) for her help with the radioimmunoassay and Livellara B (Liver Unit, Hospital Italiano de Buenos Aires) for preserving adult serum samples.

Author Contributions

Conceived and designed the experiments: PV MVP. Performed the experiments: PV EDM JMDC EM. Analyzed the data: PV MVP MCG OG AG. Contributed reagents/materials/analysis tools: EM PC. Wrote the paper: PV MVP PC. Reviewed clinical records: AG OG MCG.

References

1. Murray K, Finn L, Taylor S, Seidel K, Larson A (2005) Liver histology and alanine aminotransferase levels in children and adults with chronic hepatitis C infection. J Pediatr Gastroenterol Nutr 41: 634–638.

2. Kage M, Fujisawa T, Shiraki K, Tanaka T, Fujisawa T, et al. (1997) Pathology of chronic hepatitis C in children. Child Liver Study Group of Japan. Hepatology 26: 771–775.

3. Badizadegan K, Jonas M, Ott M, Nelson S, Perez-Atayde A (1998) Histopathology of the liver in children with chronic hepatitis C viral infection. Hepatology 28: 1416–1423.

4. Jara P, Resti M, Hierro L, Giacchino R, Barbera C, et al. (2003) Chronic hepatitis C virus infection in childhood: clinical patterns and evolution in 224 white children. Clin Infect Dis 36: 275–280.

5. Chen S, Morgan T (2006) The Natural History of Hepatitis C Virus. Infection Int J Med Sci 3: 47–52.

6. Dienstag J (2002) The role of liver biopsy in chronic hepatitis. Hepatology 36: S152–160.

7. Bravo A, Sheth S, Chopra S (2001) Liver biopsy. N Engl J Med 344: 495–500.

8. Thampanitchawong P, Piratvisuth T (1999) Liver biopsy:complications and risk factors. World J Gastroenterol 5: 301–304.

9. Afdhal N, Nunes D (2004) Evaluation of liver fibrosis: a concise review. Am J Gastroenterol 99: 1160–1174.

10. Martínez SM, Crespo G, Navasa M, Forns X (2011) Noninvasive assessment of liver fibrosis. Hepatology 53: 325–335.

11. Manning D, Afdhal N (2008) Diagnosis and quantitation of fibrosis. Gastroenterology 134: 1670–1681.

12. Gismondi M, Turazza E, Grinstein S, Galoppo M, Preciado M (2004) Hepatitis C virus infection in infants and children from Argentina. J Clin Microbiol 42: 1199–1202.

13. Sanai F, Benmousa A, Al-Hussaini H, Ashraf S, Alhafi O, et al. (2008) Is serum alanine transaminase level a reliable marker of histological disease in chronic hepatitis C infection? Liver Int 28: 1011–1018.

14. Sebastiani G, Vario A, Guido M, Alberti A (2008) Performance of noninvasive markers for liver fibrosis is reduced in chronic hepatitis C with normal transaminases. J Viral Hepat 15: 212–218.

15. Pinzani M, Rombouts K, Colagrande S (2005) Fibrosis in chronic liver diseases: diagnosis and management. J Hepatol 45: S22–36.

16. Saitou Y, Shiraki K, Yamanaka Y, Yamaguchi Y, Kawakita T, et al. (2005) Noninvasive estimation of liver fibrosis and response to interferon therapy by a serum fibrogenesis marker, YKL-40, in patients with HCV-associated liver disease. World J Gastroenterol 28: 476–481.

17. Leroy V, Monier F, Bottari S, Trocme C, Sturm N, et al. (2004) Circulating matrix metalloproteinases 1, 2, 9 and their inhibitors TIMP-1 and TIMP-2 as serum markers of liver fibrosis in patients with chronic hepatitis C: comparison with PIIINP and hyaluronic acid. Am J Gastroenterol 99: 271–279.

18. Sanvisens A, Serra I, Tural C, Tor J, Ojanguren I, et al. (2009) Hyaluronic acid, transforming growth factor-beta1 and hepatic fibrosis in patients with chronic hepatitis C virus and human immunodeficiency virus co-infection. J Viral Hepat 16: 513–518.

19. Fontana R, Goodman Z, Dienstag J, Bonkovsky H, Naishadham D, et al. (2008) Relationship of serum fibrosis markers with liver fibrosis stage and collagen content in patients with advanced chronic hepatitis C. Hepatology 47: 789–798.

20. Martinez S, Fernández-Varo G, González P, Sampson E, Bruguera M, et al. (2011) Assessment of liver fibrosis before and after antiviral therapy by different serum marker panels in patients with chronic hepatitis C. Aliment Pharmacol Ther 33: 138–148.

21. Patel K, Lajoie A, Heaton S, Pianko S, Behling CA, et al. (2003) Clinical use of hyaluronic acid as a predictor of fibrosis change in hepatitis C. J Gastroenterol Hepatol 18: 253–257.

22. Fontana RJ, Bonkovsky HL, Naishadham D, Dienstag JL, Sterling RK, et al. (2009) Serum fibrosis marker levels decrease after successful antiviral treatment in chronic hepatitis C patients with advanced fibrosis. Clin Gastroenterol Hepatol 7: 219–226.

23. Parkes J, Guha IN, Roderick P, Harris S, Cross R, et al. (2011) Enhanced Liver Fibrosis (ELF) test accurately identifies liver fibrosis in patients with chronic hepatitis C. J Viral Hepat 18: 23–31.

24. Macías J, Mira J, Gilabert I, Neukam K, Roldán C, et al. (2011) Combined use of aspartate aminotransferase, platelet count and matrix metalloproteinase 2 measurements to predict liver fibrosis in HIV/hepatitis C virus-coinfected patients. HIV Med 12: 12–21.

25. Moreno S, García-Samaniego J, Moreno A, Ortega E, Pineda J, et al. (2009) Noninvasive diagnosis of liver fibrosis in patients with HIV infection and HCV/HBV co-infection. Viral Hepat 16: 249–258.

26. Forns X, Ampurdanès S, Llovet J, Aponte J, Quintó L, et al. (2002) Identification of chronic hepatitis C patients without hepatic fibrosis by a simple predictive model. Hepatology 36: 986–992.

27. Theise N, Bordenheimer H, Ferrel L (2007) Acute and chronic viral hepatitis. In: Burt AD, Portmann BC, Ferrel LD, eds. MacSweens Pathology of the liver. London: Churchill-Livingstone, 5° edition cap 8: 418–419.

28. Consenso Argentino de Hepatitis C (2007) Documento final Consenso Argentino Hepatitis C, Asociación Argentina para el Estudio de las Enfermedades del Hígado. .

29. Poynard T, Halfon P, Castera L, Munteanu M, Imbert-Bismut F, et al. (2007) Standardization of ROC curve areas for diagnostic evaluation of liver fibrosis markers based on prevalences of fibrosis stages. Clin Chem 53: 1615–1622.

30. Gebo KA, Herlong HF, Torbenson MS, Jenckes MW, Chander G, et al. (2002) Role of liver biopsy in management of chronic hepatitis C: a systematic review. Hepatology 36: S161–172.

31. Poynard T, Ratziu V, Benhamou Y, Thabut D, J M (2005) Biomarkers as a first-line estimate of injury in chronic liver diseases: time for a moratorium on liver biopsy? Gastroenterology 128: 1146–1148.

32. Sebastiani G, Alberti A (2006) Non invasive fibrosis biomarkers reduce but not substitute the need for liver biopsy. World J Gastroenterol 12: 3682–3694.

33. Castera L, Pinzani M (2010) Biopsy and non-invasive methods for the diagnosis of liver fibrosis: does it take two to tango? Gut 59: 861–866. 2010.

34. Poynard T, Halfon P, Castera L, Charlotte F, Le Bail B, et al. (2007) Variability of the area under the receiver operating characteristic curves in the diagnostic evaluation of liver fibrosis markers: impact of biopsy length and fragmentation. Aliment Pharmacol Ther 25: 733–739.

35. Colloredo G, Guido M, Sonzogni A, Leandro G (2003) Impact of liver biopsy size on histological evaluation of chronic viral hepatitis: the smaller the sample, the milder the disease. J Hepatol 39: 239–244.

36. Regev A, Berho M, Jeffers LJ, Milikowski C, Molina EG, et al. (2002) Sampling error and intraobserver variation in liver biopsy in patients with chronic HCV infection. Am J Gastroenterol 97: 2614–2618.

37. Hermeziu B, Messous D, Fabre M, Munteanu M, Baussan C, et al. (2010) Evaluation of FibroTest-ActiTest in children with chronic hepatitis C virus infection. Gastroenterol Clin Biol 34: 16–22.

38. El-Shabrawi MH, Mohsen NA, Sherif MM, El-Karaksy HM, Abou-Yosef H, et al. (2010) Noninvasive assessment of hepatic fibrosis and necroinflammatory activity in Egyptian children with chronic hepatitis C virus infection using FibroTest and ActiTest. Eur J Gastroenterol Hepatol 22: 946–951.

39. Friedman S (2003) Liver fibrosis: from bench to bedside. J Hepatol 38: S38–53.

40. Gressner A (1998) The cell biology of liver fibrogenesis - an imbalance of proliferation, growth arrest and apoptosis of myofibroblasts. Cell Tissue Res 292: 447–452.

41. Gressner A, Weiskirchen R (2006) Modern pathogenetic concepts of liver fibrosis suggest stellate cells and TGF-beta as major players and therapeutic targets. J Cell Mol Med 10: 76–99.

42. Powell E, Edwards-Smith C, Hay J, Clouston A, Crawford D, et al. (2000) Host genetic factors influence disease progression in chronic hepatitis C. Hepatology 31: 828–833.

43. Goto T, Mikami K, Miura K, Ohshima S, Yoneyama K, et al. (2004) Mechanical stretch induces matrix metalloproteinase 1 production in human hepatic stellate cells. Pathophysiology 11: 153–158.

44. Friedman S (2008) Mechanisms of hepatic fibrogenesis. Gastroenterology 134: 1655–1669.

45. Miyoshi H, Moriya K, Tsutsumi T, Shinzawa S, Fujie H, et al. (2011) Pathogenesis of lipid metabolism disorder in hepatitis C: Polyunsaturated fatty acids counteract lipid alterations induced by the core protein. J Hepatol 54: 432–438.

46. Okuda M, Li K, Beard MR, Showalter LA, Scholle F, et al. (2002) Mitochondrial injury, oxidative stress, and antioxidant gene expression are induced by hepatitis C virus core protein. Gastroenterology 122: 366–375.

47. Taniguchi H, Kato N, Otsuka M, Goto T, Yoshida H, et al. (2004) Hepatitis C virus core protein upregulates transforming growth factor-beta 1 transcription. J Med Virol 72: 52–59.

48. Plebani M, Basso D (2007) Non-invasive assessment of chronic liver and gastric diseases. 2007. Clin Chim Acta 381: 39–49.

49. Murphy FR, Issa R, Zhou X, Ratnarajah S, Nagase H, et al. (2002) Inhibition of apoptosis of activated hepatic stellate cells by tissue inhibitor of metalloprotei-nase-1 is mediated via effects on matrix metalloproteinase inhibition: implications for reversibility of liver fibrosis. J Biol Chem 277: 11069–11076.

50. Resino S, Bellón J, Asensio C, Micheloud D, Miralles P, et al. (2010) Can serum hyaluronic acid replace simple non-invasive indexes to predict liver fibrosis in HIV/Hepatitis C coinfected patients? BMC Infect Dis 10: 244.

51. Lebensztejn DM, Sobaniec-Lotowska ME, Kaczmarski M, Voelker M, Schuppan D (2006) Matrix-derived serum markers in monitoring liver fibrosis in children with chronic hepatitis B treated with interferon alpha. World J Gastroenterol 12: 3338–3343.

52. Nobili V, Alisi A, Torre G, De Vito R, Pietrobattista A, et al. (2010) Hyaluronic acid predicts hepatic fibrosis in children with nonalcoholic fatty liver disease. Transl Res 156: 229–234.

53. Lebensztejn DM, Kaczmarski M, Sobaniec-Lotowska M, Bauer M, Voelker M, et al. (2004) Serum laminin-2 and hyaluronan predict severe liver fibrosis in children with chronic hepatitis B. Hepatology 39: 868–869.

54. Elmetwally IM, Elmahalaway AM, Abuhashem SH, ahmed AM (2009) Determination of serum fibrosis index in patients with chronic hepatitis and its relationship to histological activity index. Saudi Med J 30: 638–646.

55. Saltik-Temizel IN, Koçak N, Ozen H, Demir H (2004) Serum hyaluronic acid concentrations in children with cirrhosis. Indian J Gastroenterol 23: 129–130.

56. Hartley JL, Brown RM, Tybulewicz A, Hayes P, Wilson DC, et al. (2006) Hyaluronic acid predicts hepatic fibrosis in children with hepatic disease. J Pediatr Gastroenterol Nutr 43: 217–221.

57. Poynard T, Halfon P, Castera L, Charlotte F, Le Bail B, et al. (2007) Variability of the area under the receiver operating characteristic curves in the diagnostic evaluation of liver fibrosis markers: impact of biopsy length and fragmentation. Aliment Pharmacol Ther 25: 733–739.

58. Nelson DR, Gonzalez-Peralta RP, Qian K, Xu Y, Marousis CG, et al. (1997) Transforming growth factor-beta 1 in chronic hepatitis C. J Viral Hepat 4: 29–35.

59. Soliman GM, Mohammed KA, Taha A, barrack AA (2010) The role of plasma transforming growth factor beta-1 in the development of fibrosis in patient with HCV related steatohepatitis.. J Egypt Soc Parasitol 40: 759–772.

60. Rallón NI, Barreiro P, Soriano V, García-Samaniego J, López M, Benito JM (2011) Elevated TGF-β1 levels might protect HCV/HIV-coinfected patients from liver fibrosis. Eur J Clin Invest 41: 70–76.

4

Serum MicroRNA-21 as Marker for Necroinflammation in Hepatitis C Patients with and without Hepatocellular Carcinoma

Verena Bihrer[1◐], Oliver Waidmann[1◐], Mireen Friedrich-Rust[1], Nicole Forestier[1], Simone Susser[1], Jörg Haupenthal[1¤], Martin Welker[1], Ying Shi[1], Jan Peveling-Oberhag[1], Andreas Polta[1], Michael von Wagner[1], Heinfried H. Radeke[2], Christoph Sarrazin[1], Jörg Trojan[1], Stefan Zeuzem[1], Bernd Kronenberger[1¶], Albrecht Piiper[1]*

1 Department of Medicine I, University of Frankfurt/M., Frankfurt, Germany, 2 Institute of Pharmacology/ZAFES, University of Frankfurt/M., Frankfurt, Germany

Abstract

Background: MicroRNA-21 (miR-21) is up-regulated in tumor tissue of patients with malignant diseases, including hepatocellular carcinoma (HCC). Elevated concentrations of miR-21 have also been found in sera or plasma from patients with malignancies, rendering it an interesting candidate as serum/plasma marker for malignancies. Here we correlated serum miR-21 levels with clinical parameters in patients with different stages of chronic hepatitis C virus infection (CHC) and CHC-associated HCC.

Methodology/Principal Findings: 62 CHC patients, 29 patients with CHC and HCC and 19 healthy controls were prospectively enrolled. RNA was extracted from the sera and miR-21 as well as miR-16 levels were analyzed by quantitative real-time PCR; miR-21 levels (normalized by miR-16) were correlated with standard liver parameters, histological grading and staging of CHC. The data show that serum levels of miR-21 were elevated in patients with CHC compared to healthy controls ($P<0.001$); there was no difference between serum miR-21 in patients with CHC and CHC-associated HCC. Serum miR-21 levels correlated with histological activity index (HAI) in the liver ($r = -0.494$, $P = 0.00002$), alanine aminotransferase (ALT) ($r = -0.309$, $P = 0.007$), aspartate aminotransferase ($r = -0.495$, $P = 0.000007$), bilirubin ($r = -0.362$, $P = 0.002$), international normalized ratio ($r = -0.338$, $P = 0.034$) and γ-glutamyltransferase ($r = -0.244$, $P = 0.034$). Multivariate analysis revealed that ALT and miR-21 serum levels were independently associated with HAI. At a cut-off dC_T of 1.96, miR-21 discriminated between minimal and mild-severe necroinflammation (AUC = 0.758) with a sensitivity of 53.3% and a specificity of 95.2%.

Conclusions/Significance: The serum miR-21 level is a marker for necroinflammatory activity, but does not differ between patients with HCV and HCV-induced HCC.

Editor: Hana Algül, Technische Universität München, Germany

Funding: This work was supported by grants from the Else Kröner-Fresenius Foundation, the Deutsche Forschungsgemeinschaft (GRK 1172), and the foundations Dr. Paul und Ursula Klein, Marie Christine Held und Erika Hecker, the Scolari Foundation and the Heinrich und Erna Schaufler Foundation. The funders had no role in study design, data collection and analysis, decision to publish, or preparation of the manuscript.

Competing Interests: The authors have declared that no competing interests exist.

* E-mail: piiper@med.uni-frankfurt.de

◐ These authors contributed equally to this work.

¶ This author also contributed equally to this work.

¤ Current address: Helmholtz Institute for Pharmaceutical Research Saarland, Department of Drug Design and Optimization, University of Saarland, Saarbrücken, Germany

Introduction

Hepatocellular carcinoma (HCC) is one of the most common solid tumors, rated third in mortality worldwide [1]. Most HCCs develop in fibrotic or already cirrhotic liver which are a result of chronic infection with hepatitis B (HBV) or hepatitis C virus (HCV) [1]. Currently, there are no biomarkers for the early detection of HCC, and most patients with HCC are diagnosed at advanced stages, which are associated with poor prognosis and low survival rates due to a lack of curative treatment options. α-Fetoprotein (AFP) has mainly been used for diagnosis of HCC; however, its sensitivity and specificity are not satisfying [2].

MicroRNAs (miRNAs) are small noncoding RNAs (18–24 nucleotides) that interact with their target mRNAs to inhibit translation by promoting mRNA degradation or to block translation by binding to complementary sequences in the 3′-untranslated region of mRNAs [3]. An integral role of miRNAs in cancer pathogenesis has begun to emerge. MiRNA expression profiling reveals characteristic signatures for many tumor types [4]. Importantly, miRNAs have also been detected in human serum

Table 1. Characteristics of CHC patients, CHC patients with HCC and healthy subjects.

		CHC patients (n = 62)	CHC patients with HCC (n = 29)	Healthy subjects (n = 19)
Age (years)	Mean ± SD	46.1±11.2	61.4±9.1	33.2±10.6
Sex (n)	Male	34 (54.8%)	22 (75.9%)	11 (57.9%)
	Female	28 (45.2)	7 (24.1%)	8 (42.1%)
HAI (n)	2	7 (11.3%)	-	
	3	8 (12.9%)	-	
	4	13 (21.0%)	-	
	5	10 (16.1%)	2 (6.9%)	
	6	14 (22.6%)	1 (3.4%)	
	7	5 (8.1%)	2 (6.9%)	
	8	2 (3.2%)	2 (6.9%)	
	9	3 (4.8%)	2 (6.9%)	
	11	-	1 (3.4%)	
	Unknown	-	19 (65.5%)	
Fibrosis (n)	F0	7 (11.3%)	-	
	F1	20 (32.3%)	-	
	F2	4 (6.5%)	-	
	F3	6 (9.7%)	-	
	F4	10 (16.1%)	3 (10.3%)	
	F5	4 (6.5%)	1(3.4%)	
	F6	5 (8.1%)	9 (31.0%)	
	Unknown	6 (9.7%)	16 (55.2%)	
ALT (n)	Elevated*	44 (71.0%)	24 (82.8%)	
	Normal	18 (29.0%)	5 (17.2%)	

*>35 IU/l female; >50 IU/l male.

and plasma, where they are remarkably stable [5], raising the possibility that unique miRNA patterns in serum and plasma might be used as non-invasive disease markers. In support of this, differences have been found between miRNA patterns in serum or plasma of patients with a number of malignancies and healthy controls [5].

Analysis of the miRNA signatures of a large number of tumor samples, including lung, breast, stomach, prostate, colon, and pancreatic cancer and their respective normal adjacent tissue, revealed that miR-21 is the only miRNA upregulated in all these tumors [4], including HCC [6–9]. Considerable evidence supports the hypothesis that miR-21 is a central oncomiR [10]. miR-21 levels are also significantly elevated in serum/plasma of patients with diffuse large B-cell lymphoma, ovarian cancer, prostate cancer or breast cancer [11–13], rendering it an interesting candidate as serum/plasma marker for malignancies.

miR-21 has also been linked to fibrosis in the lung [14], heart [15] and liver [9]. In the liver the level of miR-21 correlates with hepatic fibrosis [9]. A close link between miR-21 and hepatic fibrosis is supported by the findings that transforming growth factor β (TGF-β), a critical mediator of hepatic fibrogenesis [16,17], promotes the expression of miR-21 [18], and that miR-21 decreases the expression of SMAD7 [9], a negative regulator of TGF-β signalling [17]. A recent study has reported that circulating miR-21 might be useful as biomarker for HCC [19].

Alterations of the miR-21 concentration in serum or plasma of patients with HCV-induced chronic hepatitis C (CHC) have not yet been reported. Hypothesizing that miR-21 serum levels might

be related to either malignancy, i. e. HCC, or liver fibrosis/cirrhosis or both, we here investigated the relation between miR-21 serum levels and clinical parameters in patients with CHC, CHC plus HCC, and healthy volunteers.

Methods

Patients

Patients with CHC (n = 62) as well as CHC plus HCC (n = 29), who had undergone liver biopsy for staging and grading of CHC at the Frankfurt University hospital, were prospectively enrolled in the present cohort study. An independent cohort of 47 CHC patients

Table 2. Characteristics of the independent validation cohort of CHC patients.

		CHC patients (n = 47)
Age (years)	Mean±SD	45.4±10.4
Sex (n)	Male	22 (46.8%)
	Female	25 (53.2%)
ALT (n)	Elevated*	34 (72.3%)
	Normal	13 (27.7%)

*>35 IU/l female; >50 IU/l male.

A

B

C

D

ALT levels (n = 18). Boxes represent range, median and quartiles of the number of threshold cycles (C_T) required to detect miR-21 by real-time RT-qPCR normalized to C_T of miR-16. Differences were calculated with Wilcoxon-Mann-Whitney-U-test. *$P<.05$, ***$P<.001$, compared with the healthy control group. +++$P<.001$ between CHC patients with normal or elevated ALT. (B), ROC curve analysis of serum miR-21 concentration for discriminating CHC patients and healthy controls. (C), dC_T values of CHC patients with elevated ALT and HAI≥5 (n = 31) and patients with CHC and HCC (n = 29) showing no significant difference in miR-21 levels (Wilcoxon-Mann-Whitney-U-test: $P>.3$) between both groups, n. s. = not significant. (D) Relationship between serum miR-21 levels and the serum HCV RNA in patients with CHC. The relation is not significant ($P = .29$).

was used for validation. Inclusion criteria were detectable anti-HCV antibodies and HCV-RNA for at least six months. Exclusion criteria were decompensated liver disease, malignancy other than HCC, organ transplantation, co-infection with HIV or HBV, immuno-suppression and autoimmune co-morbidities. Patients' characteristics are summarized in Table 1 and 2. The Ethics Committee of the University Hospital Frankfurt approved this study. From all enrolled patients and healthy subjects written informed consent was obtained according to the Declaration of Helsinki.

Liver Histology

Hematoxylin-eosin stained sections of formalin-fixed, paraffin-embedded liver biopsies were reviewed by experienced pathologists for evaluation of fibrosis stages (F0 = no fibrosis - F6 = cirrhosis) and the histologic activity index (HAI) in the liver according to the Ishak criteria [20].

Blood Sampling

10 mL of peripheral blood was collected at the time of liver biopsy (serum tubes, Sarstedt, Nümbrecht, Germany). Cellular components were removed by two consecutive centrifugation steps (1500 g for 10 min at 4°C and 2000 g for 3 min at 4°C, respectively). Sera were stored at −80°C until use.

Detection of miRNAs by Quantitative Real-time Reverse-Transcription (RT)-PCR

RNA was isolated from 500 μL serum using Tri®ReagentLS (Sigma-Aldrich, St. Louis, MO), chloroform and the mirVana™ RNA isolation kit (Ambion-ABI, Austin, TX). Total RNA was eluted in 100 μL and stored at −20°C. 5 μL of RNA was reverse transcribed with the TaqMan® miRNA reverse transcription kit and the TaqMan® miRNA assay specific RT primers for miR-21 or miR-16 according to the instructions of the manufacturer (ABI). Real-time PCR was performed with 3 μL of each cDNA on a StepOne™Plus Real-Time PCR System (ABI) in duplicates. The cycle treshold (C_T) defines the number of PCR cycles required for the fluorescent signal to cross the threshold.

Statistical Analysis

Data were analyzed using the BiAS software for windows (version 9.07). Statistical significance for correlations was determined using Spearman's nonparametric rank test. Differences between two groups were evaluated using the Wilcoxon-Mann-Whitney-U test. P values<0.05 were considered to be significant. For the multivariate analysis a logistic regression with Wald's test was used to evaluate whether minimal ($HAI_{A+B+C}≤3$) vs. mild to severe ($HAI_{A+B+C}>3$) necroinflammation correlated independently with the parameters. The criterion for elimination in the stepwise model was $P>0.1$.

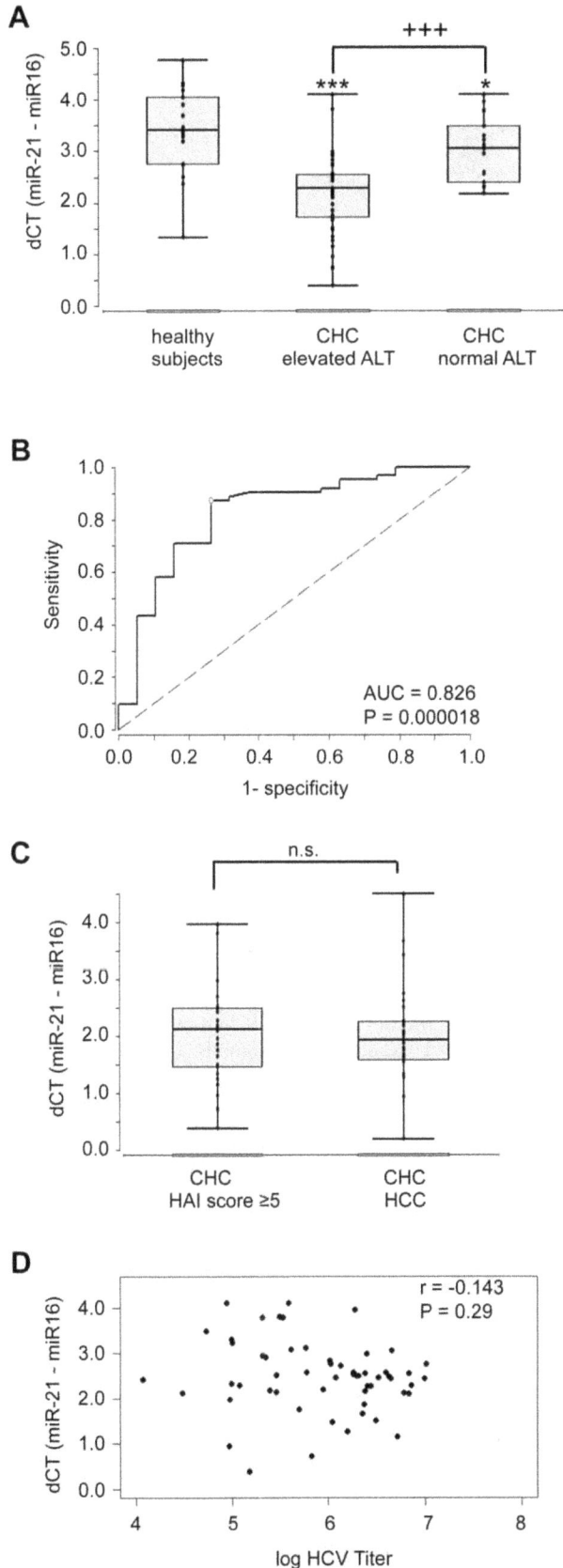

Figure 1. Increased serum miR-21 concentrations in patients with CHC and elevated levels of ALT. (A), dC_T values of miR-21 of sera from healthy control individuals (n = 19), patients with CHC and elevated serum ALT levels (n = 44) and CHC patients with normal serum

A

B

C

D

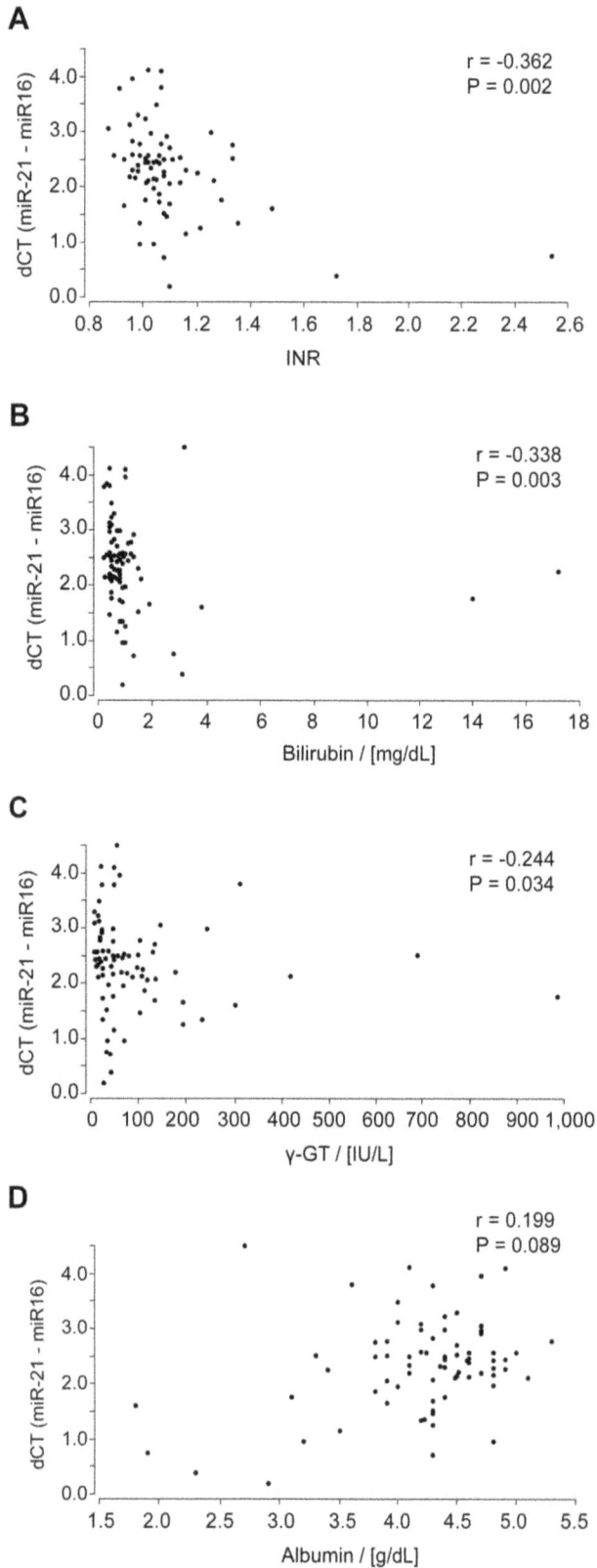

Figure 2. Relationship between serum miR-21 levels and INR (A), bilirubin (B), γ-GT (C) and serum albumin concentration (D).

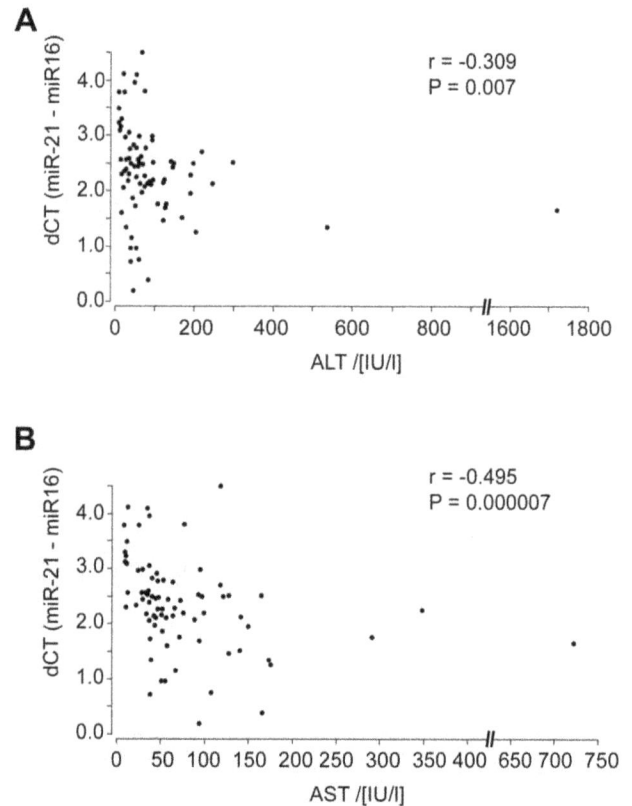

A

B

Figure 3. Correlation between serum miR-21 levels and ALT (A) or AST (B) in patients with CHC. Points represent dC_T values for miR-21 normalized to miR-16.

Results

miR-21 as well as miR-16, a miRNA found at constant levels in sera from various diseases, including chronic hepatitis B [5,13], were quantified by real-time RT-PCR in sera from patients with CHC, CHC plus HCC and healthy controls. The mean C_T values (95% confidence interval (CI)) of miR-16 were 25.1 (24.5–25.6) in healthy donors and 25.2 (24.9–25.5), 25.0 (24.4–25.6) and 25.1 (24.2–26.0) in patients with CHC, in patients with CHC and normal alanine aminotransferase (ALT) and CHC plus HCC, respectively, showing that miR-16 in serum can be used as an internal control to normalize sampling variations in RT-qPCR in our collective of sera. The dC_T (C_T-miR-21 - C_T-miR-16) value negatively correlates with the serum level of miR-21. dC_T of miR-21 was higher in sera from healthy controls (3.4, CI: 3.0–3.8) than in sera from patients with CHC and elevated serum ALT activity (2.2, CI: 2.0–2.4) ($P<0.001$, Fig. 1A), a parameter reflecting liver damage. In contrast, the dCT value for miR-21 in sera from CHC patients with normal ALT values (3.0, CI: 2.7–3.3, $P<0.05$) only slightly differed from that of the control sera (Fig. 1A). ROC curve analysis was performed on the data from all CHC patients (without HCC) and controls. The area under the ROC curve (AUC) was 0.826 (CI: 0.711–0.942) (Fig. 1B), with a P value of 0.000018. The optimal cut-off value for miR-21 (normalized to miR-16) to discriminate between healthy controls and CHC patients was 3.16, with a sensitivity of 87.1%, specificity of 73.7% and false classification rate of 19.6%.

There was no significant difference between the dC_T values of miR-21 in sera from patients with CHC plus HCC and those with CHC and matched HAI (Fig. 1C). Moreover, we investigated if

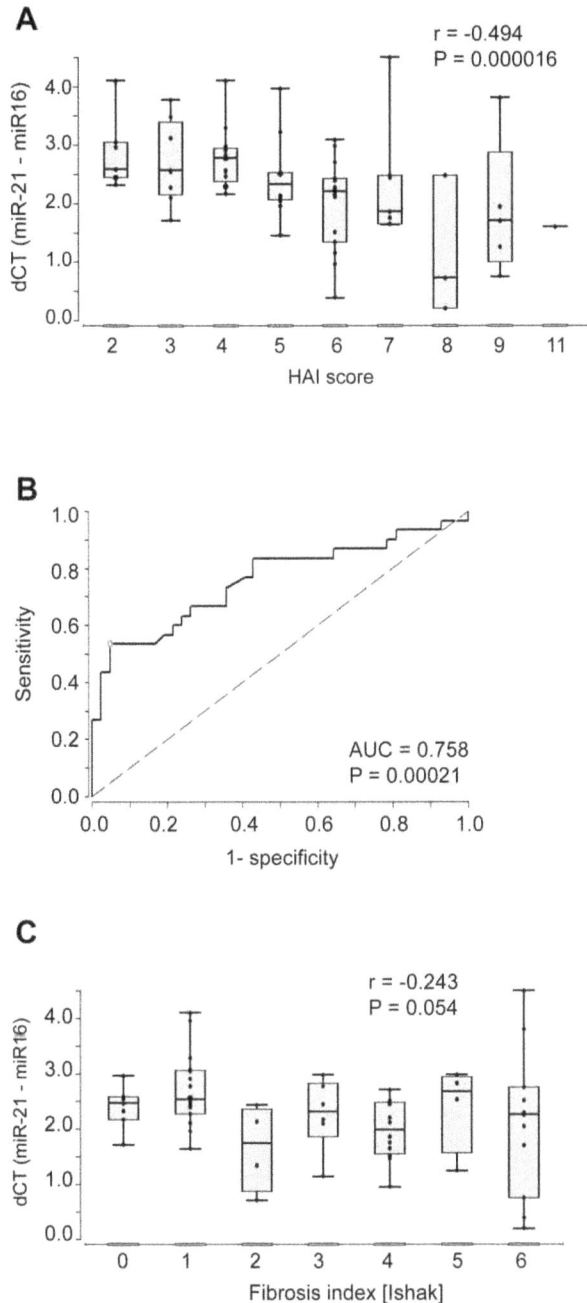

A

B

C

Figure 4. Relationship between serum miR-21 levels and the HAI score (A); (B), ROC curve analysis of serum miR-21 concentration for discriminating patients with minimal ($HAI_{A+B+C} \leq 3$) vs. moderate to severe necroinflammatory activity ($HAI_{A+B+C} > 3$) using dC_T of miR-21; (C), relationship between serum miR-21 and fibrosis index in patients with CHC.

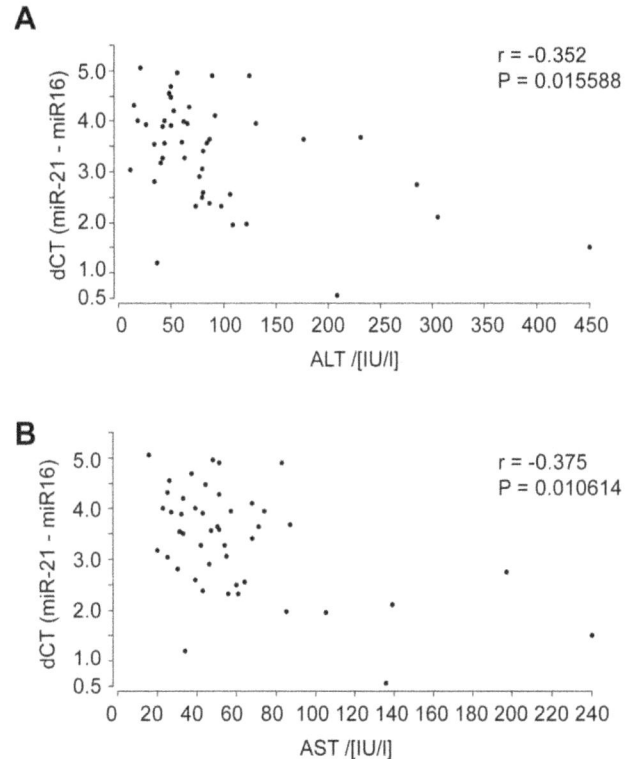

A

B

Figure 5. Validation of the relationship between the serum levels of miR-21 and ALT (A) and AST (B) in an independent cohort of 47 CHC patients.

$P = 0.002$) (Fig. 2A), serum bilirubin concentration (r = -0.338, $P = 0.003$) (Fig. 2B) and γ-GT activity (r = -0.244, $P = 0.034$) (Fig. 2C). The correlation between the serum albumin concentration and the serum miR-21 level did not reach statistical significance ($P = 0.0893$) (Fig. 2D).

To examine if the levels of miR-21 in sera from patients with CHC as well as CHC plus HCC reflects necroinflammatory activity in the liver rather than HCC, we correlated the dC_T values of serum miR-21 with ALT, aspartate aminotransferase (AST) as well as with the histologic activity index (HAI) score in the liver. The dC_T value of miR-21 in the sera negatively correlated with serum levels of ALT (r = -0.309, $P = 0.007$) (Fig. 3A) and AST (r = -0.495, $P = 0.000007$) (Fig. 3B), i. e. the serum level of miR-21 positively correlated with ALT and AST activities. The dC_T values of serum miR-21 also strongly correlated with the HAI score (r = -0.494, $P = 0.00002$) (Fig. 4A).

In order to confirm the correlation between serum miR-21 levels and hepatic necroinflammation, we examined an independent validation cohort of 47 CHC patients. As illustrated in Fig. 5, the serum levels of miR-21 correlated with ALT (r = -0.352, $P = 0.015588$) and AST (r = -0.375, $P = 0.010614$). Histological classification according to Ishak was not available for these patients.

To investigate if the serum miR-21 level might be useful to discriminate patients with minimal ($HAI_{A+B+C} \leq 3$) and mild to severe necroinflammation in the liver ($HAI_{A+B+C} > 3$), we performed multivariate analysis to examine the independency of the different parameters. Multivariate analysis revealed that only the correlations between HAI and serum ALT as well as miR-21 were independent (Table 3).

To test the suitability of miR-21 to discriminate minimal from mild to severe necroinflammation, we performed a ROC curve

there is a relation between the serum levels of miR-21 and serum HCV RNA. However, there was no correlation between the serum miR-21 and HCV RNA level ($P = 0.29$) (Fig. 1D).

To investigate the relation between the serum miR-21 level and standard liver function parameters, we correlated the relationship between the levels of miR-21 with the serum albumin concentration, international normalized ratio (INR), bilirubin and γ-glutamyl-transferase (γ-GT). There were positive correlations between the serum level of miR-21 and INR (r = -0.362,

Table 3. Uni- and multivariate analysis of factors correlated to minimal (HAI≤3) vs. mild to severe (HAI>3) necroinflammation.

	Univariate analysis			Multivariate analysis		
	Odds ratio	**95% confidence intervall**	**Wald's p-value**	**Odds ratio**	**95% confidence intervall**	**Wald's p-value**
Fibrosis stage	1.4821	1.1150–1.9701	0.006744			
Sex	0.9524	0.3266–2.7774	0.928807			
Age	1.0817	1.0203–1.1469	0.008421			
Log bilirubin	1.7982	0.2684–12.0467	0.545413			
Log ALT	17.5591	2.4437–126.1671	0.004399	17.5478	1.3734–224.2070	0.027520
Log AST	36.3935.	3.3857–391.2003	0.003012			
Log γGT	2.4165	0.6476–9.0177	0.189115			
INR	19.1873	0.2329–1580.7251	0.18933			
miR21-16	0.1507	0.0399–0.5694	0.005262	0.1734	0.0487–0.6168	0.006804

The HAI score used for this analysis was the sum of HAI-A, -B and -C.

analysis on the data. The AUC was 0.758 ($P = 0.00021$) (Fig. 4B). At the optimal cut-off value of 1.96, the sensitivity was 53.3%, the specificity 95.2% and false classification rate was 25.7%.

To investigate if the serum miR-21 level might be related to liver fibrosis, we correlated the dC_T values of serum miR-21 and the histological fibrosis index in the liver. There was a trend towards a negative correlation between the Ishak fibrosis index and the dCT of miR-21 in the sera from CHC patients ($r = -0.243$, $P = 0.054$) (Fig. 4C).

Discussion

Compared to the corresponding normal tissue miR-21 has been shown to be consistently elevated in malignant tumors, including HCC [4,7]. Importantly, this miRNA is not only upregulated in association with oncogenesis, but can act as oncogenic miRNA [21]. It inhibits targets related to apoptosis and to transformation such as programmed cell death 4 and phosphatase and tensin homolog [6,22]. miR-21 is also elevated in sera from patients with prostate carcinoma [12], mamma carcinoma [13,22] and HBV-associated HCC [23], raising the possibility that it may serve as serum marker for malignant diseases. A recent study has suggested that circulating miR-21 is a marker for HCC [19]. However, that study did not allow differentiation between patients with liver cirrhosis and HCC. We report here that the level of miR-21 in sera from patients with CHC-associated HCC was elevated compared to healthy controls. However, we also detected increased levels of miR-21 in sera from patients with CHC without HCC. Indeed, sera from patients with matched HAI score and CHC showed similar miR-21 levels than sera from patients with CHC-associated HCC. Thus, the elevation of serum miR-21 levels in our CHC patients appears to be mainly associated with chronic hepatitis rather than HCC. The link between the elevated levels of serum miR-21 and CHC is supported by our finding that miR-21 serum levels strongly correlated with ALT and AST activities in two independent cohorts of CHC patients, parameters of ongoing liver damage. Concordantly, elevated serum levels of miR-21 were found only in CHC patients showing elevated ALT levels, whereas sera from CHC patients with normal ALT levels also contain normal miR-21 serum concentrations. Moreover, the serum miR-21 levels also strongly correlated with the HAI score, supporting the suggestion that the serum miR-21 level is related to necroinflammatory activity in the liver in patients with CHC. Multivariate analysis of the data from patients with minimal or

mild to severe necroinflammation in the liver revealed that only ALT and miR-21 correlated independently with necroinflammation in the liver. Thus, the serum miR-21 concentration might be a useful parameter to differentiate patients with minimal vs. mild to severe necroinflammation in the liver which is of clinical relevance.

Mechanistically, miR-21 may leak from damaged cells similar to ALT and AST, or may be actively exported from altered tissues as a mechanism of adaptation to alterations of the state of a cell [24]. Recent evidence suggests that the majority of miRNAs in serum or plasma, including miR-21, is complexed to proteins such as Ago2, thereby explaining the high stability of endogenous miRNAs in serum/plasma [25].

There is clear evidence for a close relation between miR-21 and hepatic fibrosis. Thus, the hepatic level of miR-21 appears to correlate with the stage of liver fibrosis [9]. miR-21 is strongly expressed in tumor cells, but also in tumor-associated fibroblasts [26]. In the present study the miR-21 concentration in serum showed a strong correlation with the HAI score, whereas the relation between the serum miR-21 level and the fibrosis score did not reach statistical significance, which is in agreement with a study published during revision of the present manuscript [27]. This suggests that serum miR-21 levels are related to liver damage activity rather than to liver fibrosis in patients with CHC.

There was no correlation between the concentrations of miR-21 and HCV RNA in serum. This can be reconciled with the lack of correlation of HCV serum level and disease activity in patients with CHC [28].

Similar to the data of the present study, it has recently been reported that sera from HBV-induced chronic hepatitis contain elevated levels of miR-21 in comparison to healthy controls [23]. However, in another study with patients suffering from HBV-induced chronic hepatitis, no elevation of serum miR-21 levels was found despite strongly elevated ALT and HAI scores in these patients [29], leaving the role of serum miR-21 in HBV-induced chronic hepatitis unclear.

Recent studies reported differential levels of miR-16 in sera from patients with HCC, chronic hepatitis of different etiology and healthy controls [27,30]. In the present study, however, we did not find differences in the levels of miR-16 between sera from patients with CHC, CHC-associated HCC and healthy controls. Our data are in agreement with several other studies reporting invariant levels of miR-16 in sera from patients with several diseases [13], including HBV-induced chronic hepatitis and HCC, and healthy controls [23,29], prompting utilization of this miRNA for normalization [13]. The reasons for the different findings between the studies remain elusive.

Our recent data show that serum levels of the liver-specific miR-122 also correlate with the HAI score as well as serum AST and ALT levels [31]. Thus, miR-21 and miR-122 may originate from the inflamed liver. However, miR-21 and miR-122 differ in that miR-21, but not miR-122, correlates with bilirubin, INR and γ-GT in CHC patients. Obviously, the serum levels of miR-21 and miR-122 reflect overlapping, but not identical disease parameters in CHC patients. This might be related to the different expression pattern of miR-21 and miR-122, miR-122 being highly selective for the liver, whereas miR-21 shows significant expression in other cells and tissues. For instance, miR-21 is strongly expressed in lymphocytes [32]. Thus, release of miR-21 from several different cell types may contribute to the elevation of the serum miR-21 level in patients with chronic hepatitis. A drawback of the broader expression pattern of miR-21 compared to miR-122 is that co-morbidities are more likely to reduce the diagnostic power of the serum miR-21 level than that of miR-122.

The identification of non-invasive biomarkers for the diagnosis of diseases has become a rapidly growing area of clinical research [33]. The discovery of miRNAs circulating in the peripheral blood has opened new directions of research to identify new non-invasive ways of diagnosis of disease. In summary, the data of the present study indicate that the level of serum miR-21 is suitable to detect necroinflammatory activity in the liver and not the presence of HCC. It appears likely that serum miRNAs can provide information on different aspects of chronic hepatitis not available from the presently used routine parameters of liver damage.

Acknowledgments

We thank Ursula Karey, Dany Perner and Yolanda Martinez for excellent technical assistance.

Author Contributions

Conceived and designed the experiments: A. Piiper BK OW. Performed the experiments: VB JH. Analyzed the data: OW BK JP-O SZ A. Polta HHR. Contributed reagents/materials/analysis tools: MF-R NF MW YS JT CS MvW SS OW BK. Wrote the paper: A. Piiper.

References

1. El-Serag HB, Marrero JA, Rudolph L, Reddy KR (2008) Diagnosis and treatment of hepatocellular carcinoma. Gastroenterology 134: 1752–1763.
2. Zinkin NT, Grall F, Bhaskar K, Otu HH, Spentzos D, et al. (2008) Serum proteomics and biomarkers in hepatocellular carcinoma and chronic liver disease. Clin Cancer Res 14: 470–477.
3. Du T, Zamore PD (2005) microPrimer: the biogenesis and function of microRNA. Development 132: 4645–4652.
4. Volinia S, Calin GA, Liu CG, Ambs S, Cimmino A, et al. (2006) A microRNA expression signature of human solid tumors defines cancer gene targets. Proc Natl Acad Sci USA 103: 2257–2261.
5. Mitchell PS, Parkin RK, Kroh EM, Fritz BR, Wyman SK, et al. (2008) Circulating microRNAs as stable blood-based markers for cancer detection. Proc Natl Acad Sci USA 105: 10513–10518.
6. Meng F, Henson R, Wehbe-Janek H, Ghoshal K, Jacob ST, et al. (2007) MicroRNA-21 regulates expression of the PTEN tumor suppressor gene in human hepatocellular cancer. Gastroenterology 133: 647–658.
7. Varnholt H (2008) The role of microRNAs in primary liver cancer. Ann Hepatol 7: 104–113.
8. Ladeiro Y, Couchy G, Balabaud C, Bioulac-Sage P, Pelletier L, et al. (2008) MicroRNA profiling in hepatocellular tumors is associated with clinical features and oncogene/tumor suppressor gene mutations. Hepatology 47: 1955–1963.
9. Marquez RT, Bandyopadhyay S, Wendlandt EB, Keck K, Hoffer BA, et al. (2010) Correlation between microRNA expression levels and clinical parameters associated with chronic hepatitis C viral infection in humans. Lab Invest 90: 1727–1736.
10. Medina PP, Nolde M, Slack FJ (2010) OncomiR addiction in an in vivo model of microRNA-21-induced pre-B-cell lymphoma. Nature 467: 86–90.
11. Lawrie CH, Gal S, Dunlop HM, Pushkaran B, Liggins AP, et al. (2008) Detection of elevated levels of tumour-associated microRNAs in serum of patients with diffuse large B-cell lymphoma. Br J Haematol 141: 672–675.
12. Zhang HL, Yang LF, Zhu Y, Yao XD, Zhang SL, et al. (2011) Serum miRNA-21: Elevated levels in patients with metastatic hormone-refractory prostate cancer and potential predictive factor for the efficacy of docetaxel-based chemotherapy. Prostate 71: 326–331.
13. Asaga S, Kuo C, Nguyen T, Terpenning M, Giuliano AE, et al. (2011) Direct serum assay for microRNA-21 concentrations in early and advanced breast cancer. Clin Chem 57: 84–91.
14. Liu G, Friggeri A, Yang Y, Milosevic J, Ding Q, et al. (2010) miR-21 mediates fibrogenic activation of pulmonary fibroblasts and lung fibrosis. J Exp Med 207: 1589–1597.
15. Thum T, Gross C, Fiedler J, Fischer T, Kissler S, et al. (2008) MicroRNA-21 contributes to myocardial disease by stimulating MAP kinase signalling in fibroblasts. Nature 456: 980–984.
16. Matsuzaki K, Murata M, Yoshida K, Sekimoto G, Uemura Y, et al. (2007) Chronic inflammation associated with hepatitis C virus infection perturbs hepatic transforming growth factor beta signaling, promoting cirrhosis and hepatocellular carcinoma. Hepatology 46: 48–57.

17. Dooley S, Hamzavi J, Ciuclan L, Godoy P, Ilkavets I, et al. (2008) Hepatocyte-specific Smad7 expression attenuates TGF-beta-mediated fibrogenesis and protects against liver damage. Gastroenterology 135: 642–659.
18. Davis BN, Hilyard AC, Lagna G, Hata A (2008) SMAD proteins control DROSHA-mediated microRNA maturation. Nature 454: 56–61.
19. Tomimaru Y, Eguchi H, Nagano H, Wada H, Kobayashi S, et al. (2011) Circulating microRNA-21 as a novel biomarker for hepatocellular carcinoma. J Hepatol. doi: 10.1016/j.jhep.2011.04.026.
20. Ishak K, Baptista A, Bianchi L, Callea F, Groote JD, et al. (1995) Histological grading and staging of chronic hepatitis. J Hepatol 22: 696–699.
21. Iliopoulos D, Jaeger SA, Hirsch HA, Bulyk ML, Struhl K (2010) STAT3 activation of miR-21 and miR-181b-1 via PTEN and CYLD are part of the epigenetic switch linking inflammation to cancer. Mol Cell 39: 493–506.
22. Frankel LB, Christoffersen NR, Jacobsen A, Lindow M, Krogh A, et al. (2008) Programmed cell death 4 (PDCD4) is an important functional target of the microRNA miR-21 in breast cancer cells. J Biol Chem 283: 1026–1033.
23. Xu J, Wu C, Che X, Wang L, Yu D, et al. (2011) Circulating microRNAs, miR-21, miR 122, and miR 223, in patients with hepatocellular carcinoma or chronic hepatitis. Mol Carcinog 50: 136–142.
24. Wang K, Zhang S, Weber J, Baxter D, Galas DJ (2010) Export of microRNAs and microRNA-protective protein by mammalian cells. Nucl Acids Res 38: 7248–7259.
25. Arroyo JD, Chevilleta JR, Kroha EM, Rufa IK, Colin C, et al. (2011) Argonaute2 complexes carry a population of circulating microRNAs independent of vesicles in human plasma. Proc Natl Acad Sci USA 108: 5003–5008.
26. Yamamichi N, Shimomura R, Inada K, Sakurai K, Haraguchi T, et al. (2009) Locked nucleic acid in situ hybridization analysis of miR-21 expression during colorectal cancer development. Clin Cancer Res 15: 4009–4016.
27. Cermelli S, Ruggieri A, Marrero JA, Ioannou GN, Beretta L (2011) Circulating MicroRNAs in Patients with Chronic Hepatitis C and Non-Alcoholic Fatty Liver Disease. PLoS One 6: e23937.
28. Poynard T, Bedossa P, Opolon P (1997) Natural history of liver fibrosis progression in patients with chronic hepatitis C. The OBSVIRC, METAVIR, CLINIVIR, and DOSVIRC groups. Lancet 349: 825–832.
29. Zhang Y, Jia Y, Zheng R, Guo Y, Wang Y, et al. (2010) Plasma microRNA-122 as a biomarker for viral-, alcohol-, and chemical-related hepatic diseases. Clin Chem 56: 1830–1838.
30. Qu KZ, Zhang K, Li H, Afdhal NH, Albitar M (2011) Circulating microRNAs as biomarkers for hepatocellular carcinoma. J Clin Gastroenterol 45: 355–360.
31. Bihrer V, Friedrich-Rust M, Kronenberger B, Forestier N, Haupenthal J, et al. (2011) Serum miR-122 as a biomarker of necroinflammation in patients with chronic hepatitis C virus infection. Am J Gastroenterol 106: 1663–1669.
32. Wu H, Neilson JR, Kumar P, Manocha M, Shankar P, et al. (2007) miRNA profiling of naïve, effector and memory CD8 T cells. PLoS One 2: e1020.
33. Zen K, Zhang CY (2010) Circulating MicroRNAs: a novel class of biomarkers to diagnose and monitor human cancers. Med Res Rev [Epub ahead of print].

5

Discovery of Novel Biomarker Candidates for Liver Fibrosis in Hepatitis C Patients

Bevin Gangadharan[1]*, **Manisha Bapat**[1]⊃, **Jan Rossa**[1]⊃, **Robin Antrobus**[1], **David Chittenden**[1], **Bettina Kampa**[1], **Eleanor Barnes**[2,3], **Paul Klenerman**[2], **Raymond A. Dwek**[1], **Nicole Zitzmann**[1]

1 Oxford Antiviral Drug Discovery Unit, Oxford Glycobiology Institute, Department of Biochemistry, University of Oxford, Oxford, United Kingdom, 2 Nuffield Department of Clinical Medicine, University of Oxford, Oxford, United Kingdom, 3 Oxford NIHR Biomedical Research Centre, The John Radcliffe Hospital, Headington, Oxford, United Kingdom

Abstract

Background: Liver biopsy is the reference standard for assessing liver fibrosis and no reliable non-invasive diagnostic approach is available to discriminate between the intermediate stages of fibrosis. Therefore suitable serological biomarkers of liver fibrosis are urgently needed. We used proteomics to identify novel fibrosis biomarkers in hepatitis C patients with different degrees of liver fibrosis.

Methodology/Principal Findings: Proteins in plasma samples from healthy control individuals and patients with hepatitis C virus (HCV) induced cirrhosis were analysed using a proteomics technique: two dimensional gel electrophoresis (2-DE). This technique separated the proteins in plasma samples of control and cirrhotic patients and by visualizing the separated proteins we were able to identify proteins which were increasing or decreasing in hepatic cirrhosis. Identified markers were validated across all Ishak fibrosis stages and compared to the markers used in FibroTest, Enhanced Liver Fibrosis (ELF) test, Hepascore and FIBROSpect by Western blotting. Forty four candidate biomarkers for hepatic fibrosis were identified of which 20 were novel biomarkers of liver fibrosis. Western blot validation of all candidate markers using plasma samples from patients across all Ishak fibrosis scores showed that the markers which changed with increasing fibrosis most consistently included lipid transfer inhibitor protein, complement C3d, corticosteroid-binding globulin, apolipoprotein J and apolipoprotein L1. These five novel fibrosis markers which are secreted in blood showed a promising consistent change with increasing fibrosis stage when compared to the markers used for the FibroTest, ELF test, Hepascore and FIBROSpect. These markers will be further validated using a large clinical cohort.

Conclusions/Significance: This study identifies 20 novel fibrosis biomarker candidates. The proteins identified may help to assess hepatic fibrosis and eliminate the need for invasive liver biopsies.

Editor: Ravi Jhaveri, Duke University School of Medicine, United States of America

Funding: This work was supported by the Oxford Glycobiology Endowment and a 'Blue Skies' research grant from United Therapeutics Corp. NZ is a Senior Research Fellow of Linacre College, Oxford. PK was supported by the Wellcome Trust, The James Martin School for the 21st Century and the NIHR Biomedical Research Centre Programme (Oxford). The funders had no role in study design, data collection and analysis, decision to publish, or preparation of the manuscript.

Competing Interests: Professor Raymond Dwek is a Director and Member of the Scientific Board of United Therapeutics Corp., which supported this work in part through a "Blue Skies" research grant. A patent covering the biomarkers in this study has been filed. The patent number is 61178334.

* E-mail: Bevin.Gangadharan@bioch.ox.ac.uk

⊃ These authors contributed equally to this work.

Introduction

More than 170 million individuals, approximately 3% of the world's population, are currently infected with the hepatitis C virus (HCV) [1]. Infection with HCV is one of the leading causes of liver fibrosis which, if left untreated, can develop into cirrhosis and hepatocellular carcinoma. The current reference standard for assessing hepatic fibrosis is liver biopsy followed by histological analysis [2]. This procedure is invasive, expensive and up to 40% of patients experience severe pain. Coupled with this, if hepatic fibrosis is not homogenous the rate of false negatives from liver biopsy can be as high as 20%, with sampling error observed when biopsies under 10 mm are analysed [2,3].

Various non-invasive approaches have been proposed for assessing hepatic fibrosis including protein, glycoprotein and glycan biomarkers [2]. The FibroTest, a test based on five serum markers – apolipoprotein A1, haptoglobin, gamma glutamyltranspeptidase, alpha 2 macroglobulin and bilirubin, has been described to reduce the number of biopsies for managing HCV infection [4], but it eliminates the need for biopsy in only 26% of patients [5]. A more recent development, the Enhanced Liver Fibrosis (ELF) test, uses tissue inhibitor of metalloproteinase 1 (TIMP-1), hyaluronic acid and procollagen III amino terminal peptide (PIIIP) [6,7]. PIIIP has low diagnostic value in assessing fibrosis [8] and both PIIIP and hyaluronic acid increase in patients with viral hepatitis after interferon alpha treatment [9]. Hepascore [10] (which uses bilirubin, gamma glutamyltransferase, hyaluronic acid, alpha 2 macroglobulin) and FIBROSpect [11] (which uses hyaluronic acid, TIMP-1, and alpha 2 macroglobulin) are other fibrosis tests which use the same markers among FibroTest and ELF test. Although all these established tests are often able to discriminate between absence of fibrosis and advanced fibrosis/cirrhosis, serum markers have difficulties in classifying the intermediate stages between these two extremes often referred to as a 'gray area' [12]. In view of this, there remains a need for more reliable non-invasive markers to decrease the need for liver biopsy.

Previously we and others have used 2-DE over a wide pH 3–10 range to successfully identify several novel candidate biomarkers for liver fibrosis [13,14]. In our previous proteomics study we show that all proteins which increased or decreased in expression in early or moderate fibrosis (Ishak stages 1–3) also change in cirrhosis, but not all proteins which increased or decreased in cirrhosis also change in the earlier fibrosis stages [13]. In this study we compare plasma samples from healthy control individuals with samples from patients with cirrhosis using a narrower pH range, and then test whether any of the proteins with significantly changed expression levels also show a consistent and quantifiable change in the intermediate 'gray area', which we analysed by Western blotting using plasma samples across all Ishak fibrosis scores. We have recently shown that 2-DE with a narrow pH 3–5.6 range is a novel approach which is beneficial for biomarker discovery [15,16]. In the current study, we have increased our panel of candidate biomarkers for hepatic fibrosis by using this novel approach to compare plasma samples from healthy control individuals with samples from patients with cirrhosis. The pH 3–5.6 range was chosen since this lies outside the range of highly abundant albumin, transferrin and immunoglobulins. This enables more protein to be loaded than in our previous fibrosis marker study and enhances representation of low abundance proteins.

A selection of markers identified reliably changed in expression across all Ishak fibrosis scores when analysed using Western blotting and are novel candidates for non-invasive fibrosis markers. These markers appear to be very promising when compared to the markers in FibroTest, ELF test, Hepascore and FIBROSpect.

Materials and Methods

Patient Samples

Plasma samples were collected in P100 tubes (BD, Oxford, UK) from 50 subjects: 45 HCV-infected patients with varying degrees of hepatic fibrosis and 5 healthy control individuals. The patients were all recruited from outpatients attending for routine follow up visits at the John Radcliffe Hospital, Oxford, UK. The Ishak scores of all 45 patients were determined as previously described [17] and these scores along with other clinical details are displayed in Table S1. Collection of all plasma samples for this study was carried out by obtaining both verbal and written informed consent from each individual and this was approved by the Central Oxford Research Ethics Committee (No. 98.137). Unlike our previous study in which we used serum [13], for the current study we used plasma to discover novel fibrosis biomarkers, using recently developed P100 tubes. Unlike any other blood collection tube, this tube contains proprietary protein stabilizers that solubilize immediately as blood is collected and thus enhances preservation and recovery of proteins making them ideal for proteome analysis and biomarker discovery [18]. These samples were used for two studies: Firstly, plasma from healthy control individuals and patients with cirrhosis were compared by proteomics using 2-DE to identify candidate fibrosis biomarkers. Secondly, these candidate markers were validated by Western blotting using plasma

samples from patients across all seven Ishak scores. All the blood samples used for both 2-DE and Western blotting were acquired within 12 months of liver biopsy except for three cirrhotic patients who had biopsies more than 12 months before sampling but were clinically cirrhotic and therefore biopsies within 12 months were not required (see Table S1).

Proteomics using 2-DE with pH 3–5.6 Strips

Plasma samples from five different healthy control individuals and five different HCV-infected patients with hepatic cirrhosis (with an Ishak score [17] of 6) were initially selected for 2-DE analysis (Table 1). Samples were run by 2-DE using the approach we recently described [15,16]. Two mg of the plasma samples were made up to 375 µl in isoelectric focusing (IEF) rehydration buffer (5 M urea, 2 M thiourea, 2 mM tributyl phosphine, 65 mM DTT, 4% (w/v) CHAPS, 150 mM non-detergent sulfobetaine 256 (NDSB-256) and 0.0012% (w/v) bromophenol blue) with 1.8% (v/v) pH 3–6 ampholytes (SERVALYT®, SERVA, Heidelberg, Germany). Samples were left overnight to rehydrate 18 cm pH 3–5.6 DryStrips (GE Healthcare, Bucks, UK). Isoelectric focusing was carried out for 75 kVh at 17°C. Strips were incubated in equilibration solution (4 M urea, 2 M thiourea, 50 mM Tris-HCl (pH 6.8), 30% (v/v) glycerol, 2% (w/v) SDS, 130 mM DTT, 0.002% (w/v) bromophenol blue) for 15 min. Proteins were separated by 9–16% (w/v) SDS-PAGE gradient gels using 20 mA per gel for 1 h, followed by 40 mA per gel for 4 h at 10°C. Following electrophoresis, gels were fixed in 40% (v/v) ethanol and 10% (v/v) acetic acid and stained with the fluorescent dye OGT 1238 [19]. Gels were scanned using an Apollo II linear fluorescence scanner (Oxford Glycosciences, Abingdon, UK) to obtain 16-bit images at 200 µm resolution.

Differential Image Analysis

Scanned gel images were processed with a custom version of the Melanie II software (Oxford Glycosciences, Abingdon, UK) [19]. For image analysis, five gels of plasma from different healthy control individuals were compared with five gels of plasma from different HCV-infected patients with hepatic cirrhosis. A synthetic image was created using accurate spot matching which showed all protein spots (features) in the gels for control and cirrhotic plasma. The optical density of each feature was determined by summing pixels within the feature boundary and the volume was determined by integrating this optical density over the area of the feature. All statistical calculations were based on the percentage volume of the features and changes in protein expression were determined as a ratio of the mean percentages of feature volumes. Since some low abundant features may be undetected by the algorithm of the software, features present in at least three of five individual gels belonging to either the control or cirrhotic group of gels were considered for statistical analysis and all gels were later visualised in a montage format to confirm if the features were present in all five gels. Features which changed in expression by at least 2-fold in percentage spot volume were considered as differentially expressed and were statistically validated using a rank-sum test on percentage spot volumes with $P \leq 0.05$ (95% confidence) as previously described [19,20]. All changes in expression were further validated by visualizing the differentially expressed features across all gels in a montage format and these features were excised from the gels for mass spectrometric analysis. All gels were calibrated using landmarks of known pH and molecular weight so that the pH and molecular weights of the differentially expressed features could be determined.

Table 1. Details of the 20 plasma samples used for 2-DE and Western blotting.

Sample	Age	Sex	Ishak score	2-DE	Western blotting	MELD score for cirrhotic patients	Child-Pugh for cirrhotic patients
C1	28	F	0	Normal 1	Lane 1		
C2	41	F	0	Normal 2	Lane 2		
C3	47	M	0	Normal 3	Lane 3		
C4	28	M	0	Normal 4	Lane 4		
C5	56	M	0	Normal 5	na		
346	52	M	6	Cirrhosis 1	Lane 15	na	A
291	52	M	6	Cirrhosis 2	Lane 16	8	A
412	58	M	6	Cirrhosis 3	na	11	A
427	60	M	6	Cirrhosis 4	na	na	na
105	53	M	6	Cirrhosis 5	na	11	A
197	46	F	1	na	Lane 5		
146	49	M	1	na	Lane 6		
267	58	M	2	na	Lane 7		
446	42	F	2	na	Lane 8		
417	49	M	3	na	Lane 9		
440	46	F	3	na	Lane 10		
436	36	M	4	na	Lane 11		
447	71	M	4	na	Lane 12		
302	48	F	5	na	Lane 13		
191	57	M	5	na	Lane 14		

Sample name for 2-DE (in Figure S1) and lane number for Western blotting (in Figure 4) are shown.
na = not analysed.
Other clinical details for these samples and the other 30 plasma samples studied are in Table S1.

In-gel Digestion and Peptide Extraction

Differentially expressed features assigned for mass spectrometric analysis were excised from gels using a software-driven robotic cutter (Oxford Glycosciences, Abingdon, UK). Recovered gel pieces were dried in a SpeedVac followed by in-gel trypsin digestion and peptide extraction using the automated DigestPro workstation (Intavis, Cologne, Germany) as we recently described [16]. Digested samples were lyophilised and dissolved in 0.1% (v/v) formic acid prior to mass spectrometric analysis.

Mass Spectrometric Analysis

Tryptic peptides were analysed using a Q-TOF 1 mass spectrometer coupled to a CapLC (Waters, Hertfordshire, UK). Peptides were concentrated and desalted on a 300 µm I.D./5 mm C18 precolumn and resolved on a 75 µm I.D./25 cm C18 PepMap analytical column (LC packings, CA, USA) with a 45 min 5–95% (v/v) acetonitrile gradient containing 0.1% (v/v) formic acid at a flow rate of 200 nl/min. Spectra were acquired in positive mode. MS to MS/MS switching was controlled in an automatic data-dependent fashion with a 1 s survey scan followed by three 1 s MS/MS scans. Ions selected for MS/MS were excluded from further fragmentation for 2 min. Raw MS/MS spectra were smoothed and centred using ProteinLynx Global server 2.1.5, spectra were not deisotoped. Processed peak list (.pkl) files were searched against the SWISS-PROT database (release 56.9) using MASCOT Daemon 2.1.0 (Matrix Science, London, UK). Searches were restricted to human taxonomy (20402 sequences). Carbamidomethyl cysteine was defined as a fixed modification and oxidized methionine as a variable modification.

Data were searched allowing 0.5 Da error to accommodate calibration drift and up to 2 missed tryptic cleavage sites. A minimum ion score cut-off of 28 was applied with confident protein assignment requiring a minimum of 2 unique peptides. The MSMS of all single peptide IDs were manually validated and required a minimum of 6 y-ions (or b-ions for C-terminal peptides.) MSMS spectra quality was judged by s/n, fragment ion isotopes and fragmentation markers such as proline residues.

Biomarker Validation

Western blotting was used to validate the novel fibrosis markers identified and were compared to protein markers in FibroTest, ELF test, Hepascore and FIBROSpect also using Western blotting. Four different plasma samples from controls (Ishak score 0) and two different plasma samples from patients in each of the six Ishak stages of hepatic fibrosis (stages 1–6) were used for Western blotting (Table 1). These 16 samples were blotted for the markers in FibroTest, ELF test, Hepascore and FIBROSpect and our novel fibrosis markers. Immunoblotting was performed essentially as previously described. [20] Four plasma samples from controls (Ishak score 0) and two plasma samples from patients in each of the six Ishak stages of hepatic fibrosis (stages 1–6) were resolved on 17-well SDS-PAGE gels. Separated plasma proteins were electroblotted onto nitrocellulose membranes (Hybond ECL; GE Healthcare, Bucks, UK), blocked in 0.2% (w/v) casein for 2 h at room temperature, and probed successively with primary antibodies at 4°C and horseradish peroxidase (HRP) labeled secondary antibodies at room temperature. Bands were detected with Enhanced Chemiluminescence Plus reagent (ECL Plus) (GE

Healthcare, Bucks, UK). The primary anti human antibodies and secondary HRP conjugated antibodies used for Western blotting are listed in Method S1. The non-protein marker hyaluronic acid was measured using a competitive ELISA and total bilirubin and gamma glutamyltranspeptidase were measured by the Biochemistry department in the John Radcliffe Hospital, Oxford (see Method S1).

Ingenuity Pathways Analysis

The Ingenuity Pathways Analysis software (Ingenuity Systems, CA, USA) was used to investigate possible interactions between all proteins identified. Interactive pathways were generated to observe potential direct and indirect relations among the differentially expressed proteins.

Results

Identification of Candidate Biomarkers

A synthetic gel image representative of all features in the differential analysis comparing samples from all control and cirrhosis patients is shown in Figure 1. Original gel images for all ten gels are shown in Figure S1. Zoomed images of the gel regions depicting differential expression for selected novel candidate fibrosis biomarkers are shown in Figure 2. The image analysis software and statistical analysis found 243 statistically significant differentially expressed features of which 57 were considered suitable after validating by visualizing the differentially expressed features across all gels in a montage format. These 57 features were excised, digested with trypsin and analysed by LC-MSMS. Since some features contained more than one protein, among the 57 features a total of 85 proteins were identified and are listed in Table S2. For proteins identified with one peptide, the MSMS spectra are shown in Figure S2. Many of the proteins were identified as the same protein at different locations on the gels and so among these 85 proteins we identified 43 candidate biomarkers for hepatic fibrosis which are shown in Table S2. This table shows that in many cases the same protein spot contained more than one protein. The protein with the highest protein score has the greatest abundance and is therefore more likely to be the differentially expressed biomarker although the other proteins with lower protein score should not be ruled out. Among the 43 candidate biomarkers, 29 were top scoring proteins of which 20 were novel blood markers for fibrosis and not seen in our earlier study [13]. Table 2 shows a summary of all these 20 proteins with their function.

This analysis showed that expression of lipid transfer inhibitor protein, an isoform of beta haptoglobin at pH 5.46–5.49, haptoglobin-related protein, apolipoprotein C-III, apolipoprotein E, C4b-binding protein beta chain, retinol-binding protein 4, afamin, alpha-2-HS-glycoprotein, corticosteroid-binding globulin, leucine-rich alpha-2-glycoprotein and fibrinogen gamma chain was decreased in cirrhotic plasma, whereas expression of intact complement C3dg, immunoglobulin J chain, sex hormone-binding globulin, 14-3-3 protein zeta/delta and adiponectin increased. Features containing the glycoproteins alpha-1-antitrypsin, hemopexin and apolipoprotein J were increased and decreased at different locations on the gels suggesting potential post-translational modification of these proteins. In addition to these novel candidate markers for fibrosis, we also identified proteins already seen in our previous study [13] (decrease in albumin, α1 antichymotrypsin, complement C4, inter-α-trypsin inhibitor heavy chain H4, paraoxonase/arylesterase 1, zinc-alpha-2-glycoprotein and the elevation in immunoglobulin chains and CD5L).

Haptoglobin and its Isoform at pH 5.46–5.49 as a Novel Fibrosis Marker

Haptoglobin was chosen for further peptide sequence analysis since an isoform of its beta chain decreased more consistently than the alpha chain of haptoglobin and the other beta haptoglobin isoforms. The decrease in haptoglobin in cirrhosis was observed at approximately 17 kDa and 40 kDa (Figure 1 and Table S2) and the identified peptides in Figure S3A show that the features at these molecular weights correspond to the alpha chain and glycosylated beta chain, respectively. The beta chain of haptoglobin was seen as an array of evenly spaced features between pH 4.7 and 5.5 (Figure 2C upper panel). The alpha and beta chains did not consistently decrease in cirrhosis (Figure 2C upper panel and Figure S3B/S3C/S3D). However, one isoform for beta haptoglobin at approximately pH 5.46–5.49 decreased more consistently than the alpha chain of haptoglobin and the other beta haptoglobin isoforms (Figure 2C and Figure S3E). The pH of this isoform was determined by calibrating all gels using landmarks with known pH and molecular weights.

Complement C3dg Increases and Thioester Cleaved Complement C3 Decreases in Cirrhosis

Complement C3 has several cleavage products within its sequence and was chosen for further peptide sequence analysis to identify which cleavage product was higher in cirrhotic patient plasma. A fragment of complement C3 increased in cirrhosis and was observed on the 2-DE gel at 38 kDa with an approximate isoelectric point of pI 4.9 (Figure 2B). The peptide sequences identified by mass spectrometry are shown in Figure 3 and span from amino acids 955 to 1201. The amino acids for complement C3dg span from 955 to 1303 and its theoretical molecular weight and isoelectric point (39 kDa and pI 5) are in line with the observed gel feature indicating that the fragment of complement C3 in the feature is complement C3dg. Western blots using anti-complement C3d antibodies showed one band decreasing with increasing fibrosis stage (Figures 4 and 5), which is possibly thioester cleaved Complement C3 containing C3d.

Biomarker Validation by Western Blotting

The novel candidate markers of fibrosis identified in this study and in our previous study [13] were validated by Western blotting using plasma from patients across all Ishak fibrosis scores. The same patient plasma samples were blotted for the protein markers in the FibroTest, ELF test, Hepascore and FIBROSpect and were compared to our novel fibrosis markers. Figures 4 and 5 show our top five markers which appear to be most reliably changing in expression across the Ishak fibrosis scores: lipid transfer inhibitor protein (LTIP), complement C3d, apolipoprotein J, corticosteroid-binding globulin and finally apolipoprotein L1 which we identified in our previous study [13]. These five markers are different from the markers used in FibroTest, ELF test, Hepascore, FIBROSpect and other hepatic fibrosis markers. LTIP and complement C3d appeared to be the most superior markers showing clear expression differences between neighbouring stages. Both apolipoprotein L1 and apolipoprotein J showed a clear change in expression between the early stages of fibrosis (up to Ishak stage 3) and more advanced hepatic fibrosis (Ishak stages 4–6). Corticosteroid-binding globulin was high in healthy controls and consistently lower in Ishak stages 1–6. Figure S4 shows Western blots for the other novel markers of fibrosis we identified (afamin, adiponectin, IgJ, hemopexin, 14-3-3zeta, apolipoprotein E, apolipoprotein C-III) as well as other markers we identified in a previous study [13] (beta 2 glycoprotein-I, inter-alpha-trypsin

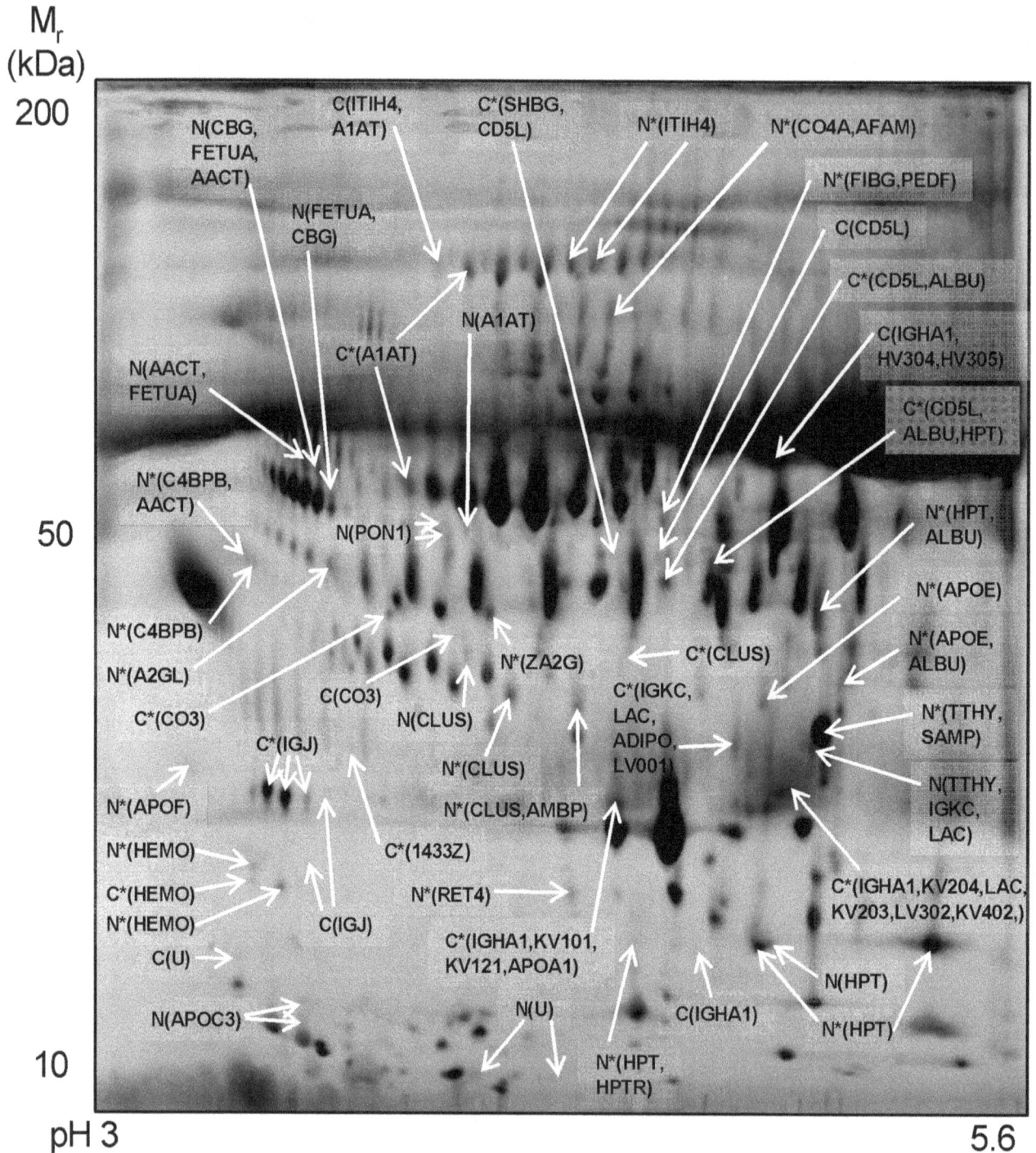

Figure 1. Synthetic 2-DE image representing all protein spots present in plasma samples in the comparison between normal healthy controls and cirrhosis patients. Gels were run using pH 3–5.6 nonlinear immobilized pH gradient DryStrips with 9–16% (w/v) SDS-PAGE gradient gels and were stained using the fluorescent dye OGT 1238. The synthetic image shown was created using accurate spot matching as previously described [19]. Differentially expressed features are indicated by arrows and the Swiss-Prot entry names are shown in parentheses. The names of selected proteins are shown in Table 2 and a full list of all proteins shown on this image can be found in Table S2. N, feature present only in gels of plasma from normal healthy controls; C, feature present only in gels of plasma from cirrhosis patients; *, features present in gels of plasma from both normal healthy controls and cirrhosis patients but expressed to a higher extent in the group indicated. For complete gel figures, see Figure S1.

inhibitor heavy chain H4, CD5L and zinc-alpha-2-glycoprotein). Although these markers were identified to be significantly changing when comparing plasma and serum of healthy and cirrhotic individuals by 2-DE, they did not appear to show a reliable trend when analysing all Ishak stages by Western blotting. Figure 4 shows Western blot, ELISA and liver function

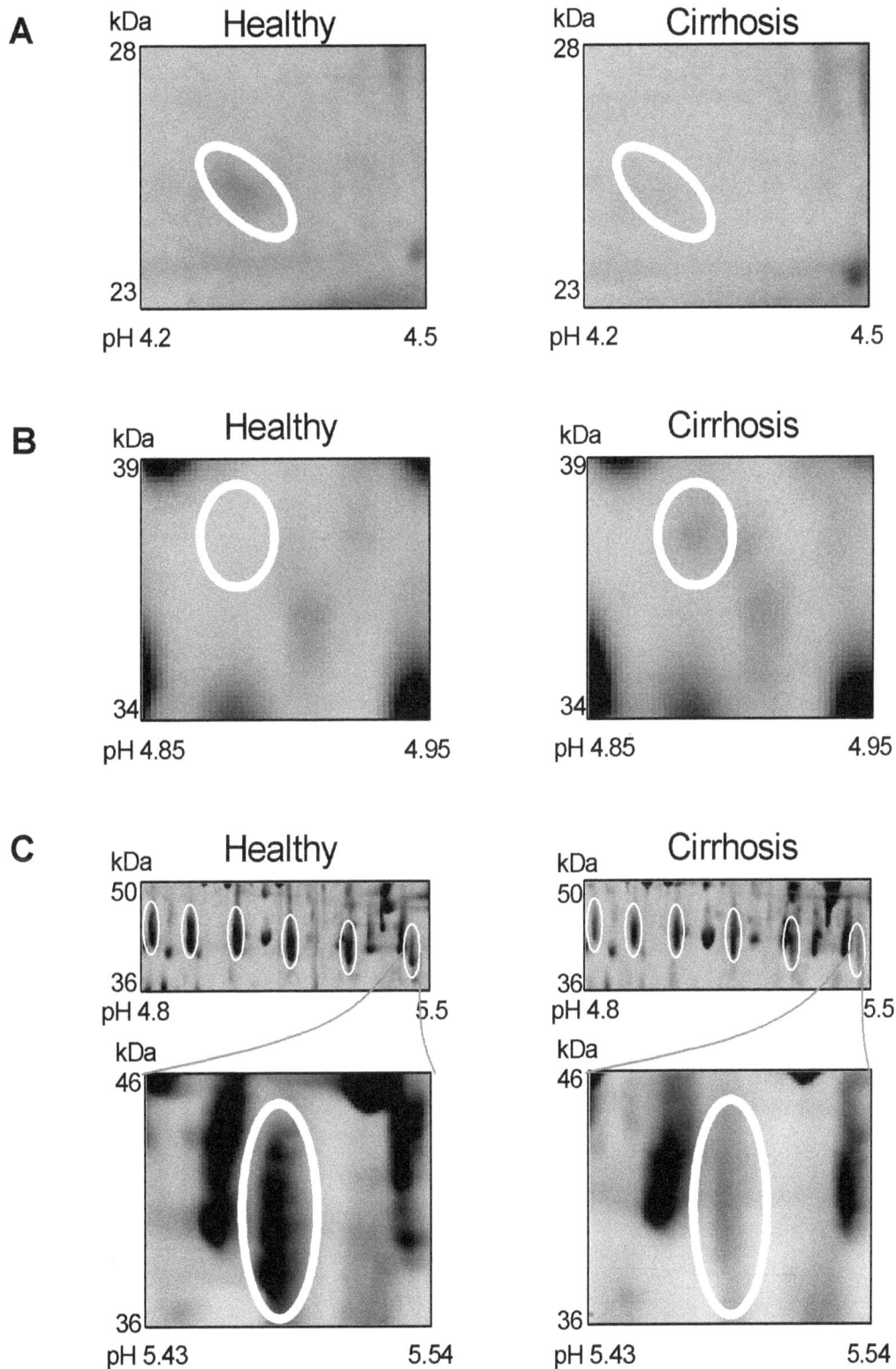

Figure 2. Magnified regions of the gels showing changes for selected potential novel fibrosis biomarkers. The relative position of the identified protein is circled. (A) LTIP is present in normal plasma but decreased in plasma from cirrhotic patients; (B) Zinc-alpha-2-glycoprotein is present in normal plasma and decreased in plasma from cirrhotic patients; (C) Decreased feature of beta haptoglobin at pH 5.46–5.49. The top panel shows evenly spaced array of beta haptoglobin spots showing no significant difference between normal plasma and plasma from cirrhotic patients. The bottom panel shows zoomed image of the beta haptoglobin spot observed at approximately pH 5.46–5.49 which is present in normal plasma and decreased in plasma from cirrhotic patients; (D) Complement C3dg is absent in normal plasma but present in plasma from cirrhotic patients.

Table 2. Differentially expressed proteins identified in the analysis between healthy control and cirrhotic plasma samples.

Spot change		Protein (Swiss-Prot entry name)	Function
Decreased in cirrhosis	⇓	Apolipoprotein C-III (APOC3)	Inhibits lipoprotein and hepatic lipases
	⇓	Corticosteroid-binding globulin (CBG)	Blood transport protein
	⇓	Alpha-2-HS-glycoprotein (FETUA)	Promotes endocytosis and possesses opsonic properties
	↓	Lipid transfer inhibitor protein LTIP (APOF)	LDL association. Inhibits cholesteryl ester transfer protein activity and regulator of cholesterol transport
	↓	β haptoglobin pH 5.46–5.49 (HPT)	Combines with free plasma hemoglobin, preventing loss of iron
	↓	Haptoglobin-related protein (HPTR)	Haptoglobin-related protein
	↓	Retinol-binding protein 4 (RET4)	Delivers retinol from liver to peripheral tissues. Prevents loss of transthyretin
	↓	Fibrinogen gamma chain (FIBG)	Yields monomers that polymerize into fibrin. Platelet aggregation cofactor
	↓	Leucine-rich alpha-2-glycoprotein (A2GL)	Role in protein-protein interactions, signal transduction, cell adhesion and development
	↓	Afamin (AFAM)	Possible role in the transport of yet unknown ligand
	↓	C4b-binding protein β chain (C4BPB)	Role in classical complement pathway
	↓	Apolipoprotein E (APOE)	Role in binding, internalisation and catabolism of lipoprotein particles
Post-translationally modified	⇓ ↓ ↑	Apolipoprotein J (CLUS)	Binds to cells, membranes and hydrophobic proteins
	⇓ ⇑ ↑	Alpha-1-antitrypsin (A1AT)	Serine protease inhibitor. Targets elastase, plasmin and thrombin
	↓ ↑	Hemopexin (HEMO)	Binds and transports heme to the liver
Increased in cirrhosis	↑	Adiponectin (ADIPO)	Involved in fat metabolism control
	↑	Sex hormone-binding globulin (SHBG)	Androgen transport protein
	↑	14-3-3 protein zeta/delta (1433Z)	Adapter protein implicated in signalling pathway regulation
	⇑ ↑	Complement C3dg (CO3)	Role in complement system
	⇑ ↑	Immunoglobulin J chain (IGJ)	Links two monomer units of IgM or IgA

Proteins shown were differentially expressed by 2-fold or more when comparing control and cirrhotic plasma gels.
⇓, feature present only in gels with plasma from normal healthy controls; ⇑, feature present only in gels with plasma from cirrhotic patients; ↓, feature present in both healthy and cirrhotic plasma but expressed to a higher extent in healthy plasma, ↑, feature present in both healthy and cirrhotic plasma but expressed to a higher extent in cirrhotic plasma.
Only novel markers of fibrosis are listed which were not seen in our previous 2-DE study. For a full list of all proteins identified, see Table S2.

test data for all the markers used in ELF test, FibroTest, Hepascore and FIBROSpect (TIMP-1, PIIIP, hyaluronic acid, haptoglobin, alpha 2 macroglobulin, apolipoprotein A1, total bilirubin and gamma glutamyltranspeptidase) using all Ishak fibrosis stages. The data in this figure and Figure 5 show that our top five markers show a consistent decrease with increasing fibrosis stage.

Discussion

Currently the primary tool for diagnosing and assessing hepatic fibrosis is by liver biopsy and a less invasive and reliable biological marker is needed. In this study we identified 44 candidate biomarkers for hepatic fibrosis of which 20 are novel blood markers of fibrosis and not seen in our earlier study [13]. The novel markers of fibrosis were validated by Western blotting with a range of fibrosis scores. This validation helped us to find five promising biomarkers, LTIP, complement C3d, apolipoprotein J, corticosteroid-binding globulin and apolipoprotein L1. All of these markers looked very promising when compared to the markers in FibroTest, ELF test, Hepascore and FIBROSpect.

We have previously applied a proteomics approach using 2-DE over the wide pH 3–10 range to identify candidate fibrosis biomarkers [13]. Although there is the limitation of a narrow dynamic range when using gel-based proteomics there is the

advantage of detecting post-translational modifications and according to a recent review [21], we have discovered more secreted human biomarkers in liver fibrosis than any other proteomics study which uses either mass spectrometry or gel-based approaches. In the study presented here, we have increased our panel of biomarkers for hepatic fibrosis and successfully identified more potential fibrosis biomarkers than our earlier proteomics study. The reason for our success in finding several more candidate markers is because we have used a new proteomics method that is more sensitive and helps to see low abundance biomarkers. We focused on the narrow pH 3–5.6 range of the plasma proteome using 2-DE. This range was chosen since it is outside the range of highly abundant albumin, transferrin and immunoglobulins and therefore this pH range allows a greater amount of plasma protein to be loaded onto the gels compared to our previous pH 3–10 study. The narrow pH range with the higher load also enhances representation of low abundance features. An alternative approach would be to deplete these highly abundant proteins prior to 2-DE. Albumin has been depleted in an earlier 2-DE fibrosis marker study by White and coworkers which has revealed the same biomarkers as identified in our previous study, but also apolipoprotein AIV [14] which was not observed in our previous or current studies. This highlights an advantage of using depletion compared to our approach and we are currently looking into immunodepletion of our samples. However our

```
  1   MGPTSGPSLL  LLLLTHLPLA  LGSPMYSIIT  PNILRLESEE  TMVLEAHDAQ
 51   GDVPVTVTVH  DFPGKKLVLS  SEKTVLTPAT  NHMGNVTFTI  PANREFKSEK
101   GRNKFVTVQA  TFGTQVVEKV  VLVSLQSGYL  FIQTDKTIYT  PGSTVLYRIF
151   TVNHKLLPVG  RTVMVNIENP  EGIPVKQDSL  SSQNQLGVLP  LSWDIPELVN
201   MGQWKIRAYY  ENSPQQVFST  EFEVKEYVLP  SFEVIVEPTE  KFYYIYNEKG
251   LEVTITARFL  YGKKVEGTAF  VIFGIQDGEQ  RISLPESLKR  IPIEDGSGEV
301   VLSRKVLLDG  VQNPRAEDLV  GKSLYVSATV  ILHSGSDMVQ  AERSGIPIVT
351   SPYQIHFTKT  PKYFKPGMPF  DLMVFVTNPD  GSPAYRVPVA  VQGEDTVQSL
401   TQGDGVAKLS  INTHPSQKPL  SITVRTKKQE  LSEAEQATRT  MQALPYSTVG
451   NSNNYLHLSV  LRTELRPGET  LNVNFLLRMD  RAHEAKIRYY  TYLIMNKGRL
501   LKAGRQVREP  GQDLVVLPLS  ITTDFIPSFR  LVAYYTLIGA  SGQREVVADS
551   VWVDVKDSCV  GSLVVKSGQS  EDRQPVPGQQ  MTLKIEGDHG  ARVVLVAVDK
601   GVFVLNKKNK  LTQSKIWDVV  EKADIGCTPG  SGKDYAGVFS  DAGLTFTSSS
651   GQQTAQRAEL  QCPQPAARRR  RSVQLTEKRM  DKVGKYPKEL  RKCCEDGMRE
701   NPMRFSCQRR  TRFISLGEAC  KKVFLDCCNY  ITELRRQHAR  ASHLGLARSN
751   LDEDIIAEEN  IVSRSEFPES  WLWNVEDLKE  PPKNGISTKL  MNIFLKDSIT
801   TWEILAVSMS  DKKGICVADP  FEVTVMQDFF  IDLRLPYSVV  RNEQVEIRAV
851   LYNYRQNQEL  KVRVELLHNP  AFCSLATTKR  RHQQTVTIPP  KSSLSVPYVI
901   VPLKTGLQEV  EVKAAVYHHF  ISDGVRKSLK  VVPEGIRMNK  TVAVRTLDPE
951   RLGREGVQKE  DIPPADLSDQ  VPDTESETRI  LLQGTPVAQM  TEDAVDAERL
1001  KHLIVTPSGC  GEQNMIGMTP  TVIAVHYLDE  TEQWEKFGLE  KRQGALELIK
1051  KGYTQQLAFR  QPSSAFAAFV  KRAPSTWLTA  YVVKVFSLAV  NLIAIDSQVL
1101  CGAVKWLILE  KQKPDGVFQE  DAPVIHQEMI  GGLRNNNEKD  MALTAFVLIS
1151  LQEAKDICEE  QVNSLPGSIT  KAGDFLEANY  MNLQRSYTVA  IAGYALAQMG
1201  RLKGPLLNKF  LTTAKDKNRW  EDPGKQLYNV  EATSYALLAL  LQLKDFDFVP
1251  PVVRWLNEQR  YYGGGYGSTQ  ATFMVFQALA  QYQKDAPDHQ  ELNLDVSLQL
1301  PSRSSKITHR  IHWESASLLR  SEETKENEGF  TVTAEGKGQG  TLSVVTMYHA
1351  KAKDQLTCNK  FDLKVTIKPA  PETEKRPQDA  KNTMILEICT  RYRGDQDATM
1401  SILDISMMTG  FAPDTDDLKQ  LANGVDRYIS  KYELDKAFSD  RNTLIIYLDK
1451  VSHSEDDCLA  FKVHQYFNVE  LIQPGAVKVY  AYYNLEESCT  RFYHPEKEDG
1501  KLNKLCRDEL  CRCAEENCFI  QKSDDKVTLE  ERLDKACEPG  VDYVYKTRLV
1551  KVQLSNDFDE  YIMAIEQTIK  SGSDEVQVGQ  QRTFISPIKC  REALKLEEKK
1601  HYLMWGLSSD  FWGEKPNLSY  IIGKDTWVEH  WPEEDECQDE  ENQKQCQDLG
1651  AFTESMVVFG  CPN
```

Figure 3. Uncleaved C3dg is elevated in hepatic cirrhosis. Using pH 3–5.6 gels, complement C3 was identified in a feature at approximately pH 4.9, MWt 38 kDa, only in gels for cirrhotic plasma. The full length sequence of complement C3 is shown with the alpha chain underlined, beta chain in italics, C3dg in bold and identified peptides highlighted in grey. Highlighted in black is the thioester site which is known to be cleaved by the fibrinolytic enzyme plasmin.

narrow pH range approach helped to identify other novel markers of fibrosis which were not observed by White and coworkers when using depletion, and all of these were different to the proteins used in FibroTest, ELF test, Hepascore and FIBROSpect and other established fibrosis tests. Also the P100 tubes used to collect the blood samples enhance preservation and recovery of proteins which may have helped to identify the novel biomarkers of fibrosis.

We confirmed some of the expression changes identified in our previous study and the new results agree with our previous findings. For example, although we had previously mentioned that zinc-alpha-2-glycoprotein and paraoxonase/arylesterase 1 could

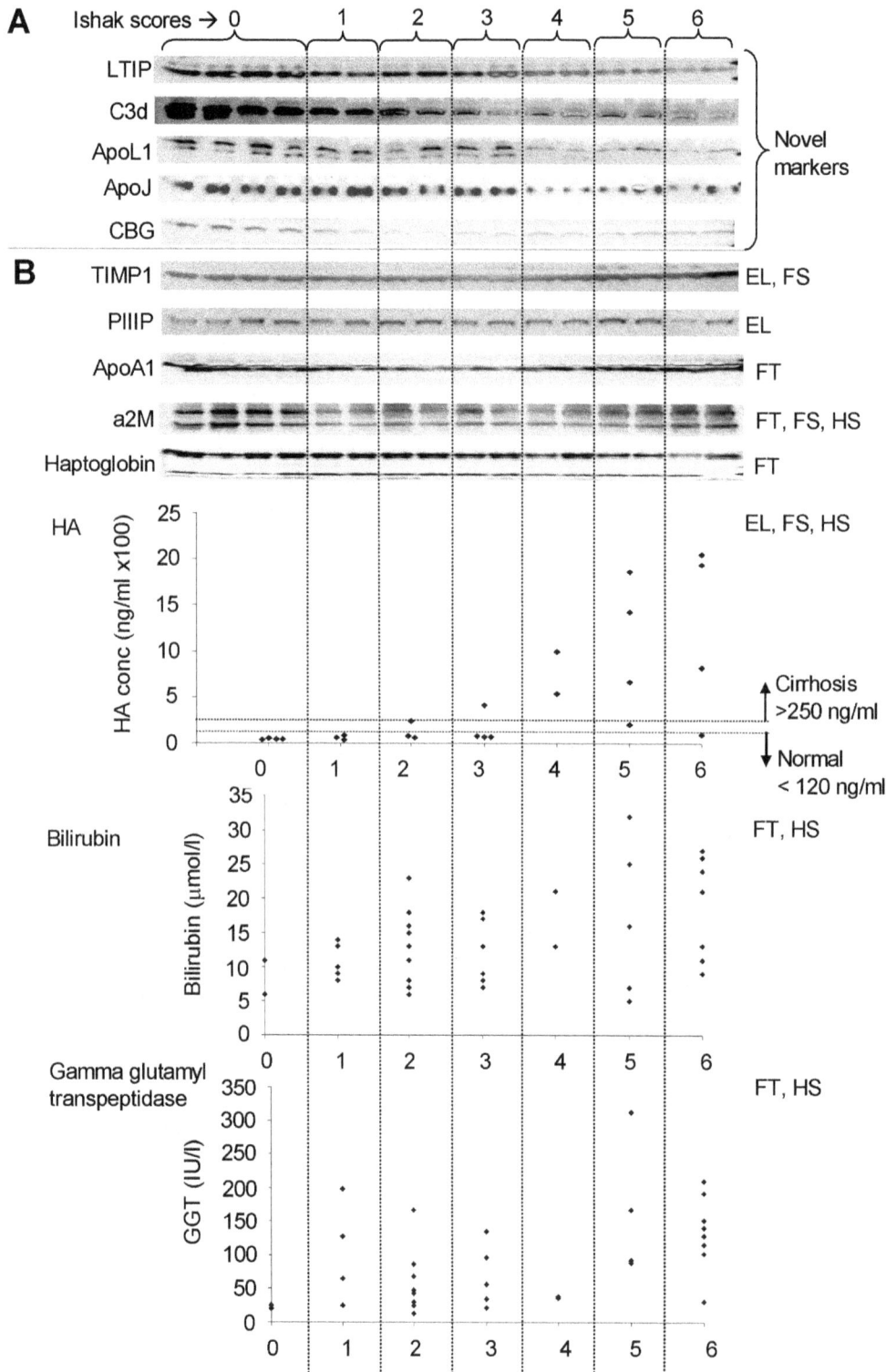

Figure 4. Validation of the novel fibrosis markers by Western blotting indicates that they are promising compared to the markers in ELF test, FibroTest, Hepascore and FIBROSpect. The novel markers of fibrosis were validated alongside the markers for the ELF test, FibroTest, Hepascore and FIBROSpect using plasma samples from individuals in each of the seven Ishak stages of hepatic scarring as indicated at the top of the figure. (A) Western blots of our novel markers of fibrosis: LTIP, complement C3d, apolipoprotein L1 (ApoL1), apolipoprotein J (ApoJ), corticosteroid-binding globulin (CBG); (B) ELF test, FibroTest, Hepascore and FIBROSpect markers. Western blots of TIMP-1, PIIIP, apolipoprotein A1 (Apo A1), alpha 2 macroglobulin (a2M) and haptoglobin, ELISA data for hyaluronic acid (HA) and levels of bilirubin and gamma glutamyltranspeptidase. For hyaluronic acid, normal individuals are recognised to have hyaluronic acid below 120 ng/ml and cirrhotic patients above 250 ng/ml as indicated with the dashed lines. The two letter codes indicate if the marker is used in ELF test (EL), FibroTest (FT), Hepascore (HS) or FIBROSpect (FS).

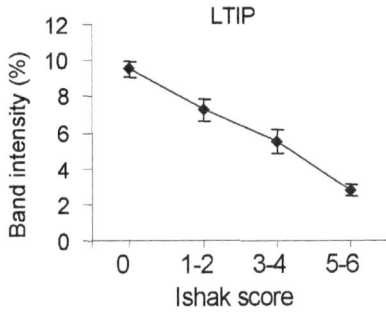

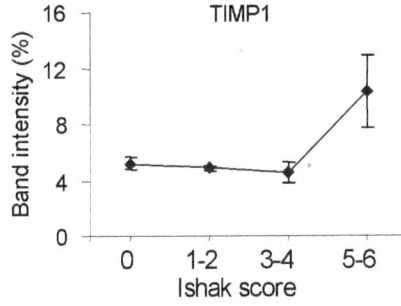

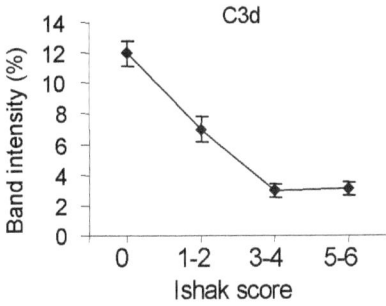

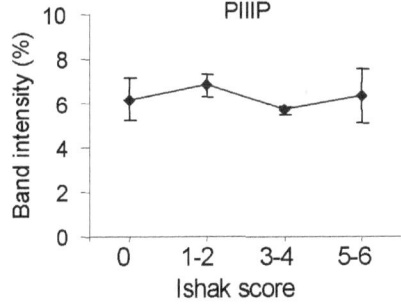

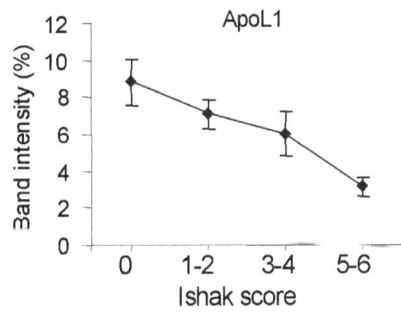

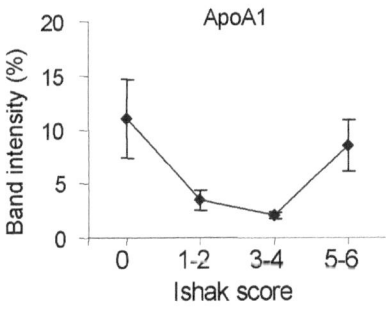

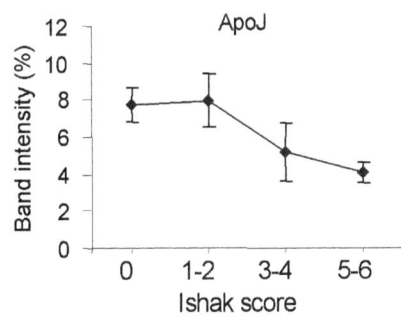

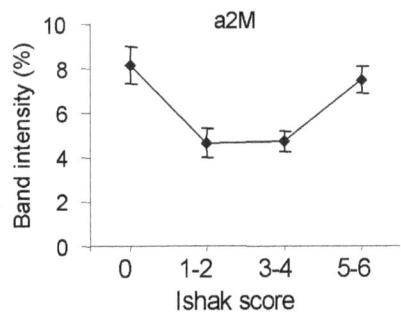

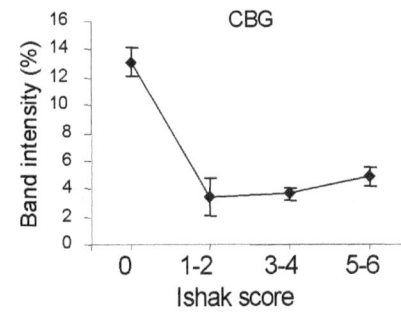

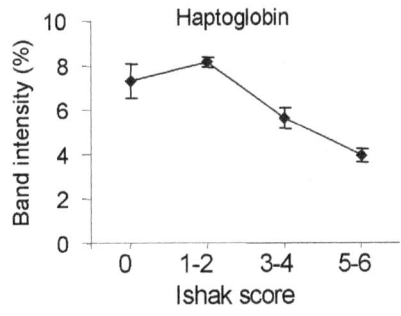

Figure 5. Western blot band densitometry. The five plots on the left show densitometry data for our five markers; from top to bottom: LTIP, complement C3d, apolipoprotein L1, apolipoprotein J and corticosteroid-binding globulin. The five plots on the right show densitometry data for all the markers that were blotted for in the ELF test (TIMP1 and PIIIP), FibroTest (apolipoprotein A1, alpha 2 macroglobulin and haptoglobin), Hepascore (alpha 2 macroglobulin) and FIBROSpect (TIMP-1, and alpha 2 macroglobulin). Each point represents the average band intensity for four patient samples. Error bars show +/− standard error.

be decreasing in cirrhosis, these proteins were identified in a feature containing another protein, haptoglobin, which was identified with higher protein score and thus we were uncertain if these proteins could be candidate biomarkers. The increased separation used in this study clearly resolves differentially expressed features where only zinc-alpha-2-glycoprotein and paraoxonase/arylesterase 1 were identified as novel markers of fibrosis.

It is unclear why the proteins we identified are markers for liver fibrosis. Below we discuss the potential involvement of our promising five novel biomarkers of hepatic fibrosis and the potential involvement of the following novel fibrosis biomarkers is shown in Table S3: apolipoprotein C-III, apolipoprotein E, hemopexin, alpha-1-antichymotrypsin (gene SERPINA3), alpha-1-antitrypsin (gene SERPINA1), C4b-binding protein beta chain. Information about the proteins, including amino acid sequence and sites of glycosylation, was derived from the ExPASy database (http://www.expasy.ch/).

We found LTIP to be decreased in cirrhosis and to be the most promising novel biomarker of fibrosis changing across the Ishak stages when validated by Western blotting, showing clear differences in expression between neighbouring stages. LTIP is a 29 kDa glyco- and apolipoprotein found in both LDL and HDL which can inhibit lipid transfer between lipoproteins. LTIP is known to inhibit cholesteryl ester transfer protein (CETP)-mediated cholesteryl ester and triglyceride transfer [22]. To our knowledge LTIP has never been identified as a biomarker for liver fibrosis or described in any virus system. An increase in CETP has already been described in primary biliary cirrhosis [23] which is consistent with the LTIP decrease observed in our study, making this glycoprotein an attractive novel biomarker candidate for hepatic scarring. The CETPs, which can be inhibited by LTIP, are functionally similar to microsomal triglyceride transfer proteins (MTP) which are also involved in triglyceride and cholesteryl ester transport, but between phospholipid surfaces. Since both MTP and CETP are involved in triglyceride and cholesteryl ester transport, inhibitors against either act as lipid-lowering agents and inhibitors against MTP can reduce CETP activity [24] although it is not known if CETP inhibitors like LTIP can affect MTP activity. MTP is essential for HCV production and is enriched in membrane vesicles in which the virus replication complex is located [25]. While it is tempting to speculate on an association between LTIP and HCV due to these relationships between HCV-MTP-CETP and LTIP-CETP, the decreased LTIP expression is more likely to be associated with hepatic scarring due to the previously reported increase in CETP in cirrhosis [23].

In addition to LTIP, other proteins in the apolipoprotein family were found to be differentially expressed: post-translational modification of apolipoprotein J and decreased expression of apolipoproteins C-III and E. Apolipoprotein J is a glycoprotein chaperone associated with elastic fibres in liver fibrosis and cirrhosis [26]. Another apolipoprotein, L1, was found to decrease in our previous study [13] indicating that several proteins in the apolipoprotein family appear to be related to hepatic fibrosis. We are currently investigating whether other apolipoproteins, which we have not identified due to low abundance or their gel location outside the pH 3–5.6 range investigated, could also serve as biomarkers. Western blots of both apolipoprotein L1 and

apolipoprotein J showed a similar trend in expression with consistently high levels in the early stages of fibrosis (up to Ishak stage 3) and consistently lower levels in more advanced hepatic scarring (Ishak stages 4–6). These markers would therefore be beneficial in differentiating patients with mild fibrosis from those with more advanced fibrosis.

We found an isoform of beta haptoglobin at pH 5.46–5.49 to be a novel marker of fibrosis which decreases in liver fibrosis. This acute phase protein is a tetramer consisting of two 16 kDa alpha chains with no potential sites of glycosylation and two 27 kDa beta chains each of which has four potential sites of N-glycosylation [27]. The array of evenly spaced features for the beta chain (Figure 2) is due to differences in glycosylation for each feature [28]. Total haptoglobin is known to decrease in fibrosis and is presently used along with other proteins to diagnose liver fibrosis [5]. Our data shows that total haptoglobin is unreliable as a fibrosis marker since both alpha and beta chains do not consistently decrease in cirrhosis (Figure S3). Furthermore, the 2-DE profile for cirrhosis patient 5 looks different to the other gels since, unlike the other cirrhotic samples, this patient had very low levels of haptoglobin. Some cirrhotic patients have very low haptoglobin and the observation was also noted in our previous study [13]. Therefore this gel is a fair representation of the expression of this protein in some cirrhotic samples. It also illustrates that haptoglobin is not consistent and its levels can be considerably different among cirrhotic patients. The isoform of beta haptoglobin identified as a novel marker of fibrosis appears to be more reliable than currently used total haptoglobin [5]. This isoform of haptoglobin has glycans which are mainly biantennary, both mono- or disialylated with hardly any tri- or tetra-antennary/sialylated structures and less sialic acid and more monosialylated structures than the other haptoglobin isoforms of lower pH [29]. The different glycosylation pattern on this isoform compared to the other isoforms is currently being investigated. Hemolytic stress in haptoglobin-hemopexin double-null mice, but not single knockout mice, causes pronounced fibrosis [30] suggesting that both haptoglobin and hemopexin, which was also identified in this study, are important for protection from liver fibrosis.

Three of the proteins identified to be differentially expressed were members of the serpin protease inhibitor family: gene names SERPINA6, SERPINA3 and SERPINA1. Corticosteroid-binding globulin (gene SERPINA6) is decreased in cirrhosis compared to healthy controls and our Western blot data showed that this marker was high in healthy controls and generally lower in Ishak stages 1–6. HCV patients with Ishak stage 0 disease would also need to be analysed to see if corticosteroid-binding globulin is beneficial in determining early hepatic scarring.

A fragment of complement C3 was found to be increased in cirrhosis. Two other proteins involved in the complement cascade, complement C4 and C4b-binding protein beta chain, were found to decrease in cirrhosis. Opposing the increase in complement C3 seen here, we have previously shown a fragment of C3 decreasing in cirrhosis [13]. In our earlier study we show that this fragment decreasing in cirrhosis contains peptides corresponding to the α-chain of C3 preceding its thioester site (the location of this site is highlighted in Figure 3). The cleavage at the thioester site was thought to be caused by plasmin, an enzyme involved in fibrinolysis, and the theoretical pI and molecular weight of the cleaved fragment were in agreement with the observed feature on the gel. This led us to suspect that the decreased levels of the thioester cleaved fragment may indicate less plasmin-mediated cleavage of the complement C3 α-chain, a finding consistent with hepatic scarring. We now further support this hypothesis by showing that C3dg, which is not cleaved since peptides were identified on either side of the thioester site (Figure 3), is elevated in cirrhosis. Complement C3dg can be cleaved at this thioester site by plasmin into C3d and C3g. Western blots were performed using anti-complement C3d antibodies to detect fragments of Complement C3 where C3dg is intact (expected increase in cirrhosis) and fragments of Complement C3 containing C3d where plasmin has cleaved the thioester site (expected decrease in cirrhosis). Results showed that there was only one band decreasing with increasing fibrosis stage (Figure 4 and 5). The increase in Complement C3 where C3dg is intact may have not been observed since it may be below the level of detection and the 2-DE data confirms that C3dg is in very low abundance (Figure 2B). The fact that the increase in C3dg is not visible by Western blotting is an advantage since if it was observed it may mask the decrease in thioester cleaved Complement C3 containing C3d making it a less reliable biomarker. To our knowledge, this is the first time it has been indicated that there is decreased thioester cleavage of complement C3 in cirrhosis.

Potential interactions between all the differentially expressed proteins were analysed using the Ingenuity Pathways Analysis software. A network diagram showing potential interactions between the proteins is shown in Figure S5. Interestingly the software recognized that some of the proteins identified were related to transforming growth factor beta-1 (TGF beta1) which is the main fibrogenic cytokine in hepatic scarring [2] suggesting that these proteins are related to pathways involved in fibrogenesis. The Ingenuity Pathways Analysis software showed that the proteins identified were most closely related to canonical pathways involved in the acute phase response which is consistent with the hepatic scarring process since inflammation has an association with fibrogenesis.

Information about the patients used in this study is shown in Table S1. The 50 patients analysed in this study varied in age and sex. It is preferable if markers are not dependent on categories such as these and so we aimed to eliminate any group specific hits from the outset. The FibroTest and Hepascore are dependent on age and gender [5,10] whereas the ELF test which initially used age was later found to be independent of this category [7,31]. For the Western blots in Figure 4, plasma samples from both males and females were analysed in most of the 7 Ishak stages of fibrosis (stages 0, 1, 2, 3 and 5) except for stages 4 and 6 where samples were only available from males (Table 1). Since our samples were from patients mixed in gender for most of the stages, the Western blot data suggest that our markers do not rely on age or sex and this will need to be confirmed using a greater number of samples.

Conclusions

This study shows how we used 2-DE gels with a narrow pH 3–5.6 range to identify candidate plasma biomarkers for liver fibrosis in hepatitis C patients. We identified 44 candidate biomarkers for hepatic fibrosis in HCV patients of which 20 were novel biomarkers of fibrosis and not seen earlier [13]. Western blot validation helped to find five promising biomarkers, which we are currently further validating, alongside the other markers we identified here and in our previous study, using dot blotting and ELISAs with a statistically relevant larger patient population. This will help us to determine the concentrations of each of our markers

in plasma and their precision and performance. We are also looking into comparing markers found by gel-free mass spectrometry-based approaches with the markers found by our gel-based approaches. In addition our markers will be investigated in other cases of hepatic fibrosis (e.g HBV and alcohol-mediated), other chronic liver diseases and other scarring diseases (e.g. cardiac and skin fibrosis). The use of dot blotting and ELISAs should confirm that one or a combination of the top five proteins already identified can be incorporated into a clinical assay which can then be used to establish a scoring system to aid in the assessment of hepatic scarring. Such an assay would also aid in assessing fibrosis reduction during therapy which would help clinicians to monitor patient improvement during current therapy and also help in clinical trials where new anti-fibrotic drugs are to be investigated. Ultimately this assay would help clinicians to determine the severity of hepatic fibrosis and eliminate the need for invasive liver biopsies.

Supporting Information

Figure S1   2 mg of plasma from five healthy individuals (Normal 1–5) and five cirrhotic patients (Cirrhosis 1–5) were separated by 9–16% 2-DE using pH 3–5.6NL IPG strips. Differentially expressed features along with their Swiss-Prot entry names are highlighted. N, feature present only in gels with plasma from normal healthy controls; C, feature present only in gels with plasma from cirrhotic patients; *, features present in both healthy and cirrhotic plasma but expressed to a higher extent in the group indicated.

Figure S2 MSMS spectra for proteins identified by a single peptide. All spectra were derived from Mascot. Peptide fragmentation patterns were generated using the observed singly charged y- or b-ions. Fragment ions minus H2O and NH3 were omitted.

Figure S3   Haptoglobin expression analysis by 2-DE and Western blotting. (A) A decrease in haptoglobin in cirrhosis was observed in gel features at approximately 17 kDa and 40 kDa. The full length sequence of haptoglobin is shown with the alpha chain underlined and beta chain in bold. Peptides identified in the features at 17 kDa are highlighted in light grey and for the feature at 40 kDa in dark grey. (B) Magnified regions of the 2D gels at approximately 40 kDa showing the array of beta haptoglobin spots (arrowed). (C) Magnified regions of the 2D gels at approximately 17 kDa showing the alpha haptoglobin spots (circled). (D)Western blot of haptoglobin using plasma from 5 healthy individuals and 10 cirrhotic patients. This confirms the data in figures C and D that there is no significant difference in the expression of both alpha and beta haptoglobin when comparing plasma from normal individuals with plasma from cirrhotic patients. (E) Upper panel = Magnified regions of the 2D gels at approximately 40 kDa showing an isoform of beta haptoglobin (circled) between pH 5.46–5.49 to the right of the beta haptoglobin array. Lower panel = Zoomed in image of the beta haptoglobin feature between pH 5.46–5.49 (circled).

Figure S4   Western blot validation. Four plasma samples from controls (Ishak score 0) and two plasma samples from patients in each of the six Ishak stages of hepatic scarring (stages 1–6) were run on 17-well SDS-PAGE gels. Separated plasma proteins were electroblotted onto nitrocellulose membranes and probed with the following primary antibodies: afamin, adiponectin, IgJ, hemopexin, 14-3-3zeta, apolipoprotein E (Apo E), apolipoprotein C3 (Apo C3), beta 2 glycoprotein-I (B2GPI), inter-alpha-trypsin inhibitor heavy chain H4 (ITIH4), CD5L and zinc-alpha-2-glycoprotein (ZAG). Bands were detected with ECL Plus. (DOC)

Figure S5 Ingenuity Pathway Analysis. Differentially expressed proteins were analysed using the Ingenuity Pathway Analysis software. Potential protein interactions are shown. Identified proteins are coloured and labelled with their gene names as shown in Table S1. Potential interacting partners which were not identified in the 2-DE study are shown in white. Solid lines (green, red, white, pink) represent direct interactions, dashed lines (yellow, grey) represent indirect interactions. Arrows (white, yellow, red, pink) from one protein node to another indicates that the node acts on the other node. Lines without arrowheads (green) represent binding. Lines with a small perpendicular line at the end (grey) represent inhibition. Proteins identified by differential analysis are shown as coloured nodes whereas unidentified proteins are white.

Method S1 Biomarker validation.

Table S1 Clinical details of all 50 plasma samples. na = not analysed. * = biopsy not performed to indicate Ishak score 0, but these individuals all declared that they had no known pathology and all were fit and well at the time of sampling. Clinical blood measurements not taken at the time of sampling are preceded with the date to show how close this value was measured to the time of sampling.

Table S2 Differentially expressed proteins identified in plasma samples of healthy controls versus cirrhotic patients. Entries in blue indicate proteins which had the highest

score within a protein spot. Among these, the protein names and entries in bold are novel and were not seen in our earlier study. [13] AN, Swiss-Prot accession number; N, feature present in plasma from healthy controls; C, feature present in plasma from cirrhosis patients. Fold change refers to proteins that were differentially expressed by 2-fold or more when comparing plasma gels from healthy controls with cirrhosis. The numerical values shown in parentheses for fold change indicate features that were present in both controls and cirrhosis but expressed to a higher extent in the indicated stage. For cases where no numerical value is shown for fold change, the feature was only present in the indicated stage. pI, isoelectric point on gel as determined by the image analysis software using calibrated landmarks; MWt, molecular weight on gel as determined by the image analysis software using calibrated landmarks. The number of MS/MS peptide matches, percentage sequence coverage and protein score were determined by the Mascot Daemon search engine. Protein functions have been adapted from the ExPASy website.

Table S3 Potential involvement of a selection of the novel proteins in hepatic scarring.

Acknowledgments

We thank Dr. Stephen Woodhouse for his valuable suggestions for the manuscript. We acknowledge Lizzie Stafford and Annie Lissington for helping to put together the clinical details for all patients and Prof. Etienne Pays for kindly providing the rat anti human apolipoprotein L1 antibody.

Author Contributions

Conceived and designed the experiments: BG NZ. Performed the experiments: BG MB JR RA DC BK. Analyzed the data: BG RA RAD NZ. Contributed reagents/materials/analysis tools: BG EB PK NZ. Wrote the paper: BG NZ.

References

1. Marcellin P (1999) Hepatitis C: the clinical spectrum of the disease. J Hepatol 31 Suppl 1: 9–16.
2. Bataller R, Brenner DA (2005) Liver fibrosis. J Clin Invest 115: 209–218.
3. Cadranel JF, Mathurin P (2002) Prothrombin index decrease: a useful and reliable marker of extensive fibrosis? Eur J Gastroenterol Hepatol 14: 1057–1059.
4. Imbert-Bismut F, Ratziu V, Pieroni L, Charlotte F, Benhamou Y, et al. (2001) Biochemical markers of liver fibrosis in patients with hepatitis C virus infection: a prospective study. Lancet 357: 1069–1075.
5. Rossi E, Adams L, Prins A, Bulsara M, de Boer B, et al. (2003) Validation of the FibroTest biochemical markers score in assessing liver fibrosis in hepatitis C patients. Clin Chem 49: 450–454.
6. Rosenberg WM, Voelker M, Thiel R, Becka M, Burt A, et al. (2004) Serum markers detect the presence of liver fibrosis: a cohort study. Gastroenterology 127: 1704–1713.
7. Guha IN, Parkes J, Roderick P, Chattopadhyay D, Cross R, et al. (2008) Noninvasive markers of fibrosis in nonalcoholic fatty liver disease: Validating the European Liver Fibrosis Panel and exploring simple markers. Hepatology 47: 455–460.
8. Gabrielli GB, Capra F, Casaril M, Squarzoni S, Tognella P, et al. (1997) Serum laminin and type III procollagen in chronic hepatitis C. Diagnostic value in the assessment of disease activity and fibrosis. Clin Chim Acta 265: 21–31.
9. Zohrens G, Armbrust T, Meyer Zum Buschenfelde KH, Ramadori G (1994) Interferon-alpha 2a increases serum concentration of hyaluronic acid and type III procollagen aminoterminal propeptide in patients with chronic hepatitis B virus infection. Dig Dis Sci 39: 2007–2013.
10. Adams LA, Bulsara M, Rossi E, DeBoer B, Speers D, et al. (2005) Hepascore: an accurate validated predictor of liver fibrosis in chronic hepatitis C infection. Clin Chem 51: 1867–1873.
11. Poordad FF (2004) FIBROSpect II: a potential noninvasive test to assess hepatic fibrosis. Expert Rev Mol Diagn 4: 593–597.
12. Pinzani M (2010) The ELF panel: a new crystal ball in hepatology? Gut 59: 1165–1167.
13. Gangadharan B, Antrobus R, Dwek RA, Zitzmann N (2007) Novel serum biomarker candidates for liver fibrosis in hepatitis C patients. Clin Chem 53: 1792–1799.
14. White IR, Patel K, Symonds WT, Dev A, Griffin P, et al. (2007) Serum proteomic analysis focused on fibrosis in patients with hepatitis C virus infection. J Transl Med 5: 33.
15. Gangadharan B, Antrobus R, Chittenden D, Rossa J, Bapat M, et al. (2011) New approaches for biomarker discovery: the search for liver fibrosis markers in hepatitis C patients. J Proteome Res 10: 2643–2650.
16. Gangadharan B, Zitzmann N (2011) Two dimensional gel electrophoresis using narrow pH 3–5.6 immobilised pH gradient strips identifies potential novel disease biomarkers in plasma or serum. Nature Protocol Exchange doi: 10.1038/protex.2011.261.
17. Ishak K, Baptista A, Bianchi L, Callea F, De Groote J, et al. (1995) Histological grading and staging of chronic hepatitis. J Hepatol 22: 696–699.
18. Matheson LA, Duong TT, Rosenberg AM, Yeung RS (2008) Assessment of sample collection and storage methods for multicenter immunologic research in children. J Immunol Methods 339: 82–89.
19. Garcia A, Prabhakar S, Hughan S, Anderson TW, Brock CJ, et al. (2004) Differential proteome analysis of TRAP-activated platelets: involvement of DOK-2 and phosphorylation of RGS proteins. Blood 103: 2088–2095.
20. Pardo M, Garcia A, Antrobus R, Blanco MJ, Dwek RA, et al. (2007) Biomarker discovery from uveal melanoma secretomes: identification of gp100 and cathepsin D in patient serum. J Proteome Res 6: 2802–2811.
21. Cheung KJ, Tilleman K, Deforce D, Colle I, Van Vlierberghe H (2008) Proteomics in liver fibrosis is more than meets the eye. Eur J Gastroenterol Hepatol 20: 450–464.
22. Lagor WR, Brown RJ, Toh SA, Millar JS, Fuki IV, et al. (2009) Overexpression of apolipoprotein F reduces HDL cholesterol levels in vivo. Arterioscler Thromb Vasc Biol 29: 40–46.
23. Hiraoka H, Yamashita S, Matsuzawa Y, Kubo M, Nozaki S, et al. (1993) Decrease of hepatic triglyceride lipase levels and increase of cholesteryl ester transfer protein levels in patients with primary biliary cirrhosis: relationship to abnormalities in high-density lipoprotein. Hepatology 18: 103–110.

24. Aggarwal D, West KL, Zern TL, Shrestha S, Vergara-Jimenez M, et al. (2005) JTT-130, a microsomal triglyceride transfer protein (MTP) inhibitor lowers plasma triglycerides and LDL cholesterol concentrations without increasing hepatic triglycerides in guinea pigs. BMC Cardiovasc Disord 5: 30.

25. Huang H, Sun F, Owen DM, Li W, Chen Y, et al. (2007) Hepatitis C virus production by human hepatocytes dependent on assembly and secretion of very low-density lipoproteins. Proc Natl Acad Sci U S A 104: 5848–5853.

26. Aigelsreiter A, Janig E, Sostaric J, Pichler M, Unterthor D, et al. (2009) Clusterin expression in cholestasis, hepatocellular carcinoma and liver fibrosis. Histopathology 54: 561–570.

27. Saldova R, Wormald MR, Dwek RA, Rudd PM (2008) Glycosylation changes on serum glycoproteins in ovarian cancer may contribute to disease pathogenesis. Dis Markers 25: 219–232.

28. He Z, Aristoteli LP, Kritharides L, Garner B (2006) HPLC analysis of discrete haptoglobin isoform N-linked oligosaccharides following 2D-PAGE isolation. Biochem Biophys Res Commun 343: 496–503.

29. Sarrats A, Saldova R, Pla E, Fort E, Harvey DJ, et al. (2010) Glycosylation of liver acute-phase proteins in pancreatic cancer and chronic pancreatitis. Proteomics Clin Appl 4: 432–448.

30. Tolosano E, Fagoonee S, Hirsch E, Berger FG, Baumann H, et al. (2002) Enhanced splenomegaly and severe liver inflammation in haptoglobin/hemopexin double-null mice after acute hemolysis. Blood 100: 4201–4208.

31. Parkes J, Guha IN, Roderick P, Harris S, Cross R, et al. (2010) Enhanced Liver Fibrosis (ELF) test accurately identifies liver fibrosis in patients with chronic hepatitis C. J Viral Hepat.

6

Progression of Biopsy-Measured Liver Fibrosis in Untreated Patients with Hepatitis C Infection: Non-Markov Multistate Model Analysis

Peter Bacchetti[1]*, **Ross Boylan**[1], **Jacquie Astemborski**[2,3], **Hui Shen**[4,5], **Shruti H. Mehta**[3], **David L. Thomas**[2], **Norah A. Terrault**[4,6], **Alexander Monto**[4,5]

1 Department of Epidemiology and Biostatistics, University of California San Francisco, San Francisco, California, United States of America, 2 Department of Medicine, Johns Hopkins University, Baltimore, Maryland, United States of America, 3 Department of Epidemiology, Johns Hopkins Bloomberg School of Public Health, Baltimore, Maryland, United States of America, 4 Department of Medicine, University of California San Francisco, San Francisco, California, United States of America, 5 Division of Gastroenterology, San Francisco Veterans Affairs Medical Center, San Francisco, California, United States of America, 6 Department of Surgery, University of California San Francisco, San Francisco, California, United States of America

Abstract

Background: Fibrosis stages from liver biopsies reflect liver damage from hepatitis C infection, but analysis is challenging due to their ordered but non-numeric nature, infrequent measurement, misclassification, and unknown infection times.

Methods: We used a non-Markov multistate model, accounting for misclassification, with multiple imputation of unknown infection times, applied to 1062 participants of whom 159 had multiple biopsies. Odds ratios (OR) quantified the estimated effects of covariates on progression risk at any given time.

Results: Models estimated that progression risk decreased the more time participants had already spent in the current stage, African American race was protective (OR 0.75, 95% confidence interval 0.60 to 0.95, p = 0.018), and older current age increased risk (OR 1.33 per decade, 95% confidence interval 1.15 to 1.54, p = 0.0002). When controlled for current age, older age at infection did not appear to increase risk (OR 0.92 per decade, 95% confidence interval 0.47 to 1.79, p = 0.80). There was a suggestion that co-infection with human immunodeficiency virus increased risk of progression in the era of highly active antiretroviral treatment beginning in 1996 (OR 2.1, 95% confidence interval 0.97 to 4.4, p = 0.059). Other examined risk factors may influence progression risk, but evidence for or against this was weak due to wide confidence intervals. The main results were essentially unchanged using different assumed misclassification rates or imputation of age of infection.

Discussion: The analysis avoided problems inherent in simpler methods, supported the previously suspected protective effect of African American race, and suggested that current age rather than age of infection increases risk. Decreasing risk of progression with longer time already spent in a stage was also previously found for post-transplant progression. This could reflect varying disease activity, with recent progression indicating active disease and high risk, while longer time already spent in a stage indicates quiescent disease and low risk.

Editor: Christian Gluud, Copenhagen University Hospital, Denmark

Funding: This work was supported by grant R01AI069952 from the United States National Institutes of Health. The studies providing data were supported by grants R01DA016078, R01DA004334, R01DA012568, R01AA012879, P30DK26743, M01RR00079, and U19AI40034 from the United States NIH and by Veterans Administration Merit grant CX000295. The funders had no role in study design, data collection and analysis, decision to publish, or preparation of the manuscript.

Competing Interests: The authors have declared that no competing interests exist.

* E-mail: peter@biostat.ucsf.edu

Introduction

Chronic infection with hepatitis C virus (HCV) has been estimated to affect 3.2 million persons in the United States and 130 million worldwide and is a leading cause of liver failure and the need for liver transplant [1,2]. One way of assessing liver damage known as fibrosis is to categorize liver biopsies into fibrosis stages using established scales that range from no damage (stage 0) to cirrhosis [3]. Although such fibrosis staging is widely used clinically, statistical analysis of biopsy-measured fibrosis progression poses considerable challenges. First, the stages are ordered but are not numeric, meaning that differences between consecutive

stages are not necessarily equivalent in any meaningful sense. Second, biopsies are too invasive and expensive to perform frequently. Many patients in research studies provide only one observed stage. When multiple observations are available, they are usually widely spaced (e.g., 5 years apart), and an observed progression could have occurred at any time between biopsies, which leaves the exact time of progression unknown. Third, observed fibrosis stage is often misclassified, both because reading of biopsy specimens is not perfectly standardized and because biopsies may not accurately represent the overall state of the entire liver [4]. Finally, most patients available for study have been infected with HCV at some unknown time in the past, and the usual practice of imputing this time based on reported histories of risk factors can be inaccurate [5].

Methods for multistate modeling [6,7], such as implemented in the "msm" package for R (available at http://cran.r-project.org/web/packages/msm/index.html), deal with many of these difficulties and have been used to analyze fibrosis stage data [8,9], but they make the strong simplifying assumption that previous history of progression does not impact current risk of progression—the so-called memoryless or Markov assumption. For HCV, however, there is considerable interest in whether slow progression up to the present predicts low risk of progression in the future. A new method for multistate modeling without Markov assumptions was recently applied to fibrosis progression following liver transplant (where time of infection of the new liver is known). Here, we apply that method [10] to data from chronically infected patients from three studies, using multiple imputation [11] to account for uncertainty about time of HCV infection.

Methods

Ethics Statement

We report here a secondary analysis of fully de-identified data, including no dates more specific than calendar year. This was approved by the University of California at San Francisco Committee on Human Research. The original source studies (see below) obtained written informed consent from participants to have their data stored and analyzed for research purposes, and they were approved by the University of California at San Francisco Committee on Human Research and the Johns Hopkins Bloomberg School of Public Health Review Board.

Objectives

We sought to assess the impact of potential risk factors on fibrosis progression, while avoiding questionable assumptions and accounting for fibrosis misclassification and uncertainty about duration of HCV infection. Particular interest focused on how history of progression up to a given time predicts current risk of progression. Human immunodeficiency virus (HIV) infection [12], African American race [9], and age [5] were predictor variables of particular interest.

Data Sources

We report here new analyses of previously-collected data from three studies: the AIDS Link to Intravenous Experience (ALIVE) study [13,14,15]; the Hepatitis C and Alcohol Study (HALS) [16]; and the San Francisco Veterans Affairs Medical Center (SFVA) liver studies cohort [17]. For this analysis, we excluded participants with chronic hepatitis B infection or hepatocellular carcinoma, and we excluded biopsy results that were after interferon treatment or liver transplant. The ALIVE study had fibrosis staged on both the Metavir [18] and Ishak [19] scales; a cross-tabulation of stages showed near-perfect correspondence of Ishak 0 with Metavir 0, Ishak 1 or 2 with Metavir 1, Ishak 3 with Metavir 2, Ishak 4 or 5 with Metavir 3, and Ishak 6 with Metavir 4 (cirrhosis). We used this correspondence to convert Ishak scores in the HALS study to Metavir scores. SFVA participants had biopsies staged from 0–4 using the Batts-Ludwig scale [20]. We treated this as equivalent to Metavir stages for analysis purposes because both are 0 to 4 ratings with similar criteria for each stage and because a study directly comparing the methods on the same biopsies found exact agreement in 49 of 50 cases [21]. All biopsies were obtained prospectively after study enrollment. (A previous analysis of SFVA data [17] excluded

pre-1997 biopsies because they lacked the needed type of data on alcohol use.)

Statistical methods

Model. To preserve the advantages of multistate modeling while avoiding questionable Markov assumptions and allowing use of covariates that change over time, we used a new method implemented in the R package *mspath*, which is available at http://cran.r-project.org/web/packages/mspath/index.html. Technical details of this method have been described elsewhere [10]. The method assumes the following outline of how disease progresses:

1. Each person starts at stage 0 at the time of HCV infection.
2. Time after infection is divided into discrete time steps (such as age in years).
3. At each time step, the person either remains at the same stage or progresses to the next higher stage.
4. The risk of progression at each time step is determined by the progression history up to that point, along with covariates, including current values of covariates that may have changed over time (termed *time-varying covariates*).

The method considers for each person every specific history of progression over time (or *path*) that could have produced the observed fibrosis stage(s). For example, a person with an observed stage of 2 at time step 5 could have 1) progressed to stage 1 at step 1, to stage 2 at step 3, stayed in stage 2 until step 5 and then been accurately observed, or 2) progressed to stage 1 at step 2, to stage 2 at step 5 and then been accurately observed, or 3) progressed to stage 1 at step 5 and then been misclassified as stage 2, and so on (too many possibilities to list, even in this simple case). Models that include effects of progression history up to a given point, and effects of time-varying covariates, can be applied to each specific path, and the likelihood of having observed the actual data is then calculated by summing over all the possible specific paths. Estimated covariate effects are obtained as those that maximize the likelihood of the observed data, a standard statistical approach to estimation. The influence of covariates on the probability of progression to the next stage is modeled on the log-odds scale, so we present estimated effects as odds ratios. We defined the time scale as current age in years minus age in years at time of HCV infection, and most models used time steps of 1.5 years (to keep computational burden manageable). In a sensitivity analysis, we re-estimated one model using 1-year time steps. We also excluded biopsies occurring 40 or more years after HCV infection (again to keep computational burden manageable).

Misclassification of stage. To account for the reality that observed stage at a given time may differ from the person's true stage at that time, we included misclassification probabilities in the models. For most models, we assumed the optimistic misclassification probabilities shown in Table 1. These are from an analysis of several studies specifically focused on misclassification of fibrosis stage from liver biopsies [4]. In a sensitivity analysis, we also re-estimated one model using the more pessimistic misclassification probabilities in Table 1, which are also from the earlier analysis [4].

Predictors based on past progression history. We investigated possible departures from the usual Markov assumptions by assessing four predictor variables that the mspath program defines for each step of each path, reflecting progression history up to that point:

Time in stage—the amount of time already spent in the current stage. A negative coefficient or odds ratio <1 for this variable indicates that risk of progression is less when a longer time has already been spent in the stage without progressing; this might

Table 1. Misclassification probabilities assumed for analyses.

	Probability of Observed Stage Given True Stage									
	Optimistic*					Pessimistic†				
	0	1	2	3	4	0	1	2	3	4
True Stage 0	0.81	0.19	0	0	0	0.74	0.26	0	0	0
1	0.07	0.73	0.19	0	0	0.24	0.54	0.22	0	0
2	0	0.10	0.80	0.09	0	0	0.19	0.65	0.16	0
3	0	0.03	0.23	0.67	0.07	0	0.10	0.45	0.37	0.08
4	0	0	0	0.08	0.92	0	0.01	0.07	0.25	0.67

*From Table 1, line 4 of reference [4].
†From Table 3 of reference [4].

occur if having recently progressed to the current stage tends to indicate that disease is active, creating higher risk of continuing progression, while having been in the stage a long time tends to indicate quiescent disease and lower risk. A positive coefficient or odds ratio >1 indicates that risk of progression is higher when a longer time has already been spent in the current stage; this might occur if underlying disease is steady and incremental so that it eventually accumulates enough to manifest as progression to the next stage.

$Log_e(c+time in stage)$, where c is a specified positive number that prevents taking the logarithm of zero the first time a path is in a new stage (we used $c =$ half the step size in all analyses). This allows a different shape for the influence of time in stage on progression risk. Its qualitative interpretation is the same as noted above for time in stage.

Total time in all previous stages—the amount of time that it took to reach the current stage. A negative coefficient or odds ratio <1 for this variable indicates that risk of progression is less if the person has previously been progressing more slowly (took longer to reach the current stage). A positive coefficient or odds ratio >1 would indicate that those previously progressing more slowly are now at higher risk. (This variable is not used in modeling progression from stage 0 to 1, because there are no previous stages.)

$Log_e(c+total time in previous stages)$, where c is the specified positive constant described above. This allows a different shape for the influence of time in previous stages on progression risk.

Other predictors. We evaluated a number of other factors that may influence fibrosis progression. The three studies selected participants in different ways from different populations, so we controlled for study in all models by including indicator variables for ALIVE and for HALS. This was important for preventing spurious apparent associations due to confounding with source study. We allowed the effects of study to be *stage-varying*, i.e., to differ for progression between different stages, because the simplifying assumption that the effect was identical for all 4 transitions between stages did not fit the data nearly as well. Other predictors were initially evaluated as having the same effect on all transitions; they are listed below:

Sex—male compared to female.

Race/ethnicity—classified as Caucasian, African America, Hispanic, and other. Because of previous findings concerning African Americans, we also evaluated this as African American compared to all other categories lumped together.

HIV—we determined coinfection with HIV at each time step, based on age at HIV infection imputed as described in the next

section. Because treatment for HIV changed dramatically over time [22], we also examined whether the effect of HIV differed in different calendar periods: before 1996 versus 1996 and later; and before 1996 versus1996–2000 versus after 2000.

Primary reported HCV infection risk factor—classified as injection drug use for participants reporting any injection drug use; otherwise, we classified it as receipt of blood transfusion or as needlestick if those were reported. All others were lumped together as "Other/none".

Tobacco smoking—collected only during study participation. We classified this as yes or no based on any reported smoking, and assumed that the earliest report also applied back to age 16.

Alcohol consumption—the HALS study collected a comprehensive alcohol consumption history, but the other studies only provided information on recent consumption collected during study participation. For each year of age of HALS participants, we categorized alcohol consumption as "None" if the age was in a period of reported alcohol abstinence, as "Moderate" if they reported drinking less than 3 drinks per day on less than 20 days per month or less than 5 drinks per day on less than 4 day per month, or as "Heavy" otherwise. For the other two studies, we approximated similar definitions using available data and assumed that the earliest measures applied back to age 21. Because this is likely to be inaccurate, primary analyses of alcohol only used HALS participants.

Injection drug use—based on reported ages of first and last injection drug use, we determined whether each participant was using injection drugs at each time step.

Body mass index—this was defined as weight in kilograms divided by the square of height in meters, which were only collected during study participation. We assumed that the earliest value also applied back to the age of HCV infection.

Current age—evaluated at each time step as a time-varying covariate.

Age at HCV infection—evaluated as a fixed covariate, multiply imputed as described in the next section.

Multiple imputation. We applied a strategy known as multiple imputation [11], because exact values were generally unavailable for age at HCV infection and age at HIV infection, and some observations had missing data for alcohol consumption, smoking, and body mass index. This approach is more valid than assuming that infection occurred at the reported age of first risk factor (which has typically been used for age at HCV infection [5]) or the common practice of simply deleting observations that have a missing value for any covariate. For risk factor modeling, we generated 5 data sets, each replacing missing covariates with values randomly imputed from models built using the non-missing data, along with imputed ages of HCV and HIV infection from external analyses (see next paragraph). We then analyzed each and combined the results of the 5 analyses using established methods to obtain overall estimates and standard errors [11]. In some cases, estimated log odds ratios in some or all imputed data sets were effectively infinite, causing methods based on standard errors in multiple imputation to break down. We therefore note likelihood ratio p-values and profile likelihood confidence bounds for some results. We use the term *deviance* to denote twice the negative log likelihood, which is the quantity used in likelihood ratio tests; a difference in deviance of 3.84 has $p = 0.05$ for comparing a base model to one with one additional parameter.

We imputed 5 values of age at HCV infection for each participant by putting their risk factor histories and age first known to be infected into an external model of risk. The model has been reported previously [5] and was based on reported injection drug use history and other characteristics; it was built using data from

4623 street-recruited injection drug users. As a sensitivity analysis, we repeated some models using 5 imputed data sets based on a model of HCV infection risk built by the same methods but using data from 2248 mostly HIV-infected women [5]. The reference [5] fully describes both models, includes figures illustrating the effects of age and calendar time, and gives the exact code that we used to obtain the fitted probabilities of infection at each age for each person in a supplemental file at http://www.biomedcentral. com/content/supplementary/1471-2334-7-145-s2.pdf. For purposes of summarizing the available data, we also imputed one additional value as the conditional mean of the probability distribution of age at HCV infection given each participant's first age known infected and risk factors. We imputed age of HIV infection using age first known to be infected and the estimated distribution of numbers of infections among injection drug users over calendar time from a national study [23], assuming no risk before age 13 or before the year 1980. We then imputed other missing predictors using the Markov-chain-Monte-Carlo method in the Statistical Analysis System's (SAS Institute, Cary, NC, version 9.1.3) MI procedure, separately for each study, with all available variables included in the process. To approximate the recommended practice of including the outcome as one of the variables used to impute missing predictors [24], we also included a variable defined as the first observed fibrosis score divided by years since imputed HCV infection.

Predictor selection. Because simultaneous inclusion of all potential risk factors in a single model would not be computationally feasible or statistically reliable, we sought to build a parsimonious multivariate model that included risk factors that had the strongest evidence for an influence on progression. We then examined the effects of the remaining potential risk factors when added to this model. Because of the high computational burden of our method, we performed some preliminary exploration of models using the additional single imputation based on conditional mean age of HCV infection, but we found that this differed too much from multiple imputation analyses using the 5 randomly imputed data sets. We therefore used full multiple imputation for confirmation of predictor selection. We included source study because it was a potential confounder of other effects, and we included log(0.75+years in stage) because it was of primary interest and appeared to strongly influence progression risk. When added to a model including stage-varying study effects and log(0.75+years in stage), African American race (versus all others) appeared to be an important predictor, based on the p-value and direction and magnitude of the estimated effect. We therefore report this primary model in detail, along with the estimated effects that other predictors had when added to this model. We also evaluated substituting each of the other 3 predictors based on progression history for log(0.75+years in stage), and adding the time-in-previous-stages predictors to the primary model.

Special handling of age variables. The estimated effects of the two age variables listed above, current age at each time step and age at HCV infection, may be subject to bias [5]. When the imputed age of HCV infection is too early, this will make progression look slower than it really was, inducing a spurious protective effect of younger age at infection. When imputed age of infection is too late, this will make progression look faster than it really was, making older age at infection appear to increase risk, which is the same spurious effect. Thus, any error in either direction creates the same bias, and multiple imputation may not do much to mitigate this problem. Little change in the estimated effect was observed with multiple imputation in a previous study [9]. For current age at each time step, the impact may be more subtle because this variable is known rather than imputed with

some error. Bias may nevertheless occur because age at infection determines which ages are assumed to be part of followup during which progression could have occurred. A too-early imputation of age at HCV infection will make progression look slower and cause spurious inclusion of some younger current ages in the post-infection followup time, while a too-late imputation will make progression look faster and will cause only older current ages to be included as post-infection. We therefore did not include current age or age at HCV infection in the primary models evaluated as described in the previous paragraph. We added each, and both, to the primary model, and we also performed some simulations to evaluate the potential bias. We used the primary fitted model without age effects to generate simulated observations of fibrosis stage, at the same times as the original observations, using an additional independent set of imputed ages at HCV infection. We did this independently for each of the 5 original imputed data sets, generating 5 new simulated data sets with realistic amounts of error in the imputed HCV infection ages and with no actual association of current age or age at HCV infection with rate of progression. We then fit the primary model plus current age and the primary model plus age at HCV infection to the simulated data; any apparent effects in these models are due to bias and therefore provide some indication of how much bias may be present. We then repeated the entire process using another independently imputed set of assumed actual HCV infection ages. Performing a large number of such simulations, however, would not be computationally practical.

Results

Study participants

There were 1082 participants available for study, with 1284 biopsies. For 20 of them, their first biopsy was ≥40 years after their mean predicted age of HCV infection. Because our limitation of followup time to 39 years is likely to exclude these from most imputed data sets, Tables 2 and 3 summarize characteristics of the remaining 1062. The randomly imputed ages of HCV infection are more variable than the means and therefore have more that were long ago, so the 5 imputed data sets ranged from 1015 to 1027 participants included.

Progression model and risk factors

Our primary fitted progression model is described by Figure 1 and the top part of Table 4. The odds ratios for years in stage are somewhat complicated to interpret. For example, for the 0 to 1 transition, the odds ratio of 0.39 implies that the estimated odds of progressing drop by a factor of 0.39 if $\log_e(0.75+\text{years in stage})$ increases by 1 unit, which means that (0.75+years in stage) increases by a factor of $e \approx 2.72$. This would be the case if years in current stage increase from 1.5 to 5.4, for example. We use Figure 1 to more simply illustrate the estimated baseline progression risk by time step based on fitted intercept terms and the odds ratios for $\log_e(0.75+\text{years in stage})$. We show the pointwise averages of the fitted curves for the five imputed data sets, because curves defined by average parameter values would be distorted by instances of effectively infinite estimated parameters for some of the imputed data sets. All the estimates had risk of progression decreasing as time already spent in the stage increased. From Table 4, we see that evidence for this phenomenon was statistically significant for the stage 0 to 1 and 2 to 3 transitions. The decrease had a large p-value for the 1 to 2 transition. The overall strength of evidence is unclear for the 3 to 4 transition, because two of the imputed data sets produced effectively infinite estimates (risk drops to zero after progression has been avoided for

Table 2. Summary of time-related characteristics, by source study.

		ALIVE N (% of 236)	HALS N (% of 202)	SFVA N (% of 624)	Total N (% of 1062)
Age at HCV Infection*	<15	6 (2.5)	8 (4.0)	10 (1.6)	24 (2.3)
	15–19	92 (39.0)	71 (35.2)	145 (23.2)	308 (29.0)
	20–24	103 (43.6)	85 (42.1)	249 (39.9)	437 (41.2)
	25–29	24 (10.2)	32 (15.8)	162 (26.0)	218 (20.5)
	≥30	11 (4.7)	6 (3.0)	58 (9.3)	75 (7.1)
Age at last biopsy	<30	2 (0.9)	6 (3.0)	2 (0.3)	10 (0.9)
	30–39	33 (14.0)	33 (16.3)	36 (5.8)	102 (9.6)
	40–49	141 (59.8)	102 (50.5)	198 (31.7)	441 (41.5)
	50–59	57 (24.2)	58 (28.7)	335 (53.7)	450 (42.4)
	≥60	3 (1.3)	3 (1.5)	53 (8.5)	59 (5.6)
Year of HCV infection*	Pre-1966	0 (0.0)	3 (1.5)	12 (1.9)	15 (1.4)
	1966–1970	42 (17.8)	28 (13.9)	156 (25.0)	226 (21.3)
	1971–1975	66 (28.0)	50 (24.8)	230 (36.9)	346 (32.6)
	1976–1980	65 (27.5)	60 (29.7)	162 (26.0)	287 (27.0)
	1981–1990	59 (25.0)	56 (27.7)	60 (9.6)	175 (16.5)
	After 1990	4 (1.7)	5 (2.5)	4 (0.6)	13 (1.2)
Year of last biopsy	1992–1995	0	00.00	11 (1.8)	11 (1.0)
	1996–1999	83 (35.2)	2 (1.0)	134 (21.5)	219 (20.6)
	2000–2003	82 (34.7)	189 (93.6)	290 (46.5)	561 (52.8)
	2004–2008	71 (30.1)	11 (5.4)	189 (30.3)	271 (25.5)
Years, infection to last biopsy*	<20	49 (20.8)	39 (19.3)	38 (6.1)	126 (11.9)
	20–24	60 (25.4)	56 (27.7)	125 (20.0)	241 (22.7)
	25–29	69 (29.2)	58 (28.7)	212 (34.0)	339 (31.9)
	30–34	43 (18.2)	40 (19.8)	173 (27.7)	256 (24.1)
	35–39	15 (6.4)	9 (4.5)	76 (12.2)	100 (9.4)

*Based on single imputation of age at HCV infection (see text).
Abbreviations: ALIVE: AIDS Link to Intravenous Experience study [13,14,15]; HALS: Hepatitis C and Alcohol Study [16]; SFVA: San Francisco Veterans Affairs Medical Center liver studies cohort [17]; HCV: hepatitis C virus.

one step) with likelihood ratio p-values of 0.021 and 0.028. The protective effect of African American race versus all other groups was in the expected direction with a small p-value. Allowing African American race to have different effects for the different transitions did not produce a statistically significant improvement in any of the 5 imputed data sets (all p≥0.70); the estimates for all transitions were protective and similar to the overall estimate except for stage 3 to 4 (odds ratio 1.35, 95% confidence interval 0.35 to 5.2, p = 0.66).

Substituting the untransformed years in stage for $\log_e(0.75+$ years in stage) produced similar models but with slightly worse fits overall (deviance greater by 1.7 on average over the 5 data sets). Substituting either variable based on total time in previous stages produced worse fits (deviance worse by at least 17 for every data set). When added to the primary model, longer time in stage 0 appeared to greatly reduce progression risk for the stage 1 to 2 transition, indicating the plausible phenomenon of slower progression through stage 0 predicting slower progression through stage 1. The evidence for this was somewhat stronger than shown in Table 4, because one of the imputed data sets had odds ratio = 0 (a degenerate estimate) with a likelihood ratio p-value <0.0001. For the 2 to 3 and 3 to 4 transitions, the effect of total time spent in previous stages was estimated to be in the opposite direction, but with wide

confidence intervals. For the 2 to 3 transition, the evidence for increased risk with longer time spent previous stages is also stronger than indicated in Table 4 because two of the five data sets produced effectively infinite odds ratios, with likelihood ratio p-values of 0.021 and 0.082.

Table 5 shows estimated effects of other potential predictors when controlled for all the terms in the primary model. The effect of African American race was slightly weaker versus Caucasians than versus all others (Table 4). Coinfection with HIV appeared only slightly risky overall, with a wide confidence interval that included substantial increased risk. Allowing the effect of HIV to change with the advent of widely available highly active anti-retroviral therapy in 1996 [22] produced a much higher estimated risk in this era, but this did not quite reach p<0.05; the estimated effect of HIV before 1996 became very uncertain. Further subdividing HIV effects by calendar time resulted in highly uncertain estimates. The estimated effect of heavy alcohol consumption was in the expected direction, but modest and not statistically significant; the upper confidence bound, however, allows for a fairly substantial increased risk.

Sensitivity analyses

Table 6 shows the main results of interest produced by repeating the primary model from Table 4 with three alterations,

Table 3. Summary of other characteristics, by source study.

		ALIVE N (% of 236)	HALS N (% of 202)	SF VA N (% of 624)	Total N (% of 1062)
Sex	Female	73 (30.9)	62 (30.7)	63 (10.1)	198 (18.6)
	Male	163 (69.1)	140 (69.3)	561 (89.9)	864 (81.4)
Race/Ethnicity	Missing	0 (0.0)	2 (1.0)	0 (0.0)	2 (0.2)
	White	15 (6.4)	84 (41.6)	419 (67.2)	518 (48.8)
	Black	215 (91.1)	60 (29.7)	134 (21.5)	409 (38.5)
	Hispanic	5 (2.1)	37 (18.3)	38 (6.1)	80 (7.5)
	Other	1 (0.4)	19 (9.4)	33 (5.3)	53 (5.0)
HIV-infected	No	155 (65.7)	160 (79.2)	560 (89.7)	875 (82.4)
	Yes	81 (34.3)	42 (20.8)	64 (10.3)	187 (17.6)
HCV risk factor	Injection drug use	236 (100)	135 (66.8)	345 (55.3)	716 (67.4)
	Transfusion	0 (0)	25 (12.4)	58 (9.3)	83 (7.8)
	Needlestick	0 (0)	5 (2.5)	36 (5.8)	41 (3.9)
	Other/none	0 (0)	37 (18.3)	185 (29.7)	222 (20.9)
Smoking	Missing	0 (0.0)	0 (0.0)	190 (30.5)	190 (17.9)
	No	20 (8.5)	73 (36.1)	54 (8.7)	147 (13.8)
	Yes	216 (91.5)	129 (63.9)	380 (60.9)	725 (68.3)
Alcohol use*	Missing	0 (0.0)	0 (0.0)	120 (19.2)	120 (11.3)
	None	34 (14.4)	4 (2.0)	107 (17.2)	145 (13.7)
	Moderate	47 (19.9)	20 (9.9)	36 (5.8)	103 (9.7)
	Heavy	155 (65.7)	178 (88.1)	361 (57.9)	694 (65.4)
Body mass index (kg/m²)*	Missing	95 (40.3)	15 (7.4)	211 (33.8)	321 (30.2)
	<25	88 (37.3)	68 (33.7)	135 (21.6)	291 (27.4)
	25–30	22 (9.3)	78 (38.6)	156 (25.0)	256 (24.1)
	30 & up	31 (13.1)	41 (20.3)	122 (19.6)	194 (18.3)
Number of biopsies analyzed	1	130 (55.1)	202 (100)	571 (91.5)	903 (85.0)
per participant	2	65 (27.5)	0 (0)	53 (8.5)	118 (11.1)
	3	41 (17.4)	0 (0)	0 (0.0)	41 (3.9)
Highest fibrosis stage observed	0	67 (28.4)	55 (27.2)	214 (34.3)	336 (31.6)
	1	126 (53.4)	112 (55.5)	170 (27.2)	408 (38.4)
	2	23 (9.8)	19 (9.4)	139 (22.3)	181 (17.0)
	3	8 (3.4)	16 (7.9)	63 (10.1)	87 (8.2)
	4	12 (5.1)	0 (0.0)	38 (6.1)	50 (4.7)

*Highest value in available data since imputed age of HCV infection.
Abbreviations: ALIVE: AIDS Link to Intravenous Experience study [13,14,15]; HALS: Hepatitis C and Alcohol Study [16]; SFVA: San Francisco Veterans Affairs Medical Center liver studies cohort [17]; HIV: human immunodeficiency virus; HCV: hepatitis C virus.

as indicated in the body of the table. The key results, decreasing risk with longer time already spent in a stage and the protective effect of African American race, remain very similar. For the case where age of HCV infection was imputed using a different model, we also evaluated the estimated effects of HIV when added to the primary model. The estimated effect of HIV at any time remained similar (odds ratio 1.24, 95% confidence interval 0.84 to 1.83, p = 0.27), as did the estimated effect of HIV in the year 1996 and later (odds ratio 1.98, 95% confidence interval 0.98 to 4.0, p = 0.058). Changing the time step to 1 year or using the more pessimistic misclassification probabilities increased the computational burden by 3- to 5-fold, to over a full day of processing time per imputed data set in some cases. This made more extensive sensitivity analyses and pursuit of likelihood ratio p-values and profile likelihood confidence intervals too difficult to be worthwhile, particularly given the reassuring initial findings.

Evaluation of age effects

Table 7 shows the results of several analyses of age effects. Both older current age at each time step and older age at HCV infection showed strong evidence of increasing progression risk. When both were included in the same model, however, current age appeared to be the important factor. There was some collinearity between the two, particularly for participants with shorter followup after HCV infection, so the uncertainty in both estimated effects is large in the model that includes both. This indicates that, in our data, neither improves the fit to the data very much when added to the model that already includes the other. Testing the linearity assumption for current age by adding a quadratic term produced a p-value of 0.27, indicating no strong evidence for non-linearity; the estimated curvature was negative, indicating a slowing in the rate of increased risk as age increases. Allowing the effect of current age to differ for the different transitions between stages did not appear to produce substantially improved fits to the data. The average

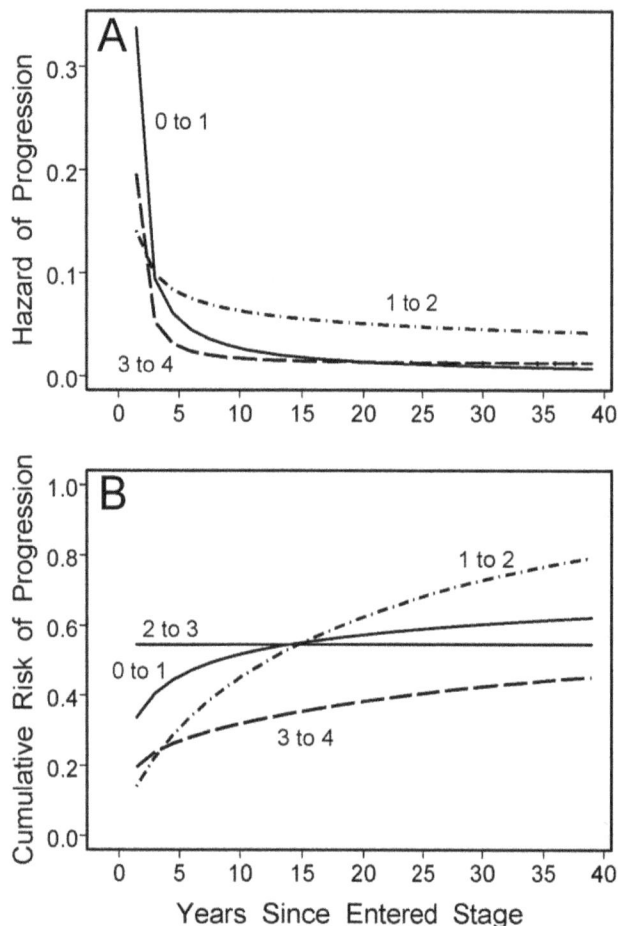

Figure 1. Baseline progression risk for the model in the top part of Table 4, for a non-black participant in the San Francisco Veterans Affairs Medical Center liver studies cohort [17]. (A) Risk of progression at a time step of 1.5 years given no progression at earlier time steps (*hazard* of progression). All transitions have decreasing hazard, reflecting the odds ratios <1 in Table 4 for years in stage. For the transition from stage 2 to 3, the estimated hazard of progression is 0.55 for the first step and 0 at all later times; this is not shown to avoid compression of the vertical scale for the other transitions. (b) Cumulative risk of progression. The cumulative risk in the first time step is equal to the hazard; at later time steps, it is equal to the previous cumulative risk plus the current hazard times (1 − previous cumulative risk). The cumulative risk therefore increases by less than the current hazard when the previous cumulative risk is already substantial.

improvement in the deviance was 4.6, which would not be unusual by chance alone with the addition of 3 parameters (4 age effects instead of one); one imputed data set had a likelihood ratio p-value of 0.060, while the others were all ≥0.20. The estimated odds ratios per 10 year increase in age were 1.17 for the stage 0 to 1 transition, 1.81 for the 1 to 2 transition, 0.98 for the 2 to 3 transition, and 1.75 for the 3 for 4 transition.

Because error in imputed ages at HCV infection could bias estimated age effects as described in the Methods, we evaluated the potential magnitude of such bias by analyzing simulated data sets that had realistic amounts of error in age at HCV infection and were generated from models with no actual age effects. Two replicates of the process, shown in Table 7, had only small estimated age effects, suggesting that most of the estimated effects for the actual data are unlikely to be due to bias.

Discussion

We analyzed a substantial amount of data on fibrosis progression using a new method that avoids many problems inherent in other methods that have been used to analyze such data. We found evidence that progression risk decreases after more time has been spent in a stage, which concords with an analysis of progression following liver transplant that used the same methods [10]; methods previously used for analyzing fibrosis progression cannot assess such effects. This finding may reflect a dynamic nature of HCV infection, with recent progression indicating active disease and a higher risk of further progression. Older age increased progression, and this appeared to be driven by current age rather than being a fixed effect of age at HCV infection (the evidence for this is not conclusive, however, as shown by the wide confidence intervals in the model in Table 7 that includes both age effects). This also accorded with the previous analysis of post-transplant progression, where progression increased with donor age. Other previous analyses have also found an age effect [25] but were limited by their methodology to evaluating presumed age at HCV infection rather than current age; they also did not recognize or assess potential bias [5]. A small simulation experiment indicated that little of our observed age effect appeared to be due to bias. We also found evidence for a protective effect of African American race, which has previously been suspected [9]. There was a suggestion of increased risk due to HIV co-infection, particularly in the era of effective anti-retroviral therapy beginning in 1996. In prior years, HIV-infected potential participants who experienced accelerated HCV progression may have also had higher mortality from opportunistic infections, causing them to be excluded from our source studies. There was also a suggestion that slower progression through stage 0 tends to be followed by slower progression through stage 1, but this did not hold for later transitions between stages. A number of other factors may influence progression, as some estimates in Table 5 may be large enough to be important (e.g., male sex, heavy alcohol consumption, and body mass index >30) and upper confidence bounds generally are not low enough to provide strong evidence against substantial increased risk.

The results here may seem to be less reliable than previous studies of similar data because of the complex methods and assumptions. The complexity, however, is inherent in the available data and the disease process. Previous studies only appear to avoid this by making strong simplifying assumptions that are implicit or not given strong emphasis. Consider, for example, the simple approach of obtaining a single fibrosis rate per year for each person by dividing current observed stage by the time since presumed infection [25]. This implicitly assumes that infection is immediate at the reported time of first risk with no inaccuracy in those reported times, fibrosis is never misclassified, each progression between stages is numerically equivalent, and the observed stage was just reached at the time of biopsy. Each of these assumptions simplifies the statistical analysis and reduces the apparent statistical variation in resulting estimates, but each is also questionable or even known to be wrong. We have attempted to deal realistically with these complexities. Notably, using multiple imputation [11] to address the unknown ages at HCV infection adds considerable complexity and results in wider confidence intervals than would have been produced by pretending that ages of HCV infection were all known, but this uncertainty really does exist. We have also used multistate models, which better match biopsy-based measurement of the disease process, and have evaluated departures from the Markov assumptions usually used in multistate modeling. We checked linearity and variation by

Table 4. Primary progression model, and estimated effects of total time in previous stages when added to the primary model.

Predictor		Transition	Odds Ratio[a]	95% confidence interval		P-value
				Lower	Upper	
Log$_e$(0.75+years in stage)		0 to 1[b]	0.39	0.23	0.65	0.0004
		1 to 2	0.72	0.37	1.42	0.35
		2 to 3[c]	0	0	0.84	0.028
		3 to 4[d]	0.52	0.06	4.6	0.56
ALIVE study	(vs SFVA study)	0 to 1	1.38	0.97	1.97	0.073
		1 to 2	0.21	0.11	0.39	<0.0001
		2 to 3[e]	20.0	0.07	+∞	0.30
		3 to 4	4.3	0.92	20.4	0.063
HALS study	(vs SFVA study)	0 to 1	1.66	1.12	2.4	0.011
		1 to 2	0.16	0.09	0.30	<0.0001
		2 to 3[f]	+∞			
		3 to 4[f]	0			
African American	(vs all others)	All	0.75	0.60	0.95	0.018
			Effects when added to above primary model			
Years in all previous stages	(per 1 year)	1 to 2[g]	0.16	0.02	1.05	0.056
	(per 5 years)	2 to 3[h]	2.1	0.31	14.3	0.45
	(per 5 years)	3 to 4	1.26	0.05	29.7	0.89

[a]Odds ratios indicate the estimated effects of the predictors on the risk of progression to the next stage at any given time step. Odds ratios below 1.0 indicate lowered risk; ratios above 1.0 indicate increased risk.Based on 4 imputed data sets; the fifth had estimated odds ratio (OR) = 0 with likelihood ratio (LR) p-value <0.0001.
[b]Based on 4 imputed data sets; the fifth had estimated odds ratio (OR) = 0 with LR p-value <0.0001.
[c]All imputed data sets had estimated OR = 0; the largest of the 5 LR p-values and the corresponding profile likelihood confidence bound are shown.
[d]Based on 3 imputed data sets; the other two estimated odds ratios were 0.13 and 0.15 with LR p-values of 0.028 and 0.021, but these were close to degenerate, with much larger estimated standard errors and deviance nearly identical at OR = 0.
[e]Although the estimated OR was finite, the estimates in all 5 imputed data sets appeared to be nearly degenerate, with large standard errors and deviance at OR = +∞ nearly as good as at the finite estimated values.
[f]Estimates in all 5 imputed data sets were degenerate. As these are not parameters of interest, we did not pursue LR p-values or profile likelihood confidence bounds.
[g]Based on 4 imputed data sets; the fifth had estimated OR = 0 with likelihood ratio p-value <0.0001.
[h]Based on 3 imputed data sets; the other two had estimated OR = +∞ with LR p-values 0.021 and 0.082.
Abbreviations: ALIVE: AIDS Link to Intravenous Experience study [13,14,15]; HALS: Hepatitis C and Alcohol Study [16]; SFVA. San Francisco Veterans Affairs Medical Center liver studies cohort [17].

stage for key predictors, and sensitivity analyses suggested that our main results did not rely on the particular size of time step, misclassification probabilities, or imputation model for age of HCV infection. We believe that all these facts add credence to our results.

Our methods permit analysis of time-varying covariates, which was important for HIV and age. The distinction between current age (time-varying) and age at HCV infection (fixed) may seem subtle, but they could have different implications for the biology of HCV disease and also for clinical prognosis. For example, detecting recent progression to higher fibrosis could be cause for alarm in an older patient even if original HCV infection was at a very young age. This is the second infectious disease for which one of us (PB) has found that careful consideration of both fixed and time-varying age effects points to a different conclusion than only considering fixed effects [26].

Limitations

Despite the specialized analyses and other strengths, this study has a number of limitations. As for many other studies using liver biopsies, selection bias is a potential concern. Restricting study to clinic populations or those already known to be HCV infected can create selection bias toward more rapid progression [27], and the SFVA and HALS groups are clinic-based or partly clinic-based.

For ALIVE, there should be little selection bias, because participants were selected from the community without respect to HCV status, enrolled participants were tested for HCV, and a random sample of those found to be chronically infected underwent biopsy [14]. For all three studies, participants had to agree to undergo liver biopsy in order to be included; this could select for more severe disease if participants were more likely to agree if they had symptoms. On the other hand, the unavoidable restriction to participants who were alive at the time of recruitment could tend to exclude more rapid progressors. Statistical methods for dealing with this, known as *left-truncation* or *late entry*, are available but would require a model that includes death from fibrosis progression as an additional stage; calculations to deal with late entry are also not available in the mspath software. Our selection of only followup before treatment with interferon could also tend to exclude more rapid progressors, although this may be mitigated by the usual clinical desire to obtain a biopsy before starting treatment. Selection bias may be most important for estimation of overall rapidity of progression rates, which we have not emphasized. For the estimated effects of risk factors to be biased, selection for greater severity would have to differ according to the levels of the risk factors. Because selection likely did differ between source studies, we took steps to fully control for the effect of study (see next paragraph).

Table 5. Estimated effects of each other predictor when added singly to the primary model from Table 4.

Predictor	Value	Odds Ratio	95% confidence interval		P-value
			Lower	Upper	
Sex	Male	1.21	0.94	1.57	0.14
Race/ethnicity[a]	African American	0.79	0.62	1.01	0.055
(vs Caucasian)	Hispanic	1.26	0.91	1.75	0.17
	Other	1.23	0.85	1.79	0.27
HIV-infected[b]	Yes	1.17	0.64	2.1	0.61
HIV-infected, by treatment era[b]	to 1995	0.68	0.17	2.7	0.58
(vs uninfected)	1996 on	2.1	0.97	4.4	0.059
HIV-infected, by treatment era[b]	to 1995	0.37	0.00	568	0.79
(vs uninfected)	1996–1999	3.0	0.57	16.1	0.19
	2000 on	1.49	0.34	6.6	0.60
Reported HCV risk factor	Transfusion	0.99	0.72	1.37	0.96
(vs injection drug use)	Needlestick	0.88	0.61	1.28	0.50
	Other/None	1.21	0.96	1.53	0.11
Smoking	Yes	1.07	0.83	1.40	0.59
Alcohol consumption[b,c]	Moderate	0.99	0.52	1.88	0.99
(vs none)	Heavy	1.16	0.72	1.89	0.54
Injection drug use[b]	Yes	0.92	0.69	1.23	0.58
Body Mass Index	per 5 Kg/m^2	1.05	0.97	1.14	0.24
Body Mass Index	25–30	1.09	0.88	1.36	0.42
(vs <25)	>30	1.19	0.95	1.50	0.14

[a]This is an alternative finer breakdown instead of an addition to the primary model.
[b]These are time-varying covariates, with potentially differing values at each time step.
[c]This model was fitted on HALS participants only, because other studies lacked complete histories.
Abbreviations: HIV: human immunodeficiency virus; HCV: hepatitis C virus; HALS: Hepatitis C and Alcohol Study [16].

The distribution of biopsy-measured fibrosis was heterogeneous across source studies. The strong influence of source study, and its variation by stage, likely result from non-biological influences. Differing misclassification of fibrosis due to differing readings of biopsies is one important possibility, but differing selection of participants is also likely to contribute to the study effects. For example, it is unlikely that the true rate of stage 4 (cirrhosis) was really the same in HALS as in the other studies; this would imply that about 10 biopsies showing cirrhosis were all misread in HALS. Because the studies were drawn from differing populations by differing methods, selection effects are bound to differ between them. The proportions of biopsies from different calendar time periods also differed between studies. The imputation models for age at HCV infection accounted for strong influences of calendar time [5]; changes over time in progression rates may also be possible, but seem less likely with our focus on pre-treatment biopsies only. We minimized the potential for source study to confound other associations by fully controlling for its influence on every transition, using a full contingent of 8 parameters for study effects. This reduced the potential influence of selection bias on other estimates, but it also added complexity to the models and may have reduced the precision of other estimates. Using fewer parameters did not seem viable, because differences between the studies varied by stage, and because any oversimplification of study effects could increase concern about selection bias and confounding.

We accounted for possible misclassification of biopsy-measured fibrosis by factoring external estimates of misclassification rates into the estimation process. This increases the statistical uncertainty in our results, but rightly so. Along with multiple rather than single imputation of age at HCV infection, this results in a better assessment of precision and is a strength of this analysis. In addition, a sensitivity analysis showed that our main findings were insensitive to the exact misclassification assumptions. Nevertheless, an ideal approach would utilize information on biopsy quality to provide a customized matrix of misclassification probabilities for each biopsy. Unfortunately, we did not have such refined estimates available. Some multistate modeling methods, including the one used here, can estimate misclassification probabilities as part of the modeling process. This, however, would be computationally very challenging and seems likely to be less accurate than estimates from studies that were focused specifically on misclassification and therefore employed multiple readings of the same biopsy or multiple biopsies of the same liver. We have therefore used the best estimates from such studies that we could obtain [4]. The median (interquartile range) biopsy length was 19mm (14–24) in HALS and 12 mm (9–19) in ALIVE, which are comparable to those in the studies used to estimate misclassification [4]. (Biopsy length was not available for the SFVA study.)

We assumed no backward transitions to lower stages; our restriction to pre-treatment biopsies may make this assumption reasonable, and no participants had spontaneously cleared HCV infection at the time of any biopsy. This assumption implies that any apparent backward transitions must be ascribed to misclassification of at least one of the biopsies. Among the 159 participants with two or three biopsies, 21% had nominal

Table 6. Results of sensitivity analyses for the primary model from Table 4 on predictors of interest.

Predictor		Transition	Odds Ratio	95% confidence interval Lower	Upper	P-value
One-year time steps instead of 1.5 year-time steps						
Log$_e$(0.75+years in stage)		0 to 1[a]	0.40	0.25	0.66	0.0003
		1 to 2	0.77	0.40	1.47	0.42
		2 to 3[b]	0			
		3 to 4[c]	0.51	0.09	2.90	0.44
African American	(vs all others)	All	0.76	0.60	0.96	0.019
Pessimistic misclassification probabilities instead of optimistic, from Table 1						
Log$_e$(0.75+years in stage)		0 to 1[a]	0.26	0.06	1.20	0.084
		1 to 2	0.77	0.37	1.59	0.48
		2 to 3[b]	0			
		3 to 4[d]	0			
African American	(vs all others)	All	0.71	0.53	0.95	0.020
Age of HCV infection imputed from alternative model						
Log$_e$(0.75+years in stage)		0 to 1[c]	0.37	0.22	0.63	0.0003
		1 to 2	0.70	0.40	1.21	0.20
		2 to 3[b]	0			
		3 to 4[e]	0.46	0.06	3.46	0.45
African American	(vs all others)	All	0.77	0.63	0.94	0.011

[a]Based on 4 imputed data sets; the fifth had estimated odds ratio (OR) = 0.
[b]All imputed data sets had estimated OR = 0.
[c]Based on all 5 imputed data sets; none had estimated OR = 0.
[d]Three of the imputed data sets had estimated OR = 0, precluding meaningful combination of just the remaining 2.
[e]Based on 4 imputed data sets; the fifth had a nearly degenerate estimated OR = 0.09 with an effectively infinite standard error, precluding synthesis with the others.
Abbreviations: HCV: hepatitis C virus.

backward transitions of one stage and 3% of two stages, rates that seem to be readily explainable by the substantial misclassification probabilities previously estimated [4]. The progression model could in principle be extended to allow backward transitions, and the mspath software allows any specification of what transitions are possible. Unfortunately, allowing backward transitions would vastly increase the number of possible paths to be evaluated, making computations infeasible. In addition, parameters govern-

Table 7. Estimated effects of age when added to the primary model from Table 4, for the original data and for simulated data with no age effects.

Predictor(s)[a]	Value	Odds Ratio	95% confidence interval Lower	Upper	P-value
Models of the original, actual data					
Current age at each time step	Per 10 years	1.33	1.15	1.54	0.0002
Age at HCV infection	Per 10 years	1.31	1.13	1.52	0.0003
Current age at each time step	Per 10 years	1.45	0.74	2.8	0.28
Age at HCV infection	Per 10 years	0.92	0.47	1.79	0.80
Models of simulated data with no actual age effects					
Current age at each time step	Per 10 years	1.08	0.88	1.31	0.46
Age at HCV infection	Per 10 years	1.07	0.90	1.27	0.45
Replication on another independently simulated set of data with no actual age effects					
Current age at each time step	Per 10 years	1.03	0.87	1.22	0.74
Age at HCV infection	Per 10 years	1.02	0.87	1.20	0.77

[a]Results separated by vertical space are from separate models; one model included both current age and age at HCV infection.
Abbreviations: HCV: hepatitis C virus.

ing the four additional transitions would have to be added, and factors influencing regression could differ from those for progression, substantially complicating the modeling. We therefore cannot evaluate the effect of allowing backward transitions on our results, but we believe that excluding them is close enough to reality that it is unlikely to introduce serious bias.

A reviewer pointed out a potential bias that could impact our estimated effects of years in prior stages, at the bottom of Table 4. For example, if a participant were known to have reached stage 2 by a given time, with an unknown time of transition from stage 0 to 1, then a shorter time in stage 0 would mean a longer time in stage 1 before progressing to stage 2, while a longer time in stage zero would mean a shorter time in stage 1 before progressing to stage 2. Either way would contribute to an apparent effect of longer time in stage 0 increasing risk of progression from stage 1 to 2. Fortunately, we observed the opposite of what this bias would produce, instead estimating a *protective* effect of longer time in stage zero. Thus, the possibility of this bias only strengthens the evidence for this effect. For the 2 to 3 and 3 to 4 transitions, we did estimate increases in risk such as this bias would produce. This bias is directly analogous to the potential bias in the estimated effect of age at infection that we described, with time in previous stages playing the role of time before (i.e., age at) HCV infection, so a similar simulation-based investigation could be undertaken. We do not consider this to be worthwhile, however, because the issue is largely overshadowed by the very wide confidence intervals for these effects.

Most of our participants had only one biopsy, which made them less informative for estimation of the effects of years in current stage and years in previous stages. Fortunately, we had enough with multiple biopsies (15%) to obtain some useful estimates, notably the protective effects of years in current stage in Table 4 for the 0 to 1 and 2 to 3 transitions. We also had relatively few participants with advanced fibrosis, which is reflected in extreme estimates or wide confidence intervals for most estimated effects that are specific to the 2 to 3 transition and the 3 to 4 transition. Some predictors may have been inaccurately measured, due to reliance on self-report and extrapolation of study values to the entire period of HCV infection, and some were missing for a considerable proportion of participants. We did not analyze HCV genotype or viral load as predictors, and complete history of alcohol consumption was only available in the HALS study. We did not evaluate the influence of measured immune status and antiretroviral treatment history directly for HIV-infected participants. This would be very complicated and could be distorted by self-selection of treatment and incomplete histories; we investigated differing HIV effects over calendar time as a feasible alternative. Our statistical methods model progression over the entire period of HCV infection, so we could not evaluate factors such as inflammation and steatosis grade that are known only at the time biopsy; these would have to be known at all times and treated as time-varying covariates, but are unlikely to have remained constant since infection. Our assumptions concerning fibrosis misclassification and our model for imputing age of HCV infection could be inaccurate, but sensitivity analyses using

alternatives showed similar results. All of our fitted models had some parameters estimated to be effectively infinite. These could not be used in standard methods for multiple imputation analysis, so we used only the finite estimates and reported the infinite estimates separately. In some cases, standard errors for other parameters had to be obtained by re-estimating models with the effectively infinite parameters held fixed; those standard errors did not appear to differ substantially from the cases where standard errors were available despite estimation of some effectively infinite parameters. Finally, the computational burden of the method we used is substantial. We were only able to complete our analyses within about a month by often running 20 or more analyses simultaneously using a specialized parallel computing facility.

Further Research

Ideally, prospective followup of persons known to be recently infected with HCV would prevent selection biases and maximize the value of information obtained from biopsies. Performing such studies, however, might be difficult and expensive. Steps to minimize misclassification (e.g., using multiple readings of each biopsy) could also make data more informative and potentially reduce the computational burden of our methods (if some misclassifications become impossible). The methods used here might provide more credible results and additional insights if applied to larger data sets with more repeat biopsies. Computational feasibility is a potential issue, but will improve with time. The non-Markov multistate modeling software that we used is freely available at http://cran.r-project.org/web/packages/mspath/index.html.

An appealing alternative to biopsy is non-invasive measurement of fibrosis via imaging or biochemical analysis of peripheral blood samples [28,29]. Some methods may already be as accurate as biopsy, but evaluation of alternatives has suffered from inappropriate use of biopsy as a gold standard [30]. Studies with frequent non-invasive measurements could be less dependent on imperfectly known times of HCV infection, because they could better focus on observed trajectories. Evaluating how recent changes in non-invasive measures predict subsequent change would permit exploration of the phenomenon we found of decreasing progression risk with longer times already spent in a stage. If the invasiveness, risk [31], and expense of biopsy curtails its use in HCV research, the methods used here may still be useful for analysis of data for other diseases that progress through stages.

Acknowledgments

Computations for this study were performed using the UCSF Biostatistics High Performance Computing System.

Author Contributions

Conceived and designed the experiments: PB RB SHM DLT NAT AM. Performed the experiments: SHM DLT NAT AM. Analyzed the data: PB RB. Contributed reagents/materials/analysis tools: JA HS DLT NAT AM. Wrote the paper: PB RB SHM DLT NAT AM. Prepared data for analysis: PB JA HS.

References

1. Armstrong GL, Wasley A, Simard EP, McQuillan GM, Kuhnert WL, et al. (2006) The prevalence of hepatitis C virus infection in the United States, 1999 through 2002. Annals of Internal Medicine 144: 705–714.
2. Williams R (2006) Global challenges in liver disease. Hepatology 44: 521–526.
3. Desmet VJ, Gerber M, Hoofnagle JH, Manns M, Scheuer PJ (1994) Classification of chronic hepatitis-diagnosis, grading and staging. Hepatology 19: 1513–1520.
4. Bacchetti P, Boylan R (2009) Estimating Complex Multi-State Misclassification Rates for Biopsy-Measured Liver Fibrosis in Patients with Hepatitis C. International Journal of Biostatistics 5: 5.
5. Bacchetti P, Tien PC, Seaberg EC, O'Brien TR, Augenbraun MH, et al. (2007) Estimating past hepatitis C infection risk from reported risk factor histories: implications for imputing age of infection and modeling fibrosis progression. BMC Infectious Diseases 7: 145.

6. Jackson CH, Sharples LD (2002) Hidden Markov models for the onset and progression of bronchiolitis obliterans syndrome in lung transplant recipients. Statistics in Medicine 21: 113–128.

7. Jackson CH, Sharples LD, Thompson SG, Duffy SW, Couto E (2003) Multistate Markov models for disease progression with classification error. Journal of the Royal Statistical Society Series D-the Statistician 52: 193–209.

8. Deuffic-Burban S, Poynard T, Valleron AJ (2002) Quantification of fibrosis progression in patients with chronic hepatitis C using a Markov model. Journal of Viral Hepatitis 9: 114–122.

9. Terrault NA, Im K, Boylan R, Bacchetti P, Kleiner DE, et al. (2008) Fibrosis Progression in African Americans and Caucasian Americans With Chronic Hepatitis C. Clinical Gastroenterology and Hepatology 6: 1403–1411.

10. Bacchetti P, Boylan RD, Terrault NA, Monto A, Berenguer M (2010) Non-Markov multistate modeling using time-varying covariates, with application to progression of liver fibrosis due to hepatitis C following liver transplant. International Journal of Biostatistics 6: 7.

11. Schafer JL (1999) Multiple imputation: a primer. Statistical Methods in Medical Research 8: 3–15.

12. Sulkowski MS, Thomas DL (2003) Hepatitis C in the HIV-infected person. Annals of Internal Medicine 138: 197–207.

13. Rai R, Wilson LE, Astemborski J, Anania F, Torbenson N, et al. (2002) Severity and correlates of liver disease in hepatitis C virus-infected injection drug users. Hepatology 35: 1247–1255.

14. Wilson LE, Torbenson M, Astemborski J, Faruki H, Spoler C, et al. (2006) Progression of liver fibrosis among injection drug users with chronic hepatitis C. Hepatology 43: 788–795.

15. Vlahov D, Anthony JC, Munoz A, Margolick J, Nelson KE, et al. (1991) The ALIVE study-A longitudinal-study of HIV-1 infection in intravenous-drug-users-description of methods. Journal of Drug Issues 21: 759–776.

16. Ishida JH, Peters MG, Jin C, Louie K, Tan V, et al. (2008) Influence of cannabis use on severity of hepatitis C disease. Clinical Gastroenterology and Hepatology 6: 69–75.

17. Monto A, Patel K, Bostrom A, Pianko S, Pockros P, et al. (2004) Risks of a range of alcohol intake on hepatitis C-related fibrosis. Hepatology 39: 826–834.

18. Bedossa P, Poynard T (1996) An algorithm for the grading of activity in chronic hepatitis C. Hepatology 24: 289–293.

19. Ishak K, Baptista A, Bianchi L, Callea F, Degroote J, et al. (1995) Histological grading and staging of chronic hepatitis. Journal of Hepatology 22: 696–699.

20. Batts KP, Ludwig J (1995) Chronic hepatitis-an update on terminology and reporting. American Journal of Surgical Pathology 19: 1409–1417.

21. Okafor O, Ojo S (2004) A comparative analysis of six current histological classification schemes and scoring systems used in chronic hepatitis reporting. Rev Esp Patol 37: 269–277.

22. Walensky RP, Paltiel AD, Losina E, Mercincavage LM, Schackman BR, et al. (2006) The survival benefits of AIDS treatment in the United States. Journal of Infectious Diseases 194: 11–19.

23. Hall HI, Song RG, Rhodes P, Prejean J, An Q, et al. (2008) Estimation of HIV incidence in the United States. Jama-Journal of the American Medical Association 300: 520–529.

24. Moons KGM, Donders R, Stijnen T, Harrell FE (2006) Using the outcome for imputation of missing predictor values was preferred. Journal of Clinical Epidemiology 59: 1092–1101.

25. Poynard T, Bedossa P, Opolon P (1997) Natural history of liver fibrosis progression in patients with chronic hepatitis C. Lancet 349: 825–832.

26. Bacchetti P (2003) Age and variant Creutzfeldt-Jakob disease. Emerging Infectious Diseases 9: 1611–1612.

27. Freeman AJ, Dore GJ, Law MG, Thorpe M, Von Overbeck J, et al. (2001) Estimating progression to cirrhosis in chronic hepatitis C virus infection. Hepatology 34: 809–816.

28. Cross T, Antoniades C, Harrison P (2008) Non-invasive markers for the prediction of fibrosis in chronic hepatitis C infection. Hepatology Research 38: 762–769.

29. Manning DS, Afdhal NH (2008) Diagnosis and quantitation of fibrosis. Gastroenterology 134: 1670–1681.

30. Mehta SH, Lau B, Afdhal NH, Thomas DL (2009) Exceeding the limits of liver histology markers. Journal of Hepatology 50: 36–41.

31. Rid A, Emanuel EJ, Wendler D (2010) Evaluating the Risks of Clinical Research. Jama-Journal of the American Medical Association 304: 1472–1479.

7

Hepatitis B Virus Infection in Human Immunodeficiency Virus Infected Southern African Adults

Trevor G. Bell[1], Euphodia Makondo[1], Neil A. Martinson[2,3], Anna Kramvis[1]*

1 Hepatitis Virus Diversity Research Programme, Department of Internal Medicine, University of the Witwatersrand, Johannesburg, South Africa, **2** Perinatal HIV Research Unit, University of the Witwatersrand, Johannesburg, South Africa, **3** Johns Hopkins University School of Medicine, Baltimore, Maryland, United States of America

Abstract

Hepatitis B virus (HBV) and human immunodeficiency virus (HIV) share transmission routes and are endemic in sub-Saharan Africa. The objective of the present study was to use the *Taormina* definition of occult HBV infection, together with stringent amplification conditions, to determine the prevalence and characteristics of HBV infection in antiretroviral treatment (ART)-naïve HIV^{+ve} adults in a rural cohort in South Africa. The presence of HBV serological markers was determined by enzyme linked immunoassay (ELISA) tests. HBV DNA-positivity was determined by polymerase chain reaction (PCR) of at least two of three different regions of the HBV genome. HBV viral loads were determined by real-time PCR. Liver fibrosis was determined using the aspartate aminotransferase-to-platelet ratio index. Of the 298 participants, 231 (77.5%) showed at least one HBV marker, with 53.7% HBV DNA^{-ve} (resolved) and 23.8% HBV DNA^{+ve} (current) [8.7% HBsAg^{+ve}: 15.1% HBsAg^{-ve}]. Only the total number of sexual partners distinguished HBV DNA^{+ve} and HBV DNA^{-ve} participants, implicating sexual transmission of HBV and/or HIV. It is plausible that sexual transmission of HBV and/or HIV may result in a new HBV infection, superinfection and re-activation as a consequence of immunesuppression. Three HBsAg^{-ve} HBV DNA^{+ve} participants had HBV viral loads <200 IU/ml and were therefore true occult HBV infections. The majority of HBsAg^{-ve} HBV DNA^{+ve} participants did not differ from HBsAg^{+ve} HBV DNA^{+ve} (overt) participants in terms of HBV viral loads, ALT levels or frequency of liver fibrosis. Close to a quarter of HIV^{+ve} participants were HBV DNA^{+ve}, of which the majority were HBsAg^{-ve} and were only detected using nucleic acid testing. Detection of HBsAg^{-ve} HBV DNA^{+ve} subjects is advisable considering they were clinically indistinguishable from HBsAg^{+ve} HBV DNA^{+ve} individuals and should not be overlooked, especially if lamivudine is included in the ART.

Editor: Sheila Mary Bowyer, University of Pretoria/NHLS TAD, South Africa

Funding: This study was supported by grants received from the South African Medical Research Council and the National Research Foundation (NRF; GUN#65530) awarded to AK. TGB received bursaries from the National Bioinformatics Network, Poliomyelitis Research Foundation (PRF) and NRF. EM received a Belgium Technical Cooperation Fellowship and bursaries from the NRF and PRF. The funders had no role in study design, data collection and analysis, decision to publish.

Competing Interests: The authors have declared that no competing interests exist.

* E-mail: Anna.Kramvis@wits.ac.za

Introduction

Hepatitis B virus (HBV) and human immunodeficiency virus (HIV) share transmission routes and represent the two most important blood-borne pathogens in terms of prevalence, morbidity and mortality in sub-Saharan Africa, where both viruses are endemic. Of the 33.3 million adults and children living with HIV globally, 22.5 million reside in sub-Saharan Africa [1]. Moreover, it is estimated that 65% to 98% of populations in sub-Saharan Africa have been exposed to HBV and 8% to 20% are chronic carriers of HBV [2], far exceeding the 4% to 6% lifetime exposure rates and 0.2% to 0.5% carrier rates in regions of low endemicity. Thus, widespread co-infections are likely to occur, with 16% to 98% of HIV^{+ve} individuals in sub-Saharan Africa being carriers of HBV or showing exposure to HBV [3].

The progression of chronic HBV to cirrhosis, end-stage liver disease (ESLD), and hepatocellular carcinoma (HCC) is more rapid in HIV^{+ve} individuals than those with HBV alone [4], with a significant increase in hepatic-related mortality rates [5]. Furthermore, HBV co-infection negatively impacts on HIV outcomes [6].

Before the introduction of antiretroviral therapy (ART), the majority of HBV/HIV co-infected individuals were more likely to die from the clinical consequences of HIV than those of HBV [3]. However, since the introduction of ART, the disease profile has changed, with increases in the proportion of mortality attributed to HBV-associated ESLD [7]. Thus, HBV/HIV co-infection can potentially impact on the safety and effectiveness of ART, requiring an integrated approach for the appropriate management of co-infected individuals [8].

There is a paucity of comprehensive and standardized data describing HBV/HIV co-infection from southern African countries, where HIV prevalence is extremely high. Existing data show large discrepancies, with exposure rate to HBV in HIV^{+ve} South Africans varying from 28% to 99.8% and HBsAg prevalence ranging from 0.4% to 23% [9–18]. Differences can be attributed to different locations, study designs, laboratory measures and/or the composition of the study populations.

HIV infection has been implicated as a risk factor for the development of occult HBV infection (OBI) [12], defined by the *Taormina* expert panel as the "*Presence of HBV DNA in liver (with* *detectable or undetectable HBV DNA in the serum) of individuals testing HBsAg negative by currently available assays. When detectable, the amount of HBV DNA in the serum is usually very low (<200 IU/ml)"* [19]. Because liver biopsies are not commonly available, especially in resource-limited environments, OBI is usually detected by the analysis of sera [19]. Furthermore, the experts differentiate between true occult (HBV viral load <200 IU ml^{-1}) and false occult where HBV DNA levels are comparable to those detected in HBsAg^{+ve} infection (overt) and are usually as a result of infection by HBV variants with S gene escape mutants, producing HBsAg that is not recognized by detection assays [19]. The clinical implications of OBI are unclear.

The prevalence of OBI in HIV infected individuals varies depending on the definition used, the sensitivity of the assay and the HBV viral loads [11–13,16,17]. Furthermore, studies performed outside Africa, in areas of low HBV and HIV endemicity, cannot necessarily be extrapolated to Africa because of differences in host factors, epidemiology, transmission patterns and genotypes of the viruses between the two regions.

The objective of the present study was to use the *Taormina* definition of OBI [19], together with stringent amplification conditions, to determine the prevalence and characteristics of HBV infection in ART-naïve HIV^{+ve} adults entering a rural cohort in Mpumalanga Province, which has a HIV prevalence of 15.4% [20]. No in-depth studies have been undertaken to determine the prevalence and characteristics of HBV/HIV co-infection in this province.

Materials and Methods

Subjects

A new rural cohort was established at Shongwe Hospital in Mpumalanga Province in South Africa and 298 ART-naïve, HIV^{+ve} adults were enrolled from July to November 2009. All had qualified for ART according to the then-current South African ART guidelines (CD4 counts <200 cells mm^{-3}) [21] and were recruited while undergoing treatment-readiness counselling. Universal HBV vaccination at 6, 10, and 14 weeks of age was introduced into the South African Expanded Programme on Immunization (EPI) in 1995 and therefore none of the participants were likely to have received this vaccination and self-reported as unvaccinated. Clinical and demographic data (including ALT levels, CD4 T-cell count, age, sex, height and weight) were obtained from hospital records, the National Health Laboratory Services (NHLS) databases and the TherapyEdge-HIV (TE)^{TM} electronic patient record. All participants signed informed consent. The study was approved by the Human Research Ethics Committee (Medical) of the University of the Witwatersrand and Mpumalanga Department of Health Research Ethics Committee.

Serology

The presence of HBsAg, anti-HBsAg and anti-HBcAg was determined for 298 sera using the Monolisa^{TM} HBsAg ULTRA, HBsAb ULTRA and HBcAb PLUS ELISA kits (Bio-Rad, Hercules, CA), respectively. HBeAg and anti-HBe tests were performed on HBV DNA^{+ve} sera using the Monolisa^{TM} HBeAg-Ab PLUS kit. Anti-HBcAg IgM was determined for 17 anti-HBc^{+ve} HBV DNA^{+ve} samples for which serum was available using the ARCHITECT® kit (Abbott Diagnostics, Wiesbaden, Germany). The M30-Apoptosense® ELISA (Peviva AB, Stockholm, Sweden) was used on all sera to quantify the apoptosis-associated cytokeratin 18Asp396 neo-epitope as a measure of hepatocyte apoptosis [22].

Measurement of liver fibrosis

The aspartate aminotransferase (AST)-to-platelet ratio index (APRI) = (AST[/ULN]*100)/platelet count [10^9 L^{-1}], a noninvasive measure of liver fibrosis in patients with chronic HBV [23], was calculated for 163 subjects for whom AST levels and platelet counts were available. APRI indicates liver fibrosis only when liver disease has reached a severely advanced stage, with significant fibrosis defined as APRI≥1.5, and no fibrosis as APRI≤0.5 [24].

Polymerase chain reaction (PCR)

DNA was extracted from 200 µl blood plasma with the QIAamp DNA Blood Mini Kit (QIAGEN Gmbh, Hilden, Germany) and eluted into 75 µl of best-quality water (BQW). Known positive and negative sera and BQW were used as controls for the extraction. Three regions of the HBV genome were amplified in a MyCycler^{TM} thermocycler (Bio-Rad, Hercules, Ca, USA) using Promega Taq DNA polymerase (Promega, Madison, WI) (Table 1). To avoid cross-contamination and false positives, the precautions and procedures of Kwok and Higuchi [25] were strictly adhered to. DNA extraction, PCR, and electrophoresis were performed in physically separated venues.

Real-time PCR quantification of HBV DNA

PCR primers, HBV-Taq1 and HBV-Taq2 covering a region of the S gene (321 to 401 from the *EcoR*I site) with a FAM/TAMRA labelled TaqMan BS-1 probe [26] were used to quantify HBV DNA in an ABI 7500 Real Time PCR System (Applied Biosystems, Foster City, Ca, USA). A serial dilution of cloned plasmid DNA containing a single genome of HBV DNA, with concentrations ranging from 2×10^1 to 2×10^{11} IU ml^{-1}, was used as template to generate the standard curve. The second WHO International Standard for HBV Nucleic Acid Amplification Techniques (product code 97/750 National Institute for Biological Standards and Controls (NIBSC); Hertfordshire, UK), which has a final concentration of 10^6 IU ml^{-1} was used as the internal standard. The standard curve, blank, positive and negative controls, and samples were all tested in duplicate. The measured IU/ml for each reaction was calculated using the Ct (cycle threshold) value of each PCR interpolated against the linear regression of the standard curve. The lower detection limit of our assay is ~20 IU ml^{-1}. The conversion formula of IU = copies/4.7 was used [11,27].

Statistical analysis

Clinical data were inspected visually. As all continuous variables showed a skewed distribution, the Mann-Whitney U test (Wilcoxon rank-sum test) was used to compare samples. Chi-squared and Fisher's exact test were used to compare categorical variables. Exhaustive multivariate logistic regression analyses were performed. The R statistical language was used throughout [28].

Results

Serological and nucleic acid testing for HBV

The study group consisted of 298 adults (114 men and 184 women) with median age, CD4 count and BMI of 34 years, 147 cells mm^{-3} and 22 kg m^{-2}, respectively. Men were older than women and had lower CD4 counts (Table 2).

The 298 participants were classified into five serogroups: 28 (9.4%) HBsAg^{+ve}, 57 (19.1%) isolated anti-HBc^{+ve}, 123(41.3%) anti-HBc^{+ve}anti-HBs^{+ve}, 11 (3.7%) anti-HBs^{+ve} alone and 79 (26.5%) serologically^{-ve} for HBV. Six percent of men (7/114) were anti-HBs^{+ve} alone compared to 2% (4/184) of women (p<0.05). The HBV serologically^{-ve} participants were significant-

Table 1. PCR primers and cycling parameters used for amplification of the three regions of the HBV genome.

Genome Region	Primer	Position[a]	Sequence	Cycles	Denaturation	Annealing	Extension	Size	Reference
Complete S PCR1F	2410(+)	2410-2439	5'-TCAATCGCCGCGTCGCAGAAGATCTCAATC-3'	40	94°C for 1 min	65°C for 1 min	72°C for 3 min	2126	[48]
Complete S PCR1R	1314(−)	1314-1291	5'-TCCAGACCXGCTGCGAGCAAAACA-3'						
Complete S PCR2F	2451(+)	2451-2482	5'-AATGTTAGTATTCCTTGGACTCATAAGGTGGG-3'	40	94°C for 1 min	66°C for 1 min	72°C for 3 min	2051	[48]
Complete S PCR2R	1280(−)	1280-1254	5'-AGTTCCGCAGTATGGATCGGCAGAGGA-3'						
Partial S PCR1F	231(+)	231-249	5'-TCACAATACCGCAGAGTCT-3'	40	94°C for 1 min	55°C for 1 min	72°C for 2 min	571	
Partial S PCR1R	801(−)	801-782	5'-AACAGCGGTATAAAGGGACT-3'						
Partial S PCR2F	256(+)	256-278	5'-GTGGTGGACTTCTCAATTTC-3'	40	94°C for 1 min	55°C for 1 min	72°C for 2 min	541	[49]
Partial S PCR2R	796(−)	796-776	5'-CGGTATAAAGGGACTCACGAT-3'						
BCP PCR1F	1606(+)	1606-1625	5'-GCATGGAGACCACCGTGAAC-3'	40	94°C for 1 min	55°C for 1 min	72°C for 2 min	369	[48]; [50][b]
BCP PCR1R	1974(−)	1974-1955	5'-GGAAAGAAGTCAGAAGGCCAA-3'						
BCP PCR2F	1653(+)	1653-1672	5'-CATAAGAGGACTCTTGGACT-3'	40	94°C for 1 min	55°C for 1 min	72°C for 2 min	307	[48]; [50][b]
BCP PCR2R	1959(−)	1959-1941	5'-GGCAAAAAACAGAGTAACTCA-3'						

[a]Nucleotide position of HBV *adw* genome (GenBank accession number (AY233276), where position 1 is the *EcoR*I cleavage site.
[b]Modifications underlined.
(+) and "F" indicate forward (sense) direction; (−) and "R" indicate reverse (anti-sense) direction; PCR1 indicates first round PCR; PCR2 indicates second round PCR.

ly younger than most HBV serologically[+ve] groups and had significantly fewer lifetime sexual partners than those with isolated anti-HBs[+ve] ($p < 0.05$). There was no significant difference in serologically-negative and -positive individuals in terms of CD4 counts, age of sexual debut, BMI, ALT and Apoptosense® levels. Only five participants were HBeAg[+ve] and they did not differ from HBeAg[−ve] individuals in either demographic or clinical features.

Screening for HBV DNA was carried out using primers targeting three non-overlapping regions of the HBV genome (Table 1). A sample was considered to be HBV DNA[+ve], only if at least two regions amplified. Sixty-seven of 298 participants (22.5%) lacked HBV DNA and all HBV serological markers, ruling out HBV exposure and/or infection and with no antibodies against HBV would be susceptible to acquiring HBV infection. The remaining 231/298 (77.5%) showed at least one marker for HBV, with 160/298 (53.7%) HBV DNA[−ve] (resolved) and 71/298 (23.8%) HBV DNA[+ve] (current) [26/298 (8.7%) HBsAg[+ve] (overt): 45/298 (15.1%) HBsAg[−ve] ("occult")] (Figure 1).

Of the entire group of 298, 26 (8.7%)/28 (9.4%) HBsAg[+ve] participants were HBV DNA[+ve] and together with the 45 (15.1%) HBsAg[−ve] HBV DNA[+ve] participants were classified into 6 serogroups (Figure 2). Within the HBsAg[−ve] groups, the frequency of HBV DNA was significantly higher in anti-HBc[+ve] alone individuals (16/57; 28.1%) compared to those anti-HBc[+ve]anti-HBs[+ve] (17/123; 13.8%) ($p < 0.05$). The relative risk of an HBsAg[−ve] individual, who was anti-HBc[+ve] alone, being HBV DNA[+ve] was twice as high as that of one with anti-HBc[+ve]anti-HBs[+ve]. The frequency of HBV DNA in the serologically[−ve] group was not significantly different to that in the anti-HBc[+ve] alone or anti-HBc[+ve]anti-HBs[+ve]. Moreover, HBV DNA was not detected in any of the 11 isolated anti-HBs[+ve] individuals. Sufficient serum was available to test for anti-HBc IgM in 17 of 57 anti-HBc[+ve] HBV DNA[+ve] participants and all tested negative. Only three HBsAg[−ve] HBV DNA[+ve] participants had viral loads < 200 IU ml^{-1}, thus meeting the *Taormina* criterion for true OBI [19]. These participants had serological patterns of groups A, D and E, respectively (Figure 2). All other HBsAg[−ve] HBV DNA[+ve] individuals had HBV viral loads > 200 IU ml^{-1}.

Comparison of demographic and clinical characteristics between HBV DNA[+ve] and HBV DNA[−ve] groups

Visual inspection of plots and linear regression models of each of the continuous variables in Tables 2 and 3 (age, age at sexual debut, lifetime sexual partners, BMI (body mass index), ALT, Apoptosense, CD4 cell count, HBV viral load) against each other, for HBV DNA[+ve] versus HBV DNA[−ve], and HBsAg[+ve] versus HBsAg[−ve] groups, revealed no significant correlation.

A multiple logistic regression model was used to determine predictors of HBV DNA positivity. In this model, only ALT levels were significant when all variables were included ($p < 0.05$; OR = 1.01; 95% CI: 1.002–1.020). When the data were split according to gender, number of lifetime sexual partners was the only predictor in the females ($p < 0.05$; OR = 1.16; 95% CI: 1.01–1.36) and ALT in the males ($p < 0.05$; OR = 1.02; 95% CI: 1.004–1.030).

As shown in Table 2, the only variable that differentiated the HBV DNA[+ve] and HBV DNA[−ve] groups was number of lifetime sexual partners ($p < 0.05$). Regardless of whether they were HBV DNA[+ve] or HBV DNA[−ve], males were older than females, had a higher ALT and lower CD4 count. In the whole cohort and the HBV DNA[−ve] group, females had a higher BMI ($p < 0.05$) and fewer sexual partners than males ($p < 0.05$). These differences were not seen in the HBV DNA[+ve] group. The age of sexual debut was

Table 2. Characteristics of treatment-naïve HIV-infected adults: comparison of HBV DNA+ve versus HBV DNA-ve individuals[a].

Characteristic	All participants (n = 292)			HBV DNA+ve participants (n = 71)			HBV DNA-ve participants (n = 221)			Significance – p-values[b]			
	All	Male[A]	Female[A]	All[D]	Male[B]	Female[B]	All[D]	Male[C]	Female[C]	A	B	C	D
Numbers (%)	292[c]	113(39%)	179(61%)	71	30(42%)	41(58%)	221	83(38%)	138(62%)	n/a	0.54	0.72	n/a
Age in years	34(28-43)	36(32-43)	32(27-40)	35(28-41)	37(34-47)	31(25-39)	33(28-41)	35(32-41)	32(27-40)	<0.0001	0.01	0.002	0.42
Age at sexual debut in years[d]	17(16-19)	17(16-20)	17(16-18)	17(16-18)	17(16-19)	16(15-18)	17(16-19)	17(16-20)	17(16-18)	0.035	0.12	0.11	0.36
Lifetime sexual partners[e]	3(1-5)	4(2-8)	2(1-4)	3(2-5)	4(2-8)	3(2-5)	3(1-5)	4(2-8)	2(1-3)	<0.0001	0.34	<0.0001	0.025
BMI in kg m^{-2}	22(20-25)	21(19-24)	23(20-26)	22(20-24)	21(20-23)	22(20-25)	22(20-26)	21(19-24)	23(20-26)	0.0051	0.37	0.007	0.43
ALT in U L^{-1}	21(12-32)	27(17-38)	18(11-27)	23(15-37)	31(19-59)	20(12-28)	20(12-31)	26(17-37)	17(11-27)	<0.0001	0.027	<0.0001	0.12
Apoptosense in U L^{-1}	110(89-150)	112(91-150)	109(89-150)	114(91-158)	117(91-160)	114(91-152)	109(89-142)	111(92-141)	109(88-147)	0.63	0.96	0.68	0.34
CD4 cells mm^{-3}	147(76-196)	99(49-171)	179(104-222)	148(74-199)	104(60-171)	180(103-245)	144(76-194)	98(46-169)	177(104-215)	<0.0001	0.006	<0.0001	0.83

[a] all values expressed as "Median (Interquartile Range)".
[b] comparing the columns marked by UPPER case letter; statistical significance is indicated by underlining.
[c] 6 of the 298 participants were not included in the analyses because they lacked a complete data set.
[d] 9 samples without data points omitted.
[e] 2 samples without data points omitted.

significantly different only when comparing males and females in the whole cohort.

Comparison of demographic and clinical characteristics between HBsAg+ve HBV DNA+ve and HBsAg-ve HBV DNA+ve groups

Data from the HBV DNA+ve participants were examined by logistic regression for predictors of HBV DNA-positivity in the absence of HBsAg. Only increasing age was weakly significant. The female subset showed that age was a significant predictor (p<0.05; OR = 1.28; 95% CI: 1.06–1.72). No predictors in the male subset were significant.

In the HBsAg-ve HBV DNA+ve group, men were older and had significantly lower CD4 cell counts compared to females (p<0.05). Although the difference in ALT levels between the HBsAg+ve HBV DNA+ve and HBsAg-ve HBV DNA+ve groups did not reach statistical significance (Table 3), individuals who were HBsAg+ve anti-HBc+ve HBV DNA+ve [group C] had significantly higher ALT levels compared to individuals who were either serologically-ve HBV DNA+ve [group A] (p<0.05) or anti-HBc+ve HBV DNA+ve [group E] (p<0.05) (Figure 2). There was no significant difference between the HBsAg+ve and HBsAg-ve DNA+ve groups when ALT levels were coded into binary groups: >29 U/L for males and >19 U/L for females. HBV viral loads did not differ significantly between HBsAg+ve and HBsAg-ve groups (Table 3).

Measurement of liver fibrosis using APRI score

Ten percent of 163 individuals, for which data were available, had elevated APRI scores (≥1.5), representing advanced fibrosis: 7.94% (10/126) HBV DNA-ve [5.3% (2/38) seronegative and 9.1% (8/88) seropositive] and 16.2% (6/37) HBV DNA+ve [26.7% (4/15) HBsAg+ve HBV DNA+ve and 9.1% (2/22) HBsAg-ve HBV DNA+ve]. The frequency of liver fibrosis was significantly higher in HBsAg+ve HBV DNA+ve individuals compared to seronegative HBV DNA-ve ones (p<0.05), but not to seropositive HBV DNA-ve ones (p = 0.07). There was no significant difference between the HBsAg+ve and HBsAg-ve HBV DNA+ve groups.

Discussion

In this group of 298 southern African ART-naïve HIV+ve individuals, 231 participants had at least one HBV marker, giving an overall exposure to HBV of 77.5%, comparable to that in HBV monoinfected individuals [2]. In addition, almost one quarter of the group was HBV DNA+ve (Figure 1) of whom almost two thirds were HBsAg-ve. Direct comparison with other South African ART-naïve HIV+ve cohorts is difficult because of the different markers were used to measure exposure. In Limpopo Province, exposure to HBV, measured by anti-HBc and/or anti-HBs positivity, was 28.2% in a rural cohort [17] and 39.2% in anti-natal HIV+ve women [16]. This differs from the 63% HBV exposure rate (measured by at least one marker: HBsAg, anti-HBs or anti-HBc) found in a rural-urban HIV+ve cohort in Limpopo [13] and the much higher exposure rate of 99.8% in hospital-admitted HIV+ve patients [12]. In Gauteng Province, a 47% exposure was seen in an urban HIV+ve cohort where ~15% were HBV-positive as follows: 4.8% HBsAg+ve [10], 7.6% anti-HBc+ve HBV DNA+ve [11] and 2.4% serologically-ve HBV DNA+ve [27].

The 9.4% HBsAg prevalence was comparable to that reported for some HIV+ve South African cohorts: 6.2% in anti-natal women in Limpopo Province [16]; 7.1% in rural Eastern Cape (6.6% in ART-treated versus 8.8% in ART-naïve, p>0.05) [9]; and 6% in a

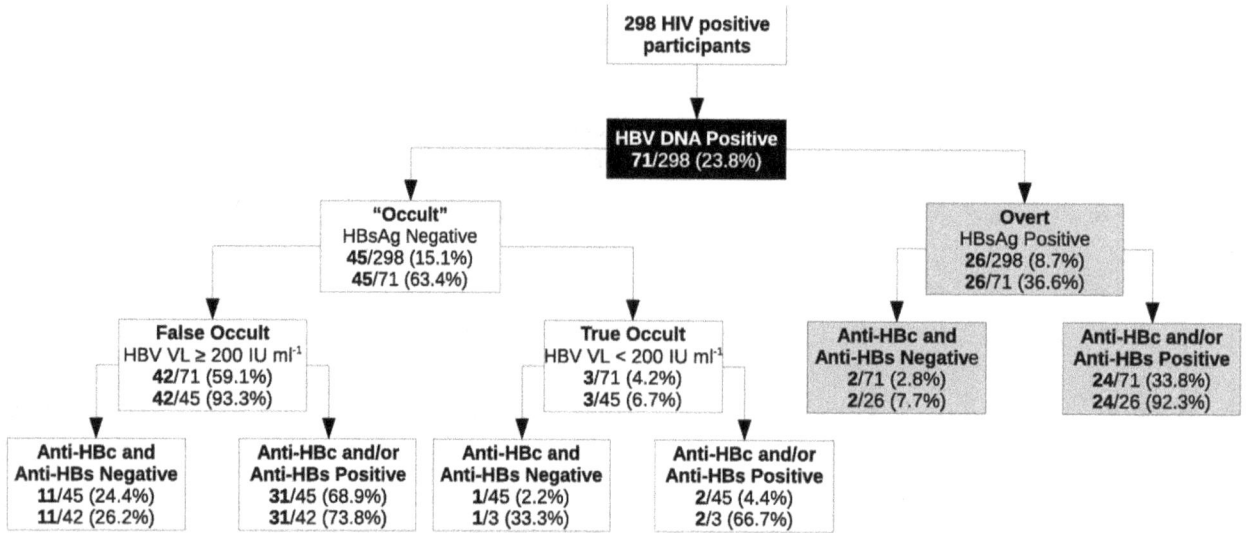

Figure 1. Serological and DNA markers for HBV detected in 71 of 298 HIV^{+ve} participants. Overt refers to HBsAg^{+ve} and "occult" to HBsAg^{-ve}. According to the *Taormina* definition, false occult infections are HBsAg^{-ve} with HBV viral load (VL) $\geq$200 IU ml^{-1} and true occult infections are HBsAg^{-ve} with HBV VL <200 IU ml^{-1} [19].

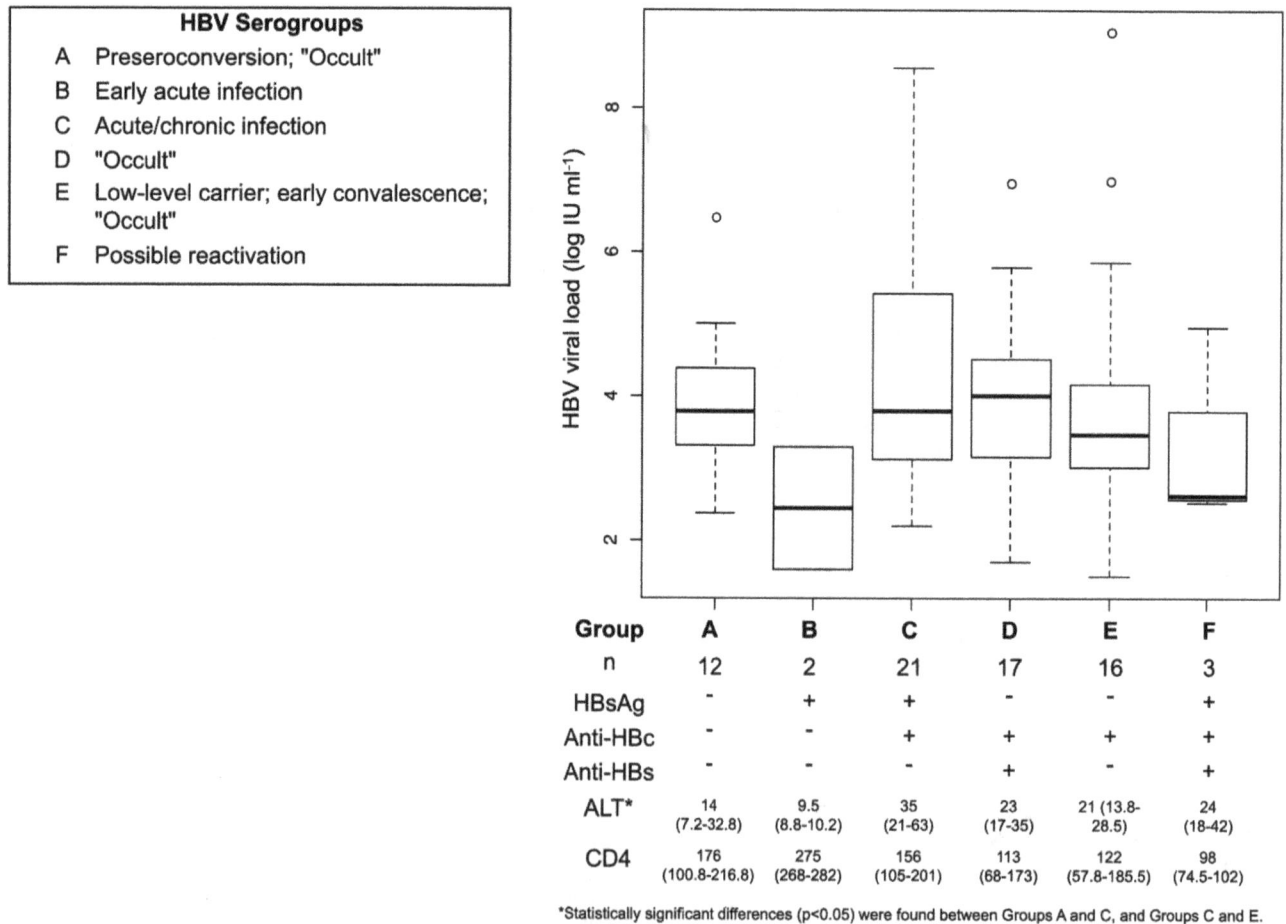

HBV Serogroups	
A	Preseroconversion; "Occult"
B	Early acute infection
C	Acute/chronic infection
D	"Occult"
E	Low-level carrier; early convalescence; "Occult"
F	Possible reactivation

Group	A	B	C	D	E	F
n	12	2	21	17	16	3
HBsAg	-	+	+	-	-	+
Anti-HBc	-	-	+	+	+	+
Anti-HBs	-	-	-	+	-	+
ALT*	14 (7.2-32.8)	9.5 (8.8-10.2)	35 (21-63)	23 (17-35)	21 (13.8-28.5)	24 (18-42)
CD4	176 (100.8-216.8)	275 (268-282)	156 (105-201)	113 (68-173)	122 (57.8-185.5)	98 (74.5-102)

*Statistically significant differences (p<0.05) were found between Groups A and C, and Groups C and E.

Figure 2. Box and whisker plot of HBV viral loads of the 71 HBV DNA^{+ve} participants separated into the six serological groups (A to F), interpreted according to Hollinger (2008) with modifications [35]. "n" indicates the number of participants in each group. ALT and CD4 cell counts for each group are indicated in the table below the plot as "Median (Interquartile Range)". Viral loads and CD4 cell counts did not differ significantly between the six serological groups. The five HBeAg^{+ve} participants belonged to serological group C.

Table 3. Characteristics of treatment-naïve HIV-infected adults: comparison of HBsAg+ve HBV DNA+ve versus HBsAg-ve HBV DNA+ve individuals[a].

Characteristic	HBV DNA+ve participants (n=71)			HBsAg+ve HBV DNA+ve (n=26)			HBsAg-ve HBV DNA-ve (n=45)			Significance-p values[b]			
	All	Male[A]	Female[A]	All[D]	Male[B]	Female[B]	All[D]	Male[C]	Female[C]	A	B	C	D
Numbers (%)	71	30(42%)	41(58%)	26	13(50%)	13(50%)	45	17(38%)	28(62%)	n/a	0.42	0.54	n/a
Age in years	35(28-41)	37(34-47)	31(25-39)	34(27-28)	35(33-39)	29(25-35)	36(29-45)	38(35-47)	34(28-40)	0.01	0.07	0.035	0.14
Age at sexual debut in years[c]	17(16-18)	17(16-19)	16(15-18)	17(16-20)	18(16-22)	17(15-18)	16(15-18)	17(16-18)	16(15-18)	0.12	0.11	0.66	0.23
Lifetime sexual partners[d]	3(2-5)	4(2-8)	3(2-5)	3(1-6)	2(1-6)	3(1-5)	4(2-5)	4(2-10)	3(2-5)	0.34	0.98	0.17	0.38
BMI in kg m^{-2}	22(20-24)	21(20-23)	22(20-25)	23(20-25)	22(20-23)	25(20-27)	21(20-23)	21(20-22)	22(20-24)	0.37	0.29	0.64	0.30
ALT in U L^{-1}	23(15-37)	31(18-59)	20(12-28)	30(19-59)	35(22-60)	21(12-39)	20(13-32)	27(15-37)	19(13-25)	0.027	0.29	0.12	0.07
Apoptosense U L^{-1}	114(91-158)	117(91-160)	114(91-152)	113(84-156)	110(75-150)	114(91-161)	114(94-158)	121(96-188)	114(91-142)	0.96	0.27	0.37	0.62
CD4 cells mm^{-3}	148(74-199)	104(60-171)	180(103-245)	152(101-202)	125(98-184)	179(132-255)	147(68-196)	87(57-165)	181(91-229)	0.006	0.13	0.016	0.52
LogHBVVL[e]	3.72 (3.04-4.41)	3.76 (2.95-4.47)	3.61 (3.08-4.35)	3.64 (2.73-4.80)	4.14 (2.74-5.44)	3.22 (2.54-4.01)	3.78 (3.15-4.35)	3.74 (2.99-4.28)	3.81 (3.19-4.44)	0.66	0.14	0.59	0.74

[a] all values expressed as "Median (Interquartile Range)".
[b] Comparing the columns marked by UPPER case letter; statistical significance is indicated by underlining.
[c] 9 samples without data points omitted.
[d] 2 samples without data points omitted.
[e] "LogHBVVL" indicates the log of the HBV viral load rounded to two decimal places [A Mann-Whitney U test was used on the untransformed viral loads (IU ml^{-1})].

country-wide study of treatment-naïve HIV+ve military personnel and their family members [14]. On the other hand, the HBsAg prevalence was higher than the 0.4% in another rural cohort in Limpopo Province [17], double the 4.8% in a Gauteng urban cohort [10], but lower than the 11.3% in hospital-admitted Limpopo Province patients [12], the 19.7% in miners [15] and the 22.9% from a rural-urban cohort in Limpopo Province [13]. This difference in HBsAg prevalence correlates with the variations reported in HBV monoinfected individuals from different locales [16,29,30].

Regardless of whether they were HBV DNA+ve or HBV DNA−ve, males were older, had higher ALT levels and lower CD4 counts than females (Table 1). These differences are because males tend to come for treatment later than females [31]. In the cohort as a whole and in the HBV DNA−ve group, males had significantly more partners than females, with BMI significantly lower. In the HBV DNA+ve group, these factors did not differ between the genders. The only factor differentiating the HBV DNA+ve versus HBV DNA−ve participants was the number of lifetime sexual partners (Table 2), suggesting sexual transmission of HBV and/or HIV. It is plausible this mode of transmission may result in a new HBV infection, superinfection and re-activation as a consequence of immunesuppression. Twenty percent of the 71 HBV DNA+ve participants had possible markers of recent infection: 12 serologically−ve HBV DNA+ve and 2 HBsAg+ve HBV DNA+ve (Figure 2). Of the 17 anti-HBc+ve HBV DNA+ve sera tested for anti-HBc IgM, none were positive.

The HBV serology of the cohort, the high frequency of HBeAg-negativity, the absence of anti-HBc IgM and the relatively low HBV viral loads (Figure 2) reflect the natural history of HBV infection in sub-Saharan Africa, where most individuals are infected at childhood by horizontal transmission [2]. This means that most individuals have been exposed to HBV, and are protected by anti-HBV antibodies, by the time they become sexually active and acquire HIV. All isolated anti-HBs+ve participants were HBV DNA−ve and the presence of anti-HBs with anti-HBc reduced the risk of being HBV DNA+ve. None of the participants had received HBV vaccination.

The HBsAg prevalence in this HIV+ve cohort was not different to HIV−ve cohorts [2,3]. This differs from observations in areas of low HBV and HIV endemicity, where HBV and HIV are acquired simultaneously and therefore HBsAg prevalence in HIV+ve individuals is significantly higher than in HIV−ve individuals [3]. Only four participants in the present study were HBsAg+ve alone: two were HBV DNA+ve, whereas the other two were HBV DNA−ve, even after repeated attempts to amplify HBV DNA, possibly indicating low viral loads undetectable by PCR. This might reflect the process of natural HBsAg clearance [32]. Although immune suppression by HIV may lead to the HBsAg+ve anti-HBc−ve profile [33], this is unlikely in these two cases, considering that ~59% of the participants were anti-HBc+ve, with a third of these having isolated anti-HBc. Moreover, HIV+ve patients with CD4<100 cells mm^3 are more likely to have isolated anti-HBc [34].

HBV DNA without HBsAg was detected in 15.1% of the participants (Figure 1). This is within the 8% to 18% range for South African HIV+ve cohorts but again direct comparison is complicated by differences in study design [11-13,16,17]. Twelve participants were serologically−ve HBV DNA+ve, which can occur before the appearance of HBsAg, in the preseroconversion phase (indicating a recent infection), or at the tail end of the infection [35]. Anti-HBsAg seroconversion, in the presence or absence of anti-HBc, decreased the relative risk of being HBV DNA+ve in the

HBsAg^{-ve} group. This agrees with findings in HBV monoinfected [36] and in HBV/HIV coinfected individuals [37].

There was no difference in the demographics of the HBV DNA^{+ve} subjects, with and without HBsAg (Table 2). In the presence of HBsAg, there was no difference between males and females, whereas in the absence of HBsAg, males were older and had lower CD4 counts than females. Thus older males with lower CD4 counts are more likely to be HBsAg^{-ve} HBV DNA^{+ve}. Lower CD4 counts have been associated with HBsAg^{-ve} viremia regardless of gender [37], however the median CD4 counts in that study were relatively higher (316 cells mm^{-3} versus 147cells mm^{-3} in the present study) [37].

In agreement with other studies [38,39], there were similar ALT levels in HBsAg^{+ve} and HBsAg^{-ve} HBV DNA^{+ve} participants and between HBV DNA^{+ve} and HBV DNA^{-ve} participants. The absence of transaminitis is as a result of the immunosuppressed state of the HIV^{+ve} subjects. Immunosuppression causes HBV reactivation and can lead to high viremia without clinical manifestation [40]. The APRI score was used to compare the frequency of liver fibrosis in the HBV^{+ve} versus HBV^{-ve} participants. The frequency of liver fibrosis was significantly higher in HBsAg^{+ve} HBV DNA^{+ve} individuals compared to seronegative HBV DNA^{-ve} ones, but not relative to seropositive HBV DNA^{-ve} ones. It is intriguing that there was no difference in the frequency of liver fibrosis between HBV DNA^{+ve} individuals, with and without HBsAg.

The reactivation of an infection, which originated in childhood, can explain why no significant difference was seen in the HBV viral loads between the HBsAg^{+ve} and HBsAg^{-ve} participants (Table 2), nor between the different serological groups (Figure 2). Following HIV infection, HBV can reactivate in anti-HBs^{+ve} only individuals, with and without the reappearance of HBsAg [41]. Group F, which had the lowest CD4 count of <100 cells mm^{-3}, and by inference was the most immunosuppressed, was HBsAg^{+ve} anti-HBc^{+ve} anti-HBs^{+ve} HBV DNA^{+ve} with a viral load >10^2 IU ml^{-1} (Figure 2). Spontaneous reverse seroconversion, where anti-HBs disappears and HBsAg reappears can also occur in the presence of CD4 counts <200 cells mm^{-3} [42]. Although HBV viral loads have been shown to be higher in HBV^{+ve} HIV^{+ve} individuals compared to HBV^{+ve} ones [43], the HBV viral loads detected in the present study were comparable to those detected in HBV mono-infected individuals [44]. This is probably because the majority of individuals were infected with subgenotype A1 [45], which is characterized by relatively low viral loads in mono-infected individuals compared to other genotypes or subgenotypes [44].

Only three HBsAg^{-ve} HBV DNA^{+ve} patients had HBV loads <200 IU ml^{-1}, meeting the *Taormina* criterion for OBI. Thus the majority of HBsAg^{-ve} HBV DNA^{+ve} would be classified as false "occult" [19]. It is possible that immunosuppression precludes true occult HBV infection. Because the majority of HBsAg^{-ve} HBV DNA^{+ve} ("occult") participants did not differ from HBsAg^{+ve} HBV DNA^{+ve} (overt) participants in terms of viral loads, CD4 counts, ALT levels and frequency of liver fibrosis, it may be more accurate to refer to these HBV infections as *HBsAg-covert* (HBsAg-*c*ryptic *o*vert) instead of false "occult" [19].

HIV infection was demonstrated to be a risk factor for HBsAg^{-ve} HBV infection [12], and pre-S mutations preventing HBsAg secretion [46], 'a' determinant mutations leading to detection escape and overlapping polymerase mutations affecting replication, may be responsible for this. This possibility was investigated and is presented in a follow-up paper, where 12 of 13 HBV S region sequences, from HBsAg^{-ve} participants, had pre-S and/or S mutations [45]. Another possible explanation for HBsAg-negativity may be that HIV co-infection prevents HBsAg secretion, as shown in co-infected hepatic cell lines [47].

Despite the possible limitations of this study, including its cross-sectional nature, the absence of HIV viral loads, no HBV mono-infected patients and patients with higher CD4 counts for comparison, a number of important conclusions can be reached. The number of lifetime sexual partners was the only factor differentiating HBV DNA^{+ve} and HBV DNA^{-ve} infections, suggesting sexual transmission of HBV and/or HIV. HBV^{+ve} HIV^{+ve} individuals were found to have significantly higher lifetime sexual partners than HBV-monoinfected individuals [18]. HBV infection in HIV^{+ve} individuals was predominantly HBsAg^{-ve}, which did not differ significantly from HBsAg^{+ve} infections in terms of viral loads, CD4 counts, ALT levels and frequency of liver fibrosis.

The detection of HBV DNA in the absence of HBsAg in this and other South African studies [11–13,17] has important implications for the clinical management of HIV in sub-Saharan Africa, where the burden of HBV/HIV co-infection is disproportionately high (24% in this study). Although the World Health Organization recommends that ART be initiated in HBV/HIV co-infected individuals irrespective of CD4 count, in South Africa we face a number of challenges. The most recent South African guidelines recommend initiation of treatment of patients with CD4 counts <350 cells mm^{-3} and HBsAg testing if ALT levels exceed 100 U L^{-1}. Considering that the highest median ALT levels (IQR) of 30 (19–59) U L^{-1} were found in the HBsAg^{+ve} HBV DNA^{+ve} group (Table 3), which also had the highest frequency of advanced fibrosis, this cut-off value is inappropriate. Moreover, 65% of the 71 participants, who were HBV^{+ve} HIV^{+ve}, lacked HBsAg and HBV could only be detected by nucleic acid testing, which is unaffordable in resource-limited environments. Although the clinical significance of HBsAg^{-ve} infection is under debate [32], it is imperative that HBV/HIV co-infection is detected before ART initiation, especially because lamivudine remains in two of the three drug regimens currently provided by the South African government and HBV can develop resistance to lamivudine. To determine the clinical relevance of *HBsAg-covert* HBV infection in our setting, prospective studies following ART initiation are in progress.

Acknowledgments

The authors thank Sisters Ntombikayise Elizabeth Agatha Nkosi and Rosalina Candlovu for enrolling participants and drawing blood samples, Dr Precious Gabashane, chief medical officer, Shongwe Hospital and all the study participants. Professor Jacky Galpin and Ms Elsabe Smit of the School of Statistics and Actuarial Science of the University of the Witwatersrand provided guidance with the statistical analyses. Some clinical data were provided by the National Health Laboratory Services (NHLS) Corporate Data Warehouse Team and by Dr Mhairi Maskew (Right-to-Care/TherapyEdge).

Author Contributions

Conceived and designed the experiments: TGB EM NM AK. Performed the experiments: TGB EM. Analyzed the data: TGB EM AK. Contributed reagents/materials/analysis tools: TGB AK. Wrote the paper: TGB AK. Set up rural cohort site: TGB NM AK.

References

1. UNAIDS (2010) UNAIDS report on the global AIDS epidemic 2010. Available: http://www.unaids.org/en/dataanalysis/. Accessed 2011 November 16.
2. Kramvis A, Kew MC (2007) Epidemiology of hepatitis B virus in Africa, its genotypes and clinical associations of genotypes. Hepatol Res 37: S9–S19.
3. Burnett RJ, Francois G, Kew MC, Leroux-Roels G, Meheus A, et al. (2005) Hepatitis B virus and human immunodeficiency virus co-infection in sub-Saharan Africa: a call for further investigation. Liver Int 25: 201–213.
4. Chung RT (2006) Hepatitis C and B viruses: the new opportunists in HIV infection. Top HIV Med 14: 78–83.
5. Thio CL, Seaberg EC, Skolasky R, Phair J, Visscher B, et al. (2002) HIV-1, hepatitis B virus, and risk of liver-related mortality in the Multicenter Cohort Study (MACS). Lancet 360: 1921–1926.
6. Chun HM, Roediger MP, Hullsiek KH, Thio CL, Agan BK, et al. (2011) Hepatitis B Virus Coinfection Negatively Impacts HIV Outcomes in HIV Seroconverters. J Infect Dis 205: 185–193.
7. Thomas DL (2006) Growing importance of liver disease in HIV-infected persons. Hepatology 43: S221–229.
8. Soriano V, Sheldon J, Ramos B, Nunez M (2006) Confronting chronic hepatitis B virus infection in HIV: new diagnostic tools and more weapons. Aids 20: 451–453.
9. Boyles TH, Cohen K (2011) The prevalence of hepatitis B infection in a rural South African HIV clinic. S Afr Med J 101: 470–471.
10. Firnhaber C, Reyneke A, Schulze D, Malope B, Maskew M, et al. (2008) The prevalence of hepatitis B co-infection in a South African urban government HIV clinic. S Afr Med J 98: 541–544.
11. Firnhaber C, Viana R, Reyneke A, Schultze D, Malope B, et al. (2009) Occult hepatitis B virus infection in patients with isolated core antibody and HIV co-infection in an urban clinic in Johannesburg, South Africa. Int J Infect Dis 13: 488–492.
12. Mphahlele MJ, Lukhwareni A, Burnett RJ, Moropeng LM, Ngobeni JM (2006) High risk of occult hepatitis B virus infection in HIV-positive patients from South Africa. J Clin Virol 35: 14–20.
13. Lukhwareni A, Burnett RJ, Selabe SG, Mzileni MO, Mphahlele MJ (2009) Increased detection of HBV DNA in HBsAg-positive and HBsAg-negative South African HIV/AIDS patients enrolling for highly active antiretroviral therapy at a Tertiary Hospital. J Med Virol 81: 406–412.
14. Matthews GV, Manzini P, Hu Z, Khabo P, Maja P, et al. (2011) Impact of lamivudine on HIV and hepatitis B virus-related outcomes in HIV/hepatitis B virus individuals in a randomized clinical trial of antiretroviral therapy in southern Africa. AIDS 25: 1727–1735.
15. Hoffmann CJ, Charalambous S, Martin DJ, Innes C, Churchyard GJ, et al. (2008) Hepatitis B virus infection and response to antiretroviral therapy (ART) in a South African ART program. Clin Infect Dis 47: 1479–1485.
16. Burnett RJ, Ngobeni JM, Francois G, Hoosen AA, Leroux-Roels G, et al. (2007) Increased exposure to hepatitis B virus infection in HIV-positive South African antenatal women. Int J STD AIDS 18: 152–156.
17. Barth RE, Huijgen Q, Tempelman HA, Mudrikova T, Wensing AM, et al. (2011) Presence of occult HBV, but near absence of active HBV and HCV infections in people infected with HIV in rural South Africa. J Med Virol 83: 929–934.
18. Mayaphi SH, Roussow TM, Masemola DP, Olorunju SA, Mphahlele MJ, et al. (2012) HBV/HIV co-infection: the dynamics of HBV in South African patients with AIDS. S Afr Med J 102: 157–162.
19. Raimondo G, Allain JP, Brunetto MR, Buendia MA, Chen DS, et al. (2008) Statements from the Taormina expert meeting on occult hepatitis B virus infection. J Hepatol 49: 652–657.
20. Shisana O, Rehle T., Simyabi L. C., Zuma K., Jooste S., Pillay-van-Wyk V., Mbelle N., Van Zyl J Parker W., Zungu N. P., Pezi S. and the SABSSM III Implementation Team (2009) South African national HIV prevalence, incidence, behavior and communication survey 2008: A turning tide among teenagers? Cape Town: HSRC Press.
21. National Department of Health SA (2004) National Antiretroviral Treatment Guidelines: Jacana, Minuteman Press.
22. Leers MP, Kolgen W, Bjorklund V, Bergman T, Tribbick G, et al. (1999) Immunocytochemical detection and mapping of a cytokeratin 18 neo-epitope exposed during early apoptosis. J Pathol 187: 567–572.
23. Lebensztejn DM, Skiba E, Sobaniec-Lotowska M, Kaczmarski M (2005) A simple noninvasive index (APRI) predicts advanced liver fibrosis in children with chronic hepatitis B. Hepatology 41: 1434–1435.
24. Lo Re V, 3rd, Frank I, Gross R, Dockter J, Linnen JM, et al. (2007) Prevalence, risk factors, and outcomes for occult hepatitis B virus infection among HIV-infected patients. J Acquir Immune Defic Syndr 44: 315–320.
25. Kwok S, Higuchi R (1989) Avoiding false positives with PCR. Nature 339: 237–238.
26. Weinberger KM, Wiedenmann E, Bohm S, Jilg W (2000) Sensitive and accurate quantitation of hepatitis B virus DNA using a kinetic fluorescence detection system (TaqMan PCR). J Virol Methods 85: 75–82.
27. Firnhaber C, Chen CY, Evans D, Maskew M, Schulz D, et al. (2012) Prevalence of hepatitis B virus (HBV) co-infection in HBV serologically-negative South African HIV patients and retrospective evaluation of the clinical course of mono- and co-infection. Int J Infect Dis 16: e268–272.
28. R Development Core Team (2011) R: A Language and Environment for Statistical Computing, R Foundation for Statistical Computing. Available: http://www.R-project.org. Accessed 2010 June.
29. Kew MC (1996) Progress towards the comprehensive control of hepatitis B in Africa: a view from South Africa. Gut 38 Suppl 2: S31–36.
30. Vardas E, Mathai M, Blaauw D, McAnerney J, Coppin A, et al. (1999) Preimmunization epidemiology of hepatitis B virus infection in South African children. J Med Virol 58: 111–115.
31. Grinsztejn B, Smeaton L, Barnett R, Klingman K, Hakim J, et al. (2011) Sex-associated differences in pre-antiretroviral therapy plasma HIV-1 RNA in diverse areas of the world vary by CD4(+) T-cell count. Antivir Ther 16: 1057–1062.
32. Togashi H, Hashimoto C, Yokozawa J, Suzuki A, Sugahara K, et al. (2008) What can be revealed by extending the sensitivity of HBsAg detection to below the present limit? J Hepatol 49: 17–24.
33. Avettand-Fenoel V, Thabut D, Katlama C, Poynard T, Thibault V (2006) Immune suppression as the etiology of failure to detect anti-HBc antibodies in patients with chronic hepatitis B virus infection. J Clin Microbiol 44: 2250–2253.
34. Sun HY, Lee HC, Liu CE, Yang CL, Su SC, et al. (2009) Factors associated with isolated anti-hepatitis B core antibody in HIV-positive patients: impact of compromised immunity. J Viral Hepat 17: 578–587.
35. Hollinger FB (2008) Hepatitis B virus infection and transfusion medicine: science and the occult. Transfusion 48: 1001–1026.
36. Chu CM, Liaw YF (2012) Prevalence of and Risk Factors for Hepatitis B Viremia After Spontaneous Hepatitis B Surface Antigen Seroclearance in Hepatitis B Carriers. Clin Infect Dis 54: 88–90.
37. Cohen Stuart JW, Velema M, Schuurman R, Boucher CA, Hoepelman AI (2009) Occult hepatitis B in persons infected with HIV is associated with low CD4 counts and resolves during antiretroviral therapy. J Med Virol 81: 441–445.
38. Lo Re V, 3rd, Kostman JR, Gross R, Reddy KR, Mounzer K, et al. (2007) Incidence and risk factors for weight loss during dual HIV/hepatitis C virus therapy. J Acquir Immune Defic Syndr 44: 344–350.
39. Shire NJ, Rouster SD, Rajicic N, Sherman KE (2004) Occult hepatitis B in HIV-infected patients. J Acquir Immune Defic Syndr 36: 869–875.
40. Gerlich WH, Bremer C, Saniewski M, Schuttler CG, Wend UC, et al. (2010) Occult hepatitis B virus infection: detection and significance. Dig Dis 28: 116–125.
41. Vento S, di Perri G, Luzzati R, Cruciani M, Garofano T, et al. (1989) Clinical reactivation of hepatitis B in anti-HBs-positive patients with AIDS. Lancet 1: 332–333.
42. Thio CL (2009) Hepatitis B and human immunodeficiency virus coinfection. Hepatology 49: S138–145.
43. Gilson RJ, Hawkins AE, Beecham MR, Ross E, Waite J, et al. (1997) Interactions between HIV and hepatitis B virus in homosexual men: effects on the natural history of infection. AIDS 11: 597–606.
44. Tanaka Y, Hasegawa I, Kato T, Orito E, Hirashima N, et al. (2004) A case-control study for differences among hepatitis B virus infections of genotypes A (subtypes Aa and Ae) and D. Hepatology 40: 747–755.
45. Makondo E, Bell TG, Kramvis A (2012) Genotyping and molecular characterization of hepatitis B virus (HBV) from antiretroviral treatment naive human immunodeficiency virus (HIV)-infected southern African adults. PlosOne (in press): e46345. doi:10.1371/journal.pone.0046345.
46. Melegari M, Bruno S, Wands JR (1994) Properties of hepatitis B virus pre-S1 deletion mutants. Virology 199: 292–300.
47. Iser DM, Avihingsanon A, Wisedopas N, Thompson AJ, Boyd A, et al. (2010) Increased intrahepatic apoptosis but reduced immune activation in HIV-HBV co-infected patients with advanced immunosuppression. AIDS 25: 197–205.
48. Vermeulen M, Dickens C, Lelie N, Walker E, Coleman C, et al. (2012) Hepatitis B virus transmission by blood transfusion during 4 years of individual-donation nucleic acid testing in South Africa: estimated and observed window period risk. Transfusion 52: 880–892.
49. Lindh M, Andersson AS, Gusdal A (1997) Genotypes, nt 1858 variants, and geographic origin of hepatitis B virus–large-scale analysis using a new genotyping method. J Infect Dis 175: 1285–1293.
50. Takahashi K, Aoyama K, Ohno N, Iwata K, Akahane Y, et al. (1995) The precore/core promoter mutant (T1762A1764) of hepatitis B virus: clinical significance and an easy method for detection. J Gen Virol 76 (Pt 12): 3159–3164.

8

A Large Population Histology Study Showing the Lack of Association between ALT Elevation and Significant Fibrosis in Chronic Hepatitis B

Wai-Kay Seto[1], Ching-Lung Lai[1,3], Philip P. C. Ip[2], James Fung[1], Danny Ka-Ho Wong[1], John Chi-Hang Yuen[1], Ivan Fan-Ngai Hung[1], Man-Fung Yuen[1,3]*

1 Department of Medicine, The University of Hong Kong, Queen Mary Hospital, Hong Kong, 2 Department of Pathology, The University of Hong Kong, Queen Mary Hospital, Hong Kong, 3 State Key Laboratory for Liver Research, The University of Hong Kong, Queen Mary Hospital, Hong Kong

Abstract

Objective: We determined the association between various clinical parameters and significant liver injury in both hepatitis B e antigen (HBeAg)-positive and HBeAg-negative patients.

Methods: From 1994 to 2008, liver biopsy was performed on 319 treatment-naïve CHB patients. Histologic assessment was based on the Knodell histologic activity index for necroinflammation and the Ishak fibrosis staging for fibrosis.

Results: 211 HBeAg-positive and 108 HBeAg-negative patients were recruited, with a median age of 31 and 46 years respectively. 9 out of 40 (22.5%) HBeAg-positive patients with normal ALT had significant histologic abnormalities (necroinflammation grading ≥7 or fibrosis score ≥3). There was a significant difference in fibrosis scores among HBeAg-positive patients with an ALT level within the Prati criteria (30 U/L for men, 19 U/L for women) and patients with a normal ALT but exceeding the Prati criteria (p = 0.024). Age, aspartate aminotransferase and platelet count were independent predictors of significant fibrosis in HBeAg-positive patients with an elevated ALT by multivariate analysis (p = 0.007, 0.047 and 0.045 respectively). HBV DNA and platelet count were predictors of significant fibrosis in HBeAg-negative disease (p = 0.020 and 0.015 respectively). An elevated ALT was not predictive of significant fibrosis for HBeAg-positive (p = 0.345) and -negative (p = 0.544) disease. There was no significant difference in fibrosis staging among ALT 1–2×upper limit of normal (ULN) and >×2 ULN for both HBeAg-positive (p = 0.098) and -negative (p = 0.838) disease.

Conclusion: An elevated ALT does not accurately predict significant liver injury. Decisions on commencing antiviral therapy should not be heavily based on a particular ALT threshold.

Editor: Anthony W. I. Lo, The Chinese University of Hong Kong, Hong Kong

Funding: The authors have no support or funding to report.

Competing Interests: The authors have declared that no competing interests exist.

* E-mail: mfyuen@hkucc.hku.hk

Introduction

Clinical course of chronic hepatitis B (CHB) is highly variable, ranging from an asymptomatic carrier state [1,2] to the development of cirrhosis, hepatic decompensation and hepatocellular carcinoma (HCC) [3]. The aim of CHB treatment is to prevent the development of these long-term complications, of which effective implementation would require identification of high-risk patients. Histologic injury and fibrosis have a good correlation with long-term risk, since repeated hepatitic flares in CHB were found to have increased necroinflammation on liver biopsies, resulting in increased fibrogenesis and eventual disease progression [4].

Serum alanine aminotransferase (ALT) is an important biochemical marker used in the assessment of hepatic injury, but is limited by its poor correlation with disease severity [5]. Serum HBV DNA levels directly reflect the degree of HBV replication, and are strongly correlated with long-term mortality [6,7].

However, patients in the immune tolerant phase have minimal changes on liver biopsy despite high HBV DNA levels [8]. Although liver biopsy remains an integral part in determining disease severity , it is an invasive procedure and not without complications [9]. Sampling error and intra-observer variations are also unavoidable [10,11].

Current treatment guidelines recommend the use of both serum ALT and HBV DNA in selecting patients for therapy, with a persistent ALT level of more than 2×upper limit of normal (ULN) required for commencing therapy in two of the three international treatment guidelines on CHB [12,13]. Certain subgroups still require consideration of liver biopsy. These include hepatitis B e antigen (HBeAg)-positive patients of 40 years and older with ALT 1–2×ULN, and HBeAg-negative patients with ALT 1–2×ULN and an elevated HBV DNA (more than $1×10^4$ copies/mL or 2000 IU/mL). A study of 4376 HBeAg-negative patients from Taiwan claimed that normal ALT levels in HBeAg-negative disease had good prognosis [14]. However, other studies have shown that between 10 to 37% of CHB patients with normal ALT already having significant necroinflammation, fibrosis and even cirrhosis on liver biopsy [10,15,16]. An Italian population study by Prati et al based on 6835 healthy individuals suggested to lower the ULN of ALT to 30 U/L for men and 19 U/L for women [17], making the definition of "normal ALT" more confusing.

Previous studies investigating the association between clinical parameters and advanced histologic abnormalities were limited by either a small sample size or a disproportional distribution of HBeAg-positive and -negative disease [18,19,20,21]. The present study aimed at studying the association between ALT and advanced histologic abnormalities in the 3 phases of HBV replication: the immune tolerant phase, the immune clearance phase and HBeAg-negative disease.

Methods

From 1994 to 2008, 1054 treatment-naive CHB patients followed up in the Department of Medicine, the University of Hong Kong, Queen Mary Hospital were screened for entry into therapeutic drug trials that required liver biopsy. Three hundred and nineteen out of these 1054 patients with similar demographics and clinical characteristics who had consented to enter these trials were recruited in the present study. In addition, we had previously investigated and reported the usage of routinely available clinical parameters to derive a score to predict significant fibrosis in CHB based on 237 out of these 319 patientss [22].

Patients were recruited if they were positive for hepatitis B surface antigen (HBsAg) for at least 6 months and had available baseline biochemical and hematological parameters on presentation. The inclusion criteria for ALT and HBV DNA for each therapeutic drug trial differed, and are listed in Table 1. Patients who had decompensated liver disease and other concomitant liver disease, including chronic hepatitis C or D virus infection, primary biliary cirrhosis, autoimmune hepatitis, Wilson's disease, and significant intake of alcohol (20 grams per day for female; 30 grams per day for male) were excluded. All patients had written consent on entry into trials for research purposes, and all trials were approved by the Institutional Review Board of the University of Hong Kong.

Clinical and biochemical parameters were recorded from all patients at the day of liver biopsy. These include the patient's age, gender, HBeAg status, albumin, bilirubin, ALT, AST, platelet count and HBV DNA level. The ULN of ALT was based on the respective therapeutic drug trials, and was ranged from 45 to 53 U/L in men and 31 to 43 U/L in women. Serum HBV DNA levels were measured by three different assays, as follow: a branched DNA assay (Versant HBV DNA 3.0 assay, Bayer Health-Care Diagnostic Division, Tarrytown, NY), with a lower limit of quantification of 2000 copies/mL (400 IU/mL) in 88 patients, Cobas Amplicor HBV Monitor Test (Roche Diagnostic, Branchburg, NJ) with a lower limit of quantification of 300 copies/ mL (60 IU/mL) in 115 patients, Cobas Taqman assay (Roche Diagnostic, Branchburg, NJ) with a lower limit of quantification of 60 copies/mL (12 IU/mL) in 116 patients.

Two different biopsy needles were used to obtain liver biopsies. An 18G sheathed cutting needle (Temno Evolution, Cardinal Health, McGaw Park, IL) was used for 88 patients, of which the biopsies obtained were 1.5 to 1.8 cm in length. For the rest of the cohort, liver biopsies were obtained using a 17G core aspiration needle (Hepafix, B. Braun Melsungen AG, Germany), with a biopsy length between 2 to 5 cm. Only pre-treatment biopsies were included. Biopsies were fixed, paraffin-embedded, and stained with hematoxylin and eosin for morphological evaluation and Masson's trichrome stain for assessment of fibrosis. The pathologist assessing the biopsy specimens was blinded to the biochemical and virologic results of the patients. Histologic grading of necroinflammation and the staging of liver fibrosis were performed using the Knodell histologic activity index (HAI) [23] and Ishak fibrosis score [24] respectively. Necroinflammation was graded from 0 to 18 while fibrosis was staged from 0 to 6. Significant necroinflammation was defined as a Knodell HAI of 7 or more. Significant fibrosis was defined as an Ishak score of 3 or more, meaning the presence of bridging fibrosis or cirrhosis.

All statistical analyses were performed using SPSS version 16.0 (SPSS Inc, Chicago, Illinois). The Mann-Whitney U-test was used for continuous variables with a skewed distribution; Pearson's chi squared test was used for categorical variables. Multivariate logistic regression was used to determine whether the identified variables associated with advanced histologic abnormalities were independent risk factors. A two-sided p value of <0.05 was considered statistically significant.

Results

The baseline characteristics of the study population are depicted in Table 2. Two hundred and eleven patients were HBeAg-positive, of which 40 , 78 and 93 patients had a normal ALT, ALT 1–2×ULN and ALT more than 2×ULN respectively. Of the 108 HBeAg-negative patients, only four (3.7%) had normal ALT levels.

The distribution of liver necroinflammation and fibrosis is shown in Figures 1 and 2. Significant necroinflammation and fibrosis were found in 54.2% (57.8% for HBeAg-positive, 47.2% for HBeAg-negative) and 27.6% (24.6% for HBeAg-positive, 33.3% for HBeAg-negative) of patients respectively. Altogether 88 patients had significant fibrosis, of which 32 (36.4%) had an ALT level of 1 to 2×ULN. Six patients (5 HBeAg-positive, 1 HBeAg-negative) had histologic evidence of cirrhosis. The distribution of significant liver fibrosis among different age groups is shown in Figure 3. For the whole study population, the proportion of significant fibrosis increased from 18.3% in patients with an age of

Table 1. Inclusion criteria concerning ALT and HBV DNA for all 319 patients.

HBeAg-positive	88 patients	ALT<10×ULN
		HBV DNA≥1.4×10^6 copies/mL
	53 patients	ALT 1.3–10×ULN
		HBV DNA≥1×10^5 copies/mL
	49 patients	ALT 1.3 – 10×ULN
		HBV DNA≥1×10^6 copies/mL
	15 patients	ALT 1.3 – 10×ULN
		HBV DNA≥3×10^6 copies/mL
	6 patients	ALT < 10×ULN
		HBV DNA≥1×10^6 copies/mL
HBeAg-negative	63 patients	ALT 1.3–10×ULN
		HBV DNA≥1×10^4 copies/mL
	24 patients	ALT 1.3–10×ULN
		HBV DNA≥3×10^6 copies/mL
	21 patients	ALT 1.3–10×ULN
		HBV DNA≥1×10^6 copies/mL

ULN = upper limit of normal.

Table 2. Baseline Characteristics of all 319 patients.

Patient Characteristic	HBeAg-positive Normal ALT (n = 40)	HBeAg-positive Elevated ALT (n = 171)	HBeAg-negative (n = 108)
Age	32 (17–43)	32 (16–60)	46 (18–63)
Male	62.5% (n = 25)	67.3% (n = 115)	71.3% (n = 77)
Albumin (g/L)	47 (43–52)	45 (29–55)	46 (40–53)
Bilirubin (umol/L)	9 (5–22)	11 (3–31)	13 (3–28)
ALT (U/L)	27 (14–55)	93 (38–636)	90 (41–576)
≤1×ULN	100% (n = 40)	-	3.7% (n = 4)
1–2×ULN	-	45.6% (n = 78)	48.1% (n = 52)
>2×ULN	-	54.4% (n = 93)	48.1% (n = 52)
AST (U/L)	23 (15–39)	56 (23–304)	55 (26–255)
Platelet (×10^9/L)	211 (148–308)	166 (89–334)	189 (80–331)
HBV DNA (log IU/mL)	8.14 (4.83–10.96)	7.89 (3.48–14.00)	5.71 (2.67–9.42)

Continous variables expressed in median (range).
ULN = Upper limit of normal.

30 years or less to 41.9% in patients older than 50 years. HBeAg-positive patients show an increasing prevalence of significant fibrosis with age (p = 0.001). A similar trend was seen in HBeAg-negative patients, except for the group of age less than 30 years (n = 14).

Patients were further analyzed according to different stages of disease. Among the 40 HBeAg-positive patients with a normal serum ALT, 9 (22.5%) had significant necroinflammation and of these 9 patients, 2 (22.2%) had significant fibrosis. These 9 patients had a median age of 29 (range: 17 to 42) and a median ALT of 26 (range: 18 to 53). However, only 17 patients (42.5%) had an ALT level within the normal reference ranges suggested by Prati et al [17] (i.e. 30 U/L for men and 19 U/L for women). Among these 17 patients, only 2 (11.8%) showed significant necroinflammation and none had significant fibrosis. A comparison of fibrosis scores between those with ALT levels within the Prati criteria and those exceeding the Prati criteria among all 40 patients is shown in Figure 4. Patients with ALT levels exceeding the Prati criteria were more likely to have significant fibrosis (p = 0.024).

One hundred and seventy-one HBeAg-positive patients had an elevated ALT. Univariate analysis of showed that age (p = 0.015), albumin (p = <0.001), ALT (p = 0.01), AST (p = 0.005) and platelet count (p = 0.012) were associated with significant necroinflammation, while age (p<0.001), ALT (p = 0.013), AST (p<0.001) and platelet count (p = 0.005) were also associated with significant fibrosis. The multivariate analysis of clinical parameters independently associated with significant necroinflammation or fibrosis is shown in Table 3. A lower serum albumin (p = 0.001) and platelet count (p = 0.037) were independently associated with significant necroinflammation, while older age, higher AST and lower platelet count were independently associated with significant fibrosis (p = 0.007, 0.047 and 0.045 respectively). A higher ALT was not independently associated with significant fibrosis (p = 0.345). The Ishak fibrosis scores among the 78 patients with an ALT level of 1–2×ULN were compared with the 93 patients with an ALT of more than 2×ULN (Figure 5). There was no significant difference noted (p = 0.098). After revising the ULN of ALT according to the Prati criteria, the fibrosis scores of patients with ALT 1–2×ULN (n = 33) were compared with patients having

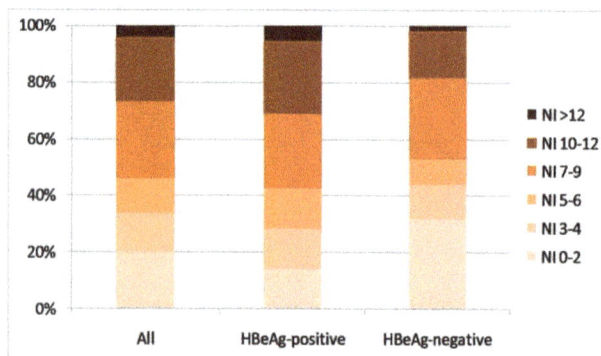

Figure 1. Distribution of liver necroinflammation (graded by Knodell histologic activity index) among 319 chronic hepatitis B patients.

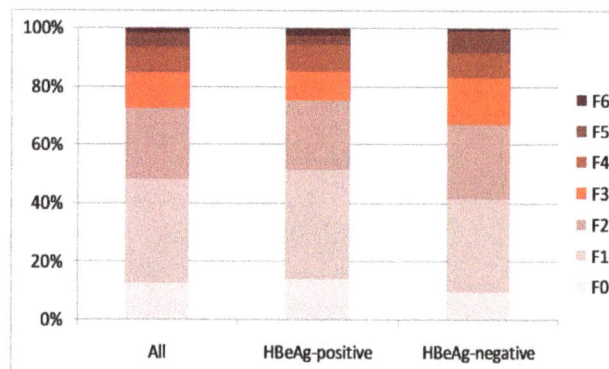

Figure 2. Distribution of liver fibrosis (staged by Ishak fibrosis score) in 319 chronic hepatitis B patients.

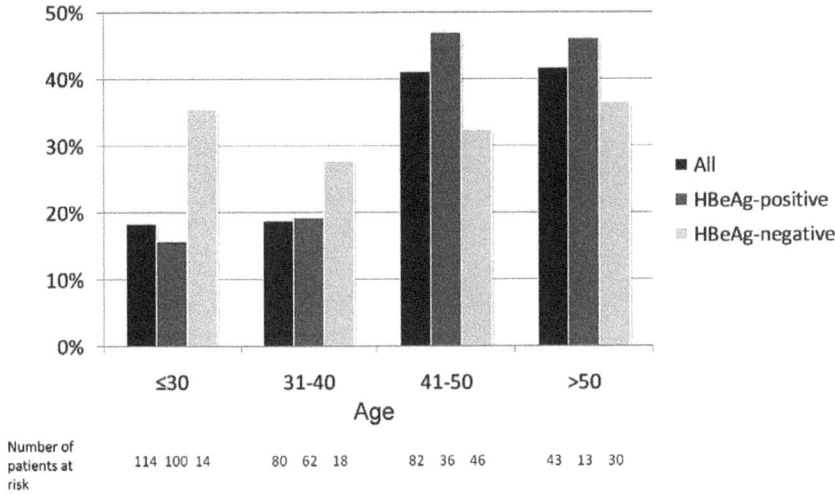

Figure 3. Distribution of significant liver fibrosis (Ishak fibrosis score ≥3) among different age groups.

ALT more than 2×ULN (n = 161). Again, there was no significant difference (p = 0.106).

From the univariate analysis of 108 HBeAg-negative patients, albumin (p<0.001), ALT (p = 0.038), AST (p = 0.013) and HBV DNA (p = 0.001) were associated with significant necroinflammation, while only platelet count (p = 0.005) and HBV DNA (p = 0.002) were associated with significant fibrosis. The multivariate analysis of clinical parameters independently associated with significant necroinflammation and fibrosis in HBeAg-negative disease are shown in Table 3. A lower serum albumin (p = 0.003) and a higher serum HBV DNA level (p = 0.004) were independently associated with significant necroinflammation, while a low platelet count (p = 0.015) and an increased HBV DNA level (p = 0.020) were independently associated with significant fibrosis. Increasing age and elevated ALT levels were not independently associated with significant fibrosis (p = 0.779 and 0.544 respectively).The Ishak fibrosis scores among patients with an ALT level of 1–2×ULN (n = 52) were compared with those having an ALT level of more than 2×ULN (n = 52) (Figure 5). There was again no significant difference (p = 0.838). After the Prati criteria revision,

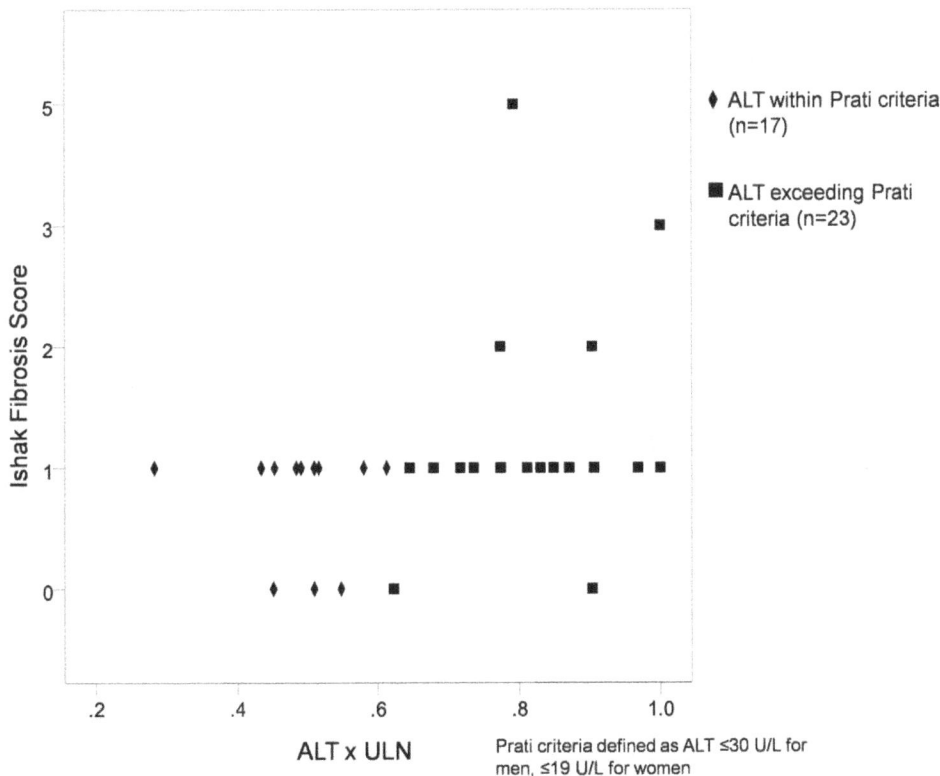

Figure 4. Comparison of Ishak fibrosis scores among HBeAg-positive patients with normal ALT (p = 0.024).

Table 3. Clinical parameters predictive of significant liver necroinflammation and fibrosis by multivariate analysis.

		Clinical Parameter	p value	Odds ratio	95% Confidence Interval
HBeAg-positive with elevated ALT (n = 171)	Knodell HAI ≥7 (n = 113)	Albumin (g/L)	0.001	0.828	0.738–0.929
		Platelet (×10^9/L)	0.037	0.993	0.986–1.000
	Ishak Fibrosis score ≥3 (n = 50)	Age (years)	0.007	1.048	1.013–1.084
		AST (U/L)	0.047	1.108	1.000–1.036
		Platelet (×10^9/L)	0.045	0.992	0.985–1.000
HBeAg-negative (n = 108)	Knodell HAI ≥7 (n = 51)	Albumin (g/L)	0.003	0.792	0.680–0.923
		DNA (log IU/mL)	0.004	1.741	1.194–2.540
	Ishak Fibrosis score ≥3 (n = 36)	Platelet (×10^9/L)	0.015	0.988	0.978–0.998
		DNA (log IU/mL)	0.020	1.513	1.066–2.147

based on the 10 and 98 patients with ALT 1–2×ULN and more than 2×ULN respectively, fibrosis score also had no significant difference (p = 0.485).

Discussion

Various treatment guidelines require a certain ALT threshold for treatment decisions. Both the guidelines from the American Association for the Study of Liver Diseases (AASLD) [12] and the Asia-Pacific Association for the Study of the Liver (APASL) [13] only consider treatment when ALT is more than 2×ULN, while treatment is optional for ALT 1 to 2 times×ULN with liver biopsy recommended. Using such an ALT threshold is open to debate, especially when previous studies had shown CHB patients with a normal ALT at the upper range had an increased risk of long-term cirrhotic complications and HCC [25,26]. Our present study investigated the association of various routinely available clinical parameters, including ALT, with liver histology for all three phases of disease in CHB: the immune tolerant phase, the immune clearance phase and HBeAg-negative disease.

In the present study, we first examined the role of normal ALT levels in predicting liver histology. 22.5% (9 out of 40) of HBeAg-

positive patients with a normal ALT had significant histologic abnormalities present. A significant proportion of these patients had abnormal ALT levels using the reference ranges suggested by Prati et al [17]. Therefore, the findings of our study support lowering the currently accepted reference ranges for ALT. In fact, an Asian study based on 1105 healthy individuals also concluded the ULN of ALT should be lowered, this time to 33 U/L for men and 25 U/L for women [27]. In addition, patients with an ALT above 0.5×ULN (defined as 53 U/L for male and 36 U/L for female in that study) were already shown to at an increased risk of cirrhotic complications [25]. Thus, HBeAg-positive patients with a serum ALT at the upper range of the traditionally-accepted normal ranges may in fact be in the immune clearance phase, and hence leading to significant fibrosis on liver histology. A previous study found 39% of HBeAg-positive patients with a normal ALT to have significant fibrosis [16]. Further population studies in different ethnic groups are needed to define the exact suitable reference ranges for ALT.

We then continued to investigate whether there was any difference in liver histology in patients with different levels of elevated ALT. Several studies had demonstrated that there was no good association between ALT levels and fibrosis [16,21,28]. Our current study also found that the degree of ALT elevation was not

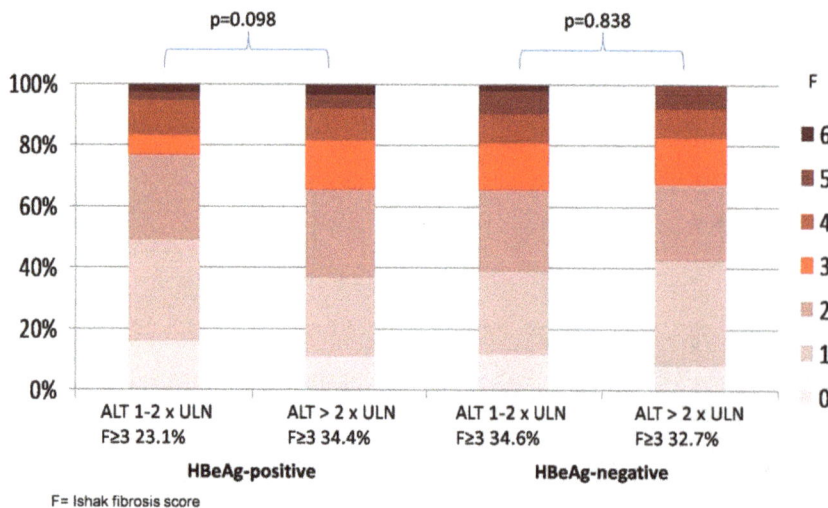

F= Ishak fibrosis score

Figure 5. Comparison of Ishak fibrosis scores between ALT 1–2×ULN and ALT >2×ULN in both HBeAg-positive and HBeAg-negative patients.

associated with significant changes in necroinflammation or fibrosis for both HBeAg-positive and -negative patients. In addition, there was no significance difference in fibrosis staging for both groups of patients with an ALT level of 1–2×ULN and more than 2×ULN (p = 0.098 and p = 0.838 respectively). Therefore, using the ALT threshold of more than 2×ULN in selecting patients for treatment has the potential of not treating patients with significant fibrosis or cirrhosis. However, this finding should be further confirmed by studies with larger number of HBeAg-positive and -negative patients with different ALT levels.

Increasing age was independently associated with significant fibrosis in HBeAg-positive patients with an elevated ALT, which is consistent with previous studies [16,19,29]. In our present study, age had no association with fibrosis in HBeAg-negative disease, with a substantial proportion of young patients of age 30 or less having significant fibrosis (35.7%, 5 out of 14). While this could be related to the small sample size for these patients, another possible explanation is that the majority of HBeAg-negative patients in our study (96.3%, 105 out of 108) had an elevated ALT (median level 90 U/L) and HBV DNA (median level 5.71 log IU/mL). This may represent a special group of patients who underwent HBeAg seroconversion at a relatively younger age (median age of HBeAg seroconversion in our locality is 35 years [25]) and yet having a more serious disease as reflected by high ALT and HBV DNA levels. Regardless of this, a study in Asia had shown the prevalence of significant fibrosis among HBeAg-negative patients with the age of less than 25 years to be 17% [29], which is much higher than figures reported in Europe [20]. This can be explained by Asian patients acquiring the infection perinatally, with liver injury starting early in life.

For HBeAg-negative disease, increased HBV DNA levels were independently associated with significant fibrosis. The findings are in line with the suggestion of suppressing HBV DNA permanently as a treatment end point [30], especially when long-term viral suppression has been shown to reverse histologic damage [31,32]. Serum HBV DNA levels had no association with fibrosis in the immune clearance phase, which can be explained by an extensive immune-mediated response leading to low viremic levels despite significant abnormalities on histology [33]. Although a study from Taiwan showed that normal ALT levels in HBeAg-negative disease are associated with a good prognosis and recommended treatment initiation only for patients with ALT levels more than 2×ULN [14], HBV DNA measurements were not incorporated in that study. A large population study has shown elevated HBV DNA levels in noncirrhotic HBeAg-negative patients with normal ALT to be associated with an increased risk of HCC [7].

Among HBeAg-positive patients with elevated ALT (n = 171), both elevated AST and low platelet count were independently associated with significant fibrosis, although the p values were only borderline significant (p = 0.047 and 0.045 respectively). These findings are however consistent with a previous study showing that both AST and platelet count are associated with significant fibrosis, from which the AST to platelet ratio index (APRI) was

derived [34]._In addition, our current findings are also in line with our previous study in which AST and platelet count were used to create a model to predict significant fibrosis [22]. Another model known as the APGA (AST/platelet/GGT/AFP) score showed promising results when correlating with liver stiffness measured by transient elastography in CHB. Further studies correlating with actual histologic specimens would be needed to determine its clinical applicability [35].

There are several limitations in our study, including its retrospective nature, the different biopsy methods used and the lack of HBeAg-negative patients with normal ALT. Although the differences in inclusion criteria would result in selection bias, our present study was able to recruit patients from different phases of disease, thus making the study more representative of the whole CHB patient population. HBV genotype and the presence of the core-promoter mutation were not checked in our present study, which could be important since previous small-scale studies found genotype C and the core-promoter mutation to be associated with significant histologic abnormalities [19,36]. However, the determination of HBV genotype and core promoter mutations requires more advanced molecular diagnostics, and may not be available for routine clinical practice. Since serum ALT and HBV DNA levels tend to fluctuate with time [37], the measurement of each clinical parameter at several time points might be more representative. An average ALT obtained by integral calculus would be one such method [38]. However, whether an average value or a single value at the time of biopsy would have better histologic correlation and prognostic determination in a cross-sectional study would require further evaluation. Our study also lacked clinical information concerning the patient's metabolic profile i.e. the presence of diabetes mellitus or insulin resistance. Nevertheless, recent studies focusing on Chinese CHB patients did not show any association between metabolic factors and liver disease severity [39,40].

In conclusion, ALT is not a useful marker for the decision of commencing antiviral therapy in CHB because of its poor correlation with significant liver injury in both HBeAg-positive and -negative patients. Patients with ALT levels less than 2×ULN should be considered for possible treatment if histology, or other non-invasive assessment such as transient elastography, shows significant fibrosis. HBeAg-positive CHB with a normal ALT might already have significant histologic abnormalities, which supports the lowering of the current ALT reference ranges. Increased HBV DNA levels and low platelet count are associated with significant fibrosis in HBeAg-negative disease.

Author Contributions

Conceived and designed the experiments: WKS CLL MFY. Performed the experiments: CLL PPCI MFY. Analyzed the data: WKS. Contributed reagents/materials/analysis tools: JF DKHW JCHY IFNH. Wrote the paper: WKS CLL MFY.

References

1. Manno M, Camma C, Schepis F, Bassi F, Gelmini R, et al. (2004) Natural history of chronic HBV in northern Italy: Morbidity and morality after 30 years. Gastroenterology 127: 756–763.

2. Martinot-Peignoux M, Boyer N, Colombat M, Akremi R, Pham BN, et al. (2002) Serum hepatitis B virus DNA levels and liver histology in inactive HBsAg carriers. J Hepatol 36: 543–546.

3. Yuen MF (2007) Revisiting the natural history of chronic hepatitis B: impact of new concepts on clinical management. J Gastroenterol Hepatol 22: 973–976.

4. Mani H, Kleiner DE (2009) Liver biopsy findings in chronic hepatitis B. Hepatology 49: S61–71.

5. Dufour DR, Lott JA, Nolte FS, Gretch DR, Koff RS, et al. (2000) Diagnosis and monitoring of hepatic injury. II. Recommendations for use of laboratory tests in screening, diagnosis, and monitoring. Clin Chem 46: 2050–2068.

6. Iloeje UH, Yang HI, Jen CL, Su J, Wang LY, et al. (2007) Risk and predictors of mortality associated with chronic hepatitis B infection. Clin Gastroenterol Hepatol 5: 921–931.

7. Chen CJ, Yang HI, Su J, Jen CL, You SL, et al. (2006) Risk of hepatocellular carcinoma across a biological gradient of serum hepatitis B virus DNA level. JAMA 295: 65–73.

8. Andreani T, Serfaty L, Mohand D, Dernaika S, Wendum D, et al. (2007) Chronic hepatitis B virus carriers in the immunotolerant phase of infection: histologic findings and outcome. Clin Gastroenterol Hepatol 5: 636–641.

9. Huang JF, Hsieh MY, Dai CY, Hou NJ, Lee LP, et al. (2007) The incidence and risks of liver biopsy in non-cirrhotic patients: An evaluation of 3806 biopsies. Gut 56: 736–737.

10. ter Borg F, ten Kate FJ, Cuypers HT, Leentvaar-Kuijpers A, Oosting J, et al. (2000) A survey of liver pathology in needle biopsies from HBsAg and anti-HBe positive individuals. J Clin Pathol 53: 541–548.

11. Regev A, Berho M, Jeffers LJ, Milikowski C, Molina EG, et al. (2002) Sampling error and intraobserver variation in liver biopsy in patients with chronic HCV infection. Am J Gastroenterol 97: 2614–2618.

12. Lok AS, McMahon BJ (2009) Chronic hepatitis B: update 2009. Hepatology 50: 661–662.

13. Liaw YF, Leung N, Kao JH, Piratvisuth T, Gane E, et al. (2008) Asian-Pacific consensus statement on the management of chronic hepatitis B: a 2008 update. Hepatol Int 2: 263–283.

14. Tai DI, Lin SM, Sheen IS, Chu CM, Lin DY, et al. (2009) Long-term outcome of hepatitis B e antigen-negative hepatitis B surface antigen carriers in relation to changes of alanine aminotransferase levels over time. Hepatology 49: 1859–1867.

15. Lai M, Hyatt BJ, Nasser I, Curry M, Afdhal NH (2007) The clinical significance of persistently normal ALT in chronic hepatitis B infection. J Hepatol 47: 760–767.

16. Kumar M, Sarin SK, Hissar S, Pande C, Sakhuja P, et al. (2008) Virologic and histologic features of chronic hepatitis B virus-infected asymptomatic patients with persistently normal ALT. Gastroenterology 134: 1376–1384.

17. Prati D, Taioli E, Zanella A, Della Torre E, Butelli S, et al. (2002) Updated definitions of healthy ranges for serum alanine aminotransferase levels. Ann Intern Med 137: 1–10.

18. Chan HL, Tsang SW, Liew CT, Tse CH, Wong ML, et al. (2002) Viral genotype and hepatitis B virus DNA levels are correlated with histological liver damage in HBeAg-negative chronic hepatitis B virus infection. Am J Gastroenterol 97: 406–412.

19. Park JY, Park YN, Kim DY, Paik YH, Lee KS, et al. (2008) High prevalence of significant histology in asymptomatic chronic hepatitis B patients with genotype C and high serum HBV DNA levels. Journal of Viral Hepatitis 15: 615–621.

20. Zacharakis G, Koskinas J, Kotsiou S, Tzara F, Vafeiadis N, et al. (2008) The role of serial measurement of serum HBV DNA levels in patients with chronic HBeAg(−) hepatitis B infection: association with liver disease progression. A prospective cohort study. J Hepatol 49: 884–891.

21. Mohamadnejad M, Montazeri G, Fazlollahi A, Zamani F, Nasiri J, et al. (2006) Noninvasive markers of liver fibrosis and inflammation in chronic hepatitis B-virus related liver disease. Am J Gastroenterol 101: 2537–2545.

22. Seto WK, Lee CF, Lai CL, Ip PP, Fong DY, et al. (2011) A new model using routinely available clinical parameters to predict significant liver fibrosis in chronic hepatitis B. PLoS One 6: e23077.

23. Knodell RG, Ishak KG, Black WC, Chen TS, Craig R, et al. (1981) Formulation and application of a numerical scoring system for assessing histological activity in asymptomatic chronic active hepatitis. Hepatology 1: 431–435.

24. Ishak K, Baptista A, Bianchi L, Callea F, De Groote J, et al. (1995) Histological grading and staging of chronic hepatitis. J Hepatol 22: 696–699.

25. Yuen MF, Yuan HJ, Wong DK, Yuen JC, Wong WM, et al. (2005) Prognostic determinants for chronic hepatitis B in Asians: therapeutic implications. Gut 54: 1610–1614.

26. Kumada T, Toyoda H, Kiriyama S, Sone Y, Tanikawa M, et al. (2010) Incidence of hepatocellular carcinoma in patients with chronic hepatitis B virus infection who have normal alanine aminotransferase values. J Med Virol 82: 539–545.

27. Lee JK, Shim JH, Lee HC, Lee SH, Kim KM, et al. (2010) Estimation of the healthy upper limits for serum alanine aminotransferase in Asian populations with normal liver histology. Hepatology 51: 1577–1583.

28. Hui AY, Chan HL, Wong VW, Liew CT, Chim AM, et al. (2005) Identification of chronic hepatitis B patients without significant liver fibrosis by a simple noninvasive predictive model. Am J Gastroenterol 100: 616–623.

29. Fung J, Lai CL, But D, Wong D, Cheung TK, et al. (2008) Prevalence of fibrosis and cirrhosis in chronic hepatitis B: implications for treatment and management. Am J Gastroenterol 103: 1421–1426.

30. Lai CL, Yuen MF (2007) The natural history and treatment of chronic hepatitis B: a critical evaluation of standard treatment criteria and end points. Ann Intern Med 147: 58–61.

31. Chang TT, Lai CL, Kew Yoon S, Lee SS, Coelho HS, et al. (2010) Entecavir treatment for up to 5 years in patients with hepatitis B e antigen-positive chronic hepatitis B. Hepatology 51: 422–430.

32. Yuen MF, Chow DH, Tsui K, Wong BC, Yuen JC, et al. (2005) Liver histology of Asian patients with chronic hepatitis B on prolonged lamivudine therapy. Aliment Pharmacol Ther 21: 841–849.

33. Yuen MF, Ng IO, Fan ST, Yuan HJ, Wong DK, et al. (2004) Significance of HBV DNA levels in liver histology of HBeAg and Anti-HBe positive patients with chronic hepatitis B. Am J Gastroenterol 99: 2032–2037.

34. Wai CT, Greenson JK, Fontana RJ, Kalbfleisch JD, Marrero JA, et al. (2003) A simple noninvasive index can predict both significant fibrosis and cirrhosis in patients with chronic hepatitis C. Hepatology 38: 518–526.

35. Fung J, Lai CL, Fong DY, Yuen JC, Wong DK, et al. (2008) Correlation of liver biochemistry with liver stiffness in chronic hepatitis B and development of a predictive model for liver fibrosis. Liver Int 28: 1408–1416.

36. Yuen MF, Tanaka Y, Ng IO, Mizokami M, Yuen JC, et al. (2005) Hepatic necroinflammation and fibrosis in patients with genotypes Ba and C, core-promoter and precore mutations. J Viral Hepat 12: 513–518.

37. Chu CJ, Hussain M, Lok AS (2002) Quantitative serum HBV DNA levels during different stages of chronic hepatitis B infection. Hepatology 36: 1408–1415.

38. Kumada T, Toyoda H, Kiriyama S, Sone Y, Tanikawa M, et al. (2007) Relation between incidence of hepatic carcinogenesis and integration value of alanine aminotransferase in patients with hepatitis C virus infection. Gut 56: 738–739.

39. Shi JP, Fan JG, Wu R, Gao XQ, Zhang L, et al. (2008) Prevalence and risk factors of hepatic steatosis and its impact on liver injury in Chinese patients with chronic hepatitis B infection. J Gastroenterol Hepatol 23: 1419–1425.

40. Peng D, Han Y, Ding H, Wei L (2008) Hepatic steatosis in chronic hepatitis B patients is associated with metabolic factors more than viral factors. J Gastroenterol Hepatol 23: 1082–1088.

9

Activation of the Connective Tissue Growth Factor (CTGF)-Transforming Growth Factor β 1 (TGF-β 1) Axis in Hepatitis C Virus-Expressing Hepatocytes

Tirumuru Nagaraja[1][9], Li Chen[2][9], Anuradha Balasubramanian[3], Jerome E. Groopman[3], Kalpana Ghoshal[4], Samson T. Jacob[4], Andrew Leask[5], David R. Brigstock[2][*][¶], Appakkudal R. Anand[1][*][¶], Ramesh K. Ganju[1][*][¶]

1 Department of Pathology, Ohio State University Wexner Medical Center, Columbus, Ohio, United States of America, 2 Center for Clinical and Translational Research, The Research Institute at Nationwide Children's Hospital, Columbus, Ohio, United States of America, 3 Division of Experimental Medicine, Beth Israel Deaconess Medical Center, Harvard Medical School, Boston, Massachusetts, United States of America, 4 Department of Molecular and Cellular Biochemistry, The Ohio State University, Columbus, Ohio, United States of America, 5 Schulich School of Medicine and Dentistry, University of Western Ontario, London, Ontario, Canada

Abstract

Background: The pro-fibrogenic cytokine connective tissue growth factor (CTGF) plays an important role in the development and progression of fibrosis in many organ systems, including liver. However, its role in the pathogenesis of hepatitis C virus (HCV)-induced liver fibrosis remains unclear.

Methods: In the present study, we assessed CTGF expression in HCV-infected hepatocytes using replicon cells containing full-length HCV genotype 1 and the infectious HCV clone JFH1 (HCV genotype 2) by real-time PCR, Western blot analysis and confocal microscopy. We evaluated transforming growth factor β1 (TGF-β1) as a key upstream mediator of CTGF production using neutralizing antibodies and shRNAs. We also determined the signaling molecules involved in CTGF production using various immunological techniques.

Results: We demonstrated an enhanced expression of CTGF in two independent models of HCV infection. We also demonstrated that HCV induced CTGF expression in a TGF-β1-dependent manner. Further dissection of the molecular mechanisms revealed that CTGF production was mediated through sequential activation of MAPkinase and Smad-dependent pathways. Finally, to determine whether CTGF regulates fibrosis, we showed that shRNA-mediated knock-down of CTGF resulted in reduced expression of fibrotic markers in HCV replicon cells.

Conclusion: Our studies demonstrate a central role for CTGF expression in HCV-induced liver fibrosis and highlight the potential value of developing CTGF-based anti-fibrotic therapies to counter HCV-induced liver damage.

Editor: Ashok Chauhan, University of South Carolina School of Medicine, United States of America

Funding: This work was supported by grants National Institutes of Health RO1 HL087576 to RKG, R01AA016003 to DRB and a collaborative seed grant from The Ohio State University and Nationwide Children's Hospital, Columbus, OH to RKG and DRB. The funders had no role in study design, data collection and analysis, decision to publish, or preparation of the manuscript.

Competing Interests: The authors have declared that no competing interests exist.

* E-mail: Ramesh.Ganju@osumc.edu (RKG); Appakkudal.Anand@osumc.edu (ARA); David.Brigstock@nationwidechildrens.org (DRB)

9 These authors contributed equally to this work.

¶ These authors also contributed equally to this work.

Introduction

Chronic hepatitis C virus (HCV) infection is a leading cause of end-stage liver disease, including liver cirrhosis and hepatocellular carcinoma, with approximately 3% of the world's population infected (130–170 million individuals) [1]. The main targets of HCV infection are human hepatocytes, where HCV not only causes an inflammatory response, but also activates pro-fibrogenic pathways that contribute to liver fibrosis [2]. Liver fibrosis is characterized by the production of pro-fibrogenic cytokines by parenchymal cells (hepatocytes) and mesenchymal cells e.g. Kupffer cells, endothelial cells, hepatic stellate cells (HSCs), which collectively contribute to the unrelenting synthesis and deposition

of extracellular matrix (ECM) components, downregulation of matrix metalloproteinases (MMPs) and increased expression/action of tissue inhibitor of metalloproteinases (TIMPs) [2,3]. Together, these molecular changes determine the progression of chronic hepatitis C to liver cirrhosis and hepatocellular carcinoma (HCC) [1].

Recently, the profibrogenic cytokine connective tissue growth factor (CTGF), a member of the CCN gene family (CTGF, cyr61/cef10, nov), has been shown to play a key role in various fibrotic disorders [3,4,5,6,7]. It is a multi-functional protein (~40 kD) produced by various cell types that acts via autocrine or paracrine pathways to regulate diverse cellular functions including growth, proliferation, apoptosis, adhesion, migration, ECM production and differentiation [8]. The receptors for CTGF on various cells have, however, not been well-characterized [9]. Data reported in recent years provides compelling evidence that CTGF is a key factor in development of hepatic fibrosis [3,10,11,12,13,14]. With regard to HCV infection, CTGF expression in liver biopsy samples has been shown to correlate independently with the fibrosis stage and plasma HCV RNA levels [11,15]. In the present study, we investigated the role of CTGF in HCV-induced liver fibrosis and the molecular mechanism of its production.

The fibrogenic mechanisms in the liver are dependent on the interplay of many pro- and anti-fibrotic cytokines. CTGF is often co-expressed with transforming growth factor β1 (TGF-β1) in various fibrotic disorders. TGF-β1 is a key profibrogenic cytokine in the liver, participating in many critical events leading to liver fibrosis, such as HSC activation, hepatocyte apoptosis, ECM formation and expression of other profibrogenic mediators. Furthermore, TGF-β1 has also been shown to facilitate epithelial-to-mesenchymal transition of hepatocytes that in turn participates in the progression of liver fibrosis [16,17,18]. Clinical studies have revealed elevated TGF-β1 serum levels in patients with chronic hepatitis B virus (HBV)/HCV infections [19,20]. Studies in several connective tissue cell types have shown that CTGF acts as a potent downstream mediator of TGF-β1, modulating its functional effects [10]. However, the cross-talk between these profibrogenic cytokines during HCV infection is not known. In the present study, we first demonstrated the upregulation of CTGF and TGF-β1 in the well-characterized Huh7.5-FL HCV replicon system and HepG2 cells transfected with HCV JFH1 RNA. We further investigated the inter-relationship between TGF-β1 and CTGF in HCV infection. Our studies reveal that HCV-stimulated CTGF is induced downstream of TGF-β1 in a MAPKinase and Smad-dependent manner and that CTGF production drives production of key fibrosis-associated markers, including procollagen I. The central role of CTGF production in HCV-infected hepatocytes highlights the potential value of developing CTGF-based anti-fibrotic therapies to counter HCV-induced liver damage.

Materials and Methods

Antibodies

The antibodies used in the study were HCV NS5B (Alexis Biochemicals, San Diego, CA), HCV Core (Abcam, Cambridge, MA), HCV NS4A, TGF-β1 (Chemicon, Temecula, CA), Phospho-Smad2, Phospho-Smad3, Smad2, Smad3, Phospho-P38, P-38, Phospho-JNK, JNK, vimentin and Slug (Cell Signaling, Danvers, MA), TGF-β receptor I, Phospho-ERK, ERK, CTGF, Procollagen I and GAPDH (Santa Cruz Biotechnology, Santa Cruz, CA) and α-SMA (Sigma, St. Louis, MO).

Cell cultures

In this study we used HCV- negative human hepatoma cell line Huh7.5 cells and Huh7.5 cells harboring full genome length HCV [Con1/FL-Neo HCV1b FL (S2204I)] (Huh7.5-FL) replicon cells (Apath, LLC; St. Louis, MO) and propagated in complete Dulbecco's modified Eagle's medium (DMEM) (Invitrogen, Carlsbad, CA). Huh 7.5 cells represent a Huh7 subline which are cured with interferon to render them highly permissive to HCV replication [21]. Huh7.5-FL cells were maintained in medium containing 750 μg/ml of Geneticin (G418) [21]. The HepG2 cell line was grown in complete Eagle's minimal essential medium and used for transfection with HCV genotype 2A (JFH1; Japanese fulminant hepatitis) RNA.

Western Blot analysis

Equivalent amounts of protein extracts were run on a 4–12% gradient polyacrylamide gel (Invitrogen). Separated proteins were transferred to nitrocellulose membranes, which were probed with specific antibodies and developed using the enhanced chemiluminescence detection system (GE Healthcare, Piscataway, NJ).

Quantitative reverse-transcriptase polymerase chain reaction (RT-PCR)

RNA extraction and real-time PCR for CTGF and TGF-β1 were performed as described before [22]. Briefly, total RNA was extracted from the Huh 7.5 or Huh7.5-FL cells, first-strand cDNA synthesized and real-time PCR reactions performed using SYBR Green Master Mix kit (Applied Biosystems, Forster City, CA). The sequences of the primers used were: CTGF forward primer: AATGCTGCGAGGAGTGGGT; CTGF reverse primer: CGGCTCTAATC ATAGTTGGGTCT; TGF-β1 forward primer: ACCTGAACCCGTGTTGCTCT; TGF-β1 reverse primer: CTAAGGCGAAA GCCCTCAAT; GAPDH forward primer: TGCACCACCAACTGCTTAGC; GAPDH reverse primer: GGCATGGACTGTGGTCATGAG; TGF-β RI forward primer ATTACCTGGACATCGGCA AC; TGF-β RI reverse primer TTGGGCACCACATCATAGAA (Operon Biotechnology, Huntsville, AL). Negative controls were a non-reverse transcriptase reaction or a non-sample reaction. GAPDH was amplified as an internal standard.

ELISA assays

Conditioned medium (DMEM containing 0.5% FCS) from Huh 7.5 or Huh7.5-FL cells were collected at different time points, centrifuged and the supernatant used for determination of biologically active TGF-β1 protein by ELISA (BD Biosciences) according to the manufacturer's instructions.

Immunofluorescence

Fixed cells were stained with primary antibodies including NH1 anti-CTGF IgY (5 μg/ml) [23], HCV NS5B, NS4A; Core or anti-TGF-β1 (1:200, Santa Cruz) followed by incubation with secondary antibodies Alexa Fluor® 568 goat-anti chicken IgY (1:1000) or Alexa Fluor® 568 goat-anti rabbit IgG (1:400) or Alexa Fluor® 488 goat-anti mouse IgG (1:400) (Invitrogen). The cells were mounted with Vectashield Mounting Medium containing DAPI (Vector Laboratories, Burlingame, CA), and examined by confocal laser microscopy (LSM510, Carl Zeiss, Jena, Germany).

Transfections and DNA Constructs

To transfect HepG2 cells with full length JFH1 RNA, pJFH1-pUC plasmid (Apath, LLC) as a DNA template and MEGAscript T7 RNA synthesis kit (Applied Biosystems) were used. 5 μg of RNA was transfected into HepG2 cells using Nucleofector V solution in an Amaxa nucleofector device (program no. T-028). Cell lysates were collected at various time points and used for the analysis of multiple proteins by Western blot analysis.

To determine Smad-dependent CTGF promoter activity, Huh7.5 and Huh7.5-FL cells were transfected with plasmids containing a secreted alkaline phosphatase (SEAP) reporter gene fused to either the wild type CTGF promoter (nucleotides −805 to +17) or individual point mutants targeting the Smad site or the basal control element (BCE-1) using Lipofectamine ™ 2000 (Invitrogen). Promoter/reporter constructs contained CCN2 promoter fragments spanning nucleotides −805 to +17 (wild type promoter) and mutations in the Smad element (TCAGA to GGATC) and GGAA element (GGAAT to TCCCG) introduced into the CCN2 promoter between nucleotides −805 to +17, but were otherwise identical to construct −805.

SEAP reporter activity was calculated after adjustment for differences among samples in transfection efficiency as determined by co-transfection with a cytomegalovirus (CMV) promoter-β-galactosidase (CMV-β-gal) reporter gene. CTGF-SEAP promoter activity assays were performed with Phospha-Light kit and β-galactosidase expression was determined by Galacto-star kit (Applied Biosystems). SEAP levels were measured using an LMax II 384 luminometer (Molecular Devices, Sunnyvale, CA).

ShRNA-mediated suppression of TGF-β1 or CTGF

Human TGF-β1 5′-ACGAGC CCTGG ACACCAACTAT-3′(sense) and 3′- ATAGTTGG TGTCCAGGGCTCGG 5′ (antisense) or CTGF 5′-CCAGCACCAGAATGTATATTAA-3′(sense) and 3′- TTAATATACATTCTGGTG CTGT-5′ (antisense) GIPZ lentiviral shRNA plasmids or negative scrambled shRNA (Open Biosystems, Huntsville, AL) were transfected into Huh7.5 or Huh7.5-FL cells using Lipofectamine ^{TM} 2000 according to the manufacturer's instructions. Transfection efficiency was monitored by co-transfection with the green fluorescent protein (GFP)-expressing plasmid, pEGFP (Invitrogen).

Cultivation of Human hepatic stellate cells (LX2 cells) with conditioned medium from Huh7.5 and Huh7.5-FL cells

To analyze the role of profibrogenic cytokines in the supernatants of Huh7.5 and Huh7.5-FL on HSCs, we incubated hepatic stellate cells (LX2) with the respective supernatants for 48 hrs, after which the HSCs were lysed and analyzed for procollagen I. LX2 cells were kindly provided by Dr. Scott Friedman (Mount Sinai School of Medicine, New York).

Statistical analysis

All the experiments were carried out in triplicate or quadruplicate. Each set of experiments was repeated at least three times with similar results in each case. Representative graphical data are presented as mean ± standard deviation. Student's t test for paired samples was used to determine statistical significance. Differences were considered significant at $p \leq 0.05$.

Results

Demonstration of active HCV replication in the HCV culture system

Firstly, we validated the presence of active HCV at the protein level in Huh7.5-FL cells stably expressing genome-length HCV. The expression of core and NS4A protein in Huh7.5-FL cells was shown by confocal microscopy (Fig. 1A) and Western blot analysis (Fig. 1B). We also validated the findings with another HCV culture system by transfecting the JFH-1 (HCV genotype-2) RNA into the HepG2 cells. The expression of HCV NS5B and core protein in HepG2 cells was confirmed by Western blot (Fig. 1C) and confocal microscopy (Fig. 1D).

CTGF expression and secretion is increased in HCV-infected hepatocytes

We first evaluated the expression of CTGF in Huh7.5 or Huh7.5-FL cells after incubation in conditioned medium (DMEM containing 0.5% FCS). After 32 hours, Huh7.5-FL cells showed a 7-fold higher expression of CTGF mRNA levels by quantitative real time-PCR (RT-PCR) in comparison to the Huh7.5 cells (Fig. 2A). The presence of a 38 kDa CTGF band in the medium

was significantly higher in Huh7.5-FL cells versus Huh7.5 cells as assessed by Western blot analysis (Fig. 2B). In addition, we demonstrated increased levels of cellular CTGF protein in Huh7.5-FL cells at 48 hours by confocal microscopy (Fig. 2C). Furthermore, we also used HepG2 cells transfected with the HCV genotype 2 (JFH1) RNA to evaluate CTGF expression. Western blot analysis of cell lysates and confocal microscopy of immuno-stained cells indicated that CTGF production was enhanced in JFH1-expressing cells, as compared to the control cells (Fig. 2D and E), thus verifying that CTGF production was stimulated in hepatocytes expressing HCV.

CTGF mediates HCV-induced expression of fibrotic markers

In the present study, we evaluated the expression of α-smooth muscle antigen (α-SMA), matrix-metalloprotease-2 (MMP-2), vimentin and slug in Huh7.5-FL cells. As compared to Huh7.5 cells, the Huh7.5-FL cells expressed higher levels of α-SMA, vimentin and slug, and showed reduced levels of MMP-2 activity (50% reduction) (Fig. 3A) at the end of the 96-hour culture period. We also evaluated the expression of α-SMA in HepG2 cells transfected with JFH1 RNA and found increased levels of α-SMA in comparison to the controls (Fig. 3B). As shown in Figure 3C, procollagen I was upregulated in Huh7.5-FL cells, but this was abrogated in cells transfected with CTGF shRNA plasmid, as compared to the scrambled shRNA transfected cells, demonstrating that CTGF directly mediates the production of procollagen.

HCV-induced CTGF expression is TGF-β1 dependent

Several studies have shown that TGF-β1 is an important mediator of CTGF expression in various cell types [10,24]. Hence, we evaluated the role of TGF-β1 in CTGF production by determining TGF-β1 mRNA and protein expression in Huh7.5 or Huh7.5-FL cells after various periods of incubation in conditioned medium. As compared to Huh7.5 cells, TGF-β1 mRNA was enhanced approximately 4-fold in Huh7.5-FL cells as assessed by quantitative RT-PCR (Fig. 4A). Furthermore, substantially higher amounts of active TGF-β1 were present in the conditioned media from Huh7.5-FL cells as compared to Huh7.5 cells at 24, 48 and 72 hours of culture in conditioned medium (Fig. 4B). Similarly, supernatant from HepG2 cells transfected with JFH1 RNA showed increased active TGF-β compared to control samples (Fig. 4C). We also confirmed the enhanced expression of TGF-β1 precursor in Huh7.5-FL versus Huh7.5 cells by confocal microscopy (Fig. 4D). In addition, we analyzed the expression of TGF-β1 precursor in HepG2 cells transfected with JFH1 RNA. Figure 4E shows the enhanced expression of TGF-β1 precursor in JFH1-transfected HepG2 cells by confocal microscopy.

To establish the functional significance of TGF-β1 in CTGF production, Huh7.5 or Huh7.5-FL cells were transfected with either TGF-β1 or non-targeting shRNA plasmid. This treatment resulted in diminished TGF-β1 precursor protein levels in cell lysates, as expected, but also a concomitant decrease in CTGF secretion (Fig. 5A). Furthermore, treatment of the Huh7.5-FL cells with TGF-β1 neutralizing antibody resulted in highly diminished CTGF levels in conditioned medium (Fig. 5B). Taken together, these data indicated that elevated CTGF expression in HCV-infected hepatocytes is mediated through TGF-β1. As shown in Figure 5A (third panel), upregulation of procollagen I was abrogated in Huh7.5-FL cells transfected with TGF-β1 shRNA when compared with Huh7.5-FL cells transfected with scrambled shRNA. We further analyzed the role of profibrogenic cytokines on fibrotic marker expression in HSCs. Conditioned medium from Huh7.5 and Huh7.5FL cells were cocultured along with LX2

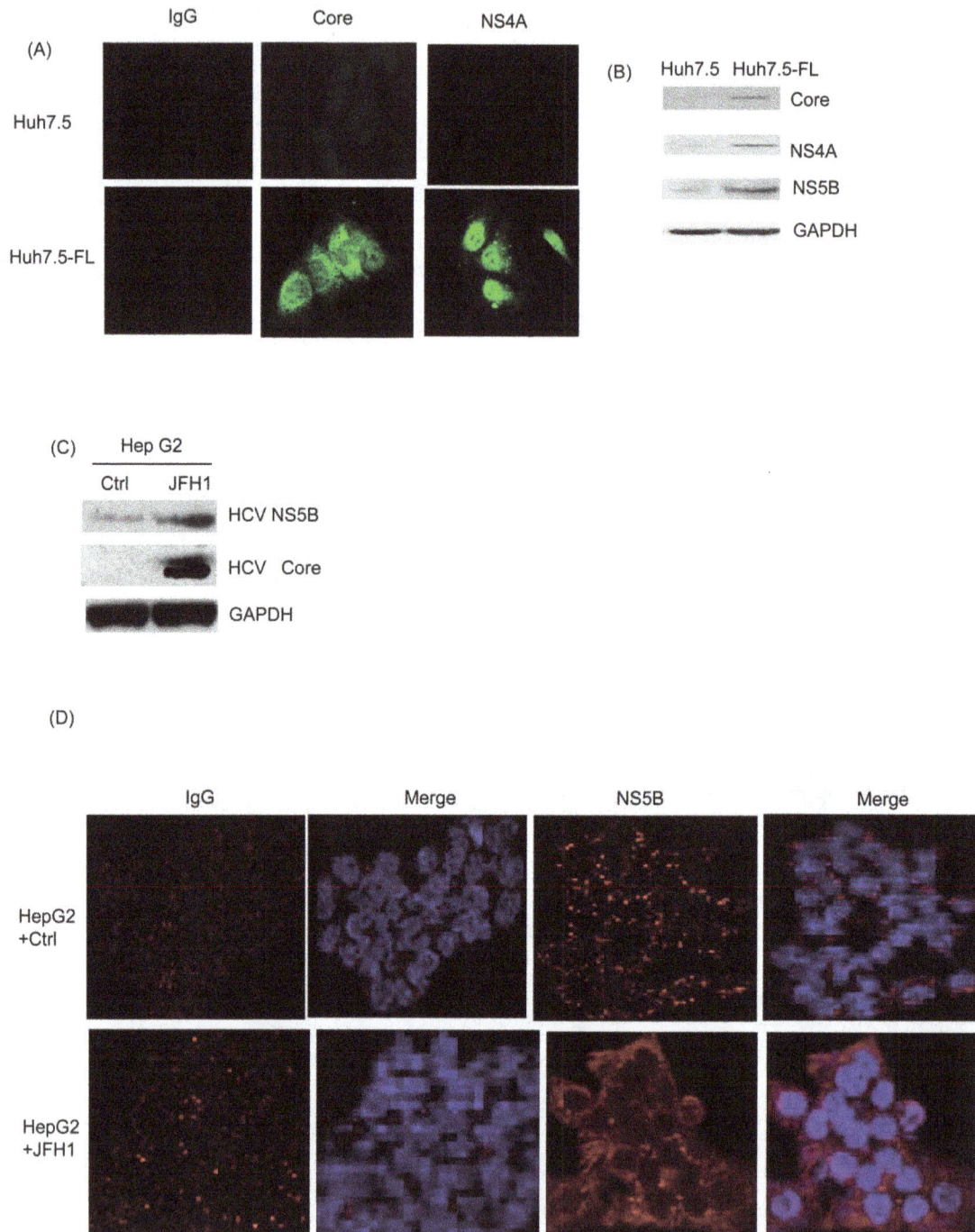

Figure 1. Detection of active HCV replication in HCV-infected cell lines. (**A**) Huh7.5 or Huh7.5-FL cells grown for 48 h were stained with antibodies against HCV proteins (HCV core or NS4A), followed by FITC-coupled secondary antibodies and detected using confocal microscopy. (**B**) Lysates of cells grown for 48 hours were analyzed for expression of HCV core, NS4A or NS5B by Western blotting. HepG2 cells were transfected with JFH-1 RNA and expression of HCV NS5B and core protein was analyzed by Western blotting (**C**) and confocal microscopy respectively (**D**). Equal protein loading in the Western blot analyses was verified using GAPDH antibody. Data are from one of three independent experiments performed in triplicate.

(Hepatic stellate cell line). As shown in figure 5C, we observed nearly two fold increase of procollagen I in LX2 cells incubated with medium from Huh7.5-FL cells compared to LX2 cells incubated with medium from Huh 7.5 cells.

Signaling pathways that mediate HCV-induced CTGF-production via TGF-β1

We further explored the HCV-induced signaling mechanisms that mediate CTGF expression downstream of TGF-β1 in Huh7.5-FL cells. Previous studies have shown that TGF-β1 mediates its functional effects by binding to the TGF-β1-receptor

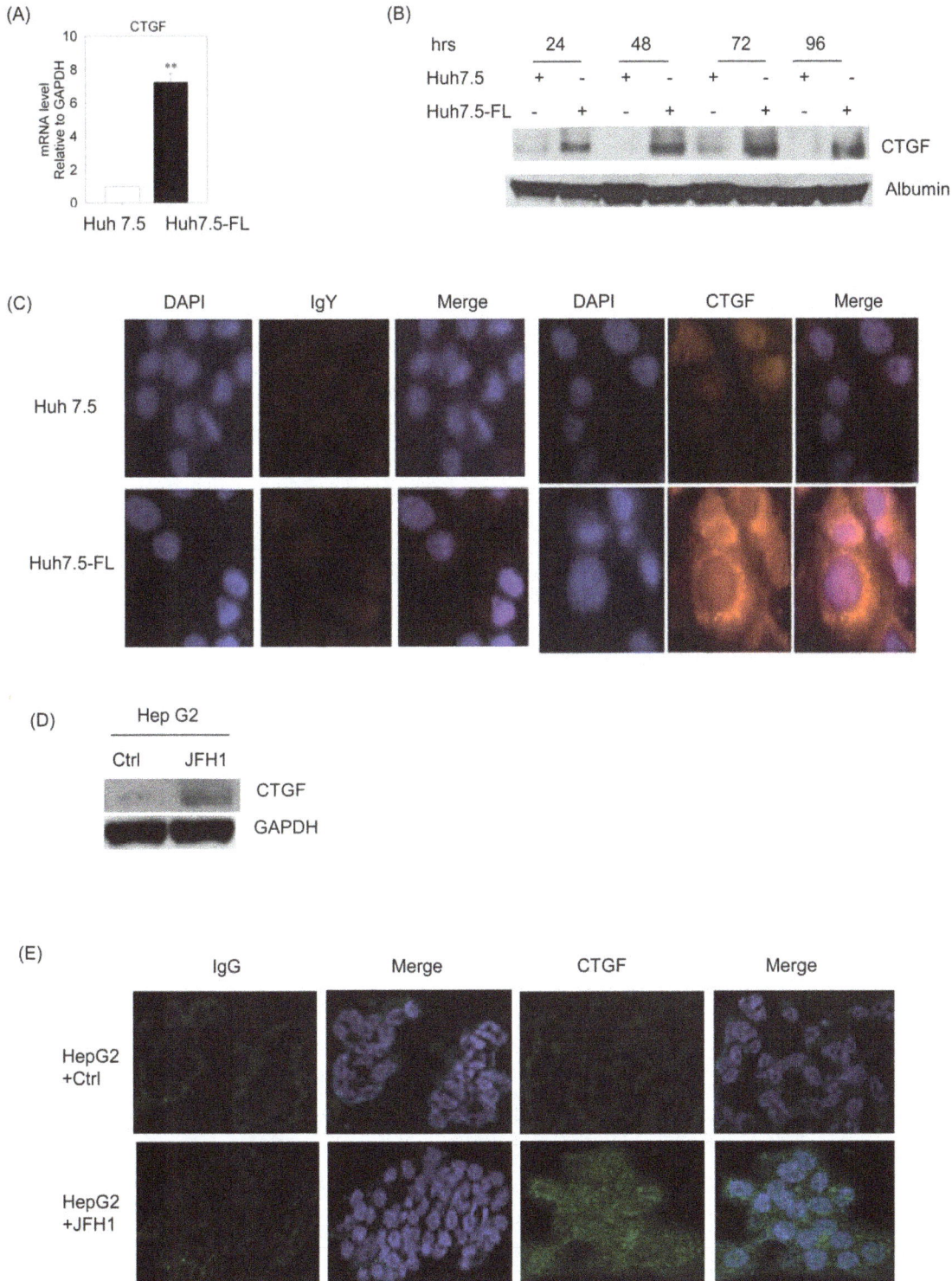

Figure 2. HCV induces CTGF expression in Huh7.5-FL cells. (A) RNA from Huh7.5 or Huh7.5-FL cells was used in the SYBR green real-time PCR to analyze CTGF expression. ** P<0.001 versus Huh7.5 cells. (B) Conditioned medium from Huh7.5 or Huh7.5-FL cells incubated for various time periods was collected, concentrated and equal amounts of protein subjected to SDS-PAGE and analyzed for CTGF by Western blotting. Albumin was used as a internal control. (C) Huh7.5 or Huh7.5-FL cells were grown for 48 hours, after which the cells were fixed, permeabilized and treated with anti-CTGF followed by FITC-coupled secondary antibodies and examined using an Olympus FV1000 confocal microscope. HepG2 cells were transfected with JFH1 RNA and CTGF expression was analyzed by (D) Western blotting and (E) confocal microscopy respectively. Equal protein loading was verified using antibodies against GAPDH. Data represent mean ± SD of 3 independent experiments.

(A)

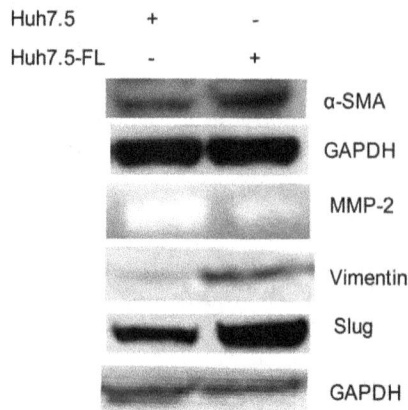

(B)

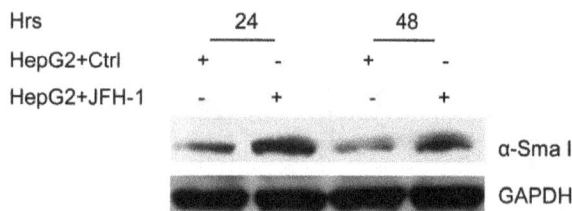

(C)

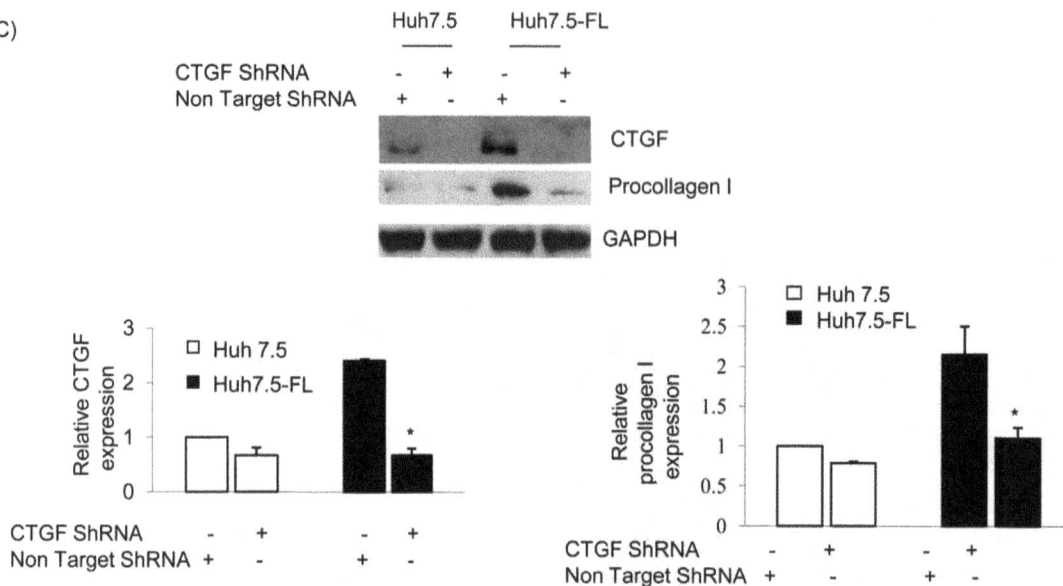

Figure 3. CTGF stimulates the expression of fibrotic markers in Huh7.5-FL cells. (**A**) Huh7.5 or Huh7.5-FL cells were incubated in conditioned medium (medium containing 0.5%FCS) for ninety-six hours and the cell lysates were blotted to examine α-SMA expression, vimentin and slug expression. Equal protein loading was verified using GAPDH antibody. The conditioned medium was used for the measurement of MMP-2 activity by zymography assay. (**B**) HepG2 cells were transfected with or without JFH-1RNA for different time points and cell lysates were blotted for α-Sma I protein. GAPDH was used as an internal control. (**C**) Lysates of Huh7.5 or Huh7.5-FL cells transfected with non targeting or CTGF shRNA for 48 hrs were blotted for CTGF, procollagen I or GAPDH. The bar graphs show the quantitative analysis of CTGF or procollagen I expression relative to that of GAPDH. * P≤0.05 versus Huh7.5-FL cells. Data represent mean ± SD of 3 independent experiments.

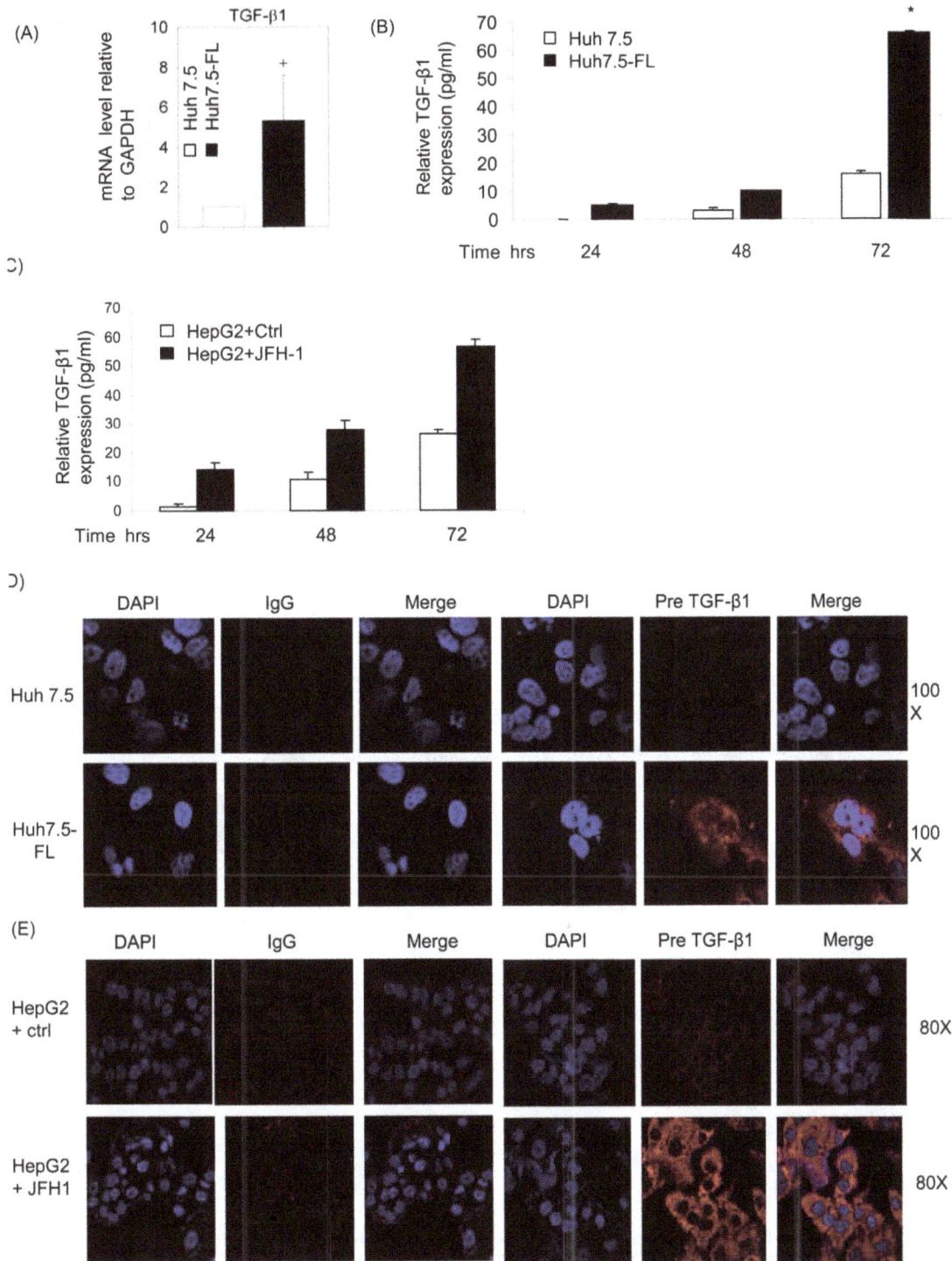

Figure 4. HCV induces TGF-β1 expression in Huh7.5-FL cells. (**A**) RNA was extracted from Huh7.5 or Huh7.5-FL cells which were incubated in conditioned medium for 32 hrs were used in SYBR green real-time PCR to analyze TGF-β1. + P<0.05 versus Huh7.5 control. (**B**) Huh7.5 or Huh7.5-FL cells were incubated for various time points and active TGF-β1 was measured in the culture supernatants by ELISA. * P≤0.05 versus Huh7.5 cells. (**C**) HepG2 cells were transfected with or without JFH-1 RNA and supernatants were collected at different time points to measure the TGF-β1 concentration in supernatant by ELISA. (**D**) Huh7.5 or Huh7.5-FL cells were fixed, permeabilized and stained with TGF-β1 antibody followed by FITC-coupled secondary antibody, and examined by confocal microscopy. (**E**) HepG2 cells transfected with or without JFH1 RNA were analyzed for TGF-β1 expression by confocal microscopy. Data are from one of three independent experiments performed in triplicate.

complex and activating the Smad-dependent pathway. In the present study, we demonstrated the increased expression of TGF-β1 receptor I (TGFβR1/ALK5) in Huh7.5-FL cells and also in

HepG2 cells transfected with JFH-1 RNA over the first 36 hours of culture by Western blot (Fig. 6A & 6D) and RT-PCR (Fig. 6B). To assess whether this difference was reflected in downstream

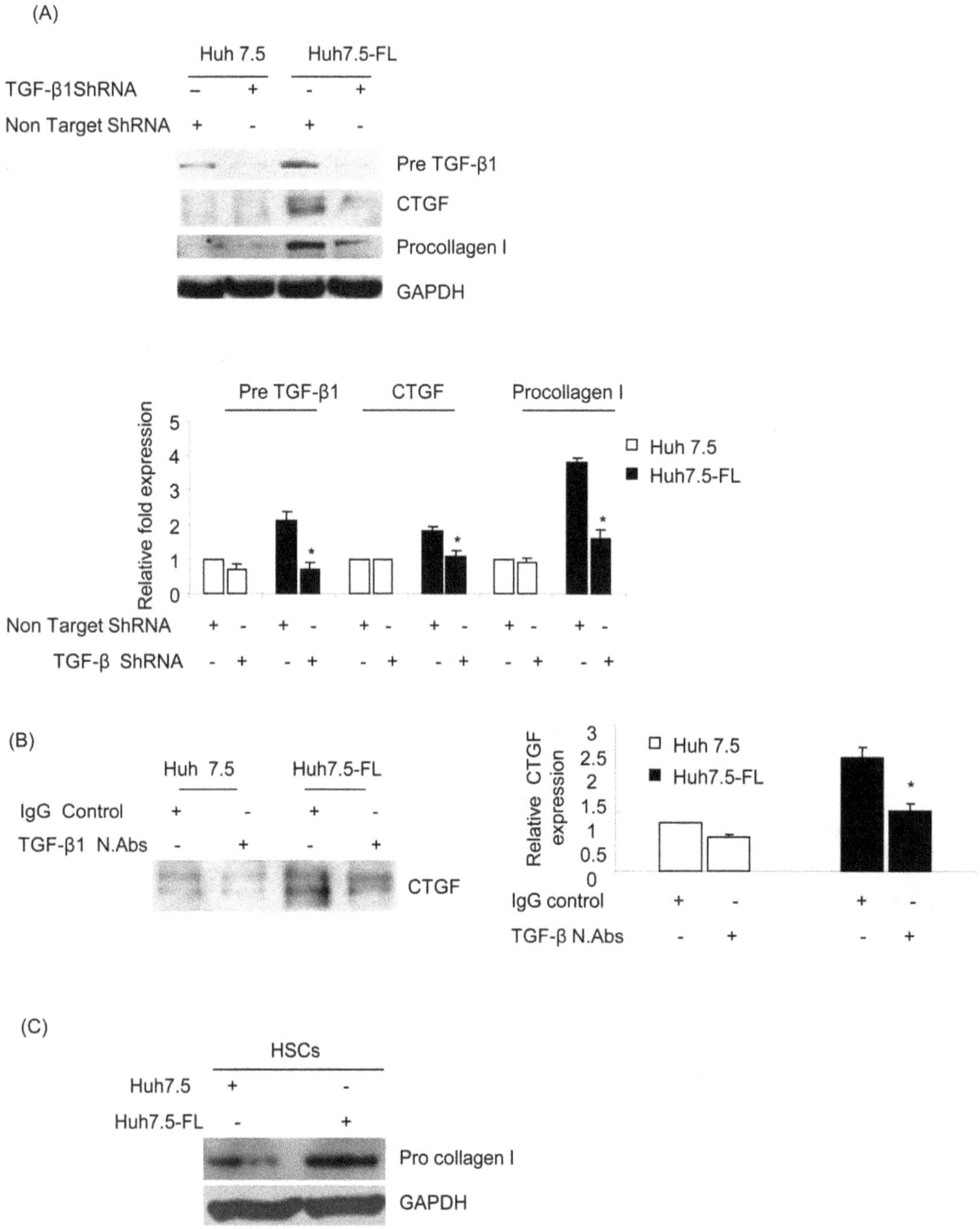

(A)

(B)

(C)

Figure 5. HCV-induced CTGF expression is TGF-β1-dependent. (A) Lysates of Huh7.5 or Huh7.5-FL cells transfected with non-targeting or TGF-β1 ShRNA for 48 hrs were blotted to determine expression of TGF-β1, CTGF or procollagen I (upper panel). Equal protein loading was determined using GAPDH antibody. The bar graph shows the quantitative analysis of TGF-β1, CTGF or procollagen I expression relative to that of GAPDH (lower panel). * P≤0.05 versus Huh7.5-FL cells. **(B)** Medium from Huh7.5 or Huh7.5-FL cells incubated for 48 hrs with anti-TGF-β1 or non-immune IgG was collected, concentrated and equal amounts of protein were used for Western blot analysis using CTGF antibody (upper panel). The bar graph shows the quantitative analysis of CTGF expression obtained by densitometry (lower panel). * P≤0.05 versus Huh7.5 cells. **(C)** Human hepatic stellate cells (LX2 cells) were co cultured with medium from Huh7.5 and Huh7.5-FL cells for 48 hrs and cell lysates were analyzed for procollagen I expression. GAPDH was used as an internal control. For all experiments, data represent mean ± SD of 3 independent experiments.

signaling events, we evaluated phosphorylation of Smad2 and Smad3 in Huh7.5 and Huh7.5-FL cells. We observed a significant increase in Smad2 and Smad3 phosphorylation in Huh7.5FL cells compared to Huh 7.5 cells (Fig. 6C) after various time points of incubation in conditioned medium. Previous studies in other cell

types showed that TGF-β-mediated induction of CTGF mRNA relies on the functional Smad element in the CTGF promoter and that, while the BCE-1 site is involved with basal CTGF promoter activity, it is also indirectly responsive to TGF-β since it is a

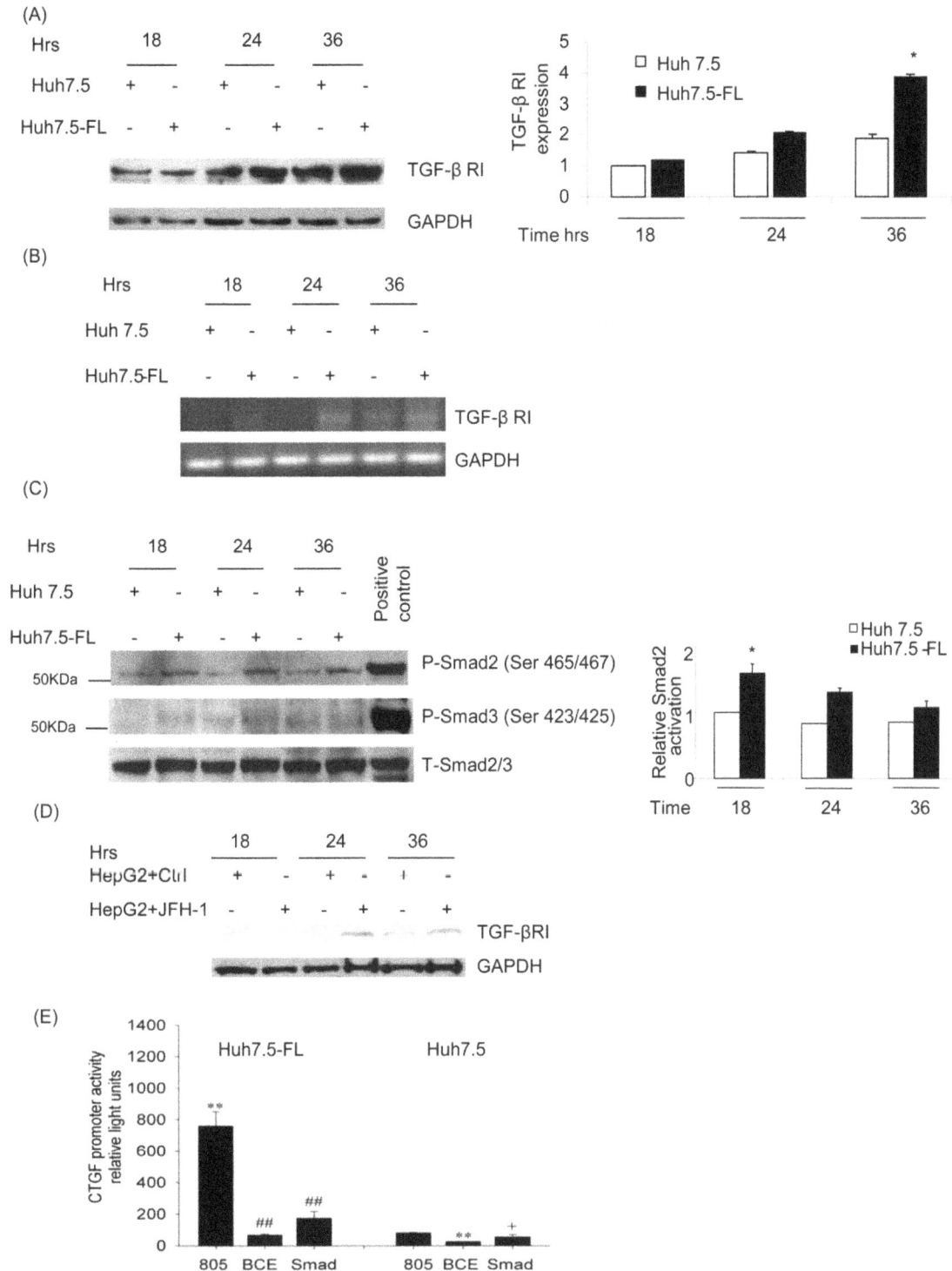

Figure 6. Expression of CTGF in Huh7.5-FL cells is Smad-dependent. Cell lysates from Huh7.5 or Huh7.5-FL cells were collected at different time points and blotted with anti-TGF-βRI (**A**) or phospho-Smad 2, phospho-Smad3 and total Smad2/3 antibodies (**C**). The bar graphs show the quantitative analyses of TGF-β RI and p-smad2 protein expression as obtained by densitometry. RNA from Huh7.5 or Huh7.5-FL cells was used in the reverse transcriptase PCR to analyze the TGF-β RI expression (**B**). (**D**) HepG2 cells were transfected with and without JFH-1 RNA. The cell lysates were collected at different time points and blotted for TGF-βRI. (**E**) Huh7.5 and Huh7.5-FL cells were transfected with different CTGF promoter/SEAP reporter constructs for 48 hrs. CTGF promoter activity was determined by measuring SEAP reporter expression. ** $P<0.001$ versus Huh7.5 cells; + $P<0.05$ versus Huh7.5 cells; and ## $P<0.001$ versus Huh7.5-FL cells. Data represent mean $\pm$ SD of 3 independent experiments.

(A)

(B)

(C)

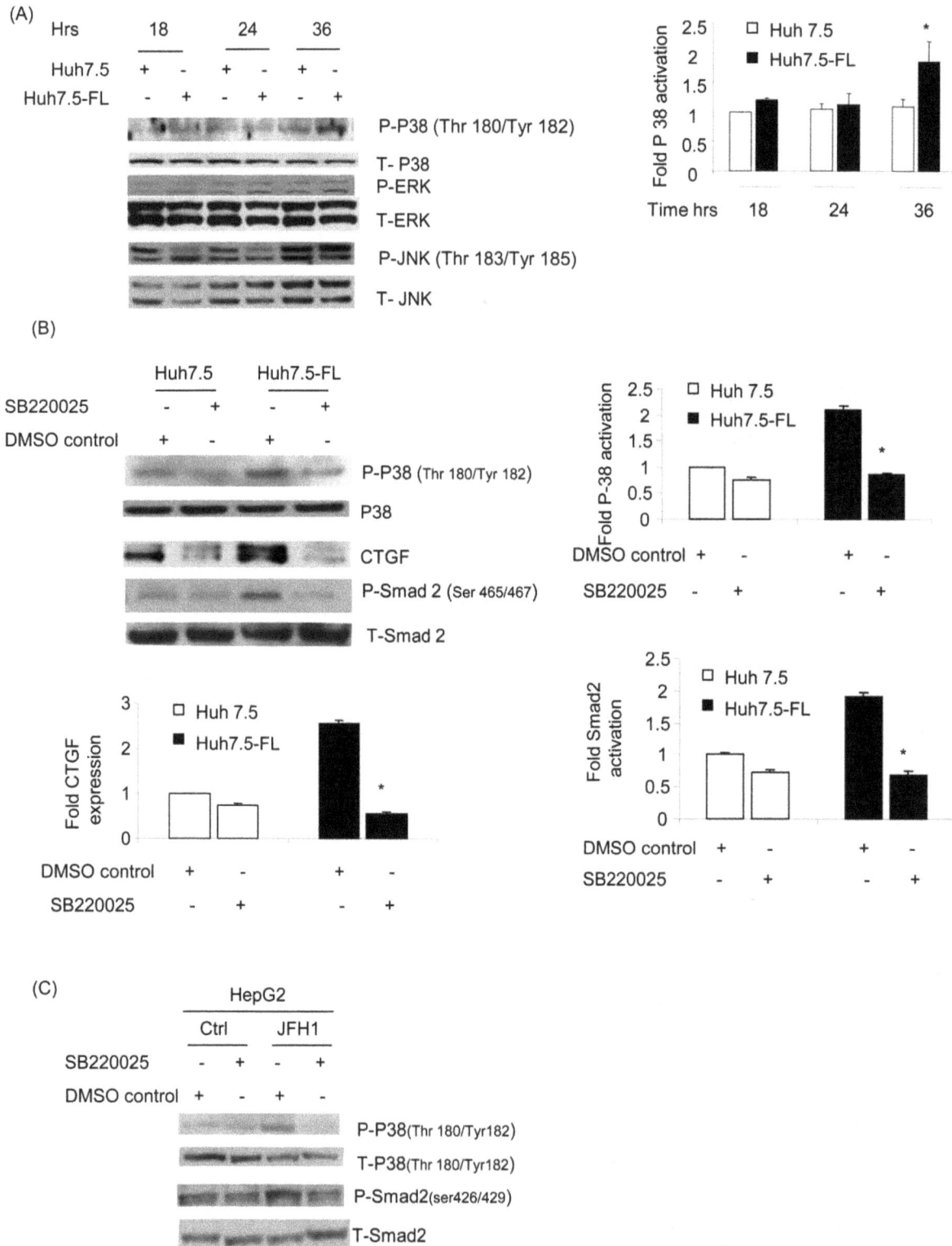

Figure 7. p38 MAP kinase mediates CTGF expression in Huh7.5-FL cells. (A) Lysates from Huh7.5 or Huh7.5-FL cells collected at the indicated time points were blotted with Phospho-p38, Phospho-JNK, Phospho-ERK, p38, JNK and ERK antibodies. The bar graph shows the quantitative analysis of p38 activation relative to the total p38 production assessed by densitometry. * $P \leq 0.05$ versus Huh7.5 cells. (B) Huh7.5 or Huh7.5-FL cells were pretreated with p38 MAPkinase inhibitor (SB220025; 50 μM) for 36 hours, after which cells were lysed and blotted with antibodies to phospho-p38, p38, CTGF, Phospho-Smad2, or Smad2. The bar graph shows the quantitative analysis of the data obtained by densitometry (left panel). * $P \leq 0.05$ versus Huh7.5-FL cells. (C) Similarly HepG2 cells were transfected with and without JFH1 RNA and cells were treated with p38 MAPkinase inhibitor (SB220025) for 24 hrs ,after which the cell lysates were analyzed for activation of p38 and Smad2. Data represent mean ± SD of 3 independent experiments.

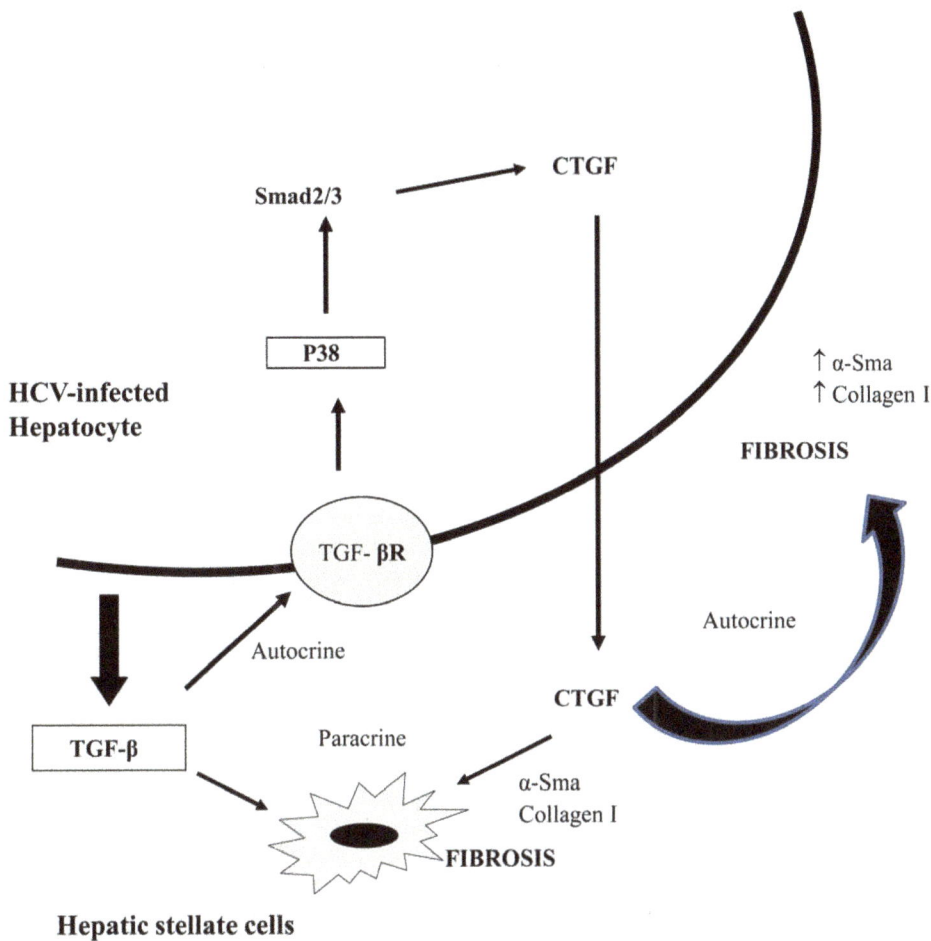

Figure 8. Proposed hypothesis on the role of CTGF in HCV-induced liver fibrosis. We hypothesize that HCV infection in hepatocytes induces TGF-β1 expression. TGF-β1, in turn mediates an enhanced expression of profibrogenic cytokine CTGF through Smad phosphorylation and p38 MAP kinase activation. CTGF may further act in a paracrine manner on hepatic stellate cells (HSCs) or in an autocrine manner on hepatocytes and drive expression of fibrotic markers including collagen and α-Sma.

response element for endothelin 1 which is induced by TGF-β and is essential for TGF-β to induce CTGF [25,26].

Next, to determine the elements in the CTGF promoter involved downstream of HCV-induced TGF-β1, we transfected Huh7.5 or Huh7.5-FL cells with CTGF promoter reporters that were either wild-type (805) or that contained point mutations in either the BCE-1 (a response element that is indirectly regulated by TGF-β1) or the Smad binding site (which is directly controlled by TGF-β1). First, we found that the level of wild-type CTGF promoter activity in lysates from the Huh7.5-FL cells was approximately 10-fold higher than in those from Huh7.5 cells (Fig. 6E), consistent with earlier data showing enhanced CTGF mRNA and protein production in the Huh7.5-FL cells (Fig. 2). Secondly, the mutant promoter activities were substantially attenuated, an effect that was particularly evident in the Huh7.5-FL cells, resulting in reduction in activity of 95% or 90% respectively (Fig. 6E).

We next investigated the involvement of the major MAPkinase pathways previously implicated in TGF-β1-induced signaling in hepatocytes. We found that p38 MAPkinase was significantly activated in Huh7.5-FL cells in comparison to the Huh7.5 cells, as demonstrated by an increase in phosphorylation at 36 hours (Fig. 7A) of incubation in conditioned medium. There was no major increase in the HCV-induced activation of JNK and ERK

1/2 in Huh7.5-FL cells, as compared to Huh7.5 cells (Fig. 7A). To further investigate the importance of p38 MAPkinase in HCV-induced CTGF production, Huh7.5 or Huh7.5-FL cells were pre-treated with SB220025, a pharmacologic inhibitor of p38 MAPkinase. The reduction in p38 MAPkinase activation (Fig. 7B, first panel) was associated with a concomitant decrease in CTGF protein in conditioned medium (Fig. 7B, third panel). These data clearly suggest the involvement of p38 MAPkinases in HCV-induced CTGF production. Furthermore, we analyzed the cross-talk between p38 MAPkinase and the Smad pathway. We found that Huh7.5-FL cells showed reduced Smad2 phosphorylation in the presence of the specific p38 MAPkinase inhibitor, when compared to control Huh7.5-FL cells (Fig. 7B, panels 4 and 5). To further confirm the role of p38 MAPkinase inhibitor, we used HepG2 cells transfected with control and JFH-1 RNA. As shown in Figure 7C, we also observed significant reduction of p-p38 as well as p-Smad2 in JFH-1 transfected cells. This finding indicates that the phosphorylation of Smad proteins is regulated by p38 MAP kinase. Together, these studies indicate that CTGF production occurs downstream of TGF-β1 and involves a signaling pathway consisting of p38 MAPkinase and Smad group of proteins.

Discussion

HCV infection is among the leading causes of chronic liver disease. Approximately one third of patients with chronic HCV infection develop significant fibrosis, and many of them develop cirrhosis with a high risk of hepatic decompensation or development of HCC [1]. However, very little is known about the mechanisms by which the virus causes hepatic fibrosis. In this study, we have elucidated for the first time the molecular mechanism of CTGF expression and its role as a mediator of fibrogenesis during HCV infection.

Previously, investigations into the pathogenesis of HCV have been hampered by the lack of *in vitro* and appropriate *in vivo* model systems. However, in the past decade, the establishment of HCV replicons and an infectious cell culture model have allowed for a better understanding of the viral life cycle, pathogenesis of HCV infection and development of antiviral strategies. These two model systems have been widely used to analyze the HCV-mediated mechanisms that lead to liver damage [21,27]. In the present study, we have shown enhanced expression of CTGF in Huh7.5-FL replicon cells (HCV genotype I) in comparison to Huh7.5 cells. Several previous studies have compared Huh7.5-FL and Huh7.5 cells to study HCV pathogenic mechanisms [28,29]. In addition, we also used HepG2 cells transfected with JFH1 (HCV genotype 2) to demonstrate increased CTGF expression. Of the six HCV genotypes, viable replicons have been reported for genotype 1 and 2 strains [30]. Hence, we have confirmed increased CTGF expression with both HCV genotypes 1 and 2.

CTGF is a multi-functional protein that drives many cellular processes, but has received special focus with respect to its fibrotic actions in several organs systems. In our study, we have shown that CTGF mediates enhanced expression of fibrotic markers during HCV infection. Specifically, increased expression of several fibrotic markers were observed in Huh7.5-FL cells and CTGF shRNA was effective in reducing procollagen I expression. CTGF produced in response to HCV may act locally on non-parenchymal cells, such as HSCs or myofibroblasts as well as hepatocytes to enhance expression of markers that are associated with fibrosis. Though recent studies have indicated an association between CTGF immunostaining intensity and stage of fibrosis in patients with chronic HCV infection and high levels of CTGF in plasma and liver biopsy samples of HCV infected patients [11,15], we provide for the first time, clear evidence for the role of CTGF-induced expression of fibrotic markers in HCV infection. Our findings demonstrating increased CTGF expression in HCV-infected hepatocytes also underscore the importance of hepatocytes in producing CTGF during HCV infection. Previous studies have indicated the contribution of parenchymal liver cells to CTGF production in normal and diseased liver [14,24].

We also investigated the signaling and transcriptional regulatory pathways involved in CTGF expression in HCV-infected hepatocytes. CTGF expression in fibrotic tissue is shown to be either TGF-β1-dependent or independent [10,24,31]. Our results show that TGF-β1 upregulates CTGF expression in HCV-infected hepatocytes. The mechanism involved in HCV-induced TGF-β1 production has been well studied. HCV has been shown to regulate TGF-β1 expression by modulating Ca^{2+} signaling and generation of reactive oxygen species (ROS), which acts through p38 MAP kinase, ERK and JNK and NF-k-B signaling pathways to induce TGF-β1 [32,33]. In the present study, we demonstrate the downstream mediators of TGF-β1 that induce CTGF production. TGF- β1 is known to mediate its functional effects through the Smad group of proteins. We have shown increased phosphorylation of Smad2 in Huh7.5-FL as well as in JFH-1 transfected HepG2 cells compared to control cells. We further demonstrated that TGF-β1-mediated CTGF- production in Huh7.5-FL cells was Smad-dependent as reduced activity was observed in CTGF promoter reporters in which the Smad or BCE sites were mutated. This is in agreement with recent studies which indicate that TGF-β1-driven CTGF gene expression in other cell types is dependent upon a functional Smad element in the CTGF promoter as well as a BCE element which responds indirectly to TGF-β1 [25]. MAPkinases are downstream signaling partners of TGF-β1 and recently MAPK signaling has been shown to directly regulate CTGF expression in fibroblasts [34]. We showed that activation of p38 MAPkinase, but not of JNK kinase or ERK kinase, is important in HCV-induced CTGF production. Previously, p38 MAPkinase was shown to be enhanced in HepG2 cells transfected with HCV core protein [13]. Together, these findings suggest HCV may mediate CTGF production by modulating Smad and p38 MAPkinase dependent pathways.

Based on our studies, we propose a HCV-induced fibrotic pathway in hepatocytes whereby there is an enhanced expression of profibrogenic cytokine CTGF mediated by TGF-β1 through Smad phosphorylation and p38 MAP kinase activation. CTGF, in turn, may act in a paracrine manner on hepatic stellate cells (HSCs) or in an autocrine manner on hepatocytes and drive expression of fibrotic markers including collagen (Fig. 8). Collectively, our data support a role for CTGF as a downstream mediator of the fibrogenic actions of TGF-β1 in promotion of ECM production. The beneficial effect of CTGF knockdown by gene silencing through shRNA has been shown independently in two models of rat liver fibrosis [35,36]. Our studies underscore the importance of CTGF in HCV-mediated fibrotic pathology and may facilitate the development of anti-fibrotic strategies in chronic-HCV infected patients.

Acknowledgments

We would like to thank Dr. Wakita (NIID, Japan) and Apath LLC (USA) for providing the HCV virus JFH1 plasmid DNA. We would also like to thank Dr. Scott Friedman for providing us the LX2 cells.

Author Contributions

Conceived and designed the experiments: TN LC AB JEG KG STJ DRB ARA RKG. Performed the experiments: TN LC AB. Analyzed the data: TN LC DRB ARA RKG. Contributed reagents/materials/analysis tools: AL. Wrote the paper: TN LC DRB ARA RKG.

References

1. Zoulim F, Chevallier M, Maynard M, Trepo C (2003) Clinical consequences of hepatitis C virus infection. Rev Med Virol 13: 57–68.
2. Gressner AM, Weiskirchen R, Breitkopf K, Dooley S (2002) Roles of TGF-beta in hepatic fibrosis. Front Biosci 7: d793–807.
3. Rachfal AW, Brigstock DR (2003) Connective tissue growth factor (CTGF/CCN2) in hepatic fibrosis. Hepatol Res 26: 1–9.
4. Brigstock DR (2002) Regulation of angiogenesis and endothelial cell function by connective tissue growth factor (CTGF) and cysteine-rich 61 (CYR61). Angiogenesis 5: 153–165.

5. Gao R, Brigstock DR (2006) A novel integrin alpha5beta1 binding domain in module 4 of connective tissue growth factor (CCN2/CTGF) promotes adhesion and migration of activated pancreatic stellate cells. Gut 55: 856–862.
6. Ponticos M, Holmes AM, Shi-wen X, Leoni P, Khan K, et al. (2009) Pivotal role of connective tissue growth factor in lung fibrosis: MAPK-dependent transcriptional activation of type I collagen. Arthritis Rheum 60: 2142–2155.
7. Surveyor GA, Brigstock DR (1999) Immunohistochemical localization of connective tissue growth factor (CTGF) in the mouse embryo between days 7.5 and 14.5 of gestation. Growth Factors 17: 115–124.

8. Brigstock DR (1999) The connective tissue growth factor/cysteine-rich 61/ nephroblastoma overexpressed (CCN) family. Endocr Rev 20: 189–206.

9. Zhao Z, Ho L, Wang J, Qin W, Festa ED, et al. (2005) Connective tissue growth factor (CTGF) expression in the brain is a downstream effector of insulin resistance- associated promotion of Alzheimer's disease beta-amyloid neuropathology. FASEB J 19: 2081–2082.

10. Grotendorst GR, Okochi H, Hayashi N (1996) A novel transforming growth factor beta response element controls the expression of the connective tissue growth factor gene. Cell Growth Differ 7: 469–480.

11. Hora C, Negro F, Leandro G, Oneta CM, Rubbia-Brandt L, et al. (2008) Connective tissue growth factor, steatosis and fibrosis in patients with chronic hepatitis C. Liver Int 28: 370–376.

12. Paradis V, Dargere D, Vidaud M, De Gouville AC, Huet S, et al. (1999) Expression of connective tissue growth factor in experimental rat and human liver fibrosis. Hepatology 30: 968–976.

13. Shin JY, Hur W, Wang JS, Jang JW, Kim CW, et al. (2005) HCV core protein promotes liver fibrogenesis via up-regulation of CTGF with TGF-beta1. Exp Mol Med 37: 138–145.

14. Tong Z, Chen R, Alt DS, Kemper S, Perbal B, et al. (2009) Susceptibility to liver fibrosis in mice expressing a connective tissue growth factor transgene in hepatocytes. Hepatology 50: 939–947.

15. Kovalenko E, Tacke F, Gressner OA, Zimmermann HW, Lahme B, et al. (2009) Validation of connective tissue growth factor (CTGF/CCN2) and its gene polymorphisms as noninvasive biomarkers for the assessment of liver fibrosis. J Viral Hepat 16: 612–620.

16. Zeisberg M, Yang C, Martino M, Duncan MB, Rieder F, et al. (2007) Fibroblasts derive from hepatocytes in liver fibrosis via epithelial to mesenchymal transition. J Biol Chem 282: 23337–23347.

17. Dooley S, Hamzavi J, Ciuclan L, Godoy P, Ilkavets I, et al. (2008) Hepatocyte-specific Smad7 expression attenuates TGF-beta-mediated fibrogenesis and protects against liver damage. Gastroenterology 135: 642–659.

18. Nitta T, Kim JS, Mohuczy D, Behrns KE (2008) Murine cirrhosis induces hepatocyte epithelial mesenchymal transition and alterations in survival signaling pathways. Hepatology 48: 909–919.

19. Dong ZZ, Yao DF, Yao M, Qiu LW, Zong L, et al. (2008) Clinical impact of plasma TGF-beta1 and circulating TGF-beta1 mRNA in diagnosis of hepatocellular carcinoma. Hepatobiliary Pancreat Dis Int 7: 288–295.

20. Nelson DR, Gonzalez-Peralta RP, Qian K, Xu Y, Marousis CG, et al. (1997) Transforming growth factor-beta 1 in chronic hepatitis C. J Viral Hepat 4: 29–35.

21. Blight KJ, McKeating JA, Rice CM (2002) Highly permissive cell lines for subgenomic and genomic hepatitis C virus RNA replication. J Virol 76: 13001–13014.

22. Chen L, Charrier AL, Leask A, French SW, Brigstock DR (2010) Ethanol-stimulated differentiated functions of human or mouse hepatic stellate cells are mediated by connective tissue growth factor. J Hepatol.

23. Charrier AL, Brigstock DR (2010) Connective tissue growth factor production by activated pancreatic stellate cells in mouse alcoholic chronic pancreatitis. Lab Invest 90: 1179–1188.

24. Gressner OA, Lahme B, Demirci I, Gressner AM, Weiskirchen R (2007) Differential effects of TGF-beta on connective tissue growth factor (CTGF/CCN2) expression in hepatic stellate cells and hepatocytes. J Hepatol 47: 699–710.

25. Leask A, Sa S, Holmes A, Shiwen X, Black CM, et al. (2001) The control of ccn2 (ctgf) gene expression in normal and scleroderma fibroblasts. Mol Pathol 54: 180–183.

26. Shi-wen X, Kennedy L, Renzoni EA, Bou-Gharios G, du Bois RM, et al. (2007) Endothelin is a downstream mediator of profibrotic responses to transforming growth factor beta in human lung fibroblasts. Arthritis Rheum 56: 4189–4194.

27. Wakita T, Pietschmann T, Kato T, Date T, Miyamoto M, et al. (2005) Production of infectious hepatitis C virus in tissue culture from a cloned viral genome. Nat Med 11: 791–796.

28. Hall CH, Kassel R, Tacke RS, Hahn YS (2010) HCV+ hepatocytes induce human regulatory CD4+ T cells through the production of TGF-beta. PLoS One 5: e12154.

29. Miura K, Taura K, Kodama Y, Schnabl B, Brenner DA (2008) Hepatitis C virus-induced oxidative stress suppresses hepcidin expression through increased histone deacetylase activity. Hepatology 48: 1420–1429.

30. Blight KJ, Norgard EA (2006) HCV Replicon Systems.

31. Gore-Hyer E, Shegogue D, Markiewicz M, Lo S, Hazen-Martin D, et al. (2002) TGF-beta and CTGF have overlapping and distinct fibrogenic effects on human renal cells. Am J Physiol Renal Physiol 283: F707–716.

32. Lin W, Wu G, Li S, Weinberg EM, Kumthip K, et al. (2011) HIV and HCV cooperatively promote hepatic fibrogenesis via induction of reactive oxygen species and NFkappaB. J Biol Chem 286: 2665–2674.

33. Presser LD, Haskett A, Waris G (2011) Hepatitis C virus-induced furin and thrombospondin-1 activate TGF-beta1: role of TGF-beta1 in HCV replication. Virology 412: 284–296.

34. Chen Y, Blom IE, Sa S, Goldschmeding R, Abraham DJ, et al. (2002) CTGF expression in mesangial cells: involvement of SMADs, MAP kinase, and PKC. Kidney Int 62: 1149–1159.

35. Georges PC, Hui JJ, Gombos Z, McCormick ME, Wang AY, et al. (2007) Increased stiffness of the rat liver precedes matrix deposition: implications for fibrosis. Am J Physiol Gastrointest Liver Physiol 293: G1147–1154.

36. Yokoi H, Mukoyama M, Nagae T, Mori K, Suganami T, et al. (2004) Reduction in connective tissue growth factor by antisense treatment ameliorates renal tubulointerstitial fibrosis. J Am Soc Nephrol 15: 1430–1440.

10

Circulating MicroRNAs in Patients with Chronic Hepatitis C and Non-Alcoholic Fatty Liver Disease

Silvia Cermelli[1], Anna Ruggieri[1,2], Jorge A. Marrero[3], George N. Ioannou[4], Laura Beretta[1]*

1 Public Health Sciences Division, Fred Hutchinson Cancer Research Center, Seattle, Washington, United States of America, 2 Department of Infectious, Parasitic and Immune-Mediated Disease, Istituto Superiore di Sanità, Roma, Italy, 3 Division of Gastroenterology, Department of Internal Medicine, University of Michigan, Ann Arbor, Michigan, United States of America, 4 Division of Gastroenterology, Department of Medicine, Veterans Affairs Puget Sound Health Care System and University of Washington, Seattle, Washington, United States of America

Abstract

MicroRNAs miR-122, miR-34a, miR-16 and miR-21 are commonly deregulated in liver fibrosis and hepatocellular carcinoma. This study examined whether circulating levels of these miRNAs correlate with hepatic histological disease severity in patients with chronic hepatitis C infection (CHC) or non-alcoholic fatty-liver disease (NAFLD) and can potentially serve as circulating markers for disease stage assessment. We first used an *in vitro* model of hepatitis C virus (HCV) infection to measure the extracellular levels of these four miRNAs. Whereas miR-21 extracellular levels were unchanged, extracellular levels of miR-122, miR-34a and to a lesser extent miR-16, steadily increased during the course of HCV infection, independently of viral replication and production. Similarly, in CHC patients, serum levels of miR-122, miR-34a and miR-16 were significantly higher than in control individuals, while miR-21 levels were unchanged. There was no correlation between the serum levels of any of these microRNAs and HCV viral loads. In contrast, miR-122 and miR-34a levels positively correlated with disease severity. Identical results were obtained in an independent cohort of CHC patients. We extended the study to patients with NAFLD. As observed in CHC patients, serum levels of miR-122, miR-34a and miR-16 were significantly higher in NAFLD patients than in controls, while miR-21 levels were unchanged. Again, miR-122 and miR-34a levels positively correlated with disease severity from simple steatosis to steatohepatitis. In both CHC and NAFLD patient groups, serum levels of miR-122 and miR-34a correlated with liver enzymes levels, fibrosis stage and inflammation activity. miR-122 levels also correlated with serum lipids in NAFLD patients. Conclusion: Serum levels of miR-34a and miR-122 may represent novel, noninvasive biomarkers of diagnosis and histological disease severity in patients with CHC or NAFLD.

Editor: John E. Tavis, Saint Louis University, United States of America

Funding: This work was supported by grant DK066840 from the National Institutes of Health. The funder had no role in study design, data collection and analysis, decision to publish, or preparation of the manuscript.

Competing Interests: The authors have declared that no competing interests exist.

* E-mail: lberetta@fhcrc.org

Introduction

Liver biopsy is often recommended in patients with unexplained elevated serum aminotransferases in order to determine the cause, to stage hepatic fibrosis and to grade hepatic inflammation. Non-invasive methods that can evaluate disease severity and the likelihood of disease progression in persons with elevated liver enzymes need to be developed. MicroRNAs are small non-coding RNAs that control translation and transcription of many genes. They are receiving growing attention because of numerous reports on their dysregulation in human diseases and their potential as diagnostic and therapeutic targets. Because of their stability and presence in almost all body fluids, miRNAs constitute a novel class of non-invasive biomarkers. Numerous studies have shown that aberrant miRNA expression is associated with the development and progression of various types of human cancer and therefore studies on circulating miRNA profiles largely focused on cancer [1–3].

This study examined whether serum levels of selected miRNAs, thought to be deregulated in liver disease, can serve as non-invasive biomarkers of diagnosis and histological severity in patients with chronic hepatitis C (CHC) or non-alcoholic fatty liver disease (NAFLD). The highly abundant liver-specific miR-122, is of particular interest. miR-122 is known to regulate metabolic pathways in the liver, including cholesterol biosynthesis [4–7]. miR-122 also positively regulates hepatitis C virus (HCV) replication and viral production [8–10]. Reduced expression of miR-122 has been observed in hepatocellular carcinoma (HCC), often in advanced tumors of poor prognosis [11–13] although an upregulation of miR-122 was also reported in HCV-derived HCC [11,14]. miRNAs encoded by the miR-15/16 cluster act as tumor suppressors and are down-regulated in several human cancers [15]. In contrast, miR-21 was identified to be consistently upregulated in many cancers [16] including HCC [17]. Upregulation of miR-21 was also found in highly fibrotic HCV-infected human livers [18]. miR-34a, a central mediator of p53 function [19], has recently emerged as another miRNA modulated in liver disease. Interestingly, while most studies report a downregulation of miR-34a in human cancers [19], miR-34a was found increased in HCC [17] as well as in a mouse model of steatohepatitis [20]. We selected these four miRNAs (miR-122, miR-16, miR-21 and miR-34a) for the present study aimed at investigating their levels in serum of patients with CHC and NAFLD with a wide spectrum of histological disease severity. In addition to this analysis on human sera, we used an *in vitro* model of HCV infection to measure extracellular levels of these same miRNAs in supernatant of HCV-infected cells.

Materials and Methods

Ethics Statement

The study protocol conforms fully to the ethical guidelines of the 1975 Declaration of Helsinki and was approved by the Institutional Review Board of the Fred Hutchinson Cancer Research Center. We used only fully de-identified samples that were transferred from formal sample repositories at the University of Michigan and the Veterans Affairs Puget Sound Health Care System. Written, informed consent was obtained from every human subject when the samples were originally collected for the repositories under the terms of study protocols approved by the Institutional Review Boards at these respective institutions.

In vitro HCV infection and HCV RNA quantitation

HCV viral stocks were generated following transfection of in vitro transcripts of the HCVJ6/JFH genotype 2a strain (kindly provided by Dr. Charles Rice) using DMRIE-C (Invitrogen). Huh7.5 cells were infected with HCVcc, at a dose of 5.6×10^3 $TCID_{50}$/ml as described [21] and cultured for 15 days, corresponding to 4 passages. Cells and supernatants were collected at five, ten and fifteen days post-infection, 48 hrs after the cells were split and seeded at a density of 2×10^5 cells/cm^2. The confluence of the cells at the time of collection was 70-80%. Intracellular and extracellular RNA was extracted using the miRNeasy extraction kit (QIAGEN). Samples were submitted to DNAse digestion,

reverse-transcription using random hexamers, and real-time PCR using the following HCV primer sequences: 5-CGGGAGAGC-CATAGTGGTCTGCG-3 and 5-CTCGCAAGCACCCTAT-CAGGCAGTA-3. To determine HCV copy numbers, standard curves were prepared by serial dilution of a plasmid bearing the amplified HCV sequence.

Patient Groups (Table S1)

The Control group was composed of 19 healthy individuals without any evidence of liver disease. The Chronic Hepatitis C (CHC) group was composed of a first set of 18 patients recruited at the University of Michigan and of an independent set of 35 patients recruited as part of an ongoing observational study of chronic liver disease at Veterans Affairs Puget Sound Health Care System. HCV infection was defined by presence of HCV RNA in serum. The Non-Alcoholic Fatty Liver Disease (NAFLD) group was composed of 34 patients also enrolled at Veterans Affairs Puget Sound Health Care System. NAFLD was defined by the presence of hepatic steatosis in at least 5% of hepatocytes, in the absence of HCV RNA and hepatitis B virus surface antigen, self-reported alcohol consumption in the preceding six months, or histological features suggestive of primary biliary cirrhosis, autoimmune hepatitis, or iron overload.

For hepatic histology assessment, formalin-fixed liver tissue was stained with hematoxylin and eosin, Masson's trichrome and special stains for iron and copper and reviewed independently by a liver pathologist, who was blinded to this study. For CHC patients, the Batts and Ludwig scoring system [22] was used to score fibrosis (0–4) and inflammation (0–4). For NAFLD patients, steatosis, ballooning

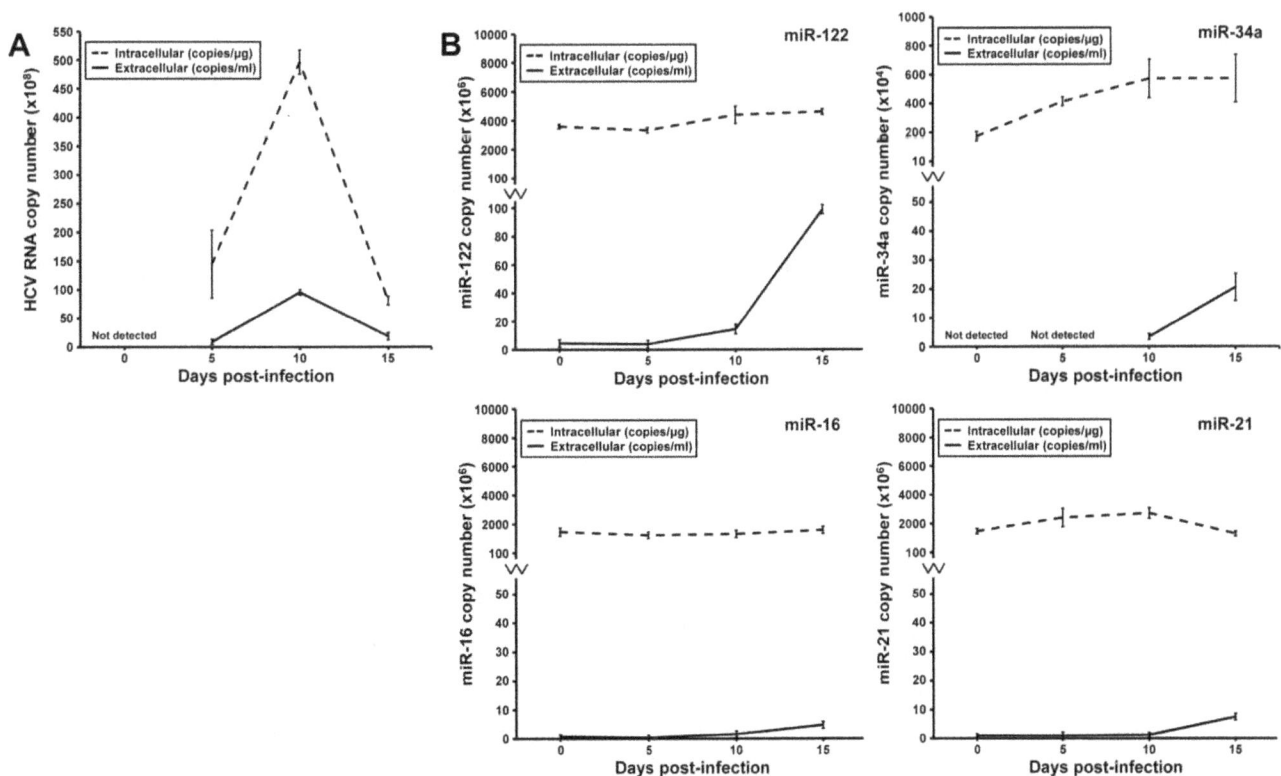

Figure 1. Differential expression of miRNAs in supernatant of HCV-infected cells. (A) Detection of intracellular and extracellular HCV RNA. (B) miR-122, miR-34a, miR-16 and miR-21 levels in uninfected and HCV-infected Huh7.5 cells at 5, 10 and 15 days post-infection. Cycle threshold (C_T) values were converted to an absolute value based on the standard curve. The expression levels are presented as the mean ± standard error of the mean (SEM) (copy number/ml of supernatant or copy number/µg of total RNA) of three independent experiments.

degeneration, inflammation, and fibrosis were scored according to the currently accepted scoring system [23]. In this scoring system, the scores for steatosis grade (0–3), lobular inflammation (0–3), and ballooning (0–2) can be summed to yield a NAFLD Activity Score (NAS) with scores ≥5 being considered diagnostic for histological steatohepatitis while scores of 1–4 are diagnostic of simple steatosis.

miRNA quantitation

Total RNA with preserved miRNAs was extracted from 100 μl of serum by miRNeasy extraction kit and using a plasma/QIAzol ratio of 1:10. Synthetic spiked-in *C. elegans* miR-238 was added to the serum and cell supernatant samples prior to RNA extraction as internal control and RNU44 was quantified in the cellular RNA samples. Expression of mature miRNAs was detected using the Taqman miRNA qRT-PCR Assay (Applied Biosystems, Carlsbad, CA). Reverse transcription and PCR reactions were run in triplicate in the Applied Biosystems 7900 System. To determine miRNA copy numbers, standard curves were prepared by serial dilution of synthetic miRNA (Integrated DNA Technologies, Coralville, IA).

Statistical Analysis

Statistical significance of differences between groups was analyzed by Wilcoxon rank sum test using TIBCO Spotfire S+ (TIBCO Spotfire, Somerville, MA). Correlation analysis was performed using two-tailed Pearson correlation test. Receiver operating characteristic (ROC) analysis was undertaken using R software version 2.9.2.

Results

Increased levels of miR-122, miR-34a and miR-16 in the supernatant of HCV-infected cells

Intracellular and extracellular levels of miR-122, miR-34a, miR-16 and miR-21 were measured in Huh7.5 cells infected with a genotype 2a chimeric HCV, after confirming the absence of confounding miRNAs in the bovine serum used to culture the cells. Copy numbers of the targeted miRNAs and of the HCV RNA were calculated at five, ten and fifteen days post-infection in

three independent experiments. HCV RNA reached the highest levels at 10 days post-infection in both the intracellular and extracellular compartments (4.9×10^{10} copies/μg and 0.9×10^{10} copies/ml, respectively) (Figure 1A). Among the four miRNAs analyzed, miR-122 was the most abundant in both the intracellular and extracellular compartments (3.7×10^{9} copies/μg of total RNA and 4.4×10^{6} copies/ml of supernatant, respectively) and miR-34a the least abundant with 1.8×10^{6} intracellular copies/μg of total RNA and undetectable extracellular levels (Figure 1B). miR-16 and miR-21 abundances were largely similar with 1.6×10^{9} intracellular copies/μg of total RNA for both miRNAs, 7.6×10^{5} copies/ml for extracellular miR-16 and 9×10^{5} copies/ml of supernatant for extracellular miR-21 (Figure 1B). Intracellular levels of miR-122, miR-16 and miR-21 remained constant during the infection while intracellular miR-34a levels increased by 2.3-fold at 5 days post-infection and by 3.2-fold at 10 and 15 days post-infection (Figure 1B). At 10 days post-infection, corresponding to the highest levels of HCV RNA, extracellular levels of miR-122 and miR-16 increased by 3.3-fold and 2.1-fold, respectively, while miR-21 remained unchanged. miR-34a levels were undetectable in supernatant of uninfected Huh7.5 cells as well as in cells infected with HCV for 5 days, but increased to detectable levels at 10 days post-infection. At 15 days post-infection, corresponding to a decline in HCV RNA levels, extracellular miR-122, miR-34a and miR-16 levels further increased by 6.9-, 6.2- and 2.9-fold, respectively and a 6-fold accumulation of miR-21 was observed (Figure 1B).

Increased serum levels of miR-122, miR-34a and miR-16 in chronic hepatitis C patients

We then investigated whether these miRNAs are detected and modulated in serum from patients with chronic hepatitis C (CHC). In healthy control sera, levels of miR-16 (3.1×10^{6} copies/ml) were higher than levels of miR-21 (1.6×10^{6} copies/ml) and miR-122 (2.8×10^{5} copies/ml), and miR-34a was undetectable, the detection limit of the assay being approximately 0.3×10^{4} copies/ml. Serum levels of miR-122 and miR-16 were significantly higher in a first set of patients with CHC (n = 18) compared to healthy

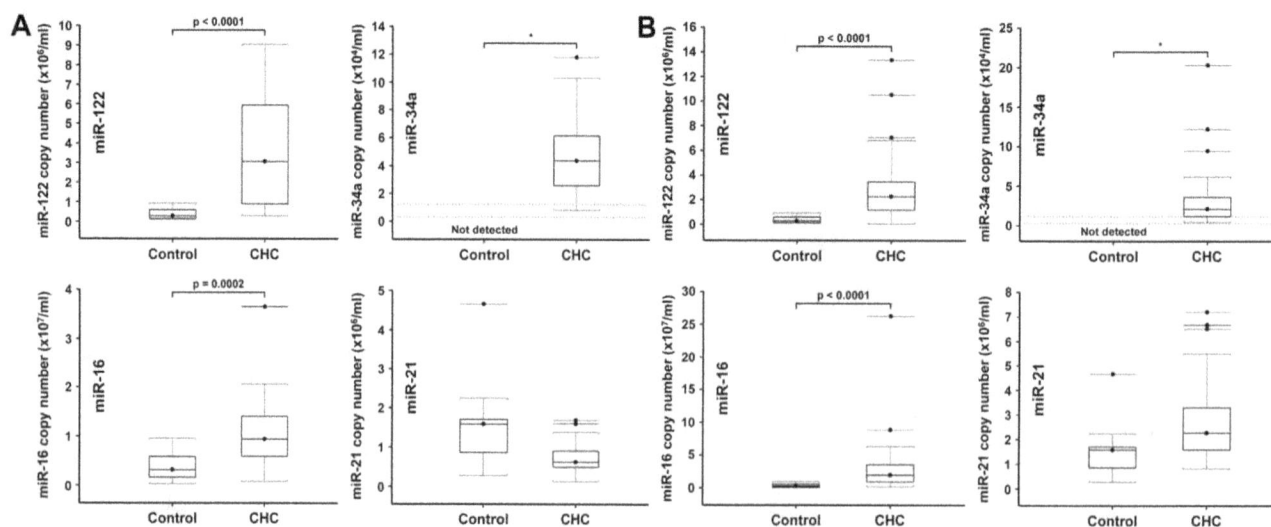

Figure 2. Up-regulation of serum miR-122, miR-34a and miR-16 in chronic hepatitis C patients. Serum levels of miR-122, miR-34a, miR-16 and miR-21 in (A) a first set of 18 CHC patients and (B) an independent set of 35 CHC patients. C_T values were converted to an absolute value based on the standard curves. Serum miRNA expression levels are expressed in copy number/ml. In the box-plot displays, the bold line indicates the median per group, the box represents 50% of the values and horizontal lines show minimum and maximum values of the calculated non-outlier values. For miR-34a, the dashed lines represent the levels corresponding to C_T values between 35 and 37 (1.2×10^{4} – 0.3×10^{4} copies/ml).

controls (n = 19) (10.8-fold (p<0.0001) and 3.0-fold (p = 0.0002), respectively) and miR-34a levels increased from undetectable levels to a median level of 4.4×10^4 copies/ml (Figure 2A). miR-21 levels were not significantly different between controls and CHC patients (Figure 2A). There was no correlation between the abundance of any of these four miRNAs and the HCV viral load measured in these patients (R from -0.08 to 0.08). We validated these results in an independent group of 35 CHC patients enrolled at a different site. Confirming the results obtained in the first set of patients, miR-122 levels were higher by 7.9-fold in CHC patients compared to controls (p<0.0001), miR-16 levels were higher by 6.3-fold (p<0.0001), miR-34a was undetectable in control sera but detected at a median of 2.1×10^4 copies/ml in the CHC group,

and miR-21 levels were unchanged (Figure 2B). Finally, there was no correlation between the serum abundance of any of these four miRNAs and the HCV viral load (R from -0.003 to 0.24).

Based on histology grading, we separated the CHC patients into patients with early stage fibrosis (F0-F1) and patients with advanced fibrosis (F3-F4). miR-122 and miR-16 serum levels were already strongly increased in the CHC-early group compared to controls (6.4-fold and p<0.0001 for both miRNAs) and miR-34a levels were detectable in all patients with early disease, with a median of 1.8×10^4 copies/ml (Figure 3A). Serum levels of miR-122 and miR-34a further increased in the CHC-advanced group compared to the CHC-early group (2.2-fold (p = 0.009) and 2.6-fold (p = 0.002), respectively) (Figure 3A). The

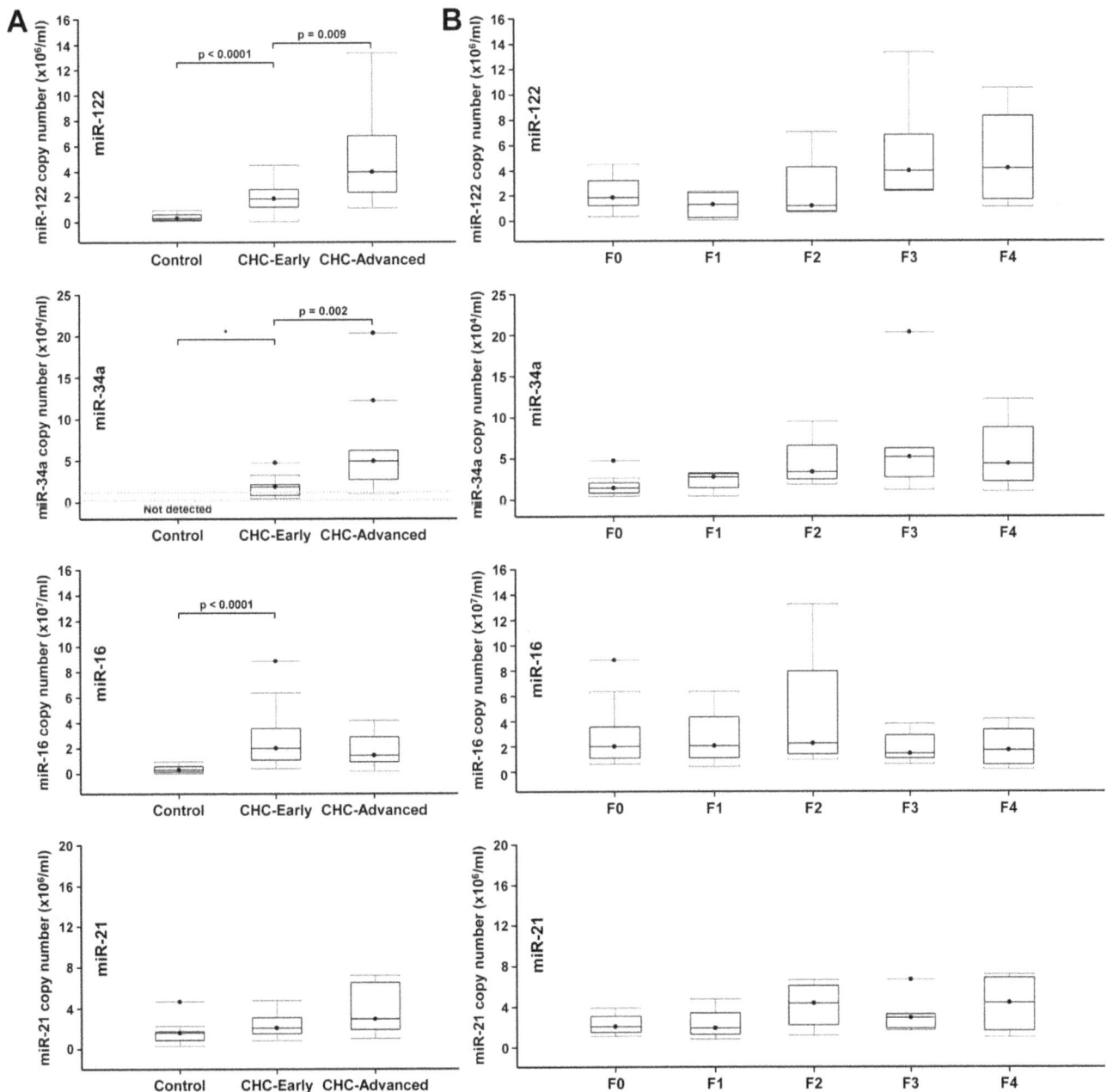

Figure 3. Serum levels of miR-122, miR-34a, miR-16 and miR-21 and histological liver disease severity in CHC patients. CHC group was subdivided into (A) CHC-early (F0-F1) and CHC-advanced groups (F3-F4) and (B) further subdivided according to individual fibrosis stage.

increase of miR-122 mostly occurred between F2 and F3 stages while the increase of miR-34a was continuous between F0–F3 (Figure 3B). In contrast to miR-122 and miR-34a, miR-16 serum levels remained unchanged in the CHC-advanced group compared to the CHC-early group (Figure 3A). There was no significant difference in miR-21 levels between the CHC-early and CHC–advanced groups although a slight increase was observed in patients with F4 stage disease (Figure 3A,B).

Increased serum levels of miR-122, miR-34a and miR-16 in patients with NAFLD.

To determine whether serum levels of miR-122, miR-34a, miR-16 and miR-21 change in patients with other chronic liver diseases, we measured these four miRNAs in sera collected from 34 patients diagnosed with NAFLD. miR-122 levels were increased by 7.2-fold in NAFLD patients compared to healthy controls (p<0.0001), miR-16 levels were increased by 5.5-fold (p<0.0001), miR-34a increased from undetectable levels to a median of 2.2×10^4 copies/ml and miR-21 was unchanged

(Figure 4A). We divided the NAFLD patients into two groups based on the NAFLD activity score (NAS): patients with simple steatosis (NAFLD-SS) defined by NAS scores 1–4 and patients with non-alcoholic steatohepatitis (NASH) defined by NAS scores 5–7. Serum levels of miR-122 and miR-16 were higher in NAFLD-SS compared to the controls (5.7-fold (p<0.0001) and 5.3-fold (p<0.0001), respectively) and miR-34a were detectable in all patients with simple steatosis with a median of 1.2×10^4 copies/ml. miR-21 levels were unchanged. miR-122 and miR-34a levels further increased in the NASH group compared to the NAFLD-SS group (2.0-fold (p = 0.05) and 2.8-fold (p = 0.009), respectively) (Figure 4B). For both miRNAs, the increase occurred mostly between NAS scores 3-4 and NAS score 5 (Figure 4C). miR-16 and miR-21 levels were similar in both groups (Figure 4B).

miR-122 and miR-34a correlation with clinical parameters and performance in disease stage assessment

Because both miR-122 and miR-34a levels correlate with disease severity, we investigated the relationship of their serum levels with

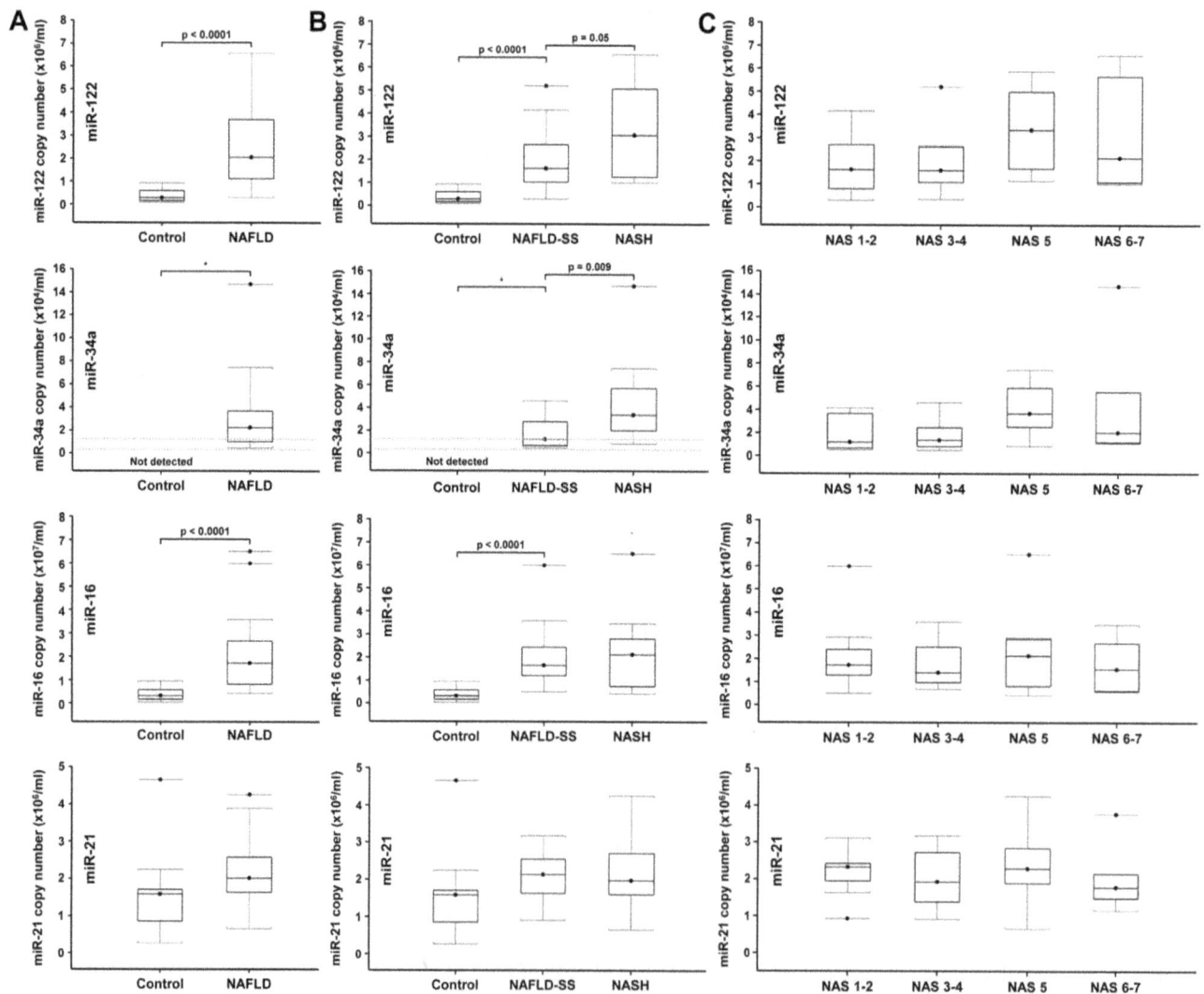

Figure 4. Serum levels of miR-122, miR-34a, miR-16 and miR-21 in NAFLD patients. (A) Expression of miR-122, miR-34a, miR-16 and miR-21 in serum from healthy controls and NAFLD patients. (B) NAFLD patients were divided into two groups based on the NAFLD activity score (NAS): NAFLD-simple steatosis (NAFLD-SS) with NAS≤4 and non-alcoholic steatohepatitis (NASH) with NAS ≥5. (C) NAFLD-SS and NASH groups were further subdivided based on individual NAS scores.

the clinicopathological parameters collected from the CHC and NAFLD patients (Table 1). In both patient groups, a strong positive correlation with alanine aminotransferase (ALT) and aspartate aminotransferase (AST) was observed for miR-122. High positive correlations were also observed for miR-122 and miR-34a with fibrosis stage and inflammation activity. In CHC patients, a positive correlation was also observed for miR-122 and miR-34a with blood glucose levels and insulin resistance. In NAFLD patients, a positive correlation was also observed between miR-122 and total cholesterol level and low-density lipoprotein (LDL).

In a pilot analysis, we evaluated whether circulating miR-122, miR-34a and miR-16 can be used to assess the disease stage in CHC and NAFLD patients. We first performed ROC curve analyses for miR-16 and miR-122 comparing healthy controls and early disease (CHC F0-F1 and NAFLD NAS 1-4) (Figure 5A,B). Because miR-34a was under the limit of detection in controls, such analysis could not be performed for miR-34a. The area under the receiver-operator characteristic curve (AUC) values for miR-122 and miR-16 in the comparison between CHC-early and control groups were 0.90 and 0.92 respectively (Figure 5A). Both miRNAs performed better than ALT (AUC = 0.85). A similar result was obtained comparing healthy controls and NAFLD-SS with AUC values of 0.93 for miR-122, 0.96 for miR-16 and 0.91 for ALT (Figure 5B). When comparing CHC-early and CHC-advanced patients, miR-34a performed better than miR-122 (AUC = 0.84 vs AUC = 0.75) (Figure 5C). Again a similar result was obtained when comparing NAFLD-SS and NASH (AUC values of 0.75 and 0.70) (Figure 5D).

Discussion

MicroRNA changes in the liver have been reported in disease processes such as hepatocarcinogenesis and liver fibrosis. There is however only limited information about their detection in blood and their correlation with histological disease severity in patients with chronic liver diseases. We first measured intracellular and extracellular levels of miR-122, miR-34a, miR-16 and miR-21 in HCV-infected Huh7.5 cells. miR-122 intracellular levels were not affected by HCV replication, in agreement with previous reports

[8]. In contrast, miR-122 strongly accumulated in the extracellular compartment of HCV-infected cells, independently of the levels of HCV replication and production. These results suggest that there is no correlation between intracellular and extracellular levels of miR-122. Similar results were observed for miR-16 although to a lesser extent. In contrast, miR-34a was increased in both the intracellular and extracellular compartments upon HCV infection and miR-21 was only slightly changed. miRNAs are associated with cell-derived vesicles or exosomes [2] but also with protein complexes [24]. miR-122 and miR-16 in particular have been reported associated with argonaute2 complexes and independent of vesicles in plasma [24]. Future experiments should investigate the mechanisms leading to the release of these microRNAs from hepatocytic cells.

In CHC patients and in patients with NAFLD, plasma levels of miR-122 were elevated compared to healthy controls. In CHC patients, miR-122 levels correlated with fibrosis stage and inflammation activity but didn't correlate with HCV viral load. An absence of correlation between intrahepatic miR-122 and HCV RNA levels was also observed in human liver biopsies [25,26]. In NAFLD patients, miR-122 levels also correlated with fibrosis stage and inflammation activity. An inverse correlation between intrahepatic miR-122 and fibrosis [18,26] and reduced intrahepatic levels of miR-122 in NASH were reported [27]. Altogether, these results are consistent with a lack of correlation between miR-122 regulation in liver tissue and in serum as observed in the HCV-infected Huh7.5 cells. Circulating miR-122 levels have been reported to be elevated in patients with chronic hepatitis B viral infection [28,29] and to correlate with liver histologic stage, inflammation grades and ALT activity [28]. Serum miR-122 levels were also higher in patients with chronic hepatitis B infection than in patients with hepatocellular carcinoma [29]. We are reporting here similar results for miR-122 in patients with chronic hepatitis C or with NAFLD, suggesting that the increase in circulating levels of miR-122 is common to chronic liver disease of all etiologies. Our study is also in agreement with a recent study reporting an increase in serum miR-122 levels in patients with chronic hepatitis C virus

Table 1. Correlation between miRNAs and specific clinical parameters.

	CHC			NAFLD		
		miR-122	mir-34a		miR-122	mir-34a
ALT (IU/L)	59 (26–394)*	0.92	0.86	76 (14–183)*	0.75	0.45
AST (IU/L)	47 (23–336)*	0.88	0.85	41.5 (15–141)*	0.55	0.46
NAS score: ≤4/≥5	NA	NA	NA	53/47**	0.38	0.46
Fibrosis stage: ≤1/≥2	60/40**	0.50	0.51	79/21**	0.33	0.41
Inflammation activity: ≤1/≥2	62/38**	0.50	0.50	62/38**	0.33	0.43
Steatosis grade: ≤1/≥2	91/9**	0.55	0.58	47/53**	0.11	0.13
Balloon Hepatocytes: ≤1/≥2	NA	NA	NA	73/27**	0.46	0.43
Total Cholesterol (mg/dL)	177 (104–274)*	−0.16	−0.10	204.5 (141–288)*	0.36	0.11
LDL (mg/dL)	107 (46–195)*	−0.09	−0.03	113 (43–182)*	0.44	0.19
HDL (mg/dL)	46 (27–74)*	−0.24	−0.34	40 (25–74)*	0.25	0.24
Triglycerides (mg/dL)	104 (51–245)*	0.10	0.20	222.5 (75–879)*	−0.14	−0.18
Glucose (mg/dL)	104 (60–292)*	0.45	0.42	111 (77–302)*	−0.19	−0.21
Insulin resist. (HOMA score)	3.5 (0.6–12.2)*	0.39	0.34	6.6 (1.4–89.9)*	0.09	0.13

*median (range);
** (%).

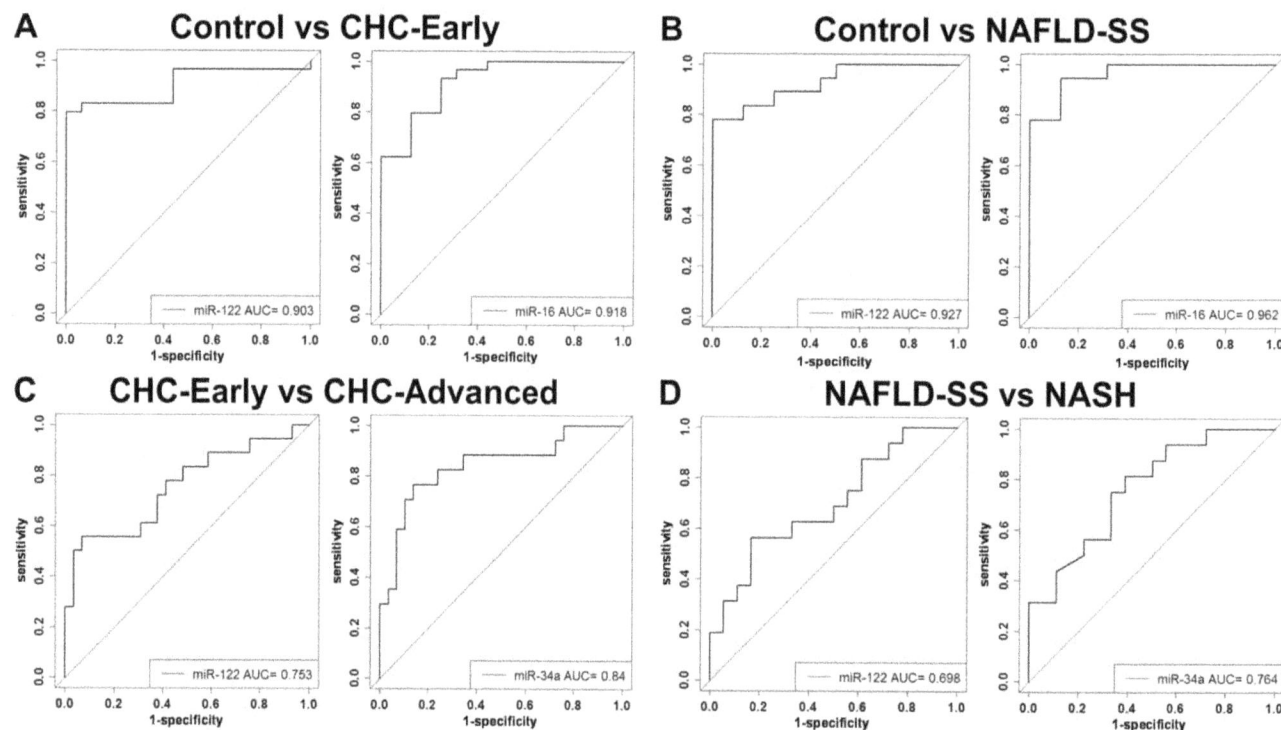

Figure 5. Receiver operating characteristic (ROC) analysis of expression of miRNAs in CHC and NAFLD patients. ROC curves with corresponding area under the ROC curve (AUC) for (A): mir-122 and miR-16 from CHC-early versus controls; (B) mir-122 and miR-16 from NAFLD-SS (NAS 1-4) versus controls; (C) miR-122 and miR-34a from CHC-early versus CHC-advanced; (D) miR-122 and miR-34a from NAFLD-SS(NAS 1-4) versus NASH (NAS 5-7).

infection, a strong correlation between serum levels of miR-122 and serum ALT and no correlation with serum HCV RNA [30]. This last report however didn't observe a significant correlation between serum miR-122 levels and fibrosis stage. In contrast to miR-122, there is only limited information about miR-34a expression in the liver and its regulation in chronic disease. We found miR-34a levels to be largely undetectable in plasma from healthy individuals but significantly increased to detectable levels in patients with CHC or NAFLD. As for miR-122, miR-34a plasma levels correlated with fibrosis severity. Further increase of miR-34a should be evaluated in HCC as miR-34a was reported linked to disease progression from normal liver through cirrhosis to HCC [31]. While a positive correlation between intrahepatic miR-21 expression and viral load, fibrosis or serum liver transaminase levels was reported [18], we only observed a marginal increase of miR-21 in late disease stages. In contrast, miR-16 was highly elevated in early disease and slightly decreased in advanced stages. Further decrease of miR-16 should be evaluated in HCC [32].

Non-invasive assessment of liver fibrosis is a very important goal in patients with chronic hepatitis C. miR-122 and miR-16 were more sensitive than ALT in detecting early stage disease in the studied sets of patients. In addition, miR-122 and miR-34a may have utility in assessing disease stage. Chronic viral infection of the liver is associated with insulin resistance and also associated with the development of hepatic steatosis. The severity of steatosis has been well correlated with the degree of hepatic fibrosis and the severity of insulin resistance [33,34]. Both miR-122 and miR-34a levels correlated with fibrosis stage, inflammation activity, steatosis grade and to a lesser extent to insulin resistance and glucose levels in CHC patients. There was overall no correlation

with serum lipids at the exception of a small negative correlation with high-density lipoprotein (HDL). This may result from the fact that in CHC patients, disease severity is associated with lower HDL levels [35]. Interest in applying non-invasive methods to assess liver fibrosis in patients with NAFLD has increased in recent years [36]. The overwhelming majority of persons with elevated ALT activity in the absence of viral hepatitis or excessive alcohol consumption are found to have NAFLD on liver biopsy in the US and Europe [37]. miR-34a and miR-122 may have utility in the identification of those NAFLD patients who have developed significant liver fibrosis. Interestingly, in contrast to CHC patients, mir-122 levels correlated with serum lipids in NAFLD patients. Overall, the prospect of using miR-122 and miR-34a as prognostic markers is of interest. Larger patient cohorts with distinct hepatic disease-causes and differential fibrosis states will have to be analyzed to further test the utility of circulating miR-122 and miR-34a as biomarkers for detection or monitoring of liver fibrosis.

Acknowledgments

We thank Dr. Charles M. Rice (Rockefeller University, New York) for the gift of the HCV J6/JFH strain and Huh7.5 cells, Dr. Muneesh Tewari and Evan M. Kroh (Division of Human Biology, Fred Hutchinson Cancer Research Center, Seattle) for helpful discussion and excellent advice, Paul J. Farley (Public Health Sciences Division, Fred Hutchinson Cancer Research Center, Seattle) and Erica V. Tartaglione (Division of Gastroenterology, Veterans Affairs Puget Sound Health Care System, Seattle) for their contributions to the project coordination.

Author Contributions

Conceived and designed the experiments: LB SC GNI. Performed the experiments: SC AR. Analyzed the data: SC LB. Wrote the paper: LB SC. Provided patient samples: JAM GNI.

References

1. Mitchell PS, Parkin RK, Kroh EM, Fritz BR, Wyman SK, et al. (2008) Circulating microRNAs as stable blood-based markers for cancer detection. Proc Natl Acad Sci U S A 105: 10513–10518.
2. Kosaka N, Iguchi H, Ochiya T (2010) Circulating microRNA in body fluid: a new potential biomarker for cancer diagnosis and prognosis. Cancer Sci 101: 2087–2092.
3. Brase JC, Wuttig D, Kuner R, Sultmann H (2010) Serum microRNAs as non-invasive biomarkers for cancer. Mol Cancer 9: 306.
4. Esau C, Davis S, Murray SF, Yu XX, Pandey SK, et al. (2006) miR-122 regulation of lipid metabolism revealed by in vivo antisense targeting. Cell Metab 3: 87–98.
5. Krutzfeldt J, Rajewsky N, Braich R, Rajeev KG, Tuschl T, et al. (2005) Silencing of microRNAs in vivo with 'antagomirs'. Nature 438: 685–689.
6. Xu H, He JH, Xiao ZD, Zhang QQ, Chen YQ, et al. (2010) Liver-enriched transcription factors regulate microRNA-122 that targets CUTL1 during liver development. Hepatology 52: 1431–1442.
7. Lewis AP, Jopling CL (2010) Regulation and biological function of the liver-specific miR-122. Biochem Soc Trans 38: 1553–1557.
8. Randall G, Panis M, Cooper JD, Tellinghuisen TL, Sukhodolets KE, et al. (2007) Cellular cofactors affecting hepatitis C virus infection and replication. Proc Natl Acad Sci U S A 104: 12884–12889.
9. Henke JI, Goergen D, Zheng J, Song Y, Schuttler CG, et al. (2008) microRNA-122 stimulates translation of hepatitis C virus RNA. EMBO J 27: 3300–3310.
10. Jangra RK, Yi M, Lemon SM (2010) Regulation of hepatitis C virus translation and infectious virus production by the microRNA miR-122. J Virol 84: 6615–6625.
11. Coulouarn C, Factor VM, Andersen JB, Durkin ME, Thorgeirsson SS (2009) Loss of miR-122 expression in liver cancer correlates with suppression of the hepatic phenotype and gain of metastatic properties. Oncogene 28: 3526–3536.
12. Zeng C, Wang R, Li D, Lin XJ, Wei QK, et al. (2010) A novel GSK-3 beta-C/EBP alpha-miR-122-insulin-like growth factor 1 receptor regulatory circuitry in human hepatocellular carcinoma. Hepatology 52: 1702–1712.
13. Filipowicz W, Grosshans H (2011) The liver-specific microRNA miR-122: biology and therapeutic potential. Prog Drug Res 67: 221–238.
14. Varnholt H, Drebber U, Schulze F, Wedemeyer I, Schirmacher P, et al. (2008) MicroRNA gene expression profile of hepatitis C virus-associated hepatocellular carcinoma. Hepatology 47: 1223–1232.
15. Aqeilan RI, Calin GA, Croce CM (2010) miR-15a and miR-16-1 in cancer: discovery, function and future perspectives. Cell Death Differ 17: 215–220.
16. Garzon R, Marcucci G, Croce CM (2010) Targeting microRNAs in cancer: rationale, strategies and challenges. Nat Rev Drug Discov 9: 775–789.
17. Mizuguchi Y, Mishima T, Yokomuro S, Arima Y, Kawahigashi Y, et al. (2011) Sequencing and bioinformatics-based analyses of the microRNA transcriptome in hepatitis B-related hepatocellular carcinoma. PLoS One 6: e15304.
18. Marquez RT, Bandyopadhyay S, Wendlandt EB, Keck K, Hoffer BA, et al. (2010) Correlation between microRNA expression levels and clinical parameters associated with chronic hepatitis C viral infection in humans. Lab Invest 90: 1727–1736.
19. Hermeking H (2007) p53 enters the microRNA world. Cancer Cell 12: 414–418.
20. Pogribny IP, Starlard-Davenport A, Tryndyak VP, Han T, Ross SA, et al. (2010) Difference in expression of hepatic microRNAs miR-29c, miR-34a, miR-155, and miR-200b is associated with strain-specific susceptibility to dietary nonalcoholic steatohepatitis in mice. Lab Invest 90: 1437–1446.
21. Parent R, Qu X, Petit MA, Beretta L (2009) The heat shock cognate protein 70 is associated with hepatitis C virus particles and modulates virus infectivity. Hepatology 49: 1798–1809.
22. Batts KP, Ludwig J (1995) Chronic hepatitis. An update on terminology and reporting. Am J Surg Pathol 19: 1409–1417.
23. Kleiner DE, Brunt EM, Van Natta M, Behling C, Contos MJ, et al. (2005) Design and validation of a histological scoring system for nonalcoholic fatty liver disease. Hepatology 41: 1313–1321.
24. Arroyo JD, Chevillet JR, Kroh EM, Ruf IK, Pritchard CC, et al. (2011) Argonaute2 complexes carry a population of circulating microRNAs independent of vesicles in human plasma. Proc Natl Acad Sci U S A 108: 5003–5008.
25. Sarasin-Filipowicz M, Krol J, Markiewicz I, Heim MH, Filipowicz W (2009) Decreased levels of microRNA miR-122 in individuals with hepatitis C responding poorly to interferon therapy. Nat Med 15: 31–33.
26. Morita K, Taketomi A, Shirabe K, Umeda K, Kayashima H, et al. (2011) Clinical significance and potential of hepatic microRNA-122 expression in hepatitis C. Liver Int 31: 474–484.
27. Wang K, Zhang S, Marzolf B, Troisch P, Brightman A, et al. (2009) Circulating microRNAs, potential biomarkers for drug-induced liver injury. Proc Natl Acad Sci U S A 106: 4402–4407.
28. Zhang Y, Jia Y, Zheng R, Guo Y, Wang Y, et al. (2010) Plasma microRNA-122 as a biomarker for viral-, alcohol-, and chemical-related hepatic diseases. Clin Chem 56: 1830–1838.
29. Xu J, Wu C, Che X, Wang L, Yu D, et al. (2011) Circulating microRNAs, miR-21, miR-122, and miR-223, in patients with hepatocellular carcinoma or chronic hepatitis. Mol Carcinog 50: 136–142.
30. Bihrer V, Friedrich-Rust M, Kronenberger B, Forestier N, Haupenthal J, et al. (2011) Serum miR-122 as a biomarker of necroinflammation in patients with chronic hepatitis C virus infection. Am J Gastroenterol.
31. Pineau P, Volinia S, McJunkin K, Marchio A, Battiston C, et al. (2010) miR-221 overexpression contributes to liver tumorigenesis. Proc Natl Acad Sci U S A 107: 264–269.
32. Qu KZ, Zhang K, Li H, Afdhal NH, Albitar M (2011) Circulating microRNAs as biomarkers for hepatocellular carcinoma. J Clin Gastroenterol In press.
33. Negro F, Sanyal AJ (2009) Hepatitis C virus, steatosis and lipid abnormalities: clinical and pathogenic data. Liver Int 29(Suppl 2): 26–37.
34. Sanyal AJ (2011) Role of insulin resistance and hepatic steatosis in the progression of fibrosis and response to treatment in hepatitis C. Liver Int 31(Suppl 1): 23–28.
35. Ramcharran D, Wahed AS, Conjeevaram HS, Evans RW, Wang T, et al. (2011) Serum lipids and their associations with viral levels and liver disease severity in a treatment-naive chronic hepatitis C type 1-infected cohort. J Viral Hepat 18: e144–152.
36. Sanyal AJ, Brunt EM, Kleiner DE, Kowdley K, Chalasani N, et al. (2011) Endpoints and clinical trial design for nonalcoholic steatohepatitis. Hepatology.
37. Ioannou GN, Boyko EJ, Lee SP (2006) The prevalence and predictors of elevated serum aminotransferase activity in the United States in 1999-2002. Am J Gastroenterol 101: 76–82.

11

ENCODE Tiling Array Analysis Identifies Differentially Expressed Annotated and Novel 5′ Capped RNAs in Hepatitis C Infected Liver

Milan E. Folkers[1,◑], Don A. Delker[1,2◑], Christopher I. Maxwell[1,2], Cassie A. Nelson[1], Jason J. Schwartz[3], David A. Nix[2], Curt H. Hagedorn[1,2,4]*

1 Department of Medicine, University of Utah, Salt Lake City, Utah, United States of America, 2 Huntsman Cancer Institute, University of Utah, Salt Lake City, Utah, United States of America, 3 Department of Surgery, University of Utah, Salt Lake City, Utah, United States of America, 4 Department of Experimental Pathology, University of Utah, Salt Lake City, Utah, United States of America

Abstract

Microarray studies of chronic hepatitis C infection have provided valuable information regarding the host response to viral infection. However, recent studies of the human transcriptome indicate pervasive transcription in previously unannotated regions of the genome and that many RNA transcripts have short or lack 3′ poly(A) ends. We hypothesized that using ENCODE tiling arrays (1% of the genome) in combination with affinity purifying Pol II RNAs by their unique 5′ m^{7}GpppN cap would identify previously undescribed annotated and unannotated genes that are differentially expressed in liver during hepatitis C virus (HCV) infection. Both 5′-capped and poly(A)+ populations of RNA were analyzed using ENCODE tiling arrays. Sixty-four annotated genes were significantly increased in HCV cirrhotic as compared to control liver; twenty-seven (42%) of these genes were identified only by analyzing 5′ capped RNA. Thirty-one annotated genes were significantly decreased; sixteen (50%) of these were identified only by analyzing 5′ capped RNA. Bioinformatic analysis showed that capped RNA produced more consistent results, provided a more extensive expression profile of intronic regions and identified upregulated Pol II transcriptionally active regions in unannotated areas of the genome in HCV cirrhotic liver. Two of these regions were verified by PCR and RACE analysis. qPCR analysis of liver biopsy specimens demonstrated that these unannotated transcripts, as well as IRF1, TRIM22 and MET, were also upregulated in hepatitis C with mild inflammation and no fibrosis. The analysis of 5′ capped RNA in combination with ENCODE tiling arrays provides additional gene expression information and identifies novel upregulated Pol II transcripts not previously described in HCV infected liver. This approach, particularly when combined with new RNA sequencing technologies, should also be useful in further defining Pol II transcripts differentially regulated in specific disease states and in studying RNAs regulated by changes in pre-mRNA splicing or 3′ polyadenylation status.

Editor: Robyn Klein, Washington University, United States of America

Funding: This study was supported by National Institutes of Healths grant CA063640 (CHH). C. Maxwell was supported by a NIH Multidisciplinary Cancer Research Training Program T32CA093247. The funders had no role in study design, data collection and analysis, decision to publish, or preparation of the manuscript.

Competing Interests: The authors have declared that no competing interests exist.

* E-mail: curt.hagedorn@hsc.utah.edu

◑ These authors contributed equally to this work.

Introduction

Microarray based gene analyses have provided a new approach to identifying disease-specific changes in gene expression. This approach has improved the understanding of molecular pathobiology by identifying genes that are differentially regulated in selected diseases and by identifying biomarkers for disease states or responses to therapy. Successful examples of this approach include identifying subtypes of diffuse large B-cell lymphomas with different prognoses and increased expression of the zeta-chain (TCR) associated 70 kDa protein kinase (*ZAP70*) in chronic lymphocytic leukemia (CLL) which is a predictor of the clinical course [1,2,3]. Examples in stratifying breast cancer include identifying a panel of transcriptional changes predicting distant metastasis in lymph-node-negative patients, predicting the response to specific therapies and survival of patients [4,5,6,7,8,9].

Progress towards stratifying patients with colon cancer using gene expression signatures was recently reported [10].

In hepatitis C infection, gene array analyses in chimpanzees identified host responsive gene pathways in acute and chronic hepatitis C infection [11]. Gene array studies have also been used to identify potential biomarkers of hepatitis C infection, interferon regulated genes which predict the response to therapy, and gene expression patterns which predict early progression to fibrosis in liver transplant recipients [12,13,14]. Unique gene expression profiles were also identified which distinguish alcoholic liver disease and hepatitis C as well as hepatitis B and hepatitis C infection [15,16]. More recent data suggests that the hepatitis C virus may regulate host non-coding RNAs (i.e., miRNAs) to promote viral replication [17].

One limit of standard oligonucleotide or cDNA microarrays is that they require prior knowledge of the sequence of the RNA that will be measured. In addition, many arrays are purposefully biased to interrogate sequences originating from 3′ ends of mRNA encoded by the 3′ terminal exon of previously annotated genes. Although these methods measure RNA transcripts from well-annotated protein coding genes and selected ncRNAs, they do not generally provide information regarding pre-mRNAs and most non-coding RNAs that can be important in physiological or pathological processes. Genomic tiling arrays or next generation sequencing provide a useful alternative for quantifying and characterizing transcription across the genome without requiring prior knowledge of gene or RNA transcript sequences. Tiling arrays are designed to cover the entire genome, selected chromosomes or contigs of the genome. Recent gene expression experiments using ENCODE (**Enc**yclopedia of **D**NA **E**lements) tiling arrays, representing 1% of the human genome, have demonstrated that much of the genome is transcribed and that most nucleotides appear to be present in at least some form of RNA transcript [18]. A recent study in *Schizosaccharomyces pombe* provides further evidence for extensive sense and antisense transcription [19]. The nature of these RNAs, the RNA polymerase responsible for their transcription and their biological function remain unknown.

Previous ENCODE studies analyzed polyadenylated [poly(A)+] RNA, but recent data suggests that many RNAs in yeast and mammals either lack or have short 3′ poly(A) ends and are underrepresented or absent in microarray analyses using poly(A)+ RNA [18,20]. To enhance the selection of Pol II transcripts we have developed an efficient method of purifying RNA polymerase II (Pol II) transcripts regardless of their 3′ polyadenylation status. Pol II RNAs have a 5′ m7GpppN cap added enzymatically to their 5′ ends during the pausing phase of transcription [21,22]. Our approach purifies Pol II transcripts by binding their 5′ caps with a high-affinity variant of the RNA cap binding protein (eIF4E$_{K119A}$) [20,23]. When compared to standard poly(A)+ dependent purifications the yield of 5′ capped RNA is 2–3 fold greater from the same quantity of total RNA starting material, suggesting that poly(A)+ purification does not recover all capped Pol II RNAs [20].

To date, no gene expression studies on hepatitis C infected liver have been performed using tiling array analyses such as ENCODE. The goal of this study was to identify differentially expressed annotated genes and novel RNAs in hepatitis C infected liver that would not typically be recorded by analyzing poly(A)+ RNA with standard gene expression arrays. In this study, we utilized 5′ capped and poly(A)+ RNA populations isolated from control and chronically infected hepatitis C (HCV) cirrhotic human liver biospecimens using ENCODE tiling arrays to measure differential expression of Pol II RNAs. Differentially expressed RNAs identified in this analysis were then measured by real-time PCR (qPCR) in additional control, mild chronic hepatitis C (no fibrosis) and chronically infected hepatitis C cirrhotic biospecimens.

Results

The ENCODE tiling array analysis of 5′ capped RNA identified 47 annotated genes with increased expression (fold change >1.5, Bonferroni adjusted p value <0.05) (Figure 1A) and 22 genes with decreased expression in a chronic hepatitis C (HCV) cirrhotic as compared to an uninfected control liver specimen (Figure 1B). Analysis of poly(A)+ RNA identified 37 genes with increased expression and 15 genes with decreased expression in HCV cirrhotic as compared to control liver. Twenty of the upregulated genes and six of the downregulated genes were

identified in both 5′ capped and poly(A)+ RNA populations (Figure 1). Of note, 8 out of 17 upregulated genes (47%) and 2 out of 9 down-regulated genes (22%) unique to poly(A)+ RNA did have a statistically significant expression difference (p<0.05) in 5′ capped RNA, but were excluded from our list because their fold change did not meet the inclusion criteria (<1.5). None of 27 upregulated or 17 downregulated genes unique to 5′ capped RNA were found to have significant differential expression in the poly(A)+ RNA (see Tables S1, S2, S3, S4, S5, S6). This is likely due to less variation in signal intensity observed with 5′ capped RNA among experimental replicates as compared to poly(A)+ RNA (the average SEM per gene was 28.1 for 5′ capped; poly(A)+ average SEM per gene was 77.2).

Thirteen of the 64 genes (20%) found to be upregulated in HCV cirrhotic liver were identified by GO-term enrichment analysis to have biologic functions related to the immune response (Table 1) [24,25]. Several of these genes were selected for qPCR analysis of liver tissue from multiple patients, including interferon regulatory factor 1 (*IRF1*), a transcription factor involved in the interferon response to HCV infection *in-vitro* [26]. On ENCODE analysis, *IRF1* was found to be upregulated in HCV cirrhotic liver in 5′ capped RNA only (fold change 2.1, p = 0.03, Figure 2A). qPCR analysis of *IRF1* in multiple patient samples confirmed the ENCODE findings of increased expression in HCV cirrhotic liver (n = 7) compared to control liver (n = 10) (fold change 2.4, p = 0.03, Figure 2B). Percutaneous liver biopsies (n = 7) from patients with chronic hepatitis C with mild inflammation and no fibrosis (Metavir grade 1, stage 0) were also analyzed and showed a significant increase in *IRF1* expression (fold change 3.5, p = 0.001, Figure 2B). These patients were not being treated with recombinant interferon at the time of liver biospecimen acquisition.

The tripartite motif-containing 22 (*TRIM22*) mRNA, encoded by an interferon regulated gene previously reported to be upregulated with HIV and hepatitis B viral infections [27,28], was also found to have increased expression in our analysis of HCV cirrhotic liver. TRIM22 was increased on ENCODE analysis in both 5′ capped (fold change 4.1, p<0.001) and poly(A)+ RNA (fold change 6.2, p = 0.001, Figure 3A); we also identified increased transcription in intronic regions within the *TRIM22* gene. qPCR analysis of *TRIM22* showed a large increased expression (fold change 9.7, p<0.001) in HCV cirrhotic liver (Figure 3B). Liver biopsies from patients with mild chronic hepatitis C and no fibrosis showed a marked increase in *TRIM22* expression (fold change 17.0, p<0.001, Figure 3B).

Connective tissue growth factor (*CTGF*) mRNA is upregulated during liver fibrosis and its protein product has recently been suggested as a non-invasive biomarker of liver fibrosis in patients infected with hepatitis C [29]. *CTGF* mRNA was upregulated in both 5′ capped (fold change 5.5, p<0.001) and poly(A)+ RNA (fold change 13, p<0.001, Figure S1A). qPCR analysis of liver tissue from multiple control and HCV cirrhotic liver specimens showed a large mean increase in *CTGF* expression (fold change 17, p = 0.004) (Figure S1B). Interestingly, qPCR analysis of liver biopsies with mild chronic hepatitis C with no fibrosis showed no increase in *CTGF* expression (fold change −5.7, p = 0.03, Figure S1B).

Several other differentially expressed genes identified in the ENCODE tiling array analysis were selected for qPCR analysis using additional patient samples. The Met proto-oncogene (*MET*) is the hepatocyte growth factor receptor and has been implicated in the development of multiple tumor types. ENCODE array analysis of 5′ capped RNA showed decreased expression of *MET* in hepatitis C cirrhotic liver (fold change −1.8, p = 0.015, Figure S2A). However, qPCR analysis of multiple patients did not

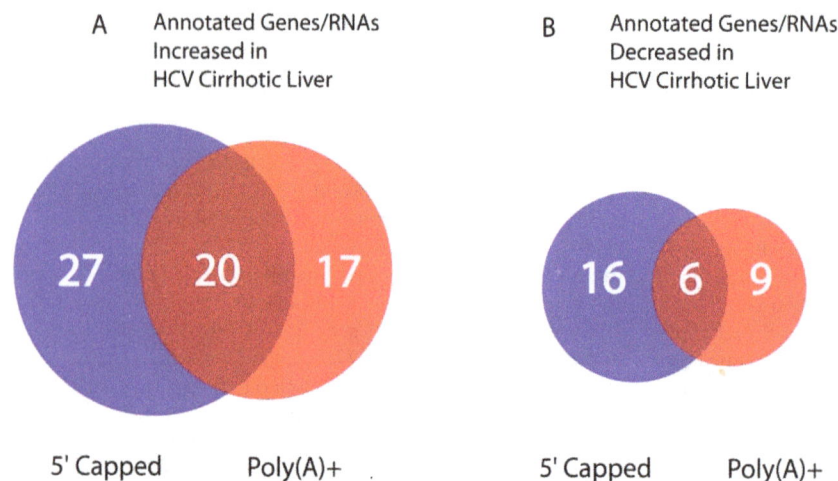

Figure 1. Differentially expressed genes in HCV cirrhotic versus control liver when analyzing 5′ or 3′ isolated RNA. Panel A. The number of genes with RNA levels that were increased in hepatitis C (HCV) cirrhotic as compared to control liver in the 5′ capped, poly(A)+, and both RNA populations are shown. **Panel B.** The number of genes with RNA levels that were decreased in HCV cirrhotic as compared to control liver in 5′ capped, poly(A)+, or both RNA populations are shown. RNA transcripts were isolated from HCV cirrhotic and control liver with the 5′ cap and poly(A)+ dependent purifications described in Methods. Four experimental replicates of HCV cirrhotic and control liver were used for this analysis. cDNA was synthesized using random hexamers and used to prepare probes (Methods). RNA transcript expression was measured by averaging fluorescent signal intensity on Agilent ENCODE gene arrays for each sample. Annotated genes with ≥1.5 fold changes and Bonferroni corrected p values <0.05 in HCV cirrhotic as compared to control liver were included in this figure.

demonstrate a significant difference in expression in HCV cirrhotic liver (Figure S2B). However, qPCR analysis of mild chronic hepatitis C biopsies with no fibrosis showed a significant increase in *MET* expression (fold change 3.7, p = 0.002, Figure S2B).

Cathepsin D (*CTSD*), a lysosomal aspartyl protease associated with several disease processes, was significantly upregulated in the ENCODE array analysis of 5′ capped RNA from hepatitis C cirrhotic liver (fold increase 1.9, p<0.001). However, when multiple patient samples were analyzed by qPCR no significant difference was identified (data not shown). The FUN14 domain containing 2 (*FUNDC2*) mRNA, encoding a protein suggested to interact with hepatitis C core protein, was downregulated in 5′ capped RNA from hepatitis C cirrhotic liver (fold change −2.1, p<0.001) [30]. However, when specimens of liver from additional patients with hepatitis C cirrhosis were analyzed by RT-PCR no significant difference was seen (data not shown). Nevertheless, RT-PCR of cDNA prepared from the same liver specimens (HCV cirrhotic 1 and Control 1) used in the ENCODE tiling array analysis did verify that *MET*, *CTSD* and *FUNDC2* were both significantly different in those specimens (data shown for MET only).

Differential gene expression associated with HCV cirrhotic liver was also observed in non-protein coding genomic regions including intronic and intergenic regions. Figure 4 illustrates the differential gene expression observed in exonic, intronic, and intergenic regions in 5′ capped and poly(A)+ RNA. Fifty percent of the upregulated and 78% of the downregulated nucleotides were found in intronic regions using 5′ capped RNA, as compared to 23% of the upregulated and 49% of the reduced nucleotides when poly(A)+ RNA was analyzed. A similar percentage of differentially expressed nucleotides were observed in intergenic regions when 5′ capped (4–10%) and poly(A)+ (8–10%) RNA samples were analyzed. Four annotated genes provide examples of higher intronic expression in 5′ capped as compared to poly(A)+ RNA: hepatocyte growth factor receptor (*MET*); tissue inhibitor of metalloproteinase 3 (*TIMP3*); mitogen-activated kinase kinase

kinase 1 (*MAP3K1*); MyoD family inhibitor domain containing (*MDFIC*); and (Figures S2 and S3).

Our ENCODE tiling array analysis of both 5′ capped and poly(A)+ RNA identified three differentially expressed transcriptionally active genomic regions where no annotated genes exist. These 5′ capped RNA transcript regions originated from chromosome 14 (Figure 5A, coordinates 53,254,000–53,256,899), chromosome 9 (Figure 6A, coordinates 131,088,154–131,089,262) and chromosome 21 (Figure S4A, coordinates 39,253,256–39,413,500). All three of these genomic regions demonstrated RNA transcription at least 10 kb from annotated genes. Although these regions were found to be transcribed in previous ENCODE tiling array analysis of HL60, HeLa, and Gm06990 human cell lines (Figure S5, http://genome.ucsc.edu/ENCODE/pilot.html), there was no prior evidence that they represented 5′ capped Pol II RNAs. Further investigation using the UCSC genome browser (http://genome.ucsc.edu) identified several ESTs (spliced and unspliced) originating from the transcribed region identified on chromosome 9 (Figure S6A). Not surprisingly, the 160kb region on chromosome 21 included several ESTs (BE870595, BG459638, BG460250, BI011795) and overlapped with one hypothetical protein (AJ011409, unpublished). It also included previously identified 5′ Rapid Amplification of cDNA Ends (RACE) products [31]. The 5′ capped RNA transcript(s) originating from the unannotated region of chromosome 14 did not overlap with any known genes in the UCSC database but was associated with a SNP (rs2884435) and several unspliced ESTs (Figure S6B).

qPCR analysis of the 5′ capped Pol II RNA(s) originating from the unannotated region on chromosome 14 confirmed the presence of a RNA transcript that was increased 7.8 fold in seven HCV cirrhotic as compared to ten control liver specimens (p<0.001) (Figure 5B). Moreover, qPCR analysis of mild chronic hepatitis C biopsies with no fibrosis showed a similar increase in expression of the transcript (fold change 11.3, p = 0.003, Figure 5B).

The 5′ capped RNA originating from the unannotated region on chromosome 9 was also confirmed to have a 4.5 fold increase by

Table 1. Differentially Expressed Genes Associated with Immune Response.

Gene Name (Ensembl)	Description	Isolation Technique	Mean Signal Intensity HCV Liver	Mean Signal Intensity Control Liver	Fold Change	Bonferroni p Value
Upregulated only in 5′ capped RNA						
*IRF1	Interferon regulatory factor 1 (IRF-1)	**5′ Capped RNA**	**674**	**323**	**2.09**	**0.033**
		Poly(A)+ RNA	2087	1363	1.53	51.505
LILRA1	Leukocyte immunoglobulin-like receptor subfamily A member 1 Precursor	**5′ Capped RNA**	**192**	**121**	**1.58**	**<0.001**
		Poly(A)+ RNA	219	171	1.28	18.386
LILRA4	Leukocyte immunoglobulin-like receptor subfamily A member 4 Precursor	**5′ Capped RNA**	**106**	**64**	**1.64**	**<0.001**
		Poly(A)+ RNA	126	102	1.24	7.956
*LILRB2	Leukocyte immunoglobulin-like receptor subfamily B member 2 Precursor	**5′ Capped RNA**	**756**	**359**	**2.1**	**0.015**
		Poly(A)+ RNA	1186	756	1.57	7.591
*LILRB4	Leukocyte immunoglobulin-like receptor subfamily B member 4 Precursor	**5′ Capped RNA**	**191**	**92**	**2.06**	**<0.001**
		Poly(A)+ RNA	378	246	1.54	0.388
RFX5	DNA-binding protein RFX5	**5′ Capped RNA**	**292**	**174**	**1.68**	**<0.001**
		Poly(A)+ RNA	899	523	1.72	0.729
TRIM34	Tripartite motif-containing protein 34	**5′ Capped RNA**	**108**	**65**	**1.67**	**<0.001**
		Poly(A)+ RNA	204	138	1.48	0.76
Upregulated only in Poly(A)+ RNA						
LEAP2	Liver-expressed antimicrobial peptide 2 Precursor	**5′ Capped RNA**	**139**	**98**	**1.42**	**0.003**
		Poly(A)+ RNA	626	712	2.96	0.001
LILRA5	Leukocyte immunoglobulin-like receptor subfamily A member 5 Precursor	**5′ Capped RNA**	**65**	**63**	**1.04**	**221.422**
		Poly(A)+ RNA	425	217	1.95	0.013
MAP4K2	Mitogen-activated protein kinase kinase kinase kinase 2	**5′ Capped RNA**	**121**	**94**	**1.29**	**0.037**
		Puly(A)+ RNA	402	226	2.13	0.021
PSMB4	Proteasome subunit beta type-4 Precursor	**5′ Capped RNA**	**390**	**393**	**−1.01**	**501.381**
		Poly(A)+ RNA	14358	4689	3.06	0.013
Upregulated in both 5′ capped and Poly(A)+ RNA						
*TRIM22	Tripartite motif-containing protein 22	**5′ Capped RNA**	**824**	**201**	**4.11**	**<0.001**
		Poly(A)+ RNA	3390	545	6.22	0.001
LAIR1	Leukocyte-associated immunoglobulin-like receptor 1 Precursor	**5′ Capped RNA**	**199**	**85**	**2.34**	**<0.001**
		Poly(A)+ RNA	337	148	2.28	0.001
Downregulated only in 5′ capped RNA						
IFNAR1	Interferon-alpha/beta receptor alpha chain Precursor	**5′ Capped RNA**	**312**	**646**	**−2.07**	**0.013**
		Poly(A)+ RNA	741	1220	−1.65	1.132
LILRB3	Leukocyte immunoglobulin-like receptor subfamily B member 3 Precursor	**5′ Capped RNA**	**83**	**138**	**−1.66**	**<0.001**
		Poly(A)+ RNA	922	980	−1.06	401.425

Pol II RNA transcripts were isolated from HCV cirrhotic and control liver via two methods. 5′ capped RNA was isolated using a high affinity variant eIF4E protein, poly(A)+ RNA was isolated with oligo-dT (Qiagen) and cDNA was synthesized with random primers (Methods). RNA transcript expression was measured by averaging fluorescent signal intensity on Agilent's ENCODE gene arrays for each sample (Methods). Differences in gene expression were visualized using Genoviz's Integrated Genome Browser software. Only annotated genes with ≥1.5 fold and Bonferroni corrected p values <0.05 between HCV cirrhotic and control liver are listed with details of their expression. Genes are listed by the specific pool of RNA analyzed. No genes with decreased expression in HCV cirrhotic liver were found in the poly(A)+ RNA. Genes which have been previously documented to have increased expression in HCV cirrhotic liver are marked with *. Only genes associated with the immune response are listed above. A complete list of differentially expressed genes is provided in supplemental materials.

qPCR analysis of seven HCV cirrhotic as compared to ten control liver specimens (p<0.001) (Figure 6B). qPCR analysis of mild chronic hepatitis C with no fibrosis showed a similar increase in expression of the transcript (fold change 4.1, p = 0.002, Figure 6B).

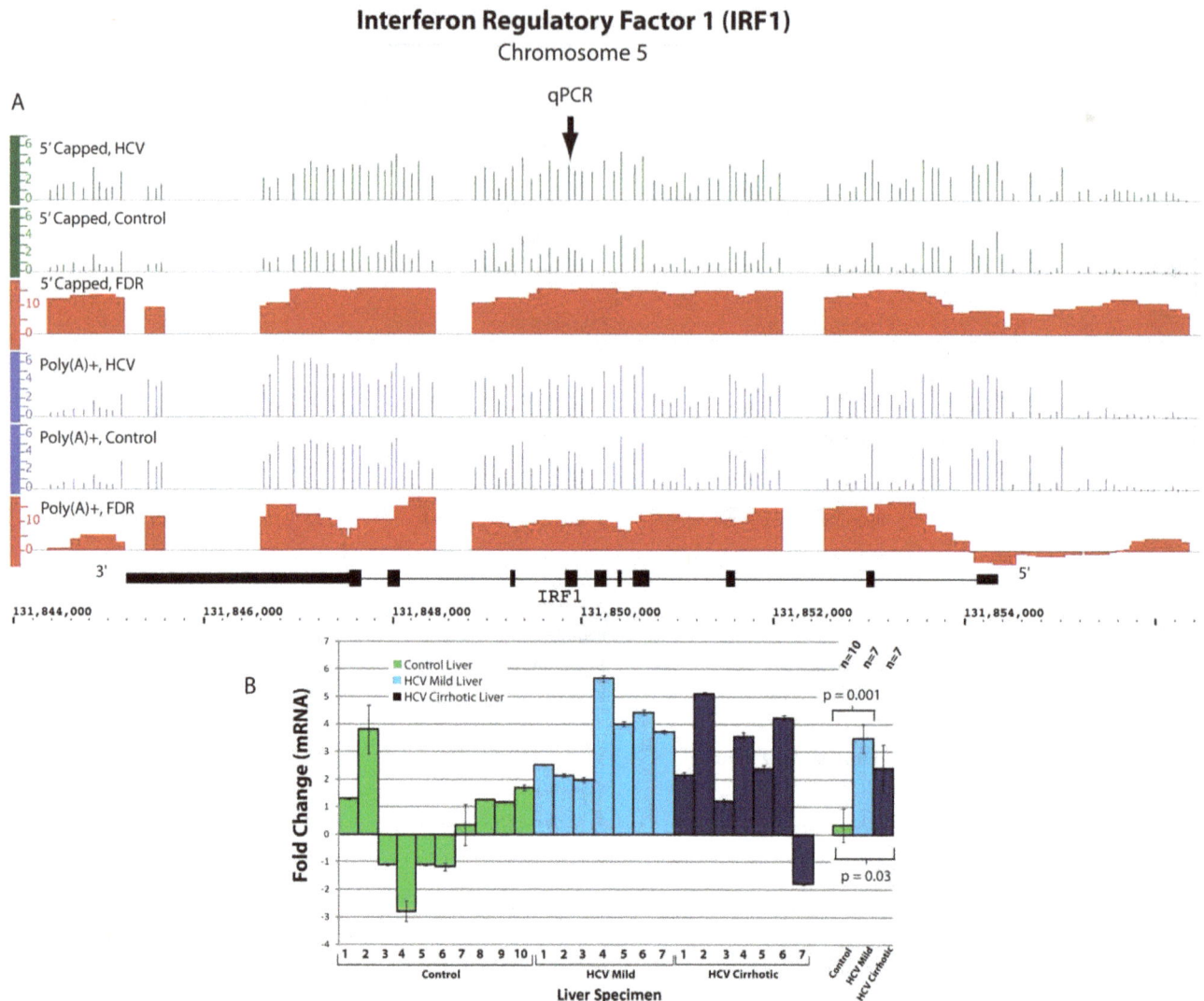

Figure 2. **Differential expression of** *IRF1* **in HCV cirrhotic as compared to control liver. Panel A.** Expression of *IRF1* as measured by signal intensity on ENCODE tiling arrays is displayed using the Integrated Genome Browser (IGB). The y-axis represents the log2 transformation of the normalized signal divided by the background signal on arrays and each bar represents the normalized signal intensity of probes hybridized to 60mer targets tiled across the gene region (Methods). Genomic regions that are tiled yet lack a signal are indicated by a baseline tick mark. Absence of a tick mark indicates no probes in that region. Gene structure, orientation, and chromosomal location are shown in black. Average RNA expression based on the analysis of 5′ capped RNA isolated from HCV cirrhotic and control liver is depicted in green for both HCV cirrhotic and control liver. Average RNA expression using poly(A)+ RNA is depicted in blue. Differences in expression between HCV cirrhotic and control liver for poly(A)+ and 5′ capped RNA populations are depicted as window level false discovery rates in red (-10Log$_{10}$ FDR) (see Methods). A transformed FDR of ≥13 (represents an untransformed FDR ≤0.05 or 5 false positives out of 100) was considered statistically significant. **Panel B.** qPCR was performed as described in Methods. Triplicate samples from seven HCV cirrhotic, seven mild HCV (no fibrosis), and ten control livers were analyzed. HCV Cirrhotic 1 and Control 1 refer to the original samples used for the ENCODE tiling array analysis. The mean ± SEM fold change for each specimen analyzed is shown and the location of the qPCR primers is indicated by qPCR in Panel A. P-values were calculated using the Student's t-test.

The region on chromosome 21 did not differ significantly among multiple patients with HCV cirrhosis using qPCR.

To further define the structure of differentially expressed RNA(s) originating from chromosome 9 and 14, we used 5′ and 3′ rapid amplification of cDNA ends (RACE) and DNA sequencing over one region on chromosome 9 and three separate regions of chromosome 14 (Chr14a, Chr14b, and Chr14c) where differential expression was observed by ENCODE analysis. Using 5′ RACE we identified the 5′ end of an unannotated RNA transcript found on chromosome 9 (Figure S6A). The 5′ end of this transcript was at a similar chromosome coordinate as other previously identified ESTs. Using 3′ RACE we identified the 3′

ends of independent RNA transcripts on the minus strand of Chr14a and Chr14b regions, respectively (Figure S6B). We also sequenced approximately 600–800 nucleotides including the poly(A)+ end of each transcript. The existence of at least a 1.50 kb transcript in the chromosome 14c region was confirmed by standard PCR product sequencing. To compare relative expression of RNA transcripts on the Chr14a and Chr14c regions we performed qPCR analysis. Interestingly, gene expression was similar in the HCV cirrhotic and control human liver samples but more than 10-fold higher in the Chr14a region compared to the Chr14c region in Huh7.5 cells, a human hepatoma cell line (data not shown).

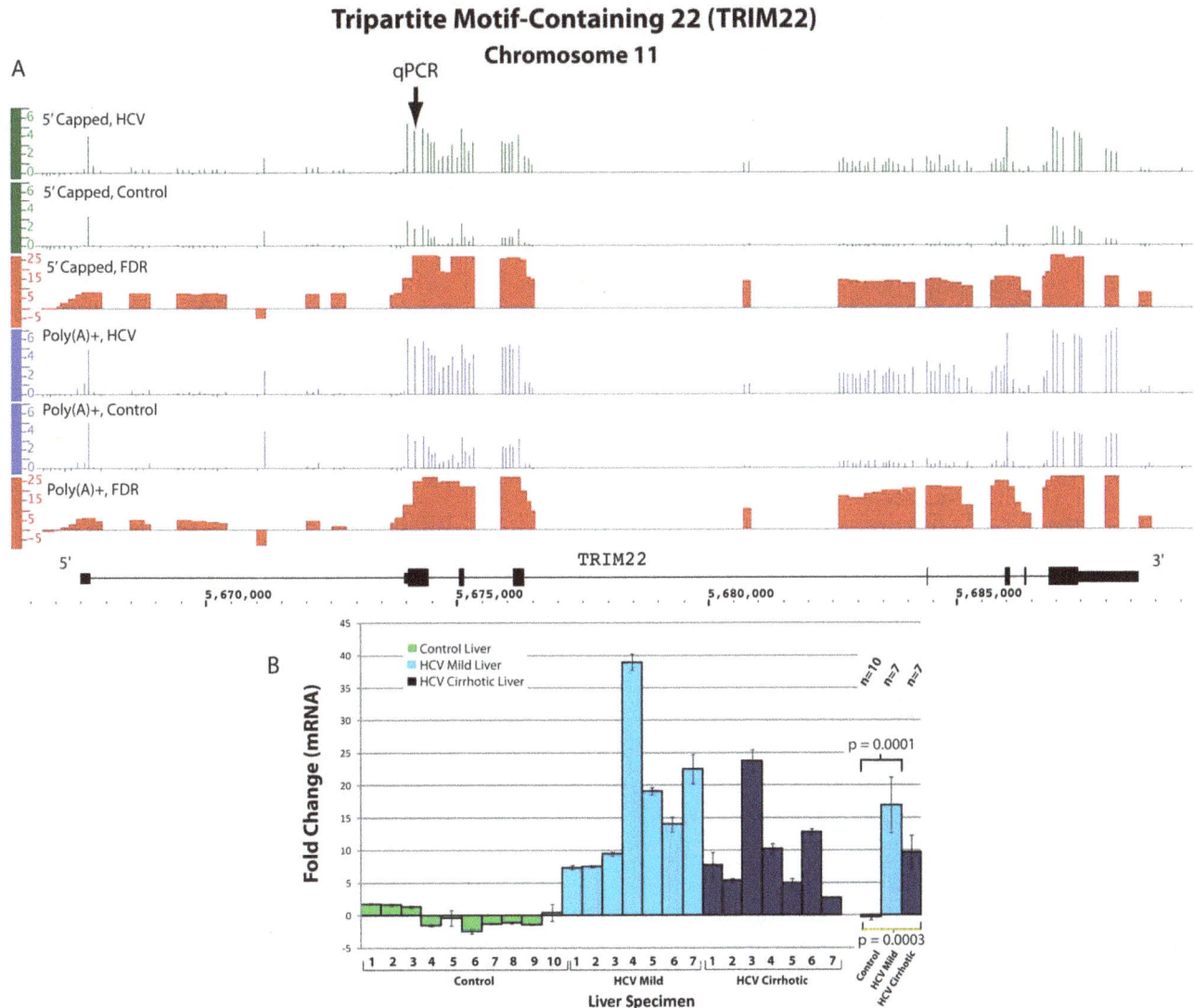

Figure 3. Differential expression of *TRIM22* in HCV cirrhotic as compared to control liver tissue. Panel A. The expression of *TRIM22* as measured by signal intensity on ENCODE tiling arrays are displayed using the IGB. The data are displayed as in Figure 2. **Panel B.** qPCR was performed as described for Figure 2 and in Methods.

Discussion

The quantitative analysis of RNA transcripts in control and diseased tissue to define differential gene expression and aid biomarker discovery has generally used cDNA derived from total or poly(A)+ RNA hybridized to oligonucleotide microarrays. Recent studies of RNA transcription in human cells using ENCODE tiling arrays and poly(A)+ RNA have surprisingly described extensive transcription in previously unannotated genomic regions [18,31,32]. A consistent observation in these studies has been unexpectedly high transcription in unannotated and intronic regions of the genome. For example, a high-resolution strand-specific analysis of the entire transcriptome of *S. pombe* showed extensive transcription including intergenic and antisense transcription [19]. In addition, studies suggest that the number of Pol II transcripts with absent or short poly(A)+ ends may be markedly underestimated (ref 18, 20). Based on these findings it seems likely that standard microarray analyses are underestimating disease specific gene expression changes. In this

study we tested this possibility by analyzing gene expression changes in hepatitis C (HCV) cirrhotic as compared to control liver in both 5′ capped and poly(A)+ populations of RNA using ENCODE tiling arrays representing 1% of the genome.

Differential gene expression between HCV cirrhotic and control liver, in most cases, was observed with a greater sensitivity and additional detail when 5′ capped RNA was analyzed as compared to poly(A)+ RNA (Table 1). Although many of the differentially expressed transcripts identified using poly(A)+ RNA had higher fold changes, the variability between experimental replicates was greater resulting in failed statistical testing. One possible explanation for the increased consistency in analyzing 5′ capped as compared to poly(A)+ RNA could be variability of the poly(A)+ ends. Short poly(A)+ ends have been demonstrated for a number of well-annotated genes in human liver, such as eNOS mRNA in vascular endothelial cells, and is a well-documented mechanism for regulating gene expression in developmental models [20,33,34]. Moreover, examples of mRNAs with a poly(A)-limiting element in their 3′ end, such as the Xenopus albumin mRNA

Differentially Expressed Exonic, Intronic, and Intergenic Regions in HCV Cirrhotic Liver

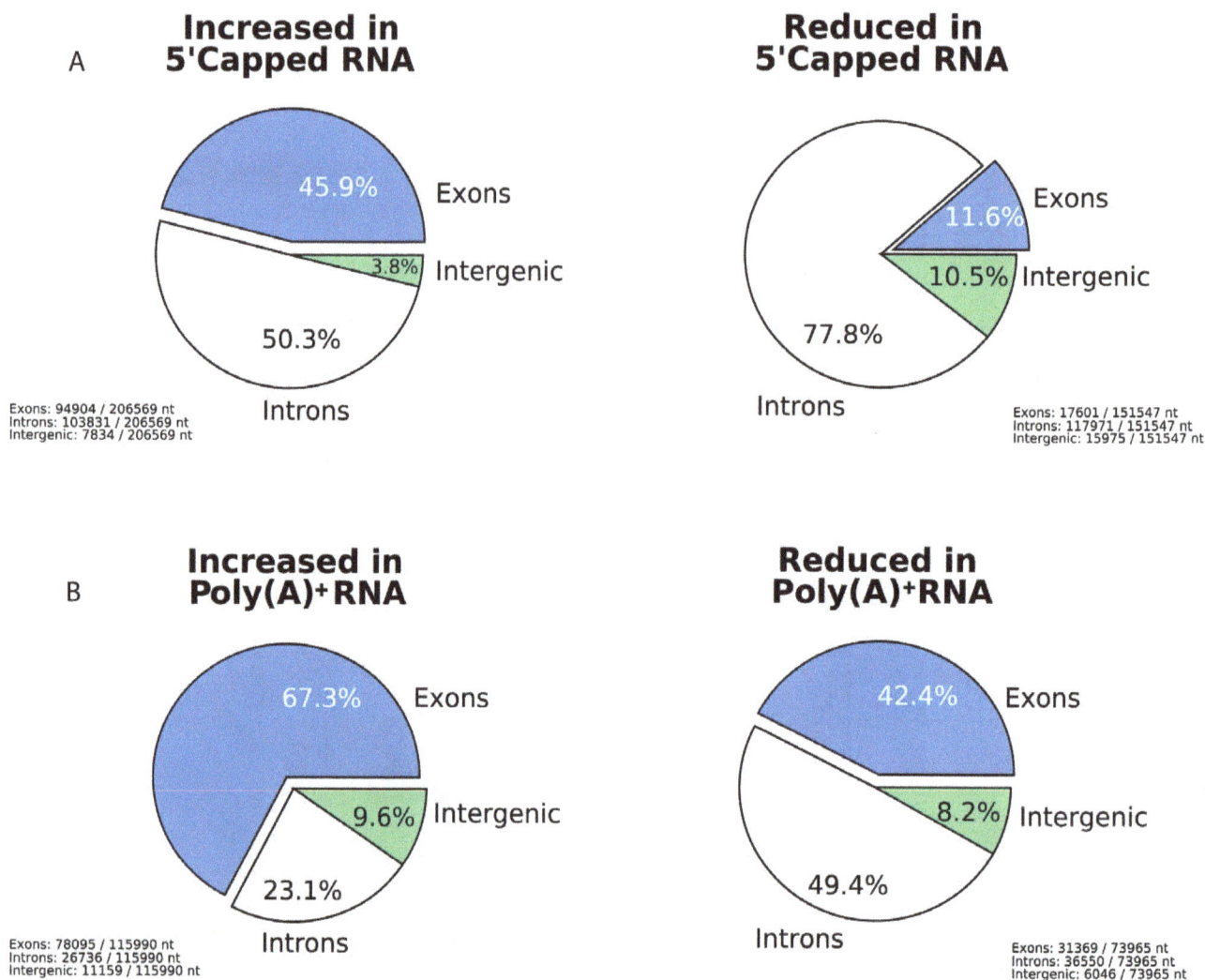

Figure 4. Differential gene expression observed in exonic, intronic, and intergenic regions in 5′ capped and poly(A)+ RNA. Pie charts depict the relative percentage of differentially expressed nucleotides in HCV cirrhotic liver as compared to control liver using 5′ capped RNA (**Panel A**) or poly(A)+ RNA analysis (**Panel B**). Charts on the left show increased expression and charts on the right show reduced expression. The percentage of differentially expressed nucleotides found in intronic, exonic, and intergenic regions are shown for 5′ capped and poly(A)+ RNA samples.

produced by liver, have poly(A)+ ends of <20 nts yet are efficiently translated [35].

Additional differences observed in the ENCODE tiling array analysis of 5′ capped and poly(A)+ RNA populations included differences in signal intensity across specific regions of each gene transcript. In most cases the signal intensities at the 3′ end of transcripts were greater when poly(A)+ RNA was analyzed as compared to 5′ capped RNA. In some cases the signal on tiling arrays was greater in the 5′ end of annotated genes when 5′ capped RNA was analyzed as compared to poly(A)+ RNA. With some gene transcripts, such as the hepatocyte growth factor receptor (MET), tissue inhibitor of metalloproteinase 3 (TIMP3), MyoD family inhibitor domain containing (MDFIC) and mitogen-activated kinase kinase kinase 1 (MAP3K1), higher levels of

transcription was observed in intronic regions when 5′ capped RNA was analyzed as compared to poly(A)+ RNA. This is consistent with the 5′ capped RNA purification that includes unspliced heterogeneous nuclear RNA (hnRNA) as well as mature spliced RNA, while the poly(A) dependent purification predominantly represents mature spliced RNA.

We identified many immune response genes that were significantly increased in HCV cirrhotic as compared to control liver, as other studies have, and found upregulated genes that were not identified previously by gene array analysis. These included IRF1, tripartite motif-containing 22 (TRIM22), and multiple leukocyte immunoglobulin-like receptors (LILRA1, LILRA4, LILRA5, LILRB2, LILRB3 and LILRB4) [14,16,36]. IRF1 transcription was significantly increased in HCV cirrhotic as

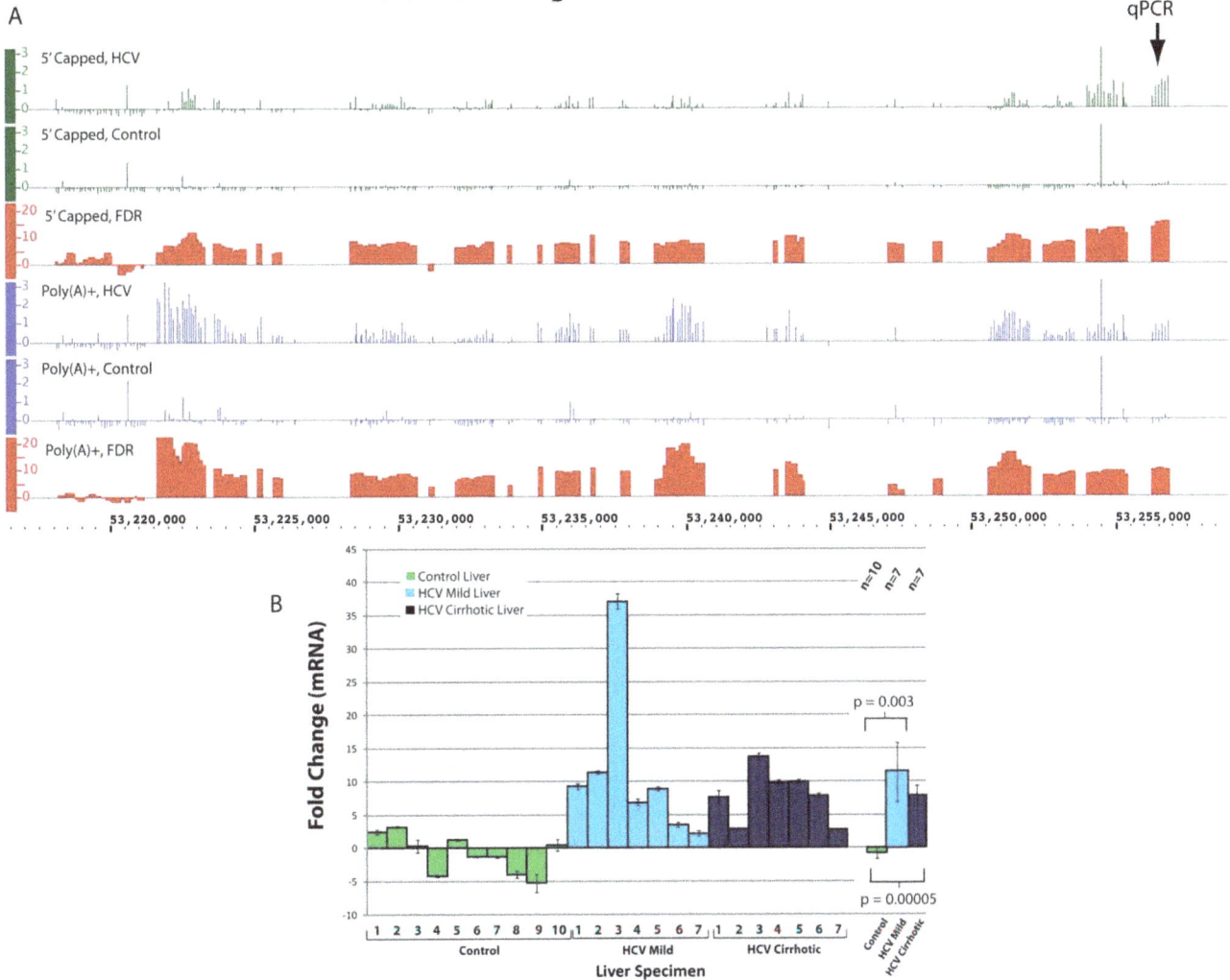

Figure 5. Differential expression of a Pol II RNA from an unannotated region of Chromosome 14. Panel A. Expression of 5′ capped and poly(A)+ RNAs as measured by signal intensity on ENCODE tiling arrays are displayed using IGB. The data is displayed as in Figure 2 except that each tick mark represents the normalized mean signal intensity of probes within a 200 nt window. **Panel B.** qPCR was performed as described in Methods. Triplicate samples from seven HCV cirrhotic, seven mild HCV (no fibrosis) and ten control livers were analyzed. HCV cirrhotic 1 and Control 1 refer to original samples used for the ENCODE tiling array analysis. The mean ± SEM fold change for all specimens analyzed is shown and the location of the qPCR primers is indicated by qPCR in Panel A.

compared to control liver when 5′ capped RNA was analyzed, but not when poly(A)+ RNA was analyzed. *IRF1* is a critical transcriptional regulatory factor that modulates interferon stimulated gene (ISG) expression and has been shown to regulate HCV subgenomic replicon activity in cultured hepatoma cells [37,38]. Interestingly, polymorphisms in the *IRF1* promoter have been reported to be associated with a better response to interferon alpha (IFN-α) therapy in patients with chronic hepatitis C [39]. Tripartite motif (TRIM) 22 was another immune response related gene that was significantly increased in HCV cirrhotic as compared to control liver in our analysis. The tripartite motif family of proteins has been associated with innate immunity to viruses by restricting viral replication [40]. *TRIM22* is dramatically upregulated by interferon signaling and decreases HIV replication (Barr et al., 2008). In addition, it has recently been shown to suppress HBV replication in culture [28]. Genome wide expression array analysis of both chimpanzee and human liver tissue have provided evidence for increased expression of TRIM22

in hepatitis C infected liver, however this is the first report to confirm its increased expression in HCV infected human liver (both cirrhotic and non-fibrotic) using real time PCR [11,12,41]. The qPCR analysis of biopsies showing mild hepatitis C without fibrosis provide evidence that the upregulation of *IRF1*, *TRIM22*, and *MET* are authentically due to HCV infection, and not due to major changes in liver tissue cell type.

Further evidence of alterations in immune response function includes the upregulation of multiple leukocyte immunoglobulin-like receptors. These receptors, also known as immunoglobulin-like transcripts (ILTs), are expressed on myelomonocytic cells and can influence both the innate and acquired immune response [42]. *LILRB2*, the most highly upregulated inhibitory ILT in our study, is also upregulated in HIV patients and may impair the antigen presentation of monocytes [43]. Increased expression of another inhibitory ILT, *LILRB4* or ILT3, also impairs antigen presentation and T cell recruitment as well as modulates the expression of proinflammatory cytokines [44]. Together, these transcriptional

Unannotated Region Chromosome 9

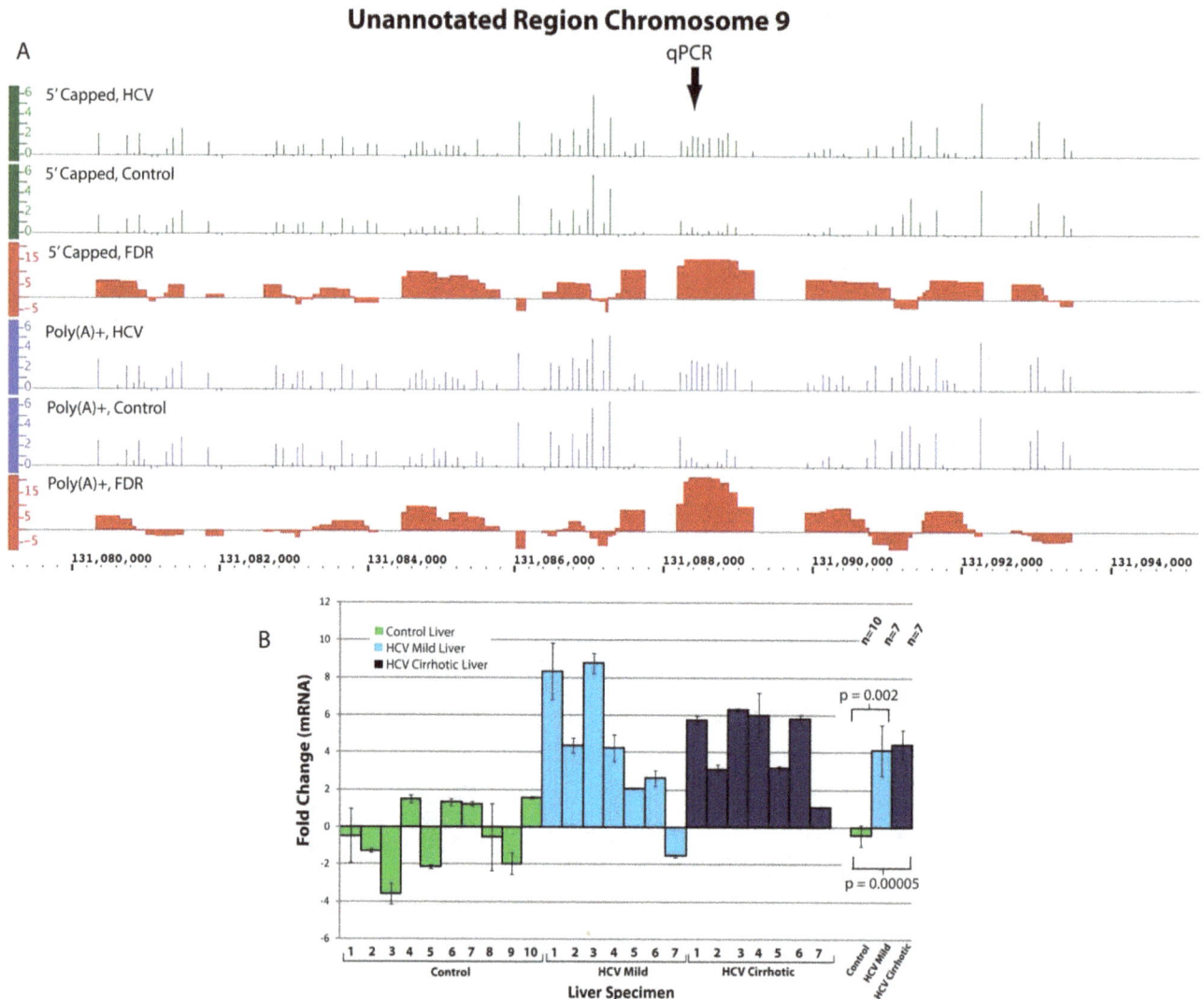

Figure 6. Differential expression of a Pol II RNA from an unannotated region of Chromosome 9. Panel A. Expression of 5′ capped and poly(A)+ RNAs as measured by signal intensity on ENCODE tiling arrays are displayed using IGB. The data is displayed as in Figure 5. **Panel B.** qPCR was performed as described in Methods. Triplicate samples from seven HCV cirrhotic, seven mild HCV (no fibrosis) and ten control livers were analyzed. HCV cirrhotic 1 and Control 1 refer to original samples used for the ENCODE tiling array analysis. The mean ± SEM fold change for all specimens analyzed is shown and the location of the qPCR primers is indicated by qPCR in Panel A.

changes observed in immune response genes are consistent with viral infection. It should be noted that a number of interferon-inducible genes previously reported to be upregulated with HCV infection were not interrogated in our ENCODE tiling array analysis (representing 1% of the genome) included *STAT1*, *IRF9*, *IFI27*, *CXCL9*, *CXCL19* and *CXCL11* [41,45,46].

A number of gene expression studies of HCV infected liver biospecimens, done with annotated gene arrays and qPCR, have been reported. They include studies that identified potential molecular makers for HCV-associated liver disease and transcript profiles predictive of both early stage fibrosis and end stage HCV induced liver disease (cirrhosis) [14,47]. These studies provided evidence that during late stages of HCV induced liver disease many of the changes in gene expression observed between HCV-infected liver as compared to control liver biospecimens are due to liver fibrosis and not HCV infection. Gene transcripts found to be upregulated in both early and late stage disease include many interferon-stimulated genes like *STAT1*, *IRF9*, *IFI27* and *CXCL10*

while transcripts involved in growth factor signaling and tissue remodeling like *CTGF*, *MMP7* and *IL8* are more commonly upregulated during fibrosis [47,48,49]. In our tiling arrays studies, 1% of the genome was interrogated at a high degree of resolution that included approximately 400 protein coding genes. Therefore a direct comparison of gene transcripts interrogated in our dataset compared to whole annotated gene datasets is limited. Nevertheless, our gene expression results are consistent with the activation of interferon signaling pathways in both mild hepatitis C (without fibrosis) and HCV cirrhotic biospecimens as observed by the significant upregulation of both liver *IRF1* and *TRIM22* mRNA transcripts. In addition, *CTGF*, considered a biomarker of fibrosis and cirrhosis, was only upregulated in HCV cirrhotic biospecimens but not in mild hepatitis C without fibrosis similar to previous reports. With the goal of improving the selection of patients for current hepatitis C therapies, liver gene expression signatures predictive of response to therapy have been identified [13,45,50]. These gene signatures have included interferon stimulated transcripts including *IFI5*, *IFI6* and *IFNAR1* that are differentially expressed between responders and non-responders. Recently *IL28B* genotype has been found to be a strong predictor of response to therapy and spontaneous clearance of HCV [51,52,53,54,55]. A recent report indicates that low interferon induced gene expression in liver biopsies is a stronger predictor of treatment response than *IL28B* genotype in patients with hepatitis C [56]. The approach we describe may be useful in developing future panels of gene expression biomarkers for patients with chronic hepatitis C or other liver disorders that predict clinical outcomes such as the risk for hepatocellular carcinoma.

We also identified novel unannotated regions showing increased transcription in both HCV cirrhotic and mild hepatitis C as compared to control liver including multiple RNA transcripts on chromosome 14 and an unannotated RNA transcript on chromosome 9. It is unknown at this time whether these transcripts represent protein coding RNAs or non-coding regulatory RNAs. The use of a sequence analysis tool (BESTORF, www.softberry.com) to predict potential coding fragments in these unannotated sequences, did not identify any open reading frames greater than 40 amino acids. This finding suggests that these transcripts may represent non-coding RNAs. In addition to the presence of open reading frames (ORF), both expression level and cross-species sequence homology are important indicators of the protein coding or non-coding nature of RNA transcripts [57]. Based on the low expression level of the novel transcript found in the chromosome 14c region, it's low sequence homology to other species, and our inability to identify a poly(A)+ tail in this transcript, it may indeed represent a non-coding RNA. Although the other two RNA transcripts on chromosome 14 (14a and 14b) and one on chromosome 9 were expressed at a higher level, their low cross species homology suggests they are also non-coding RNAs. These unannotated expressed regions were evaluated for possible miRNAs using the informatics program MIREVAL [58]. Although this analysis identified multiple possible miRNA precursor hairpin structures in the chromosome 14 transcript, none of these regions encoded known miRNAs in the miRBase database [59]. Our evidence that these transcriptionally active regions represent novel Pol II transcripts is supported by transcription at these same chromosomal coordinates in published ENCODE analysis of poly(A)+ RNA from human cell lines [18]. These uncharacterized Pol II transcripts may represent genes that are part of the host antiviral defense or those required for specific steps in replication or release of mature virions. We are currently further defining these RNAs and testing their biological role in an HCV cell culture system.

We conclude that analyzing 5′ capped RNAs in eukaryotic cells and biospecimens aids the definition of the complete Pol II transcriptome and increases the sensitivity of identifying differentially expressed Pol II genes in physiological and pathophysiological states. This approach should also prove useful in identifying subsets of mRNAs that are regulated post-transcriptionally by changes in pre-mRNA splicing or 3′ polyadenylation states [33,60,61,62]. Analyzing differentially selected RNAs, such as 5′ capped and poly(A)+ RNA, with next generation RNA sequencing technologies should be very useful in fully defining the Pol II transcriptome and identifying previously undefined Pol II transcripts that are differentially expressed in disease states. In addition, such novel transcripts may prove useful as biomarkers and may provide insight into the role of ncRNAs in the development and progression of specific diseases.

Methods

RNA isolation

Total RNA was prepared using TRIzol (Invitrogen). A single sample from one hepatitis C cirrhotic and one control liver

specimen were used for the initial ENCODE tiling array analysis. A total of seven hepatitis C cirrhotic liver explants, ten control liver specimens and seven percutaneous biopsies showing mild hepatitis C with no fibrosis were used for qPCR analysis. RNA species with 5′ m^{7}GpppN caps were purified using a recombinant GST fusion high-affinity variant of eIF4E (eIF4E$_{K119A}$) which binds m^{7}Gpp with a tenfold higher affinity as compared to wild-type eIF4E [23,63]. The 5′ capped RNAs were purified as previously described using GST-eIF4E$_{K119A}$ recombinant protein bound to glutathione-agarose beads in microfuge tubes by batch purification [20,64]. The efficiency of this purification is 70% as compared to 30% when wild-type eIF-4E is used in such purifications (manuscript in preparation). The quantity of 5′ capped RNA was measured by NanoDrop analysis and its integrity confirmed with an Agilent 2100 Bioanalyzer. Total RNA from the same liver explants was used as a starting material to purify 5′ capped and poly(A)+ RNA. The poly(A)+ RNA was purified with oligo(dT) beads (Oligotex®, Qiagen) as previously described [20]. The quantity and integrity of poly(A)+ RNA was determined by the same measures used for 5′ capped RNA.

Human liver pathological specimens

Liver explant pathological specimens from patients undergoing liver transplantation for chronic hepatitis C with cirrhosis (n = 7) and unused donor (control) liver tissue (n = 10) were collected with IRB approval. HCV cirrhotic liver samples were from both female and male patients as were the donor liver specimens. Percutaneous liver biopsy specimens from patients with chronic hepatitis C found to have mild inflammation and no fibrosis (mild HCV; Metavir grade 1, stage 0) (n = 7) were obtained with IRB approval. All HCV liver samples were flash frozen in liquid nitrogen generally within 5 to 10 minutes after biopsy or organ removal.

ENCODE tiling arrays

Four experimental replicate samples of 5′ capped RNA isolated from hepatitis C cirrhotic liver and control liver were used to produce cDNA using a commercially available kit (Just cDNA Double-Stranded cDNA Synthesis Kit, Stratagene, La Jolla, CA). Random hexamers were used to prime first strand cDNA synthesis from both 5′ capped and poly(A)+ RNA samples. The cDNA product was labeled using an Agilent Genomic DNA Labeling Kit PLUS by incorporating fluorescently labeled nucleotides (Cy3-dUTP or Cy5-dUTP) using the exo-Klenow fragment. Following termination of the labeling reaction, fluorescently labeled cDNA probes were purified by isopropanol precipitation. Precipitated pellets were dried and then rehydrated in distilled water. The concentration of purified oligonucleotides was determined using a NanoDrop ND-1000 spectrophotometer. A fraction of the labeled DNA (100 ng) was assayed with an Agilent BioAnalyzer to validate the size distribution of the labeled cDNA probes.

Fluorescently labeled cDNA probes were heat denatured after being combined with cot-1 DNA, Agilent aCGH blocking agent and Agilent Hi-RPM hybridization solution. Microarray hybridizations were performed using Agilent SureHyb chambers incubated at 65°C for 40 hours with a rotational speed of 20 rpm. Following incubation, the microarray slide was washed for 5 minutes in aCGH/ChIP-on-chip Wash Buffer 1 (0.5X SSPE, 0.005% N-lauroylsarcosine; room temperature) and 5 minutes in a CGH/ChIP-on-chip Wash Buffer 2 (0.1X SSPE, 0.005% N-lauroylsarcosine; 31°C). Microarray slides (Agilent ID# 014792) were briefly dipped in a solution of acetonitrile and dried. Two microarray slides each were used for labeled cDNA generated from 5′ capped and poly(A)+ RNA from two experimental replicate samples (HCV cirrhotic and control liver). These slides were then stripped and used again with the other two experimental replicate samples.

Microarray slides were scanned in an Agilent Technologies G2505B Microarray Scanner at 5 μm resolution for the simultaneous detection of Cy-3 and Cy-5 signals. Data captured from the scanned microarray image was saved as a TIFF image file and loaded into Agilent Feature Extraction Software version 10.1.1.1. The software automatically positions a grid and finds the centroid positions of each feature on the microarray. This information was used to perform calculations that include feature intensities, background measurements and statistical analyses. Data generated by the software was recorded as tab-delimited text files which were processed using the *TiMAT2* open-source software package (http://timat2.sourceforge.net) and results were visualized and our graphics produced using the *Integrated Genome Browser* (IGB) [65].

Bioinformatic Analysis

Data quality. The quality of data was assessed by calculating all pair Pearson correlation coefficients for each set of biological replicas using the unadjusted raw median intensity from the Agilent scan files ($R^2 * 100$: 5′ capped hepatitis C cirrhotic: 98.6%, 85.2%, 85.4%, 89.5%, 89%, 97.7%; 5′ capped control: 97.6%, 95.7%, 90.6%, 94%, 85.3%, 90%; poly(A)+ hepatitis C cirrhotic: 93.7%, 61.3%, 82.9%, 75.1%, 91.4%, 91.1%; poly(A)+ Control: 91.2%, 91.6%, 90.1%, 91.8%, 94.5%, 94.3%). The mean R^2*100 correlation was 89%.

Whole Genome Static Maps. Scaled static maps were made for comparison in *IGB* for each of the four datasets (5′ capped control, 5′ capped hepatitis C cirrhotic, poly(A)+ control, and poly(A)+ hepatitis C cirrhotic liver) using the *TiMAT2* analysis package. Agilent's ENCODE probe sequences were remapped to the NCBI 36.1 human genome build. For each sample, the four biological replica raw median probe intensities were quantile normalized and median scaled to 50 [66]. For each probe, an average was calculated for the replicas, divided by 50, and log2 transformed.

Whole Genome Dynamic Difference Maps. To identify regions of change between the different RNA samples (5′ capped HCV cirrhotic compared to 5′ capped control and poly(A)+ HCV cirrhotic compared to poly(A)+ control liver), a sliding window approach was taken to minimize noise using the *TiMAT2* package. The four test (HCV cirrhotic) and four control remapped raw median probe intensities were quantile-normalized and median scaled to 50. Probe level summaries were calculated by taking the log2 ratio between the mean treatment and mean control. Window level summaries were calculated by identifying 260 bp windows that contain 2 or more probes. These windows were scored by first calculating all the relative difference pairs between the treatment and the control replica probes, and second, by calculating the pseudo median of these relative difference pairs. For display purposes, the pseudo median relative difference scores were converted to log2 (ratios). To estimate window level FDRs, a null distribution of random label permutation pseudo median scored windows was created. The FDR estimation associated each real pseudo median window score was calculated by dividing the number of null distribution windows that met or exceeded the score (false positives) by the number of real windows that exceeded the score (true positives and false positives). For display purposes, the FDRs were -10Log10(FDR) transformed. This FDR estimation was used to score both enriched and reduced windows. Regions enriched (or reduced) in the HCV cirrhotic compared to control liver were created by joining overlapping and adjacent windows (max gap 200 bp) with an FDR of ≥13

(-10Log10(0.05)). The majority of such regions correspond with known annotation. To identify potentially novel transcribed regions, the window arrays were first filtered against those that intersected any known exonic sequence, using a known gene set created by combining UCSC's Known Genes and the Ensembl gene database [67,68].

Gene-Centric Analysis. A near identical approach was used to identify genes differentially transcribed in the HCV cirrhotic vs. control datasets. Instead of a sliding window, normalized probe intensities falling within the exons of each gene model were compared using the pseudo median and random label statistics. Those genes with an FDR ≥13 and a log2 ratio >0.65 were considered differentially transcribed.

Bayesian Analysis. Differential gene expression for well-annotated genes was determined by the regularized *t*-test, which uses a Bayesian procedure [69]. Briefly, the expression level of each gene was assumed to be from a normal distribution with μ and σ^2. Using a conjugate prior, the mean of the posterior (MP) estimate of μ is the sample mean. The MP estimate of σ^2 is $\sigma^2 = \frac{v_0\sigma_0^2 + (n-1)s^2}{v_0 + n - 2}$, where n is the sample size, s^2 is the sample variance, v_0 is the degrees of freedom of the prior (a value of 10 is used in the analysis), σ_0^2 is the mean of sample variances of genes in the neighborhood of the gene under consideration. The neighborhood was the 50 genes with sample means immediately above and below the sample mean of the gene under consideration; that is, the neighborhood consists of the 101 genes centered on the gene. After the MP estimates of μ and σ^2 are obtained, the *t*-test of unequal variances was used to calculate a P-value of differential expression.

Real-time PCR (qPCR). Ten control, seven hepatitis C cirrhotic liver and seven mild HCV (no fibrosis) specimens were used for further analysis of differential gene expression in hepatitis C infected liver tissue. cDNA was prepared from these pathological specimens and assayed for transcript levels of selected genes to determine if the same changes in gene expression observed in the ENCODE array analysis of one control and disease sample were observed in multiple patients with hepatitis C as compared to controls. Total RNA from control, hepatitis C cirrhotic and mild HCV liver was extracted using TRIzol followed by an RNA cleanup procedure using a RNeasy Mini kit (Qiagen, Valencia, CA). RNA was treated with DNase I (Invitrogen, Carlsbad, CA) to remove genomic DNA. First-strand cDNA was synthesized using Moloney Murine Leukemia Virus reverse transcriptase (SuperScript III; Invitrogen) with 20 ng/μl of RNA at 55°C (60 min) with random hexamers or oligo(dT) primers. Each PCR reaction was carried out in a 96-well optical plate (Roche Applied Science) in a 20 μl reaction buffer containing LightCycler 480 Probes Master Mix (100 mM Tris-HCl, 100 mM KCl, 400 μM of each dNTP (with dUTP instead of dTTP), 64 mM MgCl₂, FastStart Taq DNA Polymerase, 0.3 μM of each primer, 0.1 μM hydrolysis probe and approximately 50 ng of cDNA (done in triplicate). Triplicate incubations without template were used as negative controls. Thermal cycling was done in a Roche LightCycler 480 System (Roche Applied Science). The qPCR thermo cycling was 95°C for 5 min, 45 cycles at 95°C for 10 sec, 59°C for 30 sec and 72°C for 1 sec. The relative quantity of each RNA transcript was calculated with the comparative Ct (cycling threshold) method using the formula $2^{\Delta Ct}$. ΔCt represents the difference between target gene expression in control samples and target gene expression in HCV samples. A reference gene (β-actin, *ACTB*) was used as the control and statistical significance was evaluated using the Student's T-test.

RACE Analysis. To define RNA transcript(s) structure from the differentially expressed unannotated regions on chromosomes 9 and 14, 5′ and 3′ rapid amplification of cDNA ends (RACE) were performed using cDNA made from total RNA and oligo (dT) primer or 5′ capped RNA and random primers. We designed gene specific primers on the minus and plus strand of one region on chromosome 9 and three different regions on chromosome 14 (Chr14a, Chr14b, and Chr14c) that were found to be differentially expressed in HCV cirrhotic liver by ENCODE tiling array analysis. To verify the chromosome location of each RACE PCR product, each PCR product was gel purified and cloned using a TA cloning vector. Cloned products were then sequenced with an Applied Biosystems 3130xl Genetic Analyzer.

Supporting Information

Figure S1 Differential expression of CTGF in hepatitis C (HCV) cirrhotic as compared to control liver. Panel A. Expression of Connective tissue growth factor (CTGF) as measured by signal intensity on ENCODE tiling arrays is displayed using IGB. The data are displayed as in Figure 2. Panel B. Real-time PCR (qPCR) was performed as described in Methods. Triplicate samples from seven HCV cirrhotic, seven mild HCV (no fibrosis) and ten control livers were analyzed. HCV cirrhotic 1 and Control 1 refer to original samples used for the ENCODE tiling array analysis. The mean + SEM fold change for all specimens analyzed is shown.

Figure S2 Differential expression of MET in hepatitis C (HCV) cirrhotic as compared to control liver. Panel A. MET (mesenchymal-epithelial transition factor) is a proto-oncogene that encodes the tyrosine kinase MET and is also known as c-Met or hepatocyte growth factor receptor (HGFR). Expression of MET as measured by signal intensity on ENCODE tiling arrays is displayed using IGB. The data are displayed as in Figure 2. FDRs are depicted as negative because this gene showed less expression in hepatitis C cirrhotic as compared to control liver. Panel B. qPCR was performed as described in Methods. Triplicate samples from seven HCV cirrhotic, six mild HCV (no fibrosis), and ten control livers were analyzed. HCV cirrhotic 1 and Control 1 refer to original samples used for the ENCODE tiling array analysis. The mean + SEM fold change for all specimens analyzed is shown. Note that due to limited quantities of cDNA from mild HCV percutaneous liver biopsy specimens, duplicates were performed for four biospecimens and triplicates for two (note SEM bars for assays done in triplicate).

Figure S3 Increased intronic RNA expression from 5′ capped RNA compared to poly(A)+ RNA in HCV cirrhotic and normal human liver. Panel A, Tissue inhibitor of metalloproteinase 3 (TIMP3); Panel B, Mitogen-activated protein kinase kinase kinase 1 (MAP3K1); and Panel C, MyoD family inhibitor domain containing (MDFIC) gene transcripts. Expression of 5′ capped and poly(A)+ RNAs as measured by signal intensity on ENCODE tiling arrays are displayed using IGB.

Figure S4 Differential expression of a Pol II RNA transcript(s) originating from an unannotated region of Chromosome 21 in HCV cirrhotic as compared to control liver. Panel A. Expression of the unannotated region identified by signal intensity on ENCODE tiling arrays is displayed using IGB. The data are displayed as in Figure 5. Panel B. Liver specimens from seven HCV cirrhotic and seven control livers were analyzed by qPCR in

triplicate. HCV cirrhotic 1 and Control 1 refer to original samples used for the ENCODE tiling array analysis. The mean + SEM fold change for all specimens analyzed are shown for the qPCR1 primer set. Results for the second primer set (qPCR2) also did not show a significant difference between HCV cirrhotic and control specimens (not shown).

Figure S5 Differentially expressed unannotated genomic regions in HCV cirrhotic liver compared with ENCODE data from human cell lines. The data from high density tiling array analysis of GM06690 cells (nontumorigenic B lymphocytes), HeLa cells, and HL60 (human promyelocytic leukemia, predominantly neutrophilic promyelocyte precursors) cells was loaded into IGB and aligned with the ENCODE tiling array data that we obtained in this study. The signal intensity on the ENCODE tiling arrays are displayed in IGB as in Figure 5. The aligned data provide evidence that the changes in RNA signals observed in HCV cirrhotic liver as compared to control liver in the unannotated region of chromosome 14, 9, and 21 were also observed in the ENCODE array analysis of GM06690, HL60, and HeLa cells (http://genome.ucsc.edu/ENCODE/pilot.html). The strongest signals were observed in the GM06690 cells suggesting that at least some of the signal in this region observed in HCV cirrhotic liver was due to lymphoid cells that home to and infiltrate the liver during chronic hepatitis C.

Figure S6 Structural characterization of differentially expressed unannotated Pol II transcripts on chromosome 9 and 14. Schematic drawing showing an unannotated RNA transcript on chromosome 9 and 14 identified by Agilent ENCODE tiling array analysis of 5′ capped (green bars) and polyA+ (blue bars) RNA. Panel A. Chromosome 9 The solid green block represents sequenced 5′ RACE product, with the 5′ capped end shown in black. The arrow at the top of the figure depicts location of qPCR assay. Human ESTs are depicted in solid black blocks in the format of the UCSC Genome Browser. The 5′ end of multiple ESTs on the plus strand line up with the 5′ end of our 5′ RACE product supporting the existence of a novel RNA transcript in this region. Repeating elements, also shown in black, depict highly repetitive nucleotide sequences not tiled on the ENCODE array. Affymetrix ENCODE tiling array data from a lymphoblastoid cell line (GM06990, ENCODE pilot project) is presented at the bottom of the figure (purple bars). Panel B. Chromosome 14 Three differentially expressed regions upregulated in HCV cirrhotic liver (14a, 14b, and 14c) are shown in the format of the Integrated Genome Browser (IGB). Solid green blocks show regions of sequenced 3′ RACE and PCR products, with the poly(A)+ ends shown in red. Two distinct transcripts on the minus strand of 14a and 14b regions, respectively, were confirmed by DNA sequencing. One transcript 1.5 kb in length was confirmed by DNA sequencing in the 14c region. Two black lines at the top of the figure depict location of qPCR assays. Human ESTs are depicted in solid black blocks in the format of the UCSC Genome Browser. Affymetrix ENCODE tiling array data from a lymphoblastoid cell line (GM06990, ENCODE pilot project) is presented at the bottom of the figure (purple bars).

Table S1 Upregulated genes in HCV cirrhotic liver, identified only by analyzing 5′ capped RNA. RNA transcripts were isolated from hepatitis C infected and control liver as described in Methods. cDNA was prepared using random hexamers and probes prepared as described in Methods. RNA transcript expression was measured by averaging fluorescent signal intensity on Agilent ENCODE arrays for each sample. Only annotated genes with >1.5 fold differences and Bonferoni corrected p-values <0.05 between hepatitis C infected and control liver are listed. Differentially expressed genes are categorized by function. Mean signal intensity, fold change, and p-values for each gene as determined by analyzing poly(A)+ RNA is included for comparison. Genes that have been previously documented to have increased expression in HCV infected liver are highlighted marked with*.

Table S2 Upregulated genes in HCV cirrhotic liver identified only by analyzing poly(A)+ RNA. Annotated genes tiled on ENCODE arrays with >1.5 fold change and Bonferoni corrected p-values <0.05 are listed by function. Genes that have been previously documented to have increased expression in HCV infected liver, hepatocellular carcinoma, or cirrhosis due to other causes are marked with *.

Table S3 Upregulated genes in HCV cirrhotic liver identified by analyzing both 5′ capped and poly(A)+ RNA. Annotated genes with a >1.5 fold change and Bonferoni corrected p-value <0.05 are listed by function. Genes that have been previously reported to be increased in HCV infected liver, hepatocellular carcinoma or cirrhosis due to other causes are marked with*.

Table S4 Downregulated genes in HCV cirrhotic liver identified only by analyzing 5′ capped RNA. Annotated genes with a >1.5 fold change and Bonferoni corrected p-values <0.05 are listed by function. Genes that have been previously reported to be changed

in hepatitis C infected liver, hepatocellular carcinoma, or cirrhosis are marked with *.

Table S5 Downregulated genes in HCV cirrhotic liver identified only by analyzing poly(A)+ RNA. Annotated genes with a >1.5 fold change and Bonferoni corrected p-values <0.05 are listed by function.

Table S6 Downregulated genes in HCV cirrhotic liver identified by analyzing both 5′ cap and poly(A)+ RNA. Annotated genes with a >1.5 fold change and Bonferoni corrected p-values <0.05 are listed by function.

Acknowledgments

We thank B. Cairns for helpful suggestions and members of the Huntsman Cancer Institute Genomics Core Facility for assistance in this study. We thank L. Wang and B. Cairns for their critical review of the manuscript, L. Wang for several control liver biospecimens and S. Young for her illustrations.

The raw data has been submitted to the NCBI Gene Expression Omnibus (GEO) under accession number GSE18904.

Author Contributions

Conceived and designed the experiments: CH. Performed the experiments: MF DAD CAN. Analyzed the data: MF DAD CIM CAN DN CH. Contributed reagents/materials/analysis tools: JJS CH. Wrote the paper: MF DAD CIM CH.

References

1. Alizadeh AA, Eisen MB, Davis RE, Ma C, Lossos IS, et al. (2000) Distinct types of diffuse large B-cell lymphoma identified by gene expression profiling. Nature 403: 503–511.
2. Rassenti LZ, Jain S, Keating MJ, Wierda WG, Grever MR, et al. (2008) Relative value of ZAP-70, CD38, and immunoglobulin mutation status in predicting aggressive disease in chronic lymphocytic leukemia. Blood 112: 1923–1930.
3. Rosenwald A, Alizadeh AA, Widhopf G, Simon R, Davis RE, et al. (2001) Relation of gene expression phenotype to immunoglobulin mutation genotype in B cell chronic lymphocytic leukemia. J Exp Med 194: 1639–1647.
4. Chang HY, Nuyten DS, Sneddon JB, Hastie T, Tibshirani R, et al. (2005) Robustness, scalability, and integration of a wound-response gene expression signature in predicting breast cancer survival. Proc Natl Acad Sci U S A 102: 3738–3743.
5. Chang JC, Wooten EC, Tsimelzon A, Hilsenbeck SG, Gutierrez MC, et al. (2003) Gene expression profiling for the prediction of therapeutic response to docetaxel in patients with breast cancer. Lancet 362: 362–369.
6. Khan J, Wei JS, Ringner M, Saal LH, Ladanyi M, et al. (2001) Classification and diagnostic prediction of cancers using gene expression profiling and artificial neural networks. Nat Med 7: 673–679.
7. Sotiriou C, Pusztai L (2009) Gene-expression signatures in breast cancer. N Engl J Med 360: 790–800.
8. van de Vijver MJ, He YD, van't Veer LJ, Dai H, Hart AA, et al. (2002) A gene-expression signature as a predictor of survival in breast cancer. N Engl J Med 347: 1999–2009.
9. Wang Y, Klijn JG, Zhang Y, Sieuwerts AM, Look MP, et al. (2005) Gene-expression profiles to predict distant metastasis of lymph-node-negative primary breast cancer. Lancet 365: 671–679.
10. Garman KS, Acharya CR, Edelman E, Grade M, Gaedcke J, et al. (2008) A genomic approach to colon cancer risk stratification yields biologic insights into therapeutic opportunities. Proc Natl Acad Sci U S A 105: 19432–19437.
11. Bigger CB, Brasky KM, Lanford RE (2001) DNA microarray analysis of chimpanzee liver during acute resolving hepatitis C virus infection. J Virol 75: 7059–7066.
12. Smith MW, Walters KA, Korth MJ, Fitzgibbon M, Proll S, et al. (2006) Gene expression patterns that correlate with hepatitis C and early progression to fibrosis in liver transplant recipients. Gastroenterology 130: 179–187.

13. Chen L, Borozan I, Feld J, Sun J, Tannis LL, et al. (2005) Hepatic gene expression discriminates responders and nonresponders in treatment of chronic hepatitis C viral infection. Gastroenterology 128: 1437–1444.
14. Smith MW, Yue ZN, Korth MJ, Do HA, Boix L, et al. (2003) Hepatitis C virus and liver disease: global transcriptional profiling and identification of potential markers. Hepatology 38: 1458–1467.
15. Lederer SL, Walters KA, Proll S, Paeper B, Robinzon S, et al. (2006) Distinct cellular responses differentiating alcohol- and hepatitis C virus-induced liver cirrhosis. Virol J 3: 98.
16. Honda M, Yamashita T, Ueda T, Takatori H, Nishino R, et al. (2006) Different signaling pathways in the livers of patients with chronic hepatitis B or chronic hepatitis C. Hepatology 44: 1122–1138.
17. Peng X, Li Y, Walters KA, Rosenzweig ER, Lederer SL, et al. (2009) Computational identification of hepatitis C virus associated microRNA-mRNA regulatory modules in human livers. BMC Genomics 10: 373.
18. Birney E, Stamatoyannopoulos JA, Dutta A, Guigo R, Gingeras TR, et al. (2007) Identification and analysis of functional elements in 1% of the human genome by the ENCODE pilot project. Nature 447: 799–816.
19. Dutrow N, Nix DA, Holt D, Milash B, Dalley B, et al. (2008) Dynamic transcriptome of Schizosaccharomyces pombe shown by RNA-DNA hybrid mapping. Nat Genet 40: 977–986.
20. Choi YH, Hagedorn CH (2003) Purifying mRNAs with a high-affinity eIF4E mutant identifies the short 3′ poly(A) end phenotype. Proc Natl Acad Sci U S A 100: 7033–7038.
21. Rasmussen EB, Lis JT (1993) In vivo transcriptional pausing and cap formation on three Drosophila heat shock genes. Proc Natl Acad Sci U S A 90: 7923–7927.
22. Shatkin AJ, Manley JL (2000) The ends of the affair: capping and polyadenylation. Nat Struct Biol 7: 838–842.
23. Spivak-Kroizman T, Friedland DE, De Staercke C, Gernert KM, Goss DJ, et al. (2002) Mutations in the S4-H2 loop of eIF4E which increase the affinity for m7GTP. FEBS Lett 516: 9–14.
24. Ashburner M, Ball CA, Blake JA, Botstein D, Butler H, et al. (2000) Gene ontology: tool for the unification of biology. The Gene Ontology Consortium. Nat Genet 25: 25–29.
25. Zeeberg BR, Feng W, Wang G, Wang MD, Fojo AT, et al. (2003) GoMiner: a resource for biological interpretation of genomic and proteomic data. Genome Biol 4: R28.

26. Sumpter R, Jr., Wang C, Foy E, Loo YM, Gale M, Jr. (2004) Viral evolution and interferon resistance of hepatitis C virus RNA replication in a cell culture model. J Virol 78: 11591–11604.

27. Barr SD, Smiley JR, Bushman FD (2008) The interferon response inhibits HIV particle production by induction of TRIM22. PLoS Pathog 4: e1000007.

28. BoGao, ZhijianDuan, WeiXu, SidongXiong (2009) Tripartite motif-containing 22 inhibits the activity of hepatitis B virus core promoter, which is dependent on nuclear-located RING domain. Hepatology NA 9999.

29. Kovalenko E, Tacke F, Gressner OA, Zimmermann HW, Lahme B, et al. (2009) Validation of connective tissue growth factor (CTGF/CCN2) and its gene polymorphisms as noninvasive biomarkers for the assessment of liver fibrosis. J Viral Hepat 16: 612–620.

30. Li K, Wang L, Cheng J, Zhang L, Duan H, et al. (2002) [Screening and cloning gene of hepatocyte protein interacting with hepatitis C virus core protein]. Zhonghua Shi Yan He Lin Chuang Bing Du Xue Za Zhi 16: 351–353.

31. Wu JQ, Du J, Rozowsky JS, Zhang ZD, Urban AE, et al. (2008) Systematic analysis of transcribed loci in ENCODE regions using RACE sequencing reveals extensive transcription in the human genome. Genome Biology 9: R3.

32. Denoeud F, Kapranov P, Ucla C, Frankish A, Castelo R, et al. (2007) Prominent use of distal 5′ transcription start sites and discovery of a large number of additional exons in ENCODE regions. Genome Research 17: 746–759.

33. Richter JD (2008) Breaking the code of polyadenylation-induced translation. Cell 132: 335–337.

34. Weber M, Hagedorn CH, Harrison DG, Searles CD (2005) Laminar shear stress and 3′ polyadenylation of eNOS mRNA. Circ Res 96: 1161–1168.

35. Peng J, Schoenberg DR (2005) mRNA with a <20-nt poly(A) tail imparted by the poly(A)-limiting element is translated as efficiently in vivo as long poly(A) mRNA. RNA 11: 1131–1140.

36. Ura S, Honda M, Yamashita T, Ueda T, Takatori H, et al. (2009) Differential microRNA expression between hepatitis B and hepatitis C leading disease progression to hepatocellular carcinoma. Hepatology 49: 1098–1112.

37. Kanazawa N, Kurosaki M, Sakamoto N, Enomoto N, Itsui Y, et al. (2004) Regulation of hepatitis C virus replication by interferon regulatory factor 1. J Virol 78: 9713–9720.

38. Itsui Y, Sakamoto N, Kurosaki M, Kanazawa N, Tanabe Y, et al. (2006) Expressional screening of interferon-stimulated genes for antiviral activity against hepatitis C virus replication. J Viral Hepat 13: 690–700.

39. Wietzke-Braun P, Maouzi AB, Manhardt LB, Bickeboller H, Ramadori G, et al. (2006) Interferon regulatory factor-1 promoter polymorphism and the outcome of hepatitis C virus infection. Eur J Gastroenterol Hepatol 18: 991–997.

40. Nisole S, Stoye JP, Saib A (2005) TRIM family proteins: retroviral restriction and antiviral defence. Nat Rev Microbiol 3: 799–808.

41. Helbig KJ, Lau DT, Semendric L, Harley HA, Beard MR (2005) Analysis of ISG expression in chronic hepatitis C identifies viperin as a potential antiviral effector. Hepatology 42: 702–710.

42. Brown D, Trowsdale J, Allen R (2004) The LILR family: modulators of innate and adaptive immune pathways in health and disease. Tissue Antigens 64: 215–225.

43. Vlad G, Piazza F, Colovai A, Cortesini R, Della Pietra F, et al. (2003) Interleukin-10 induces the upregulation of the inhibitory receptor ILT4 in monocytes from HIV positive individuals. Hum Immunol 64: 483–489.

44. Chang CC, Liu Z, Vlad G, Qin H, Qiao X, et al. (2009) Ig-like transcript 3 regulates expression of proinflammatory cytokines and migration of activated T cells. J Immunol 182: 5208–5216.

45. Asselah T, Bieche I, Narguet S, Sabbagh A, Laurendeau I, et al. (2008) Liver gene expression signature to predict response to pegylated interferon plus ribavirin combination therapy in patients with chronic hepatitis C. Gut 57: 516–524.

46. Bieche I, Asselah T, Laurendeau I, Vidaud D, Degot C, et al. (2005) Molecular profiling of early stage liver fibrosis in patients with chronic hepatitis C virus infection. Virology 332: 130–144.

47. Asselah T, Bieche I, Laurendeau I, Paradis V, Vidaud D, et al. (2005) Liver gene expression signature of mild fibrosis in patients with chronic hepatitis C. Gastroenterology 129: 2064–2075.

48. Mas VR, Fassnacht R, Archer KJ, Maluf D (2010) Molecular mechanisms involved in the interaction effects of alcohol and hepatitis C virus in liver cirrhosis. Mol Med 16: 287–297.

49. Shackel NA, McGuinness PH, Abbott CA, Gorrell MD, McCaughan GW (2002) Insights into the pathobiology of hepatitis C virus-associated cirrhosis: analysis of intrahepatic differential gene expression. Am J Pathol 160: 641–654.

50. Hayashida K, Daiba A, Sakai A, Tanaka T, Kaji K, et al. (2005) Pretreatment prediction of interferon-alfa efficacy in chronic hepatitis C patients. Clin Gastroenterol Hepatol 3: 1253–1259.

51. Aparicio E, Parera M, Franco S, Perez-Alvarez N, Tural C, et al. (2010) IL28B SNP rs8099917 is strongly associated with pegylated interferon-alpha and ribavirin therapy treatment failure in HCV/HIV-1 coinfected patients. PLoS One 5: e13771.

52. Ge D, Fellay J, Thompson AJ, Simon JS, Shianna KV, et al. (2009) Genetic variation in IL28B predicts hepatitis C treatment-induced viral clearance. Nature 461: 399–401.

53. Thomas DL, Thio CL, Martin MP, Qi Y, Ge D, et al. (2009) Genetic variation in IL28B and spontaneous clearance of hepatitis C virus. Nature 461: 798–801.

54. Tanaka Y, Nishida N, Sugiyama M, Kurosaki M, Matsuura K, et al. (2009) Genome-wide association of IL28B with response to pegylated interferon-alpha and ribavirin therapy for chronic hepatitis C. Nat Genet 41: 1105–1109.

55. Suppiah V, Moldovan M, Ahlenstiel G, Berg T, Weltman M, et al. (2009) IL28B is associated with response to chronic hepatitis C interferon-alpha and ribavirin therapy. Nat Genet 41: 1100–1104.

56. Dill MT, Duong FH, Vogt JE, Bibert S, Bochud PY, et al. (2010) Interferon-Induced Gene Expression Is a Stronger Predictor of Treatment Response than IL28B Genotype in Patients with Hepatitis C. Gastroenterology.

57. Kikuchi K, Fukuda M, Ito T, Inoue M, Yokoi T, et al. (2009) Transcripts of unknown function in multiple-signaling pathways involved in human stem cell differentiation. Nucleic Acids Res 37: 4987–5000.

58. Ritchie W, Theodule FX, Gautheret D (2008) Mireval: a web tool for simple microRNA prediction in genome sequences. Bioinformatics 24: 1394–1396.

59. Griffiths-Jones S, Saini HK, van Dongen S, Enright AJ (2008) miRBase: tools for microRNA genomics. Nucleic Acids Res 36: D154–158.

60. Beilharz TH, Humphreys DT, Clancy JL, Thermann R, Martin DI, et al. (2009) microRNA-mediated messenger RNA deadenylation contributes to translational repression in mammalian cells. PLoS One 4: e6783.

61. Schwertz H, Tolley ND, Foulks JM, Denis MM, Risenmay BW, et al. (2006) Signal-dependent splicing of tissue factor pre-mRNA modulates the thrombogenicity of human platelets. J Exp Med 203: 2433–2440.

62. Suh N, Crittenden SL, Goldstrohm A, Hook B, Thompson B, et al. (2009) FBF and its dual control of gld-1 expression in the Caenorhabditis elegans germline. Genetics 181: 1249–1260.

63. Friedland DE, Wooten WN, LaVoy JE, Hagedorn CH, Goss DJ (2005) A mutant of eukaryotic protein synthesis initiation factor eIF4E(K119A) has an increased binding affinity for both m7G cap analogues and eIF4G peptides. Biochemistry 44: 4546–4550.

64. Bajak EZ, Hagedorn CH (2008) Efficient 5′ cap-dependent RNA purification: use in identifying and studying subsets of RNA. Methods Mol Biol 419: 147–160.

65. Nicol JW, Helt GA, Blanchard SG, Jr., Raja A, Loraine AE (2009) The Integrated Genome Browser: Free software for distribution and exploration of genome-scale data sets. Bioinformatics.

66. Bolstad BM, Irizarry RA, Astrand M, Speed TP (2003) A comparison of normalization methods for high density oligonucleotide array data based on variance and bias. Bioinformatics 19: 185–193.

67. Birney E, Andrews TD, Bevan P, Caccamo M, Chen Y, et al. (2004) An overview of Ensembl. Genome Res 14: 925–928.

68. Hsu F, Kent WJ, Clawson H, Kuhn RM, Diekhans M, et al. (2006) The UCSC Known Genes. Bioinformatics 22: 1036–1046.

69. Baldi P, Long AD (2001) A Bayesian framework for the analysis of microarray expression data: regularized t -test and statistical inferences of gene changes. Bioinformatics 17: 509–519.

12

Longitudinal Liver Stiffness Assessment in Patients with Chronic Hepatitis C Undergoing Antiviral Therapy

Stella M. Martinez[1], Juliette Foucher[2], Jean-Marc Combis[3], Sophie Métivier[4], Maurizia Brunetto[5], Dominique Capron[6], Marc Bourlière[7], Jean-Pierre Bronowicki[8], Thong Dao[9], Marianne Maynard-Muet[10], Damien Lucidarme[11], Wassil Merrouche[2], Xavier Forns[1], Victor de Lédinghen[2]*

1 Liver Unit, Hospital Clinic, IDIBAPS and CIBERehd, Barcelona, Spain, 2 Centre d'Investigation de la Fibrose hépatique, Hôpital Haut-Lévêque, CHU Bordeaux, Pessac, France, 3 Clinique Ambroise Paré, Toulouse, France, 4 Service d'hépato-gastro-entérologie, CHU Purpan, Toulouse, France, 5 Hepatology Unit, University Hospital of Pisa, Pisa, Italy, 6 Department of Hepato-Gastroenterology, Amiens University Hospital, Amiens, France, 7 Service d'hépato-gastroentérologie, Hôpital Saint-Joseph, Marseille, France, 8 Service d'hépatogastroentérologie, INSERM 954, CHU de Nancy, Vandoeuvre-les-Nancy, France, 9 Service d'Hépatogastroentérologie et de Nutrition, CHU Côte de Nacre, Caen, France, 10 Department of Gastroenterology and Hepatology, Hôpital de la Croix Rousse, Lyon, France, 11 Service de Pathologie Digestive, Université Nord de France, Groupe Hospitalier de l'Institut Catholique Lillois/Faculté Libre de Médecine Lille, Lille, France

Abstract

Background/Aims: Liver stiffness (LS) measurement by means of transient elastography (TE) is accurate to predict fibrosis stage. The effect of antiviral treatment and virologic response on LS was assessed and compared with untreated patients with chronic hepatitis C (CHC).

Methods: TE was performed at baseline, and at weeks 24, 48, and 72 in 515 patients with CHC.

Results: 323 treated (62.7%) and 192 untreated patients (37.3%) were assessed. LS experienced a significant decline in treated patients and remained stable in untreated patients at the end of study ($P<0.0001$). The decline was significant for patients with baseline LS ≥ 7.1 kPa ($P<0.0001$ and P 0.03, for LS ≥ 9.5 and ≥ 7.1 kPa vs lower values, respectively). Sustained virological responders and relapsers had a significant LS improvement whereas a trend was observed in nonresponders (mean percent change -16%, -10% and -2%, for SVR, RR and NR, respectively, P 0.03 for SVR vs NR). In multivariate analysis, high baseline LS ($P<0.0001$) and ALT levels, antiviral therapy and non-1 genotype were independent predictors of LS improvement.

Conclusions: LS decreases during and after antiviral treatment in patients with CHC. The decrease is significant in sustained responders and relapsers (particularly in those with high baseline LS) and suggests an improvement in liver damage.

Editor: James Fung, The University of Hong Kong, Hong Kong

Funding: This is an independent study, supported in part by Roche. Stella Martinez was granted by Fundación Banco Bilbao Vizcaya Argentaria (BBVA). The funders had no role in study design, data collection and analysis, decision to publish, or preparation of the manuscript.

Competing Interests: Victor de Lédinghen receives consulting fees from Merck, Roche, Gilead, Janssen, Echosens and Bayer. Xavier Forns receives unrestricted grant support from Roche and MSD. Juliette Foucher is on the advisory board for Janssen. Thông Dao is a board member for Schering Plough and receives consulting fees from Roche and Gilead. Jean Marc Combis is employed by Clinique Ambroise Paré.

* E-mail: victor.deledinghen@chu-bordeaux.fr

Introduction

Liver fibrosis is a key determinant of morbidity and mortality in the natural history of CHC. There is evidence that antiviral therapy can improve liver histology not only by reversing liver damage in sustained responders, but also by slowing the progression in relapser patients. [1,2].

Liver biopsy has been currently considered the reference standard to assess the extent of fibrosis, though it is associated with risk of complications and has limitations due to observer variability and sampling error.[3–5] Thus, several routine laboratory tests combined in scores and indices such as Forns' score, APRI index and FIB-4 index, [6–9] or other panels like FibroTest (α2-macroglobulin, haptoglobin, apolipoprotein A1, gammaglutamyl transpeptidase and total bilirubin) [10] and more recently the ELF score (aminoterminal propeptide of type III procollagen (PIIINP), hyaluronic acid (HA) and tissue inhibitor of matrix metalloproteinase type 1 (TIMP-1)) [11] have been validated as useful tools to accurately detect significant fibrosis or cirrhosis in clinical practice. FibroTest, ELF score, Forns Score or other tests that include markers of extracellular matrix have been also validated in the evaluation of response to interferon-based therapy. [12–15].

More recently, transient elastography has emerged as a useful, rapid and reproducible tool to measure liver stiffness as an accurate marker to predict liver fibrosis degree.[16–20] Furthermore, the utility of elastography has also been evaluated in monitoring progression of fibrosis in the setting of hepatitis C virus recurrence after liver transplantation. [21].

In addition, changes in liver stiffness both during and after antiviral treatment have been previously examined by several other studies.[22–24].

The aims of this large prospective longitudinal multicentre study were to assess the effects of antiviral treatment and virologic response in liver stiffness and compare these changes with untreated patients with CHC. In addition, other biochemical and indirect tests of liver fibrosis were also assessed.

Patients and Methods

Ethics Statement

All patients provided written informed consent for blood samples and to data handling in accordance with a protocol specifically approved by the appropriate institutional review boards (IRB) which included: Hospital Clinic of Barcelona IRB and University Hospital of Bordeaux IRB for the centers in France.

Study Population

From July 2008 through March 2009, we conducted this prospective multicentre study at ten participating sites in three European countries (Spain, France and Italy).

A total of 515 consecutive patients with CHC were enrolled in this study. The diagnosis of CHC was established by the presence of hepatitis C virus (HCV) RNA using polymerase chain reaction assays. Patients with human immunodeficiency virus or hepatitis B virus co-infection, or with other causes of chronic liver disease were not included.

Transient Elastography

Liver stiffness measurement was performed using transient elastography (FibroScan, Echosens, Paris France) by the previously described technique. Briefly, with the patient lying in dorsal decubitus with the right arm at maximal abduction, a transducer probe on the axis of a vibrator is placed on the skin, between the rib bones at the level of the right lobe of the liver. Mild amplitude and low-frequency vibrations (50 Hz) are transmitted to the liver tissue, inducing an elastic shear wave that propagates through the underlying liver tissue. The operator in each center was a nurse who had previously performed at least 100 determinations in patients with chronic liver disease and who was unaware of patients status. Ten successful measurements were performed on each patient and the success rate was calculated as the number of validated measurements divided by the total number of measurements. The results were expressed in kilopascals (kPa). The median value of successful measurements was considered representative of the liver stiffness in a given patient, according to the manufacturer's recommendations (interquartile range (IQR) less than 30% of the median value and success rate >60%). [25,26].

Serum Fibrosis Marker Panels

Blood samples were collected at baseline and during the study at weeks 24, 48 and 72. Laboratory tests included complete blood cell counts, HCV RNA serum concentration, HCV genotype, aspartate aminotransferase (AST), alanine aminotransferase (ALT), gamma glutamyl transpeptidase (GGT) and cholesterol. Marker panels of fibrosis including APRI and FIB-4 index were calculated as previously described.[7–9].

Liver Histology

Indication of a liver biopsy was not mandatory in treated or untreated patients. It was offered to individuals as part of the evaluation for diagnosis and prognosis of the disease, in the setting of routine clinical practice in each center, independently of the final treatment decision. Percutaneous liver biopsies were performed under local anesthesia and ultrasound guidance with a Tru-Cut 14 gauge needle (Angiomed, Bard, Karlsruhe, Germany). Specimens were fixed in formalin, embedded in paraffin and stained with hematoxylin-eosin and Massons trichrome. A minimum length of 10 mm and the presence of 6 portal tracts were required for diagnosis. Histological grade and stage were determined according to METAVIR scoring system [27] by a pathologist who was blinded for patients' data. Liver fibrosis was considered significant when it spread out of the portal tract (stages 2, 3 or 4).

Study Protocol

Treated patients included those who had stiffness values higher than 7.1 kPa (less likely to have absent or mild fibrosis according to previously suggested cut-off) [16] and those who wanted to receive antiviral treatment independent of their low liver stiffness values. Patients with stiffness values below 7.1 kPa or those who refused or had a contraindication for antiviral treatment remained untreated.

Liver stiffness measurements were obtained at baseline and at weeks 24, 48 (end of treatment) and 72 (end of follow-up) for G1-infected patients and at baseline and weeks 24 and 48 for G2/3-infected patients.

Treatment

Antiviral treatment was the standard of care, with weekly pegylated interferon alfa-2a (180 ug) or alfa-2b (1.5 ug/kg) plus ribavirin (0.8–1.2 g daily) for 24 or 48 weeks, according to HCV genotype. The use of hematopoietic growth factors, epoetin alfa or darbepoetin and filgrastim, was allowed to treat anemia or neutropenia, respectively. Sustained virologic response (SVR) was defined by undetectable serum HCV RNA by qualitative polymerase chain reaction assay (Cobas Amplicor, HCV Roche, Branchburg, New Jersey, USA; v 2.0, detection limit 50 IU/mL) at 24 weeks after the end of therapy. According to stopping and futility rules, patients with a decrease of HCV RNA level $<2 \log_{10}$ IU at week 12 or a detectable HCV RNA at 24 weeks were considered to have treatment failure, and therapy was discontinued.

Statistical Analysis

Descriptive values are expressed as percentages and the mean ($\pm$SD) or median (range). Quantitative data were compared using Students t-test or the non-parametric Mann–Whitney rank-sum test, as appropriate. The Chi-square test was used to evaluate categorical variables. The odds ratio, together with its 95% confidence interval (CI) and the corresponding P-value, was calculated for relative risks by using logistic regression. P values below 0.05 were considered statistically significant. The Wilcoxon matched pairs signed-rank test was used to evaluate changes between baseline and end of follow-up evaluations. To test for any associations with liver stiffness improvement, defined as a decrease of 20% or more from baseline LS values, variables with a P value of less than 0.1 on univariate testing were entered into a multivariate regression analysis. The Pearson's correlation coefficient was used to analyse the correlations between values of liver elastography and ALT, FIB-4 index and APRI. The general linear model (GLM) for analyzing repeated measures technique was used to examine the changes of liver stiffness over time. All statistical analyses were performed with SPSS software (version 16.0, SPSS Inc, Chicago, IL).

Results

Baseline clinical, laboratory and virologic characteristics of the patients are shown in Table 1. A total of 515 patients were evaluated: 323 treated patients (62.7%) and 192 untreated patients (37.3%). The mean age of the treated patients was 48.5 years, 66% were male and 56.7% were infected with HCV genotype 1. The mean age of untreated patients was 53.9 years, 35.9% were male and the vast majority (76.6%) were infected with HCV genotype 1. Treated patients had significantly higher baseline levels of serum ALT, AST and GGT, as well as higher histologic activity and fibrosis.

Baseline Comparison of Liver Stiffness

Treated patients had significantly higher baseline LS than untreated patients (10.6±8.9 and 5.9±2.7, respectively, $P<0.0001$). Liver biopsies were carried out in 319 patients (189 patients in the treatment cohort). The stage of liver fibrosis was distributed as follows: F0, n = 45 (14.1%); F1, n = 112 (35.1%); F2, n = 101 (31.7%); F3, n = 26 (8.2%); F4, n = 35 (11%). The prevalence of significant fibrosis (F≥2) in this cohort was 50.9%. The areas under the receiver operating characteristic (ROC) curve of the FibroScan were 0.70 (95%CI, 0.62–0.74), 0.86 (95%CI, 0.81–0.92) and 0.87 (0.95%CI, 0.80–0.94), for F≥2, F≥3 and F = 4, respectively. Areas under ROC curve of APRI and FIB4 were 0.70 (95%CI, 0.63–0.75) and 0.65 (95%CI, 0.60–0.71), 0.78

(95% CI 0.72–0.85) and 0.70 (95%CI, 0.60–0.80), 0.80 (95%CI, 0.71–0.90) and 0.70 (95%CI,0.60–0.80), for F≥2, F≥3 and F = 4, respectively.

Changes in Liver Stiffness during Treatment and According to Virologic Response

Mean liver stiffness values at each study time point for untreated and treated patients are shown in Table 2. After antiviral treatment, 202 patients (62.5%) achieved a sustained virologic response, while 121 patients (37.4%) did not. Among the latter, 66 patients (20.4%) had undetectable HCV-RNA at the end of treatment but then relapsed during follow-up. The mean interval between baseline elastography and end of study was 521.0±185.3 and 734.7±83.0 days for treated and untreated patients, respectively ($P<0.0001$).

A significant decrease in LS values was observed only in treated patients whereas in untreated patients these measurements remained stable from basal assessment to the end of the study period ($P<0.0001$). The LS dynamic profile of treated versus untreated patients is shown in Figure 1, and is based on the GLM repeated measures analytical approach ($P<0.0001$).

The evolution of liver stiffness according to treatment and virologic response and the mean percentage of change over time in the 72-week period are shown in Table S1 (supporting material) and Figure 2, respectively. The dynamic profile according to virologic response is shown in Figure S1 (supplementary material).

Table 1. Baseline characteristics of the patients.

Variable	Antiviral treatment cohort	Untreated	P value
	n = 323	n = 192	
Age (yrs)	48.5±11.2	53.9±11.7	<0.001
Sex (male)	214 (66.3)	69 (35.9)	<0.001
Body mass index (kg/m^2)	24.6±3.4	23.4±3.3	0.07
AST/ULN	1.9±1.4	1.1±0.6	<0.001
ALT/ULN	2.7±2.7	1.4±1.1	<0.001
GGT/ULN	1.5±1.4	1.2±1.1	0.001
Platelet count (10^3/mm^3)	206.6±67.6	239.6±55.9	<0.001
HCV RNA log$_{10}$ (IU/mL)	5.8±0.9	5.8±0.8	0.5
HCV genotype			<0.001
1	186 (57.6)	147 (76.6)	
2	41 (12.7)	20 (10.4)	
3	76 (23.5)	9 (4.7.)	
4	17 (5.3)	13 (6.8)	
Other	3 (0.9)	3 (1.5)	
Fibrosis stage	n = 189	n = 130	<0.001
F 0–1	78 (41.3)	79 (60.8)	
F 2	60 (31.7)	41 (31.5)	
F 3	19 (10.1)	7 (5.4)	
F 4	32 (16.9)	3 (2.3)	
Histologic activity			0.05
A 0–1	123 (65.1)	97 (74.5)	
A 2	58 (30.7)	31 (24)	
A 3	8 (4.2)	2 (1.6)	

Results are expressed as the mean ± standard deviation or n (%).
ULN, upper limit of normal.

Table 2. Liver stiffness variations during study and after follow-up and according to virologic response.

FibroScan (kPa)	Baseline	24 weeks	P	48weeks or EOT◇	P	72 weeks or 24 weeks of follow up◇	P
Treated	10.6±8.9◆	9.0±7.2	<0.001	8.8±7.0	<0.001	8.5±6.6	<0.001
SVR	9.3±5.9*	7.7±4.1	<0.001	7.7±4.7	<0.001	7.4±4.4	<0.001
RR	12.9±12.9*	11.4±9.9	0.009	10.9±9.5	0.01	10.1±8.7	<0.001
NR	12.4±11.3*	11±10.2	0.001	10.6±10.2	0.02	11.3±9.1	0.05
Untreated	5.9±2.7◆	6.3±3.4	0.3	6±3.3	0.8	6±3.2	0.7

Results are expressed as the mean.
*P 0.006 SVR vs RR and NR.
◆P<0.0001.
◇for untreated or treated patients, respectively.

Compared with baseline, a significant reduction in liver stiffness was experienced by treated patients versus untreated (mean percentage change −12% vs 3%, P<0.0001). This decline was statistically significant for those patients with baseline LS ≥ 7.1 kPa versus those below this cut-off value (mean percent changes −22%, P<0.0001 and −18%, P 0.03, for baseline LS ≥9.5 kPa and ≥7.1 kPa, respectively). In the analysis according to the final virologic response, the baseline LS in sustained responders was significantly lower than in relapser responder and nonresponder patients (P 0.006). At week 24 and 48 all treated patients (sustained virological responders, relapsers and nonresponders) had significant LS decreases from baseline, with no different mean percentage changes between them. However, only sustained and relapser responders had a significant LS improvement at the end of study,(mean percentage change −16%, −10%

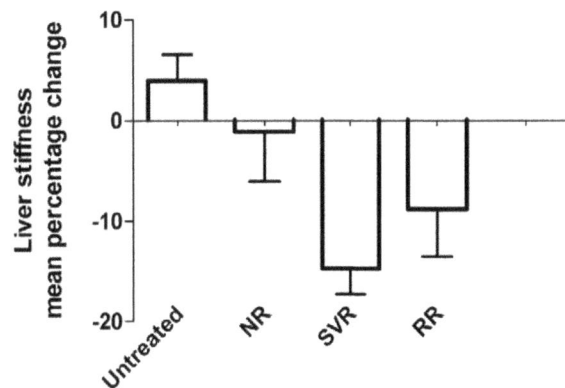

Figure 2. Mean percentage of change in liver stiffness from baseline to end of study according to treatment and virologic response.

and −2, for SVR, RR and NR, respectively, P 0.03 for SVR vs NR).

Among the 110 treated patients with baseline liver stiffness above the cut-off for advanced fibrosis and cirrhosis, values decreased below the cut-off level in 52 (47%) of them; interestingly the majority of them (70%) were sustained virological responders (Figure 3). The mean percent change in the sustained responders with LS values above cut-off for prediction of F3 (9.5 kPa) and F4 (12.5 kPa) was −25.5% and −30.8%, which resulted in a change to a lower stage of fibrosis in 80 and 60% of them, respectively.

ALT, AST and GGT serum values and FIB 4 index and APRI calculations had a significant correlation with LS at baseline (r = 0.33, 0.47, 0.34, 0.5, 0.6, respectively, P 0.0001). Similarly, ALT, FIB-4 index and APRI determinations demonstrated the evolution of LS according to treatment and virologic response, with significant differences at the end of study between SVR vs NR and RR (P<0.001). Serum ALT correlated significantly with LS in each time point of the study for each group of virologic response except for relapsers at 24 weeks post- therapy, where ALT (but not LS) showed a rebound (Figure S 1 B, supporting material).

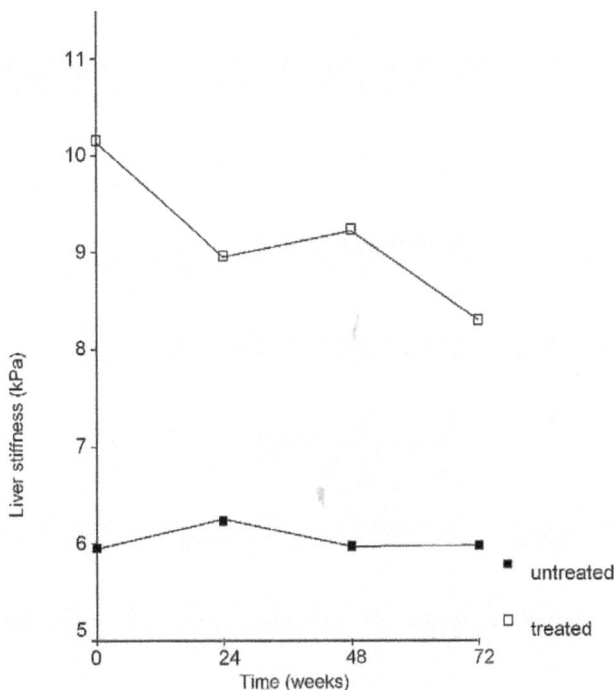

Figure 1. Liver stiffness evolution in treated vs untreated patients: Significant changes over time in treated vs untreated patients.

Predictors of Liver Stiffness Improvement

By univariate analysis, the following variables were associated with liver stiffness decline: male gender, low platelet count and time of follow-up, high body weight, body mass index (BMI), AST,

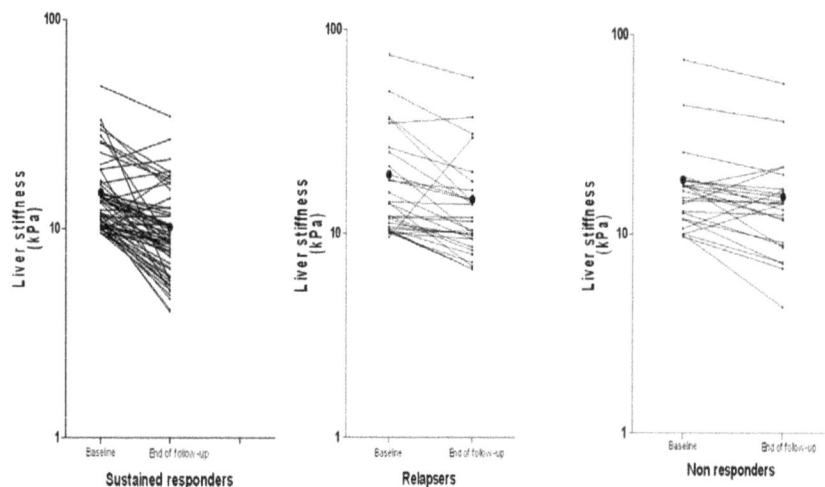

Figure 3. Liver stiffness evolution in patients with measurements above the cut-off value for advanced fibrosis and cirrhosis according to virologic response. The y axis is in logarithmic scale. The black dots indicate the mean liver stiffness value at each time points.

ALT, GGT, histologic activity, baseline LS values, non-1 genotype, diabetes and antiviral treatment. In the final model of multivariate analysis, baseline higher LS values (odds ratio (OR) 1.14, 95% CI 1.0–1.2, $P<0.0001$), ALT levels (OR 1.0, 95%CI 1.001–1.009, $P=0.01$), antiviral therapy (OR 0.5, 95%CI 0.3–0.9, $P=0.003$) and non-1 genotype (OR 1.06, 95%CI 0.4–1, $P=0.03$) were independent predictors of LS improvement (Table 3).

Discussion

The primary aim of this study was to assess liver stiffness changes following treatment with pegylated interferon and ribavirin. The results demonstrate a significant stiffness decrease with antiviral treatment in comparison with untreated patients. According to the type of response, significant changes were detected only in sustained responders and relapsers. Previous

studies had also shown a significant decrease in liver stiffness values in sustained responders.[22–24].

The improvement in liver stiffness at the end of study was particularly notable for those patients with higher pre-treatment liver stiffness values. As expected, two of the independent baseline predictors of the improvement were LS and ALT levels. The good correlation between LS and serum ALT levels during and after antiviral therapy, at least for sustained responders, as well as the association of LS improvement with ALT levels at baseline, is consistent with previous studies in which liver stiffness dynamic profiles ran in parallel with serum ALT in patients with CHC or in the course of acute hepatitis. [28,29] Although ALT has some association with inflammatory activity in the liver, its association with variations in stiffness may reflect, to some extent, the influence of necroinflammatory changes on LS measurements, as was shown in the study by Fraquelli. [30] Moreover, according to

Table 3. Factors associated with liver stiffness improvement.

Variables	Univariate analysis			Multivariate analysis		
	Odds ratio	95% CI	P	Odds ratio	95% CI	P
Male gender	1.54	0.08–2.7	0.01			
BMI≤25 Kg/m2	0.9	0.5–1.7	0.03			
Diabetes	0.6	0.2–2.2	0.001			
Genotype 1	0.6	0.4–0.9	0.004	0.6	0.4–1.0	0.03
Antiviral treatment	0.4	0.2–0.7	<0.001	0.5	0.3–0.8	0.003
Time between TE and end of FU	1	0.9–1	0.02			
Weight	1.02	0.9–1.0	0.01			
Platelet count	1	0.9–1	0.05			
AST	1	1.0–1.02	<0.001			
ALT	1.5	1.00–2.0	<0.001	1.005	1.0–1.01	0.01
GGT	1.0	0.8–1.2	0.001			
Liver stiffness	1.2	1.1–1.2	<0.001	1.14	1.0–1.2	<0.001
Histologic activity	1.6	0.9–2–8	0.08			

BMI, body mass index; FU, follow-up.

univariate analysis, the histologic activity was also associated with stiffness improvement. The lack of correlation between liver stiffness and ALT at the follow-up measurement in the group of relapser patients might suggest that ALT changes are seen earlier than liver stiffness, which may more directly reflect necroinflammation/edema of reactivation once antiviral pressure is withdrawn.

The fact that nearly 50% of the patients with LS values above the cut-off for advanced fibrosis decreased to values of non-advanced fibrosis at follow-up may be in agreement with previous studies that demonstrate liver fibrosis regression by histological parameters in concordance with noninvasive tests assessment of fibrosis degree in patients receiving interferon-based therapy. [1,2,31] These results were even more striking in the subset of sustained virological responders, with a reduction of the predicted fibrosis stage in 80% and 60% of patients who had at baseline an estimated F3 and F4 according to the proposed cut-offs values, respectively. Indeed, the decrease in LS values in patients who achieved SVR were higher than 20% of baseline levels in a significant proportion of individuals with advanced liver fibrosis. The fact that stiffness decrease remained significant at follow-up only in sustained responders and relapsers may suggest its association with liver fibrosis regression.

Our study has some limitations. First, accuracy to diagnose significant fibrosis was lower than in other published reports. Since the study was not specifically designed to assess the performance of FS to evaluate liver fibrosis, the lower accuracy value may partially reflect "real-life" problems in diagnostic performance (liver biopsies were not evaluated by a single pathologist, biopsies not reaching a minimum desirable length might have been included). Nevertheless, accuracy to diagnose advance fibrosis and cirrhosis was excellent. A second limitation is that at any conclusions are necessarily constrained by the lack of available liver biopsies to definitively confirm their degree of regression at follow-up. Thus, based on our results and on previous observations, confounders other than liver fibrosis, mainly inflammatory activity, may partially influence these findings. A final limitation of our study is the short time of follow-up of patients, which may explain similar LS dynamics between sustained responders and relapsers, and no increase in LS values in untreated patients. Strengths of the current study were the large number of CHC patients enrolled from multiple centers who received the same combination antiviral therapy in a prospective study.

In summary, this study of a large cohort of patients with CHC confirms that a significant improvement in LS is associated with antiviral therapy in sustained responders and relapsers. Further evaluation of transient elastography in the long- term follow-up of changes in liver fibrosis in these patients is needed.

Acknowledgments

The authors thank Dr Juan Gonzalez-Abraldes for his contribution in the statistical analyses. In addition, the authors thank all investigators: Amiens: Eric N'Guyen-Khac; Barcelona: Concepción Bartres; Bordeaux: Pierre-Henri Bernard, Julien Vergniol, Sandrine Villars; Caen: Catherine Guillemard, Isabelle Olivier, Benoit Dupont, Annie Cuquemelle; Lyon: François Bailly, Fabien Zoulim; Marseille: Valérie Oulès, Laurence Lecomte; Pisa: Barbara Coco; Toulouse: Hervé Desmorat, Karl Barange, Christophe Bureau, Jean-Pierre Vinel.

Author Contributions

Conceived and designed the experiments: VDL. Performed the experiments: SMM JF JMC SM M. Brunetto DC M. Bourlière JPB TD MMM DL WM XF VDL. Analyzed the data: SMM. Contributed reagents/materials/analysis tools: SMM JF JMC SM M. Brunetto DC M. Bourlière JPB TD MMM DL WM XF VDL. Wrote the paper: SMM VDL.

References

1. Poynard T, McHutchison J, Manns M, Trepo C, Lindsay K, et al. (2002) Impact of pegylated interferon alfa-2b and ribavirin on liver fibrosis in patients with chronic hepatitis C. Gastroenterology 122: 1303–13.
2. Shiffman ML, Hofmann CM, Thompson EB, Ferreira-Gonzalez A, Contos MJ, et al. (1997) Relationship between biochemical, virological, and histological response during interferon treatment of chronic hepatitis C. Hepatology 26: 780–5.
3. Perrault J, McGill DB, Ott BJ, Taylor WF (1978) Liver biopsy: complications in 1000 inpatients and outpatients. Gastroenterology 74: 103–6.
4. Regev A, Berho M, Jeffers LJ, Milikowski C, Molina EG, et al. (2002) Sampling error and intraobserver variation in liver biopsy in patients with chronic HCV infection. Am J Gastroenterol 97: 2614–8.
5. Bedossa P, Dargère D, Paradis V (2003) Sampling variability of liver fibrosis in chronic hepatitis C. Hepatology 38: 1449–57.
6. Forns X, Ampurdanès S, Llovet JM, Aponte J, Quintó L, et al. (2002) Identification of chronic hepatitis C patients without hepatic fibrosis by a simple predictive model. Hepatology 36: 986–92.
7. Wai CT, Greenson JK, Fontana RJ, Kalbfleisch JD, Marrero JA, et al. (2003) A simple noninvasive index can predict both significant fibrosis and cirrhosis in patients with chronic hepatitis C. Hepatology 38: 518–26.
8. Sterling RK, Lissen E, Clumeck N, Sola R, Correa MC, et al. (2006) Development of a simple noninvasive index to predict significant fibrosis in patients with HIV/HCV coinfection. Hepatology 43: 1317–1325.
9. Vallet-Pichard A, Mallet V, Nalpas B, Verkarre V, Nalpas A, et al. (2007) FIB-4: an inexpensive and accurate marker of fibrosis in HCV infection. Comparison with liver biopsy and fibrotest. Hepatology 46: 32–6.
10. Imbert-Bismut F, Ratziu V, Pieroni L, Charlotte F, Benhamou Y, et al. (2001) Biochemical markers of liver fibrosis in patients with hepatitis C virus infection: a prospective study. Lancet 357: 1069–75.
11. Rosenberg WM, Voelker M, Thiel R, Becka M, Burt A, et al. (2004) Serum markers detect the presence of liver fibrosis: a cohort study. Gastroenterology 127: 1704–13.
12. Poynard T, McHutchison J, Manns M, Myers RP, Albrecht J (2003) Biochemical surrogate markers of liver fibrosis and activity in a randomized trial of peginterferon alfa-2b and ribavirin. Hepatology 38: 481–92.
13. Martinez SM, Fernández-Varo G, González P, Sampson E, Bruguera M, et al. (2011) Assessment of liver fibrosis before and after antiviral therapy by different serum marker panels in patients with chronic hepatitis C. Aliment Pharmacol Ther 33: 138–48.
14. Fontana RJ, Bonkovsky HL, Naishadham D, Dienstag JL, Sterling RK, et al. (2009) Serum fibrosis marker levels decrease after successful antiviral treatment in chronic hepatitis C patients with advanced fibrosis. Clin Gastroenterol Hepatol 7: 219–26.
15. Patel K, Benhamou Y, Yoshida EM, Kaita KD, Zeuzem S, et al. (2009) An independent and prospective comparison of two commercial fibrosis marker panels (HCV FibroSURE and FIBROSpect II) during albinterferon alfa-2b combination therapy for chronic hepatitis C. J Viral Hepat 16: 178–86.
16. Castéra L, Vergniol J, Foucher J, Le Bail B, Chanteloup E, et al. (2005) Prospective comparison of transient elastography, Fibrotest, APRI, and liver biopsy for the assessment of fibrosis in chronic hepatitis C. Gastroenterology 128: 343–50.
17. Ziol M, Handra-Luca A, Kettaneh A, Christidis C, Mal F, et al. (2005) Noninvasive assessment of liver fibrosis by measurement of stiffness in patients with chronic hepatitis C. Hepatology 41: 48–54.
18. de Lédinghen V, Douvin C, Kettaneh A, Ziol M, Roulot D, et al. (2006) Diagnosis of hepatic fibrosis and cirrhosis by transient elastography in HIV/hepatitis C virus-coinfected patients. J Acquir Immune Defic Syndr 41: 175–9.
19. Foucher J, Chanteloup E, Vergniol J, Castéra L, Le Bail B, et al. (2006) Diagnosis of cirrhosis by transient elastography (FibroScan): a prospective study. Gut 55: 403–8.

20. Castera L, Forns X, Alberti A (2008) Non-invasive evaluation of liver fibrosis using transient elastography. J Hepatol 48 : 835–847.

21. Carrión JA, Torres F, Crespo G, Miquel R, García-Valdecasas JC, et al. (2010) Liver stiffness identifies two different patterns of fibrosis progression in patients with hepatitis C virus recurrence after liver transplantation. Hepatology 51: 23–34.

22. Ogawa E, Furusyo N, Toyoda K, Takeoka H, Maeda S, et al. (2009) The longitudinal quantitative assessment by transient elastography of chronic hepatitis C patients treated with pegylated interferon alpha-2b and ribavirin. Antiviral Res 83: 127–34.

23. Wang JH, Changchien CS, Hung CH, Tung WC, Kee KM, et al. (2010) Liver stiffness decrease after effective antiviral therapy in patients with chronic hepatitis C: Longitudinal study using FibroScan. J Gastroenterol Hepatol 25: 964–9.

24. Vergniol J, Foucher J, Castéra L, Bernard PH, Tournan R, et al. (2009) Changes of non-invasive markers and FibroScan values during HCV treatment. J Viral Hepat 16: 132–40.

25. Sandrin L, Fourquet B, Hasquenoph JM, Yon S, Fournier C, et al. (2003) Transient elastography: a new noninvasive method for assessment of hepatic fibrosis. Ultrasound Med Biol 29: 1705–13.

26. Lucidarme D, Foucher J, Le Bail B, Vergniol J, Castera L, et al. (2009) Factors of accuracy of transient elastography (fibroscan) for the diagnosis of liver fibrosis in chronic hepatitis C. Hepatology 49: 1083–9.

27. The French METAVIR Cooperative Study Group (1994) Intraobserver and interobserver variations in liver biopsy interpretation in patients with chronic hepatitis C. Hepatology 20: 15–20.

28. Coco B, Oliveri F, Maina AM, Ciccorossi P, Sacco R, et al. (2007) Transient elastography: a new surrogate marker of liver fibrosis influenced by major changes of transaminases. J Viral Hepat 14: 360–9.

29. Arena U, Vizzutti F, Corti G, Ambu S, Stasi C, et al. (2008) Acute viral hepatitis increases liver stiffness values measured by transient elastography. Hepatology 47: 380–4.

30. Fraquelli M, Rigamonti C, Casazza G, Conte D, Donato MF, et al. (2007) Reproducibility of transient elastography in the evaluation of liver fibrosis in patients with chronic liver disease. Gut 56: 968–73.

31. Cammà C, Di Bona D, Schepis F, Heathcote EJ, Zeuzem S, et al. (2004) Effect of peginterferon alfa-2a on liver histology in chronic hepatitis C: a meta-analysis of individual patient data. Hepatology 39: 333–42.

13

Cost Effectiveness of Fibrosis Assessment Prior to Treatment for Chronic Hepatitis C Patients

Shan Liu[1]*, **Michaël Schwarzinger**[2], **Fabrice Carrat**[3], **Jeremy D. Goldhaber-Fiebert**[4]

1 Department of Management Science and Engineering, Stanford University, Stanford, California, United States of America, **2** Equipe ATIP-AVENIR/UMR-S 738 INSERM, Paris Diderot University, Paris, France, **3** UMR-S 707 INSERM, Pierre et Marie Curie University, Paris, France, **4** Department of Medicine, Center for Health Policy and Center for Primary Care and Outcomes Research, Stanford University, Stanford, California, United States of America

Abstract

Background and Aims: Chronic hepatitis C (HCV) is a liver disease affecting over 3 million Americans. Liver biopsy is the gold standard for assessing liver fibrosis and is used as a benchmark for initiating treatment, though it is expensive and carries risks of complications. FibroTest is a non-invasive biomarker assay for fibrosis, proposed as a screening alternative to biopsy.

Methods: We assessed the cost-effectiveness of FibroTest and liver biopsy used alone or sequentially for six strategies followed by treatment of eligible U.S. patients: FibroTest only; FibroTest with liver biopsy for ambiguous results; FibroTest followed by biopsy to rule in; or to rule out significant fibrosis; biopsy only (recommended practice); and treatment without screening. We developed a Markov model of chronic HCV that tracks fibrosis progression. Outcomes were expressed as expected lifetime costs (2009 USD), quality-adjusted life-years (QALYs), and incremental cost-effectiveness ratios (ICER).

Results: Treatment of chronic HCV without fibrosis screening is preferred for both men and women. For genotype 1 patients treated with pegylated interferon and ribavirin, the ICERs are $5,400/QALY (men) and $6,300/QALY (women) compared to FibroTest only; the ICERs increase to $27,200/QALY (men) and $30,000/QALY (women) with the addition of telaprevir. For genotypes 2 and 3, treatment is more effective and less costly than all alternatives. In clinical settings where testing is required prior to treatment, FibroTest only is more effective and less costly than liver biopsy. These results are robust to multi-way and probabilistic sensitivity analyses.

Conclusions: Early treatment of chronic HCV is superior to the other fibrosis screening strategies. In clinical settings where testing is required, FibroTest screening is a cost-effective alternative to liver biopsy.

Editor: Ravi Jhaveri, Duke University School of Medicine, United States of America

Funding: Ms. Liu was supported by a Stanford Graduate Fellowship. Dr. Goldhaber-Fiebert was supported in part by a U.S. National Institutes of Health National Institute on Aging Career Development Award (K01 AG037593-01A1: PI; Goldhaber-Fiebert). The funders had no role in study design, data collection and analysis, decision to publish, or preparation of the manuscript.

Competing Interests: The authors have declared that no competing interests exist.

* E-mail: shanliu@stanford.edu

Introduction

Viral hepatitis C (HCV) is a serious liver disease affecting 180 million people worldwide [1]. In the U.S., 1.3% to 1.9% of the population has been infected with HCV, and 2.7 to 3.9 million people live with chronic infection [2]. Chronic HCV causes liver fibrosis, cirrhosis, and hepatocellular carcinoma (HCC), and is the most common cause of liver transplantation in the US [1].

Current practice guidelines in the U.S. recommend treatment for chronic HCV patients with significant fibrosis progression [1]. For pre-treatment evaluations of patients, liver biopsy is the current gold standard to ascertain liver histology and measure fibrosis progression. However, its expense, risk of side-effects, and potential inaccuracy from sampling and observation errors reduce its utility for frequent liver fibrosis screening [3,4,5]. Non-invasive tests of liver fibrosis – including serum markers such as FibroTest (FibroSure) and imaging methods such as FibroScan (transient elastography) – offer potentially viable alternatives [6]. These tests

are clinically validated in most common liver diseases caused by hepatitis C, hepatitis B, and alcohol abuse.

Few published studies have addressed the cost-effectiveness of non-invasive tests as alternatives to liver biopsy for determining when to initiate treatment for HCV. A number of studies have investigated test characteristics; some have estimated at a threshold of 0.3, sensitivities and specificities of FibroTest of 74–82% and 57–65% [6], respectively, though this changes with the definition of underlying disease and FibroTest cutoff; others have examined the cost-effectiveness of various treatment options, though generally without considering combinations of screening and treatment. One existing cost-effectiveness analysis of non-invasive screening tests fails to adhere to recommended standards including evaluating options over a lifetime horizon and including quality-of-life considerations [7,8]. Consequently uncertainties remain about the indications, accuracy, and cost-effectiveness of FibroTest and other non-invasive liver fibrosis screening technologies [3]. Furthermore, recent development in new protease inhibitors to treat HCV, such as telaprevir (Incivek™, Vertex), used in conjunction with pegylated interferon and ribavirin, have significantly improved treatment success rates compared to the standard treatment [9]. The cost-effectiveness of the new treatment is unknown.

We performed a model-based cost-effectiveness analysis of six FibroTest and liver biopsy screening strategies followed by treatment for eligible U.S. chronic HCV patients. We assessed FibroTest's viability as a tool to determine when to initiate treatment by addressing the questions: How should FibroTest be used in the context of chronic HCV, if at all? And how should HCV treatment be offered in combination with periodic screening?

Materials and Methods

Model

The Markov model simulates the lifetime disease progression of a cohort of treatment-naïve men and women who have chronic HCV infections with various stages of liver fibrosis. Progression through fibrosis stages is characterized by the Metavir Scoring system, with possible transitions occurring every 6 months. States include healthy (HCV negative), no fibrosis (F0), portal fibrosis with no septa (F1), portal fibrosis with few septa (F2), numerous septa without cirrhosis (F3), compensated cirrhosis (F4), decompensated cirrhosis (DC), HCC, and liver transplant. Without treatment, complete recovery (returning to the healthy state) is only possible from F0. A proportion of patients who start at F0 are "non-progressors" and do not progress to more severe fibrosis stages. A proportion of patients with decompensated cirrhosis and with HCC receive liver transplants. Death can occur from any state (Figure 1). The model extends a prior, empirically calibrated, model [10]. In the base case, starting age in the model is 40 years old with cohorts age 40 through 70 considered in sensitivity analyses.

We considered six strategies aimed at detecting fibrosis and beginning treatment to prevent liver disease and death [8,11]. The strategies considered (Figure 2) are:

(A) FibroTest Only. Patients are screened by FibroTest. If the test score is less than 0.31 (mild fibrosis, F0–F1), then repeat FibroTest annually. If the score is between 0.31 and 0.58 (intermediate), then repeat FibroTest every six months. If the

test score is greater than 0.58 (significant fibrosis, F2–F4), then begin treatment with no liver biopsy in patients without medical contraindication.

(B) FibroTest and Biopsy. Patients are screened by FibroTest. If the test score is less than 0.31, then repeat FibroTest annually with no liver biopsy. If the test score is between 0.31 and 0.58, then follow up with liver biopsy. If liver biopsy indicates significant fibrosis, then begin treatment in patients without medical contraindication. If liver biopsy indicates mild fibrosis, then restart the testing strategy annually. If the test score is greater than 0.58, then begin treatment with no liver biopsy in patients without medical contraindication.

(C) FibroTest Rule In. Patients are screened by FibroTest. If the test score is less than 0.58, then repeat FibroTest annually with no liver biopsy. If the test score is greater than or equal to 0.58, then follow up with liver biopsy. If liver biopsy indicates significant fibrosis, then begin treatment in patients without medical contraindication. If liver biopsy indicates mild fibrosis, then restart testing strategy annually.

(D) FibroTest Rule Out. Patients are screened by FibroTest. If the test score is less than 0.31, then repeat FibroTest annually with no liver biopsy. If the test score is greater than or equal to 0.31, then follow up with liver biopsy. If liver biopsy indicates significant fibrosis, then begin treatment in patients without medical contraindication. If liver biopsy indicates mild fibrosis, then restart testing strategy annually.

(E) Liver Biopsy Only (currently recommended practice). All patients receive liver biopsy. Those with results showing significant fibrosis without medical contraindication are treated, otherwise they are re-biopsied every 3 years.

(F) Immediate Treatment. All patients without medical contraindication are treated without screening for fibrosis.

Do Nothing (HCV natural progression without fibrosis screening or treatment) is only considered in the context of sensitivity analyses.

Standard treatment includes peginterferon alfa (2a or 2b) and ribavirin for 48 weeks for genotype 1 patients and 24 weeks for patients with genotypes 2 or 3. For genotype 1, an assessment of early viral response (EVR) is modeled at 12 weeks. EVR is defined as a 2 log reduction or complete absence of serum HCV RNA at week 12 of treatment compared with the baseline level. Failure to achieve an EVR is the most accurate predictor of not achieving

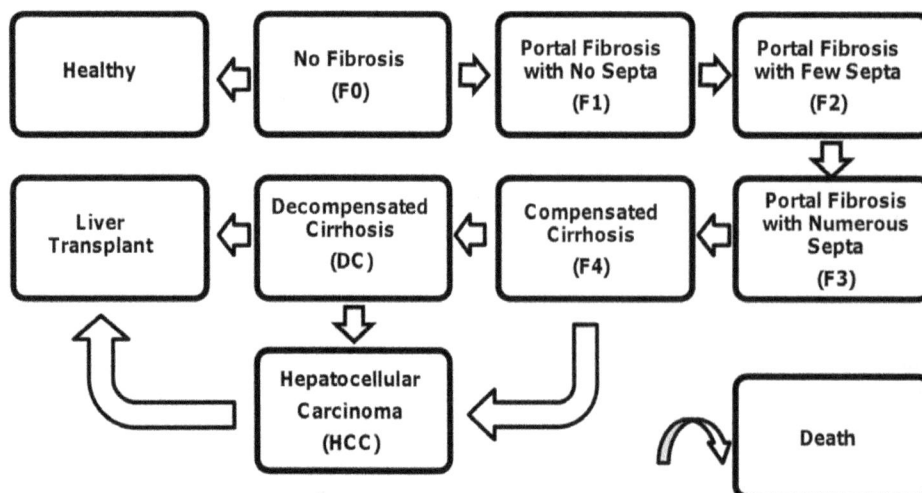

Figure 1. HCV Natural History Model.

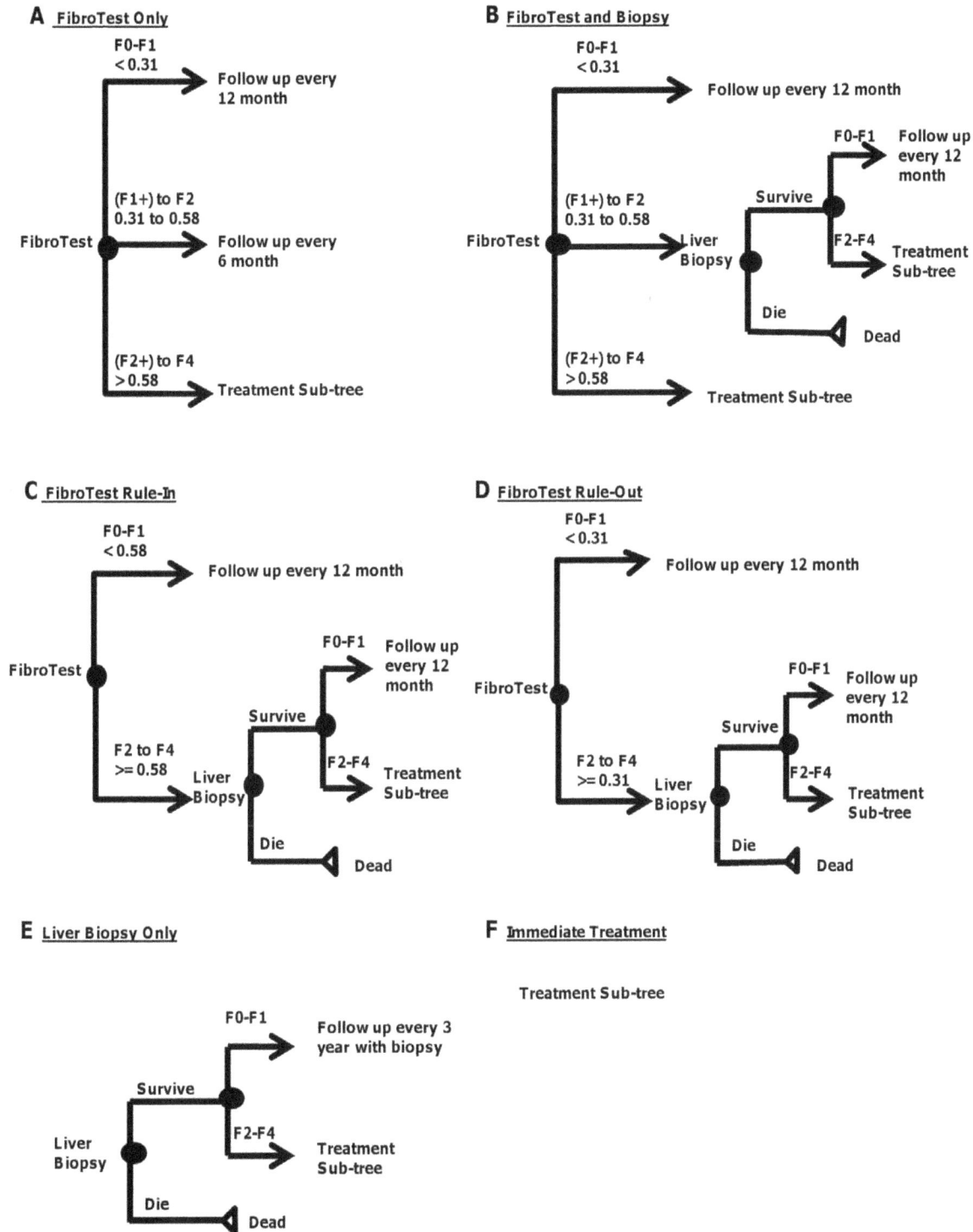

Figure 2. Model Structure; Six Strategies: (A) FibroTest Only; (B) FibroTest and Biopsy; (C) FibroTest Rule-In; (D) FibroTest Rule-Out; (E) Liver Biopsy Only; (F) Immediate Treatment. Note: Panels A–F represent separate clinical strategies that we compare by applying them in our natural history model. "Die" in the figures is to highlight the possibility of death from liver biopsy.

sustained viral response (SVR) [1]. Non-responders are taken off treatment and resume fibrosis progression. Patients who have undergone complete treatment and achieved SVR transition to a recovered health states stratified by fibrosis severity, and other patients resume fibrosis progression. SVR is defined as the absence

of HCV RNA from serum 24 weeks following discontinuation of treatment. (Figure 3 A, C)

We also examined the cost-effectiveness of fibrosis screening in the presence of a new HCV protease inhibitor — telaprevir (Incivek™ Pharmaceuticals) — for treatment naïve genotype 1

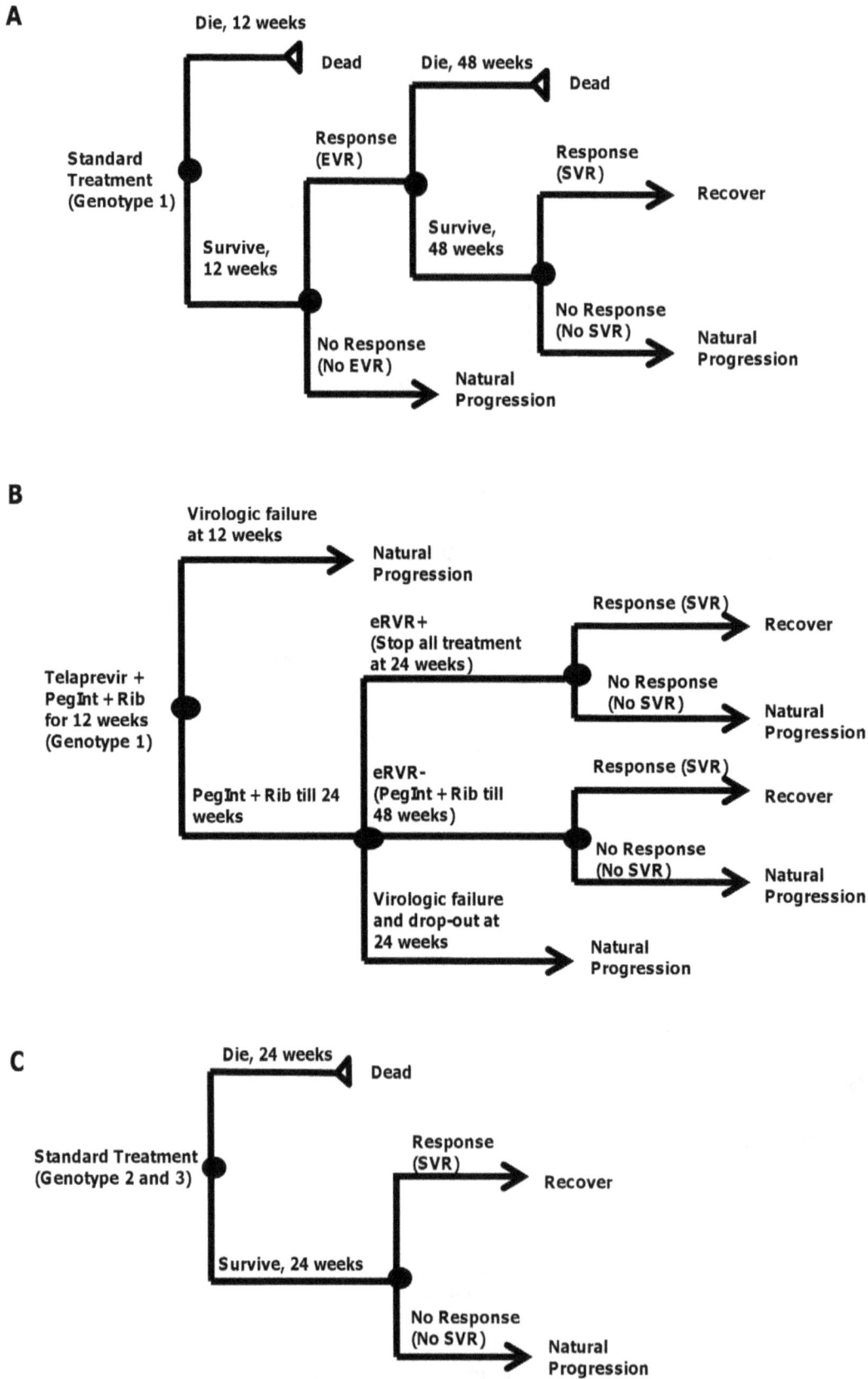

Figure 3. Treatment Sub-tree: (A) Genotype 1 (Standard Treatment); (B) Genotype 1 (Triple Therapy); (C) Genotypes 2 and 3. Note: "Die" in the figures is to highlight the possibility of death from treatment.

patients using response guided therapy in a scenario analysis. Patients receive a 12 weeks course of telaprevir with peginterferon and ribavirin, followed by peginterferon and ribavirin alone for either 12 or 36 weeks depending on extended rapid viral response (eRVR). eRVR is defined as undetectable HCV RNA at week 4 and week 12 (Figure 3 B).

For each strategy, we calculated discounted quality-adjusted life expectancy and total lifetime costs, comparing strategies with incremental cost-effectiveness ratios.

Data and Sources

We estimated model parameters from extensive review of the published literature and expert opinions.

Fibrosis

We found wide variations in the literature for the initial distribution of fibrosis stages for chronic HCV patients presented at treatment evaluations. Given the lack of nationally representative data for the US, we derived the prevalence of each fibrosis stage from a large cohort of urban HCV patients (Detroit, Michigan), with 18% F0, 24% F1, 17% F2, 13% F3, 28% F4, and

varied the prevalence over a broad range in sensitivity analyses [12].

Epidemiology

Empirical studies that accurately characterize all phases of HCV natural history and fibrosis progression are lacking due to the asymptomatic acute infection period and long duration (20 to 40 years) between initial infection and progression to end-stage liver disease [1,10,13,14]. Estimates of liver fibrosis progression rates for chronic HCV are heterogeneous [15]. Calibration of a model of HCV to infection prevalence and mortality from liver cancer in the U.S. yields plausible progression rates [16] (see section I in Appendix S1). We incorporated these calibrated rates (stratified by age and gender) in our analysis, and employed the upper and lower ranges in sensitivity analyses (Table 1). Mortality rates from causes other than HCV were derived from 2004 U.S. life tables [17].

FibroTest Characteristics

FibroTest is a risk algorithm based on a panel of six blood serum biochemical markers combined with a patient's age and

Table 1. Model Parameter Values: Epidemiology and Cohort Assumptions.*

	Base	Min	Max	Source
Proportion of F0 patients who are non-progressors	0.2420	0.0960	0.7410	[10]
6 months transition probabilities relating to fibrosis progression				[10,16]
Remission (from F0)	0.0060	0.0035	0.0085	
F4 to decompensated cirrhosis (DC)	0.0198	0.0159	0.0247	
Cirrhosis (both F4 and DC) to HCC	0.0104	0.0085	0.0139	
Progression, men by age				[10,16]
40–49	0.0266	0.0134	0.0464	
50–59	0.0606	0.0358	0.0773	
60–69	0.1046	0.0606	0.1601	
≥70	0.1397	0.0732	0.2126	
Progression, women by age				[10,16]
40–49	0.0139	0.0065	0.0286	
50–59	0.0320	0.0139	0.0564	
60–69	0.0554	0.0208	0.1113	
70–79	0.0741	0.0397	0.1298	
≥80	0.0997	0.0416	0.1626	
Liver transplant 6 month probability				[49]
Liver transplant from DC	0.0253	0	0.2254	
Liver transplant from HCC	0.0780	0.0253	0.2254	
Disease mortality (6 month rate)				
Liver transplant mortality	0.0760	0.0719	0.0807	[50]
Post liver transplant mortality	0.0256	0.0250	0.0260	[50]
Decompensated cirrhosis mortality	0.1530	0.0645	0.1975	[10]
HCC mortality	0.2165	0.1595	0.2495	[10]
Liver biopsy mortality (use as probability)	0.0003	0	0.0033	[51]
Treatment mortality (annual rate)	0.0005	0.00025	0.0008	[52]
Cohort starting age[a]	40	40	70	Assumed
Discount rate (annual)	0.03	0	0.05	[7]

*All references included in Table 1–3 are from published literature unless explicitly stated as our assumptions.
[a]We run the same model with cohorts at different starting age to identify the most cost-effective strategy at each age.

gender that results in a score from 0 to 1 [18] . FibroTest's manufacturer suggests that a score below 0.31 indicates mild fibrosis (F0–F1); 0.32 and 0.58 indicates F1 to F2; and above 0.58 indicates significant fibrosis (F2–F4) [18]. We obtained test characteristics [19] and defined plausible ranges for these test characteristics based on published studies [6,20,21,22,23,24, 25,26,27]. (Table 2)

Treatment Response

A longitudinal study of peginterferon alfa-2b and ribavirin for chronic HCV patients who have undergone EVR assessment at 12 weeks provided the probability of achieving EVR and the probability of SVR for those who achieved EVR [28]. For the new HCV drug telaprevir, we used effectiveness data from the Phase III ADVANCE study [9]. (Table 2)

Patients' initiation of and adherence to treatment can influence the optimal disease management strategy. We modeled full treatment initiation assuming our target population consisted of patients without treatment contraindication. The percentage of eligible patients was varied in sensitivity analysis as research has shown many patients with HCV are not currently treated for reasons including medical and psychiatric co-morbidities, substance abuse, patient refusal or loss to follow-up [29].

Health Outcomes

Chronic HCV negatively impacts patients' quality of life. To include this important aspect of the disease, we obtained health-state utilities by combining several published studies [10,30,31, 32,33]. There is significant variability among the HCV health-state utility research. We combined estimates to form a consistent set of utilities for all fibrosis stages, HCC, transplant, and post-

SVR (see section II in Appendix S1). We modeled utility decrements from biopsy as a one-time disutility of −0.05 (equivalent to a loss of 18 days), standard treatment for one year as −0.11 (equivalent to a loss of 40 days) [30], and assumed −0.165 for one year of triple therapy (equivalent to a loss of 60 days). Decrements were scaled by the actual time on treatment. Because of the variability in estimates, in sensitivity analyses, we widely varied these utilities (see sections II, IV in Appendix S1). (Table 3)

Costs

We included the costs of FibroTest, liver biopsy, treatment, and annual medical care for patients with chronic HCV. FibroTest and liver biopsy costs were obtained from the published literature [8,34]. Treatment costs include drug cost and medical care cost. To estimate drug costs, we assumed patients received peginterferon alfa-2b 150 mcg once weekly ($584/week, PegIntron™, Schering Corp.; and similarly $580/week, 180 mcg once weekly of peginterferon alfa-2a, Pegasys®, Roche), plus ribavirin 1,000 mg daily ($370.87/week, Rebetol®, Schering Corp.) [35,36], converting these average wholesale prices to average manufacturer prices using a 0.41 conversion factor [37]. We assumed a medical care cost related to treatment of $10,740 per year based on chronic HCV medical claims data [38]. The cost of telaprevir is reported as $49,200 ($4,100 per week for 12 weeks) for the additional cost of adding telaprevir to standard treatment in a three drug regime [39]. (Table 3)

We estimated the annual care of fibrosis (no treatment) based on medical expenditures in the year following hepatitis C diagnosis [40]. We assumed that patients who obtained SVR post-treatment incurred half of the pre-treatment annual care cost in their

Table 2. Model Parameter Values: Screening and Treatment Response Characteristics.

	Base	Min	Max	Source
Screening Test Characteristics				
FibroTest (FibroSure)				
Probability for patients with F0–F1				[6,8,19,20]
Test + (>0.58)	0.13	0.06	0.15	
Test − (<0.31), specificity at 0.31	0.68	0.57	0.72	
Probability for patients with F2–F4				
Test + (>0.58), sensitivity at 0.58	0.56	0.35	0.59	
Test − (<0.31)	0.16	0.12	0.29	
Liver biopsy screening frequency (year)	3	3	5	[47]
Treatment Response Probability				
Standard treatment (peginterferon and ribavirin)				
Probability(EVR at 12 week), genotype 1	0.71	0.66	0.76	[28]
Probability(SVR | EVR), genotype 1	0.63	0.57	0.69	[28]
Probability(SVR), genotype 2 and 3	0.80	0.60	1.00	[1,10,28,34]
Triple therapy (peginterferon+ribavirin+telaprevir), genotype 1[a]				[9]
Probability(virologic failure at 12 week)	0.03			
Probability(eRVR+, 24 week treatment | non-failure at 12 week)	0.60			
Probability(eRVR−, 48 week treatment | non-failure at 12 week)	0.35			
Probability(SVR|eRVR+, 24 week treatment)	0.89			
Probability(SVR|eRVR−, 48 week treatment)	0.67			
Noncompliance	0	0	0.63	[29]

[a]The effectiveness listed for triple therapy are for patients with fibrosis stage F0 to F2; for patients with fibrosis stage F3 and F4, SVR is reduced by 20%.

Table 3. Model Parameter Values: Quality Weights and Cost.

	Base	Min	Max	Source
Quality (utilities)[a]				[10,30,31,32,33]
Mild chronic HCV (F0, F1)	0.98	0.70	1.00	
SVR following mild HCV	1.00	0.74	1.00	
Moderate chronic HCV (F2, F3)	0.85	0.66	1.00	
SVR following moderate HCV	0.93	0.71	1.00	
Compensated cirrhosis (F4)	0.79	0.46	1.00	
SVR following F4	0.93	0.60	1.00	
Decompensated cirrhosis	0.72	0.26	0.91	
HCC	0.72	0.15	0.95	
Liver transplant[b]	0.81	0.64	1.00	
Liver biopsy decrement[c]	−0.05	−0.20	0	Assumed
Treatment decrement (standard treatment)[c]	−0.11	−0.20	0	
Treatment decrement (triple therapy)[c]	−0.055	−0.11	0	Assumed
Cost (2009 USD)				
Screening test				
Liver biopsy	$1,415	$974	$1,623	[8,34]
FibroTest (FibroSure)	$236	$100	$295	[8]
Treatment (peginterferon and ribavirin + medical care)				[10,35,38,41]
No EVR, genotype 1 (12 weeks)	$7,383	$5,605	$9,020	
SVR, genotype 1 (48 weeks)	$29,530	$22,420	$36,080	
SVR, genotype 2 and 3 (24 weeks)	$14,765	$11,812	$22,950	
Treatment (telaprevir drug cost for 12 weeks)	$49,200	$36,828	$59,040	[39,53]
Cost of annual care[d]				[10,38,40,41,42]
HCV no fibrosis (F0)	$1,610	$150	$2,000	
HCV portal fibrosis (F1, F2)	$1,610	$150	$2,000	
HCV bridging fibrosis (F3)	$1,610	$150	$2,000	
Compensated cirrhosis (F4)	$1,610	$150	$2,000	
Decompensated cirrhosis (DC)	$10,930	$5,470	$16,400	
HCC	$43,510	$21,760	$65,270	
Liver transplant, first year	$143,290	$71,650	$214,930	
Liver transplant, subsequent	$25,020	$12,510	$37,540	

[a]The quality of life weight for a given age and HCV disease state is computed as the product of the utility associated with the HCV disease state and a mean age-specific quality weight obtained from published data [54,55].
[b]Assumed the utility in the post liver transplant state is the same as the utility in F0 state.
[c]Unlike other utilities these decrement are short-term—only the time period when the intervention occurs.
[d]Baseline healthcare cost by age is included in the model [56].

associated recovered states [41] and varied this assumption widely in sensitivity analyses [10,38,40,41,42].

In cost calculations, we adopted a payer perspective, including all direct health care costs, but excluding patient time and transport. We discounted future costs and QALYs by 3% annually. Costs are inflation adjusted using the Consumer Price Index to 2009 [43].

Results

Among liver fibrosis screening options, strategies using FibroTest are more cost-effective than using Liver Biopsy Only (the current recommended practice) for both men and women with HCV genotype 1, 2, and 3.

As the current practice in the U.S. is to ascertain that a patient has significant fibrosis progression prior to initiating

HCV treatment, especially relevant for genotype 1 patients, we first considered the cost-effectiveness of screening-based strategies only, finding that FibroTest Only costs less and is more effective than Liver Biopsy Only. FibroTest and Biopsy has an ICER of $347,600 compared to FibroTest Only for men and $396,000/QALY for women with genotype 1 (Figure 4), both exceeding thresholds typically used to define cost-effectiveness ($50,000–$100,000/QALY). For patients with genotypes 2 and 3 (Figure 5), FibroTest and Biopsy has an ICER of $29,900/QALY for men and $31,100/QALY for women compared to FibroTest Only. FibroTest and Biopsy is only cost-effective for genotype 2 and 3 patients due to the greater likelihood of their response to treatment. Consequently, the extra liver biopsy and opportunity to initiate treatment based on its results offer more benefits to genotype 2 and 3 patients compare to genotype 1 patients.

A

B

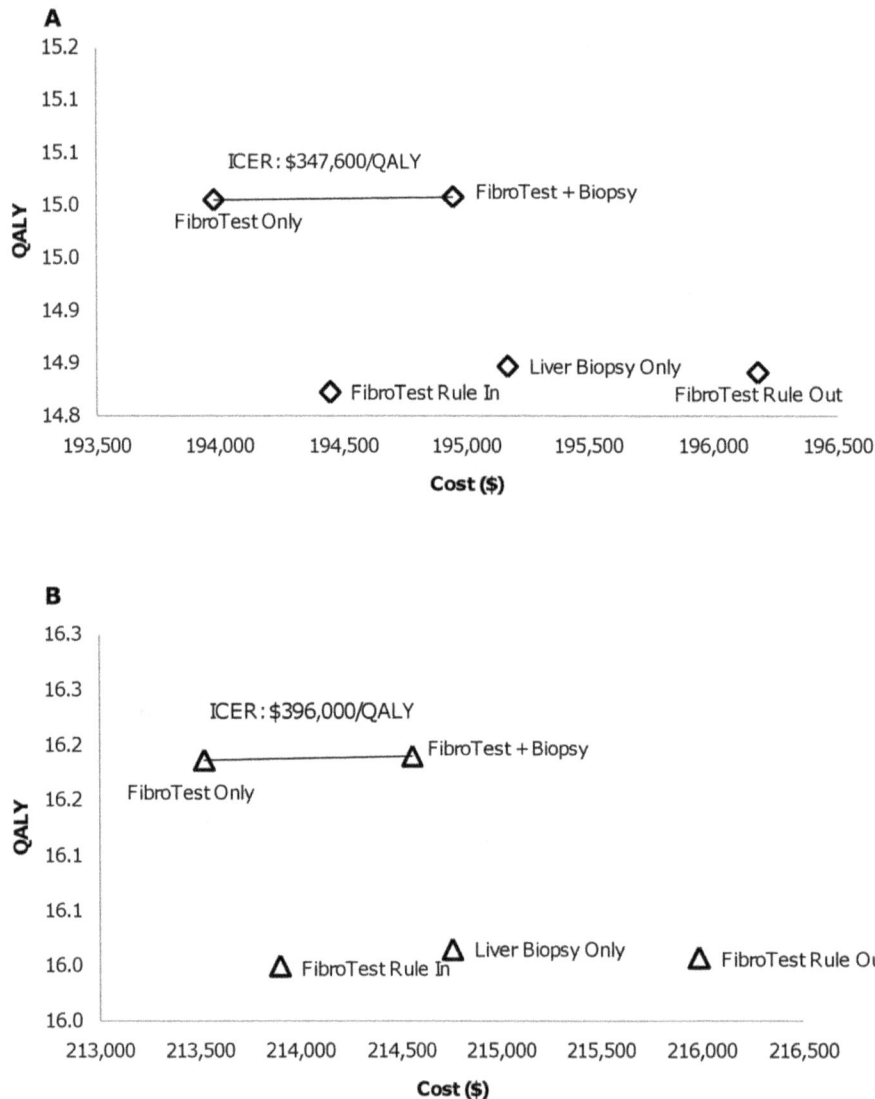

Figure 4. Cost-effectiveness Results by Gender, Genotype 1 under Standard Treatment (exclude Immediate Treatment): (A) Men; (B) Women.

If potential management options for chronic HCV included forgoing screening altogether and initiating treatment regardless of fibrosis stage, we find such a strategy cost-effective compared to fibrosis screening (Table 4), with ICERs of $5,400/QALY for men and $6,300/QALY for women with genotype 1 compared to FibroTest Only. All other screening strategies provide less health benefits and cost more. For patients with genotypes 2 or 3, all screening strategies provide less health benefits and cost more.

The current gold standard, Liver Biopsy Only, provides less health benefit and costs more than strategies using FibroTest or Immediate Treatment across a broad range of assumptions. However, if we consider only screening strategies that include liver biopsy as part of their algorithm, for genotype 1, Liver Biopsy Only is cost-effective compared to FibroTest Rule In (ICER of $29,800/QALY for men and $57,200/QALY for women). For genotypes 2 or 3, Liver Biopsy Only has an ICER below $10,000/QALY compared to FibroTest Rule In.

If telaprevir were added to standard treatment in response-guided triple therapy for genotype 1 patients, we find that Immediate Treatment remains cost-effective compared to FibroTest Only based on our assumption of the cost and disutility of telaprevir triple therapy, with an ICER of $27,200/QALY for men and $30,000/QALY for women. (Figure 6) Considering only screening-based strategies but using the new triple therapy, FibroTest Only is cost-effective with an ICER of $21,200/QALY for men and $26,100/QALY for women compared to FibroTest Rule In. (Table 5)

Additional base case results can be found in section III in Appendix S1.

Sensitivity Analyses

Immediate Treatment consistently provided greater health benefit per unit cost compared to the other strategies in one-way sensitivity analyses for all model parameters. In two-way and three-way sensitivity analyses, Immediate Treatment remained the preferred strategy (section IV in Appendix S1). The same conclusion holds for scenario analyses examining patient cohorts aged 50 to 70 years old, increased mortality risks from other

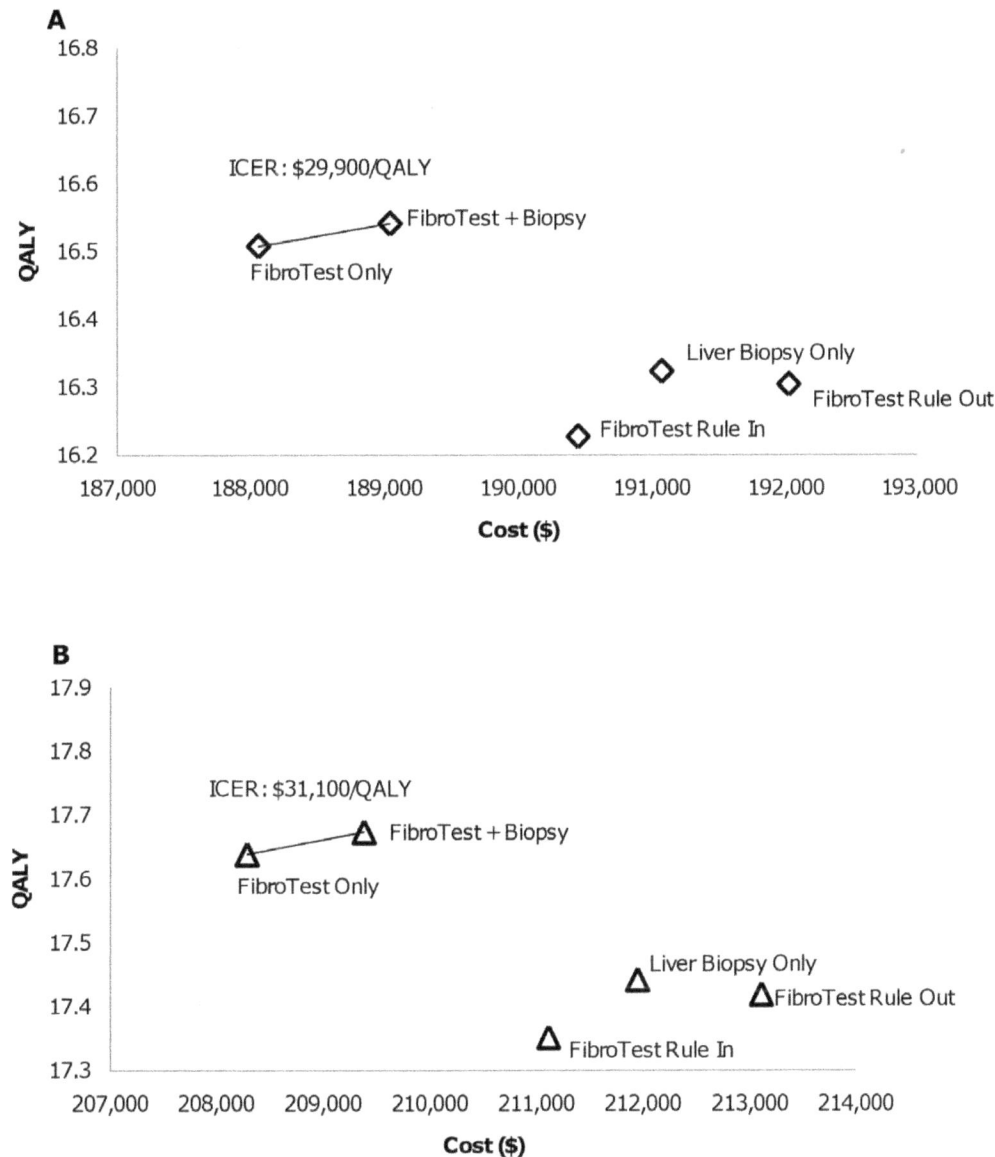

Figure 5. Cost-effectiveness Results by Gender, Genotype 2 and 3 (exclude Immediate Treatment): (A) Men; (B) Women. Note: The incremental cost-effectiveness ratio (ICER) is defined as the ratio of the additional costs of an intervention and its additional effects as compared to the next best alternative. i.e. The ICER shown on the figures is between FibroTest Only and FibroTest and Biopsy.

causes, slower disease progression rates, improved FibroTest characteristics, reduced SVR for patients with F3 and F4, and a broad range of health utilities estimates (section IV in Appendix S1). For example, while some would argue that older genotype 1 patients should be managed conservatively (i.e., a strategy like "Do Nothing"), we found that for those 70 year-olds with base case fibrosis stage assumption, treatment is still cost-effective though its ICER is higher (Table 6, $31,600/QALY, men).

If treatment was ultimately not given to 100% of eligible patients due to loss to follow-up post screening or medical contraindications discovered post-screening, Immediate Treatment is even more strongly preferred as periodic screening requires resource investment even for those patients who ultimately do not begin treatment.

Immediate Treatment is preferred to screening-based approaches in a probabilistic sensitivity analysis (PSA) (section IV in Appendix S1). Across 10,000 population simulations, at a willingness-to-pay threshold of $50,000/QALY, Immediate Treatment is the preferred strategy more than 99% of the time for both men and women and for all genotypes under standard treatment. For genotype 1 patients under triple therapy using telaprevir, at a willingness-to-pay threshold of $50,000/QALY, Immediate Treatment is the preferred strategy more than 90% of the time for men, and more than 78% of the time for women.

Discussion

For eligible men and women with chronic HCV of genotype 1, 2, and 3 in the United States, treatment without screening to determine liver fibrosis stage is cost-effective compared to periodic fibrosis screening strategies. Because there may be additional benefits to fibrosis staging prior to treatment (i.e., initiating hepatocellular carcinoma screening for patients with advanced fibrosis) and thus some clinicians may not consider treatment

Table 4. Cost-Effectiveness Results by Gender and Genotype, Standard Treatment.

Genotype 1		Cost (US, $)	QALY	ICER ($/QALY)
Men	FibroTest Only	193,979	15.01	–
	FibroTest Rule In	194,447	14.82	dominated
	Immediate Treatment	194,514	15.10	5,400
	FibroTest and Biopsy	194,950	15.01	dominated
	Liver Biopsy Only	195,169	14.85	dominated
	FibroTest Rule Out	196,182	14.84	dominated
Women	FibroTest Only	213,525	16.19	–
	FibroTest Rule In	213,901	16.00	dominated
	Immediate Treatment	214,101	16.28	6,300
	FibroTest and Biopsy	214,557	16.19	dominated
	Liver Biopsy Only	214,760	16.01	dominated
	FibroTest Rule Out	215,987	16.01	dominated
Genotype 2&3		**Cost (US, $)**	**QALY**	**ICER ($/QALY)**
Men	Immediate Treatment	187,547	16.69	–
	FibroTest Only	188,070	16.51	dominated
	FibroTest and Biopsy	189,048	16.54	dominated
	FibroTest Rule In	190,455	16.23	dominated
	Liver Biopsy Only	191,077	16.32	dominated
	FibroTest Rule Out	192,021	16.30	dominated
Women	Immediate Treatment	207,829	17.81	–
	FibroTest Only	208,296	17.64	dominated
	FibroTest and Biopsy	209,388	17.67	dominated
	FibroTest Rule In	211,118	17.35	dominated
	Liver Biopsy Only	211,953	17.44	dominated
	FibroTest Rule Out	213,109	17.42	dominated

(ICER: incremental cost-effectiveness ratios. dominated: strategy costs more but achieves less QALY than the previous strategy or a combination of strategies).

without testing viable, among screening strategies, using FibroTest alone is the next best alternative, and is more effective and less costly than fibrosis screening with liver biopsies. Compared to FibroTest alone, using FibroTest with biopsy reserved for patients with intermediate results has an ICER above $100,000/QALY for genotype 1 and below $50,000/QALY for other HCV genotypes. These finding are robust to multiple assumptions and sensitivity analyses.

This study addresses two important questions — whether to use and how to use non-invasive makers of fibrosis instead of liver biopsy to determine a patient's need for treatment, and the optimal timing to initiate treatment. Many clinicians have shown aversion to non-invasive biomarkers due to the tests' low sensitivity and specificity. Some are concerned that biomarkers fail to make accurate distinctions between mild and severe fibrosis and believe that biopsy may inform treatment decisions in these mid-zones. On the other hand, the apparent failure of serologic markers to distinguish between intermediate stages can be the consequence of classification errors from biopsy - several published studies suggest that when biopsy and marker results are discordant, diagnostic failure of biopsy is much more common than diagnostic failure of biomarkers [44]. Decisions to perform biopsy may depend more on physician preference than on the ability of liver biopsy to influence treatment decisions [45,46,47]. We acknowledge the on-going debate around the validity of FibroTest versus that of liver biopsy. However, we find that despite the uncertainties associated

with FibroTest's test characteristics, FibroTest Only strategy is preferred over liver biopsy across a broad range of sensitivities and specificities because of its advantage in cost, side effect, and frequency of follow-up. Patients afraid of liver biopsy's side effects may be more accepting of non-invasive tests and consequently these tests may also increase adherence to periodic fibrosis assessment if treatment is withheld. Furthermore, treating all patients (F0–F4) is often cost-effective and therefore distinguishing between mild and significant fibrosis may not be not essential.

Our results contribute to the current debate regarding liver biopsy. Many clinicians recognize liver biopsy's disadvantages. In addition to its cost and risk of adverse effects, liver biopsy is subject to sampling errors (biopsy with a length of 25 mm has a misclassification rate of 25%) [48]. Repeating biopsy every 3–5 years may also be unrealistic due to provider variability and patient non-adherence. Despite this, the National Institute of Health (NIH) 2002 Consensus Statement indicates that liver biopsy still provides unique information on fibrosis and histology, and no panel of serologic markers can provide an accurate assessment of intermediate stages of fibrosis [14]. Similarly, the 2009 American Association for the Study of Liver Diseases (AASLD) guideline recommends liver biopsy in making treatment decisions [1]. However, it recognizes the usefulness of non-invasive tests in defining the presence or absence of advanced fibrosis. Both of the guidelines agree that liver biopsy is not necessary in managing genotype 2 or 3 patients, since their treatment success

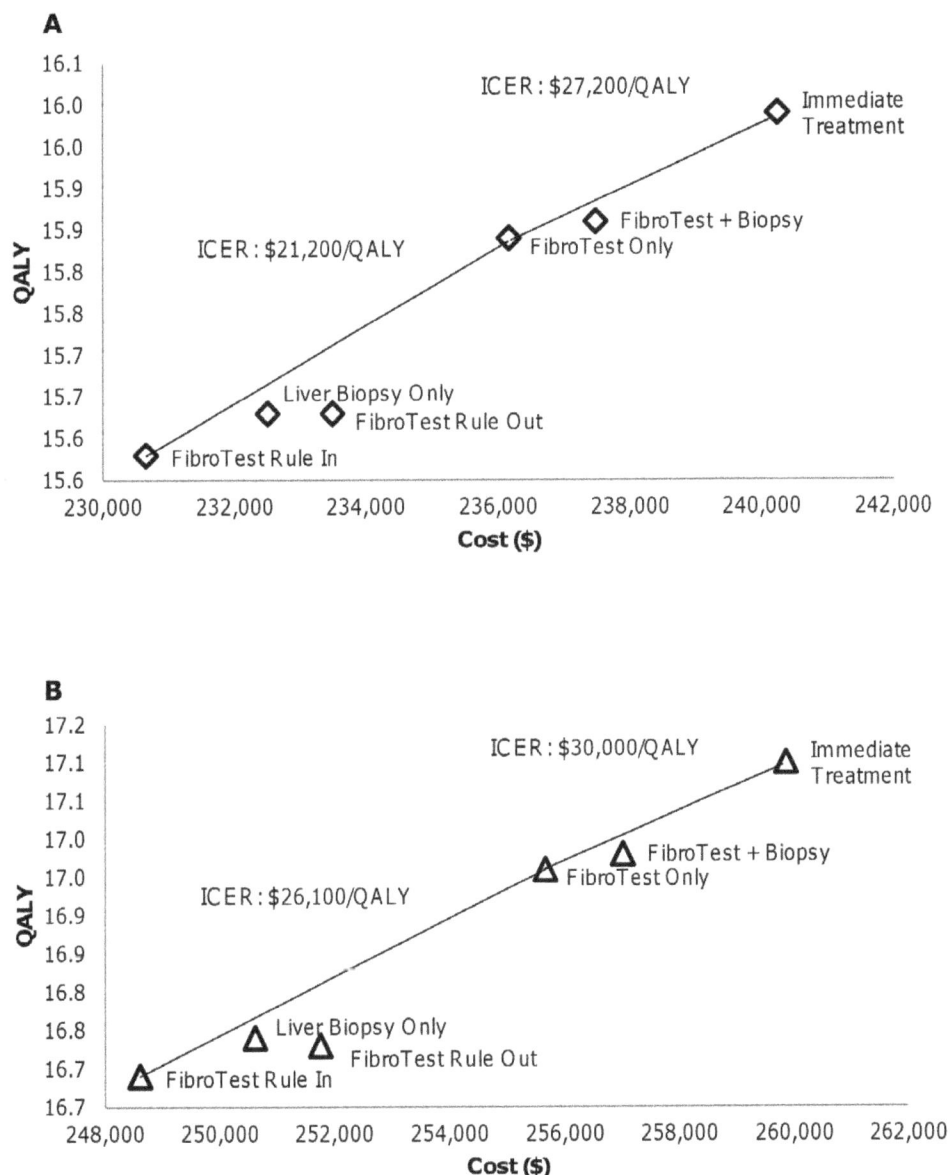

Figure 6. Cost-effectiveness Results by Gender, Genotype 1 under Triple Therapy with Telaprevir: (A) Men; (B) Women.

rate is substantially higher than genotype 1 patients. In support of future amendments to these guidelines, we find that even for genotype 1 patients, both immediate treatment and non-invasive screening appear cost-effective compared to liver biopsy. Furthermore, with the anticipated improvement in treatment success rate for genotype 1 patients, guidelines may soon be revised.

Our results suggest that re-examination of the necessity of screening prior to treatment decision may be appropriate. If treatment is generally effective, additional information obtained via screening may not provide sufficient additional value in guiding clinical decisions, since even with fibrosis stage uncertainty, treatment is likely to be sufficiently beneficial [45,46]. Our research helps to map out this trade-off between fibrosis stage accuracy and treatment success rate. Though no randomized controlled trials proving that HCV antiviral therapy is associated with long-term clinical benefits, there is a broad literature that strongly suggests this relationship. The lack of long-term evidence

may be due to the slow progression of the disease and the short history of the new combination therapy. We found immediate treatment to be cost-effective, given the current treatment effectiveness and anticipated improvements in the future [9]. Our results anticipate new anti-HCV drugs such as telaprevir and boceprevir becoming available that may significantly improve SVR for genotype 1 patients. Even with significantly increased drug costs and potentially increased risk of side-effects, our analyses support immediate treatment without fibrosis screening.

Our analyses and conclusions were robust to a variety of assumptions. Importantly, our conclusions were not sensitive to uncertainties regarding the speed of fibrosis progression and proportion of non-progressors in the cohort. As cost-effectiveness is also influenced by health utilities of HCV health states used in the model, our main conclusion remained robust despite uncertainties regarding these estimates. We also note depending on who is the payer, the cost of treatment can be much lower than our current

Table 5. Cost-Effectiveness Results by Gender and Genotype, Triple Therapy with Telaprevir.

Genotype 1		Cost (US, $)	QALY	ICER ($/QALY)
Men	FibroTest Rule In	230,651	15.58	–
	Liver Biopsy Only	232,502	15.63	dominated
	FibroTest Rule Out	233,499	15.63	dominated
	FibroTest Only	236,167	15.84	21,200
	FibroTest and Biopsy	237,482	15.86	dominated
	Immediate Treatment	240,240	15.99	27,200
Women	FibroTest Rule In	248,603	16.69	–
	Liver Biopsy Only	250,611	16.74	dominated
	FibroTest Rule Out	251,762	16.73	dominated
	FibroTest Only	255,660	16.96	26,100
	FibroTest and Biopsy	257,002	16.98	dominated
	Immediate Treatment	259,853	17.10	30,000

(ICER: incremental cost-effectiveness ratios. dominated: strategy costs more but achieves less QALY than the previous strategy or a combination of strategies).

assumptions (i.e. Federal Supply Schedule for government payers) in which case immediate treatment would appear even more favorable.

Previous research examined the economic outcomes of non-invasive testing in the diagnosis of significant liver fibrosis compared with liver biopsy and recommended against non-invasive testing [8]. The conclusion is made with the assumption that "misdiagnosis" leading to early treatment is harmful to health. The assumption is problematic by disregarding all future benefits and cost. By evaluating a one-time use of non-invasive test, the study ignored one major advantage of non-invasive test that enables more frequent monitoring of fibrosis progression than liver biopsy.

Our study has several limitations. The model does not stratify the population by race, and thus the fibrosis progression and

treatment response rates are biased towards whites reflecting the participants in the clinical studies of our source data. Because needed information on genotypes other than 1, 2, and 3 was limited, the model only considers clinical scenarios for genotypes 1, 2, and 3, which is appropriate for a U.S. analysis where these types are most common. We did not consider co-infection with HIV and/or hepatitis B. We defined alternative screening strategies by possible combinations of FibroTest and liver biopsy. Our strategy set is not comprehensive, and we note other screening patterns exist. We did not consider other non-invasive markers and imaging methods such as FibroScan to evaluate liver stiffness. However, for non-invasive tests that are conducted at similar intervals, that have comparable test characteristics and that have comparable costs to FibroTest, our conclusion are also

Table 6. Incremental Cost-Effectiveness Ratios ($/QALY) by Cohort Starting Age, Genotype 1 under Standard Treatment, Base Case Fibrosis Stage Distribution.

Men, Age	40	50	60	70
Do Nothing	–	–	–	–
FibroTest Only	ED	ED	ED	ED
FibroTest and Biopsy	D	D	D	D
FibroTest Rule In	D	D	D	ED
FibroTest Rule Out	D	D	D	D
Liver Biopsy Only	D	D	D	D
Immediate Treatment	$12,100/QALY	$14,800/QALY	$19,900/QALY	$31,600/QALY
Women, Age	40	50	60	70
Do Nothing	–	–	–	–
FibroTest Only	ED	ED	ED	ED
FibroTest and Biopsy	D	D	D	D
FibroTest Rule In	D	D	ED	ED
FibroTest Rule Out	D	D	D	D
Liver Biopsy Only	D	D	D	D
Immediate Treatment	$13,100/QALY	$15,900/QALY	$20,700/QALY	$31,000/QALY

(D: dominated, ED: Extended-Dominated by a combination of Do Nothing and Immediate Treatment).

applicable. We also found that treatment without screening to determine liver fibrosis stage would be cost-effective compared to periodic screening strategies. This result was robust to a wide range of sensitivities, specificities, and test costs, and should, therefore, hold for many other non-invasive markers.

Depending on who bears the cost of new antiviral drugs, patients may prefer to wait to initiate treatment until there is evidence of significant fibrosis progression. The model did not include possible future advances in treatment in the base case analysis and allow patients to delay treatment for a later date. The analyses also did not include the benefits of fibrosis screening to patients being able to make an informed choice and, therefore, potentially having a stronger commitment to treatment adherence.

HCV is a serious liver disease affecting up to 4 million Americans. While current recommendations favor liver biopsies prior to treatment initiation, we find that, for the hundreds of thousands of Americans with chronic HCV, other strategies are likely more effective and cost-effective. Management of chronic HCV in the U.S. could be improved by a shift towards strategies that initiate immediate treatment without fibrosis screening or else periodic screening with a non-invasive method followed by treatment for those found likely to have significant fibrosis.

Acknowledgments

The authors thank Professor Margaret Brandeau of Stanford University for helpful comments on the project.

Author Contributions

Conceived and designed the experiments: SL MS FC JDG-F. Performed the experiments: SL. Analyzed the data: SL MS JDG-F. Wrote the paper: SL JDG-F.

References

1. Ghany MG, Strader DB, Thomas DL, Seeff LB (2009) Diagnosis, Management, and Treatment of Hepatitis C: An Update. Hepatology 49: 1335–1374.
2. Armstrong GL, Wasley A, Simard EP, McQuillan GM, Kuhnert WL, et al. (2006) The prevalence of hepatitis C virus infection in the United States, 1999 through 2002. Annals of Internal Medicine 144: 705–714.
3. Bedossa P, Carrat F (2009) Liver biopsy: The best, not the gold standard. Journal of Hepatology 50: 1–3.
4. Sporea I, Popescu A, Sirli R (2008) Why, who and how should perform liver biopsy in chronic liver diseases. World Journal of Gastroenterology 14: 3396–3402.
5. Melita SH, Lau B, Afdhal NH, Thomas DL (2009) Exceeding the limits of liver histology markers. Journal of Hepatology 50: 36–41.
6. Shaheen AAM, Wan AF, Myers RP (2007) FibroTest and FibroScan for the prediction of hepatitis C-related fibrosis: A systematic review of diagnostic test accuracy. American Journal of Gastroenterology 102: 2589–2600.
7. Gold MR (1996) Cost-effectiveness in health and medicine. New York: Oxford University Press. xxiii, 425 p.
8. Carlson JJ, Kowdley KV, Sullivan SD, Ramsey SD, Veenstra DL (2009) An evaluation of the potential cost-effectiveness of non-invasive testing strategies in the diagnosis of significant liver fibrosis. Journal of Gastroenterology and Hepatology 24: 786–791.
9. Jacobson IM, McHutchison JG, Dusheiko G, Di Bisceglie AM, Reddy KR, et al. Telaprevir for previously untreated chronic hepatitis C virus infection. N Engl J Med 364: 2405–2416.
10. Salomon JA, Weinstein MC, Hammitt JK, Goldie SJ (2003) Cost-effectiveness of treatment for chronic hepatitis C infection in an evolving patient population. Jama-Journal of the American Medical Association 290: 228–237.
11. Rockey DC, Bissell DM (2006) Noninvasive measures of liver fibrosis. Hepatology 43: S113–S120.
12. Siddiqui FA, Ehrinpreis MN, Janisse J, Dhar R, May E, et al. (2008) Demographics of a large cohort of urban chronic hepatitis C patients. Hepatology International 2: 376–381.
13. Seeff LB (2002) Natural history of chronic hepatitis C. Hepatology 36: S35–S46.
14. NIH Consensus Statement on Management of hepatitis C: 2002. Jun 10–12; 19(3): 1–46. Available: http://consensus.nih.gov/2002/2002HepatitisC2002116main.htm. Accessed 2009 Oct 1. National Institutes of Health.
15. Thein HH, Yi QL, Dore GJ, Krahn MD (2008) Estimation of stage-specific fibrosis progression rates in chronic hepatitis C virus infection: A meta-analysis and meta-regression. Hepatology 48: 418–431.
16. Salomon JA, Weinstein MC, Hammitt JK, Goldie SJ (2002) Empirically calibrated model of hepatitis C virus infection in the United States. American Journal of Epidemiology 156: 761–773.
17. Arias E (2007) National Vital Statistics Reports: United States Life Tables, 2004. Available: http://www.cdc.gov/nchs/data/nvsr/nvsr56/nvsr56_09.pdf. Accessed 2009 Jun 1. Center for Disease Control, Division of Vital Statistics.
18. Practice of FibroTest for hepatitis C. BioPredictive website. Available: http://www.biopredictive.com/intl/physician/fibrotest-for-hcv/. Accessed 2009 Jun 1.
19. Poynard T, Imbert-Bismut F, Munteanu M, Messous D, Myers RP, et al. (2004) Overview of the diagnostic value of biochemical markers of liver fibrosis (FibroTest, HCV FibroSure) and necrosis (ActiTest) in patients with chronic hepatitis C. Comparative Hepatology.
20. Halfon P, Bourliere M, Deydier R, Botta-Fridlund D, Renou C, et al. (2006) Independent prospective multicenter validation of biochemical markers (Fibrotest-Actitest) for the prediction of liver fibrosis and activity in patients with chronic hepatitis C: The fibropaca study. American Journal of Gastroenterology 101: 547–555.

21. Imbert-Bismut F, Ratziu V, Pieroni L, Charlotte F, Benhamou Y, et al. (2001) Biochemical markers of liver fibrosis in patients with hepatitis C virus infection: a prospective study. Lancet 357: 1069–1075.
22. Rossi E, Adams L, Prins A, Bulsara M, de Boer B, et al. (2003) Validation of the FibroTest biochemical markers score in assessing liver fibrosis in hepatitis C patients. Clinical Chemistry 49: 450–454.
23. Cales P, de Ledinghen V, Halfon P, Bacq Y, Leroy V, et al. (2008) Evaluating the accuracy and increasing the reliable diagnosis rate of blood tests for liver fibrosis in chronic hepatitis C. Liver International 28: 1352–1362.
24. Sebastiani G, Vario A, Guido M, Noventa F, Plebani M, et al. (2006) Stepwise combination algorithms of non-invasive markers to diagnose significant fibrosis in chronic hepatitis C. Journal of Hepatology 44: 686–693.
25. Poynard T, Morra R, Halfon P, Castera L, Ratziu V, et al. (2007) Meta-analyses of FibroTest diagnostic value in chronic liver disease. BMC Gastroenterol 7: 40.
26. Boursier J, Bacq Y, Halfon P, Leroy V, de Ledinghen V, et al. (2009) Improved diagnostic accuracy of blood tests for severe fibrosis and cirrhosis in chronic hepatitis C. European Journal of Gastroenterology & Hepatology 21: 28–38.
27. Halfon P, Bacq Y, De Muret A, Penaranda G, Bourliere M, et al. (2007) Comparison of test performance profile for blood tests of liver fibrosis in chronic hepatitis C. Journal of Hepatology 46: 395–402.
28. Davis GL, Wong JB, McHutchison JG, Manns MP, Harvey J, et al. (2003) Early virologic response to treatment with peginterferon alfa-2b plus ribavirin in patients with chronic hepatitis C. Hepatology 38: 645–652.
29. Narasimhan G, Sargios TN, Kalakuntla R, Homel P, Clain DJ, et al. (2006) Treatment rates in patients with chronic hepatitis C after liver biopsy. Journal of Viral Hepatitis 13: 783–786.
30. Grieve R, Roberts J, Wright M, Sweeting M, DeAngelis D, et al. (2006) Cost effectiveness of interferon or peginterferon with ribavirin for histologically mild chronic hepatitis C. Gut 55: 1332–1338.
31. Sherman KE, Sherman SN, Chenier T, Tsevat J (2004) Health values of patients with chronic hepatitis C infection. Archives of Internal Medicine 164: 2377–2382.
32. Chong CAKY, Gulamhussein A, Heathcote EJ, Lilly L, Sherman M, et al. (2003) Health-state utilities and quality of life in hepatitis C patients. American Journal of Gastroenterology 98: 630–638.
33. McLernon DJ, Dillon J, Donnan PT (2008) Health-state utilities in liver disease: A systematic review. Medical Decision Making 28: 582–592.
34. Tan JA, Joseph TA, Saab S (2008) Treating Hepatitis C in the Prison Population Is Cost-Saving. Hepatology 48: 1387–1395.
35. Thomson Corporation (2009) Red book: pharmacy's fundamental reference. Montvale NJ: Thomson PDR. pp v.
36. AHFS Drug Information. Bethesda (MD): American Society of Health-System Pharmacists.
37. Levinson D (2005) Medicaid drug price comparisons: Average manufacturer price to published prices. Department of Health and Human Services. Office of the Inspector General. Available: http://www.oig.hhs.gov/oei/reports/oei-05-05-00240.pdf. Accessed 2009 Oct 1.
38. Armstrong EP, Charland SL (2004) Burden of illness of hepatitis C from a managed care organization perspective. Current Medical Research and Opinion 20: 671–679.
39. Pollack A (2011) Second Drug Wins Approval for Treatment of Hepatitis C. Available: http://www.nytimes.com/2011/05/24/business/24drug.html?_r=1. Accessed 2011 Jun 1. The New York Times.
40. Poret AW, Ozminkowski R, Goetzel R, Pew J, Balent J (2002) Cost Burden of Illness for Hepatitis C Patients with Employer-Sponsored Health Insurance. Disease Management 5: 95–107.

41. Mitra D, Davis KL, Beam C, Medjedovic J, Rustgi V (2010) Treatment Patterns and Adherence among Patients with Chronic Hepatitis C Virus in a US Managed Care Population. Value in Health.

42. Bennett WG, Inoue Y, Beck JR, Wong JB, Pauker SG, et al. (1997) Estimates of the cost-effectiveness of a single course of interferon-alpha 2b in patients with histologically mild chronic hepatitis C. Annals of Internal Medicine 127: 855–&.

43. U.S. Department Of Labor, Bureau of Labor Statistics Consumer Price Index. Available: ftp://ftp.bls.gov/pub/special.requests/cpi/cpiai.txt. Accessed 2010 Jun 1.

44. Poynard T, Munteanu M, Imbert-Bismut F, Charlotte F, Thabut D, et al. (2004) Prospective analysis of discordant results between biochemical markers and biopsy in patients with chronic hepatitis C. Clinical Chemistry 50: 1344–1355.

45. Wong JB, Bennett WG, Koff RS, Pauker SG (1998) Pretreatment evaluation of chronic hepatitis C - Risks, benefits, and costs. Jama-Journal of the American Medical Association 280: 2088–2093.

46. Andriulli A, Persico M, Iacobellis A, Maio G, Di Salvo D, et al. (2004) Treatment of patients with HCV infection with or without liver biopsy. Journal of Viral Hepatitis 11: 536–542.

47. Wong JB, Koff RS, Thera IHI (2000) Watchful waiting with periodic liver biopsy versus immediate empirical therapy for histologically mild chronic hepatitis C - A cost-effectiveness analysis. Annals of Internal Medicine 133: 665–675.

48. Bedossa P, Dargere D, Paradis V (2003) Sampling variability of liver fibrosis in chronic hepatitis C. Hepatology 38: 1449–1457.

49. Hutton DW, Tan D, So SK, Brandeau ML (2007) Cost-effectiveness of screening and vaccinating Asian and pacific islander adults for hepatitis B. Annals of Internal Medicine 147: 460–469.

50. United Network for Organ Sharing. Available: http://www.unos.org/. Accessed 2011 Jan 1.

51. Poynard T, Ratziu V, Bedossa P (2000) Appropriateness of liver biopsy. Canadian Journal of Gastroenterology 14: 543–548.

52. Fattovich G, Giustina G, Favarato S, Ruol A, Macarri G, et al. (1996) A survey of adverse events in 11241 patients with chronic viral hepatitis treated with alfa interferon. Journal of Hepatology 24: 38–47.

53. Federal Supply Schedule, Drug Pharmaceutical Prices 2011. Available: http://www.pbm.va.gov/DrugPharmaceuticalPrices.aspx. Accessed 2011 Jun 24. United States Department of Veterans Affairs.

54. Nyman JA, Barleen NA, Dowd BE, Russell DW, Coons SJ, et al. (2007) Quality-of-life weights for the US population - Self-reported health status and priority health conditions, by demographic characteristics. Medical Care 45: 618–628.

55. Sullivan PW, Ghushchyan V (2006) Preference-based EQ-5D index scores for chronic conditions in the United States. Medical Decision Making 26: 410–420.

56. Meara E, White C, Cutler DM (2004) Trends in medical spending by age, 1963–2000. Health Affairs 23: 176–183.

14

Liver Stiffness Measurement and Biochemical Markers in Senegalese Chronic Hepatitis B Patients with Normal ALT and High Viral Load

Papa Saliou Mbaye[1], Anna Sarr[2], Jean-Marie Sire[3,4], Marie-Louise Evra[2], Adama Ba[1], Jean Daveiga[5], Aboubakry Diallo[6], Fatou Fall[1], Loic Chartier[7], François Simon[3], Muriel Vray[7]*

1 Department of Hepatology and Gastroenterology, Principal Hospital, Dakar, Senegal, 2 Department of Hepatology and Gastroenterology, Abass Ndao Hospital, Dakar, Senegal, 3 INSERM U941, University of Medicine Paris-Diderot, Saint-Louis Hospital, Paris, France, 4 Medical Laboratory, Pasteur Institute, Dakar, Senegal, 5 Department of Hepatology and Gastroenterology, Saint-Jean de Dieu Hospital, Thies, Senegal, 6 Department of Hepatology and Gastroenterology, Grand-Yoff Hospital, Dakar, Senegal, 7 Epidemiology Unit of Infectious Diseases, Pasteur Institute, INSERM, Paris, France

Abstract

Background and Aims: Despite the high prevalence of chronic hepatitis B (CHB) in Africa, few studies have been performed among African patients. We sought to evaluate liver stiffness measurement by FibroScan® (LSM) and two biochemical scores (FibroTest®, Fibrometer®) to diagnose liver fibrosis in Senegalese CHB patients with HBV plasma DNA load $\geq$3.2 $\log_{10}$ IU/mL and normal alanine aminotransferase (ALT) values.

Methods: LSM and liver fibrosis biochemical markers were performed on 225 consecutive HBV infected Senegalese patients with high viral load. Patients with an LSM range between 7 and 13 kPa underwent liver biopsy (LB). Two experienced liver pathologists performed histological grading using Metavir and Ishak scoring.

Results: 225 patients were evaluated (84% male) and LB was performed in 69 patients, showing F2 and F3 fibrosis in 17% and 10% respectively. In these patients with a 7–13 kPa range of LSM, accuracy for diagnosis of significant fibrosis according to LB was unsatisfactory for all non-invasive markers with AUROCs below 0.70. For patients with LSM values below 7 kPa, FibroTest® (FT), and Fibrometer® (FM) using the cut-offs recommended by the test promoters suggested a fibrosis in 18% of cases for FT (8% severe fibrosis) and 8% for FM. For patients with LSM values greater than 13 kPa, FT, FM suggested a possible fibrosis in 73% and 70%, respectively.

Conclusion: In highly replicative HBV-infected African patients with normal ALT and LSM value below 13 kPa, FibroScan®, FibroTest® or Fibrometer® were unsuitable to predict the histological liver status of fibrosis.

Editor: Young Nyun Park, Yonsei University, Republic of Korea

Funding: The ANRS (National Institute of Research on AIDS and Viral Hepatitis) funded this study. The funders had no role in study design, data collection and analysis, decision to publish, or preparation of the manuscript.

Competing Interests: The authors have declared that no competing interests exist.

* E-mail: vray@pasteur.fr

Introduction

More than 350 million patients worldwide infected with hepatitis B virus (HBV) are living with chronic hepatitis B (CHB) [1]. Senegal ranks among the countries with the highest prevalence in the world; 17% of blood donors test positive in plasma for hepatitis B virus surface antigen (HBsAg). Primarily infected during early childhood, this population shows a high rate of precore mutation, around 90% (HBeAg-negative) [2]. Without treatment, 15 to 40% of subjects with chronic HBV infection will develop cirrhosis and face a risk of developing hepato-cellular carcinoma [3]. European updated guidelines for chronic hepatitis B recommended assessing liver fibrosis in patients with HBV plasma DNA load above 2,000 IU/mL or elevated ALT [4]. American guidelines differ concerning HBeAg status; they recommend liver biopsy (LB) for HBeAg-negative patients with persistent HBV DNA above 2,000 IU/mL and ALT level $\leq$2 ULN [5].

Treatment is recommended when LB shows moderate/severe necroinflammation or significant fibrosis by METAVIR scoring [4–5]. Nevertheless, LB is an invasive procedure and has rare but potentially life-threatening complications [6–7]. Also, despite being considered the "gold standard" there can be marked inter- and intra-observer variability leading to incorrect staging in up to 33% of biopsies [8–10]. Moreover, it is difficult to perform in developing countries because of its cost and the limited number of histopathologists.

In resource-poor contexts, surrogate markers that enable the non invasive measurement of fibrosis in CHB patients and serve as an alternative to liver biopsy are badly needed. These markers include a physical device that measures liver stiffness by elastometry (FibroScan®) and biochemical scores developed in industrialized countries. FibroScan®, FibroTest®, Fibrometer®, APRI, Hepascore and Fib-4 have been evaluated in Caucasian populations with chronic hepatitis C (CHC) and, show good correlation with liver fibrosis stage [11–17]. Strategies combining biochemical fibrosis scores or one biochemical score with liver stiffness measurement (LSM) by FibroScan® have decreased the need for LB in patients with viral hepatitis; [18–20] such strategies currently have already been widely implemented for hepatitis C patients, particularly in France [21].

The picture is not so clear with CHB [21–27]. Whilst studies have shown a correlation between hepatitis B virus (HBV) viral load and liver fibrosis in HBeAg negative patients [28] there is less evidence of a correlation between biochemical scores and liver stiffness measurement for CHB, particularly in countries with high CHB prevalence, with only one study involving CHB African patients [29]. We conducted a study of HBV-infected Senegalese patients with normal ALT values but elevated HBV DNA loads with the following objectives:

1- To compare the results of LSM and biochemical scores (FibroTest®, Fibrometer®).

2- To compare liver biopsy with LSM and biochemical scores (FibroTest®, Fibrometer®) for predicting liver fibrosis in patients with LSM between 7 and 13 kPa.

Materials and Methods

Patients were consecutively enrolled by private practitioners and by four public hospitals in Dakar, Senegal's capital city, from December 2006 to June 2008. Treatment-naïve patients above 18 years old, with positive HBsAg over six months, symptom-free, HIV, HCV and HDV negative, and with a serum HBV DNA level ≥3.2 $\log_{10}$ IU/mL were eligible for enrolment. All study participants underwent LSM, FT and FM on the same day. The study's scientific committee limited the LB to patients with LSM values ranging between 7 kPa and 13 kPa. This decision was based on published studies of CHC patients, in which patients with LSM≤7 kPa were assumed to have ≤F1 METAVIR stage. Conversely, people with LSM≥13 kPa were assumed to have F4 METAVIR stage, and thus no indication of LB [30].

The protocol was in accordance with Declaration of Helsinki ethical guidelines and was approved by the Senegalese ethics committee. Patients fulfilling the inclusion criteria were enrolled after providing written and informed consent. Patients eligible for treatment were prescribed Lamivudine free of charge and included in a national hepatitis B program.

Liver stiffness measurements (LSM) of FibroScan®

LSM was performed in the right lobe of the liver through the intercostal spaces, with the patient lying in the dorsal decubitus position, right arm in maximal abduction. After receiving expert training, four physicians performed LSM. Several successful acquisitions were performed on each patient. The result was expressed as the median value of 10 successful acquisitions. The inter-quartile range (IQR) was also assessed.

Liver histology and fibrosis quantification

LB was performed within six months of non-invasive markers evaluation.

Liver biopsies were obtained using 16G disposable needles (Hepafix; B. Braun, Melsungen, Germany). Fibrosis staging was considered reliable when the liver specimen length was ≥15 mm or the portal tract number ≥10 [31].

Liver specimens were stained with hematoxylin-phloxin-saffran and picrosirius red and interpreted by two highly experienced liver pathologists (MC, JLS), who were unaware of LSM, clinical, and biological data.

Liver fibrosis was scored on a 0–4 scale according to the METAVIR scoring system [32]. Necroinflammatory activity, based on assessment of interface activity and lobular necrosis, was graded on a 4-point scale [32].

Serum markers of fibrosis

Two non invasive serum methods were assessed: FibroTest® [12], and Fibrometer® [13]. The following parameters were determined on blood sampled the same day as LSM onto a Vitros automat (Ortho Clinical Diagnostics, Issy-les-Moulineaux, France): aspartate aminotransferase (AST), alanine aminotransferase (ALT), γ-glutamyl transpeptidase, total bilirubin, platelet count, HBe antigen, urea and prothrombin time.

Alpha2-macroglobulin, apolipoprotein A1, haptoglobin, hyaluronic acid and hepatitis B viral load were performed in a specialized laboratory (Biomnis, Lyon, France). Scores for the FibroTest® (FT) were calculated by Biopredictive (Paris, France). Biolivescale (Pr Calès, Angers, France) generously provided scores for the Fibrometer® (FM). All patients in whom haemolysis could influence the biochemical scores were excluded from the analysis.

Both FT and FM markers were evaluated blindly to the results of LSM and LB. Results were evaluated in both quantitative and METAVIR scores from F0 to F4.

Virological analyses

The HBV DNA quantification was assayed using the Cobas AmpliPrep/Cobas Taqman HBV test, v1.0 assay (Roche Diagnostics, Meylan, France), with a detection threshold of 12 IU/mL (1.1 $\log_{10}$ IU/mL).

Statistical analysis

Quantitative variables were expressed as mean±standard-deviation (SD) or median and interquartile range [IQ1–IQ3] and discrete variables by percentages. Differences among percentages were analyzed using the Fisher's exact test.

LSM was categorized in three classes: <7 kPa, between 7 and 13 kPa, and ≥13 kPa. The number of patients with an IQR>33% of the results of the examination was given.

Agreement between the two pathologists for METAVIR of liver specimens was evaluated using the Kappa coefficient with the interpretation scale of Landis-Koch [33].

A comparison of METAVIR staging from LB to LSM and biochemical markers was conducted only on patients with LSM values between 7 and 13 kPa.

With LB as the gold standard, the diagnostic performance of each non-invasive marker was evaluated by performing the Area under the ROC curve (AUROC) with 95% confidence interval (CI). AUROCs were compared with the rocgold procedure [34].

Statistical analysis was performed using the STATA 10 software.

Results

Patients

Eight hundred seventy four consecutive patients who were HBsAg positive for over six months were screened by seven hepatologists in Dakar. Eighty-three patients with ALT values above the normal were ineligible based on study criteria.

Among the 791 with normal ALT values, 277 patients had HBV DNA level ≥3.2 $\log_{10}$ IU/mL and 226 underwent LSM.

Only one patient failed to undergo LSM because of fatty thorax (Figure 1).

Patient characteristics

The population was primarily male (84%) with a mean age of 30 years. The median viral load was 3.6 $\log_{10}$ IU/mL, and 91% of patients were HBeAg negative. LSM ranged from 3.3 to 39.1 kPa, with median value of 6.6 kPa. Twenty seven patients (12%) had IQR values greater than 33%. One hundred and thirty three patients (59%) had values of less than 7 kPa, 80 (36%) had values between 7 and 13 kPa, and 12 (5%) had values greater than 13 kPa (Table 1).

Fifty-one percent of the patients scored ≥ 2 (with F1–F2 considered to be F2) for the FT, while 69 percent of the patients scored $\geq$F2 for the FM. Using this threshold of F2 to initiate treatment, the serum markers were in concordance in 139 patients (70%) and differed in 60 patients (30%).

The proportion of patients with values equal to F1–F2, i.e. in the grey zone, was 26% (58/220) and 50% (102/204) for FT and FM markers, respectively.

The proportion of patients identified as F3–F4 was 18% (40/220: 26 F3, 2 F3–F4 and 12 F4) for FT and 2.5% (5/204) for FM markers.

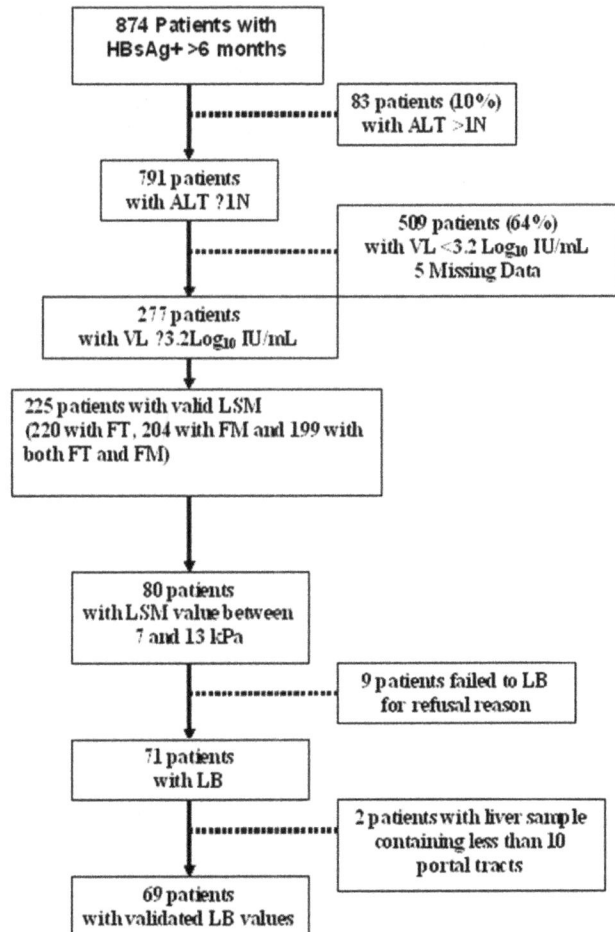

Figure 1. Flow chart.

Table 1. Main characteristics of the 225 patients with CHB.

Demographics	
Sex, Male (n,%)	188 (84)
Age* (yrs)	30±8
BMI* (kg/m2)	21.4±3.3
HBV infection	
HBe antigen positive (n,%)	21 (9)
HBV viral load* (Log IU/mL)	4.0±1.1
≥4.2 Log IU/ml (n,%)	50 (22)
Biochemical data	
Platelets* (10^3/mm^3)	195±53
Prothrombin time* (% of normal)	85±6
<80 (n,%)	66 (29)
Total bilirubin* (mol/L)	13.4±6.0
γglutamyl transpeptidase* (IU/L)	31±24
AST* (IU/L)	35±22
ALT* (IU/L)	36±10
Non Invasive Fibrosis Markers	
LSM values (kPa)**	**6.6 (5.4–8.7)**
IQR>33% (n,%)	27 (12)
<7 (n,%)	133 (59)
[7–13[(n,%)	80 (36)
≥13 (n,%)	12 (5)
FibroTest®*	**0.32 (0.21–0.49)**
<F2 (n,%)	107 (49)
≥F2*** (n,%)	113 (51)
Fibrometer®*	**0.45 (0.34–0.58)**
<F2 (n,%)	64 (31)
≥F2*** *(n,%)	140(69)

*mean±SD,
**Median [IQ1–IQ3],
***F1–F2 considered as ≥F2.

Comparison between histology and non invasive markers

A liver biopsy was performed in 71 of the 80 patients with LSM values between 7 and 13 kPa. The other nine patients declined to be biopsied. For two patients, the LB result was not retained because the LB specimens contained less than 10 portal tracts. Therefore, comparison between LB and LSM, FT and FM could be made in 69 patients.

For 64 patients (93%), the period between liver biopsy and non-invasive markers evaluation was less than two months, with all patients biopsied within a delay of less than 6 months.

The median biopsy length was 30 mm [25–34], with a median of 24 [20–30] portal tracts.

Fifty (72%) of the 69 patients had absent/mild fibrosis (METAVIR F0–F1), 12 (17%) had significant fibrosis (F2) and 7 (10%) had severe fibrosis (F3). There was no report of F4 stage.

In patients identified with a fibrosis stage equal to F2 at LB, LSM ranged from 7.1 to 11 kPa. In patients with a fibrosis stage equal to F3, LSM values ranged from 7.8 to 12 kPa.

The grades of activity were classified as A0 in 43 cases (62%), A1 in 20 cases (29%) and A2 in six cases (9%).

The Kappa coefficient between the two pathologists for significant fibrosis was 0.71±0.11.

Figure 2 shows box-plots of LSM and the two biochemical scores versus METAVIR fibrosis stages. There was no clear correlation between the values of the LSM and two biological markers and the LB METAVIR Scores.

The AUROC values for FibroScan®, FibroTest® and Fibrometer® were 0.61 [CI95%: 0.45–0.77], 0.55 [CI95%: 0.39–0.71], and 0.68 [CI95%: 0.53–0.82], respectively. No differences were observed when patients with an IQR for LSM greater than 33% were excluded from the analysis.

Comparison of AUROCs of all non-invasive markers two by two detected no significant difference.

When considering the 12 patients with LSM values greater than 13 as having a fibrosis stage equal or greater than F2, the performances of the three non-invasive markers were improved, especially for LSM with an AUROC value of 0.76 [0;64–0.88].

Comparison of FibroTest® and Fibrometer® results expressed as METAVIR scoring stages and LSM values

Table 2 reports results of FT and FM expressed as METAVIR-like scores and LSM values.

– For patients with LSM<7 kPa, 43% of patients were classified as F1–F2 or ≥F2 by FT and 57% by FM. Among the 116 patients with both FT and FM results, 39 patients (34%) were classified as F1–F2 or with stages requiring a treatment (≥F2). No patients had Metavir stage ≥F3 by FM. Conversely, seven patients, all men, displayed a Metavir score ≥F3 (2 patients F3–F4 and 5 patients F4) by FT. Table 3 summarizes for these seven patients the parameters used to calculate FT scores and FM scores. For six out of seven subjects, haptoglobin value was very low (<0.1 g/L). Haemolysis was not reported for these patients. In contrast, among the 121 patients with LSM<7 kPa

and Metavir stages by FT<F3, only six (5%) had haptoglobin value <0.1 g/L.

– For patients with LSM values over 13 kPa, 73% and 70% of patients had an FT and FM equivalent of ≥F2–F3, respectively, with one patient having a FT measure of ≤F1 (F1–F2 by FM), one patient measuring F1–F2 by both serum markers, and one patient measuring F3 by FT but F1–F2 by FM.

– Among the 73 patients with LSM values between 7 and 13 kPa, nine (12%) were classified ≤F1 by the two markers, and 40 (55%) were classified ≥F1–F2 for both markers (figure 3).

Conversely for patients classified as F3–F4 for FT or FM, the median LSM value was 8 and 10.5 kPa, respectively. For patients with FT or FM Metavir stages ≤F1–F2, LSM values were less than 13 kPa; the median LSM was less than 7 kPa. No clear relationship was identified between LSM values and FT or FM scores.

Discussion

In the present study conducted on 874 patients with HBV infection, only 10% displayed an ALT value exceeding the normal level. For most HBV-infected patients with normal ALT, monitoring remains problematic. Liver enzymes are generally the only markers routinely available in developing countries, and thus patients with normal ALT go untreated.

In Senegal, 17% of the population is considered to be HBV infected, and more than 60% of all children are infected with HBV by five years old [35]. The high prevalence of mutant precore in this Senegalese population could be explained by the virus's long evolution and selective strain bottleneck. This high prevalence of mutant precore limits the use of HBe antigen detection as a surrogate marker of HBV replication [2]. Since techniques of

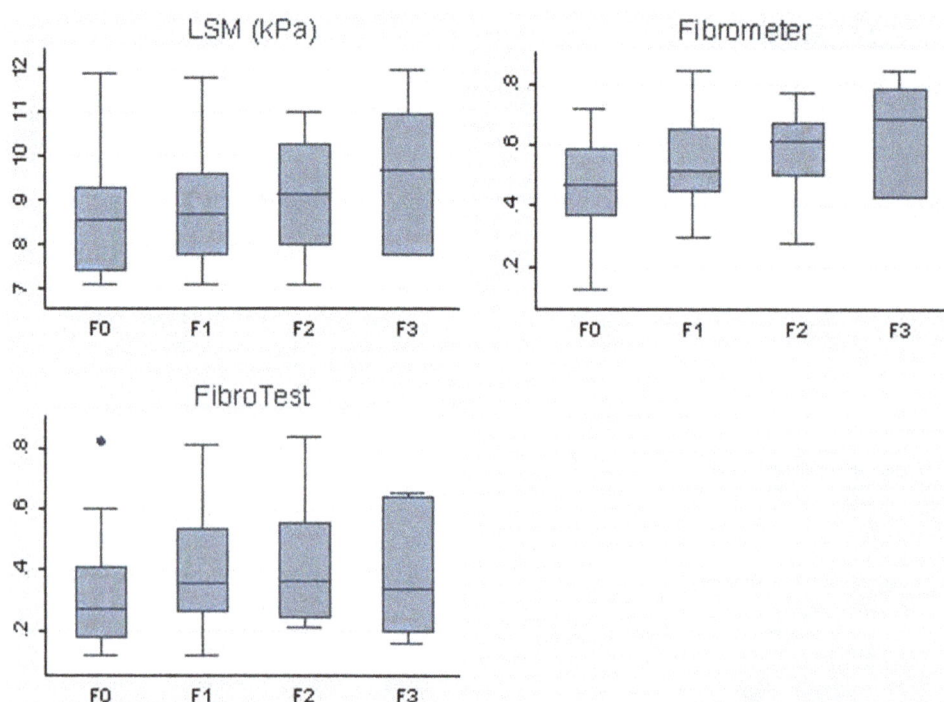

Figure 2. Box plots of LSM, FibroTest® and Fibrometer® scores according METAVIR stages from Liver Biopsy.

Table 2. Results of FT, FM METAVIR scoring stages according to Liver Stiffness Measurement values.

LSM (kPa)		≤F1	F1–F2	F2–F3	F3–F4	Total
		n (%)	n (%)	n (%)	n (%)	n
<7						
	FT	74 (57)	32 (25)	15 (12)	8 (6)	129
	FM	52 (43)	59 (49)	9 (8)	0 (0)	120
7–13						
	FT	32 (40)	24 (30)	20 (25)	4 (5)	80
	FM	12 (16)	40 (55)	18 (25)	3 (4)	73
≥13						
	FT	1 (9)	2 (18)	6 (55)	2 (18)	11
	FM	0 (0)	3 (30)	5 (50)	2 (20)	10

measuring viral load for HIV monitoring are available in many African countries, they could also be used in HBV quantification.

Patients with significant viral loads should undergo a liver fibrosis assessment before considering antiviral treatment. In this study among the patients with normal ALT values, 36% had a viral load greater than 3.2 $\log_{10}$ IU/mL, and 22% had values greater than 4.2 $\log_{10}$ IU/mL, reflecting an active infection, as LB results confirmed. Liver biopsy, however, remains difficult to perform in resource-poor countries, and non invasive markers are thus crucial to identifying patients who need treatment. The FibroScan® could be made more readily available, because the device is easy to use and the equipment simple to maintain. In contrast, expensive biochemical tests like FibroTest® or Fibrometer® are less likely to be used, since most patients cannot afford them and local laboratories often cannot perform such specialized tests.

Among the 69 patients with LSM between 7 and 13 kPa and an LB, 27% had significant fibrosis and therefore should have received treatment despite normal ALT. We found no cases at the cirrhosis stage. The quality of the biopsy was high because of large specimen sizes; the Kappa coefficient confirmed the consistent agreement between the two pathologists. The accuracy of the non invasive markers was rather low, with values of AUROC less than 0.70 for all three markers.

Various studies have already been performed using these markers in hepatitis C infected patients, with good results in diagnosing significant fibrosis and an AUROC of more than 0.80 in most studies [17,19,36]. Nevertheless, accuracy is always lower in distinguishing absent/mild fibrosis (F0 or F1) from moderate fibrosis to cirrhosis (F2, F3, F4). For CHB patients, previous studies have been published on non-invasive markers, including one in Africa [29]. Leroy et al. compared patients with CHB versus those with hepatitis C for the performance of several non-invasive markers, including FT and FM, and recorded poorer results in CHB patients in diagnosing early stages of fibrosis [17]. Marcellin et al. showed that the performance of LSM in predicting liver fibrosis in patients with CHB is comparable to that observed in CHC patients. However, cut-off values differed slightly [23]. One explanation could be that nodular fibrosis in CHB patients was less extensive than that observed in CHC patients at the same METAVIR stage. Sebastiani et al. showed a poorer performance of non invasive markers in CHC patients with normal transaminases [37].

A recent study conducted in another west African country, Burkina Faso, reported better results for FibroTest®, Fibrometer® and FibroScan® markers to diagnose significant fibrosis with AUROCs of approximately 0.80 for Fibrometer® and FibroTest® and 0.87 for the FibroScan® [29].

One explanation of the discrepancy between our results and those from the Burkina study may be the larger proportion of significant fibrosis among the Burkinabe population due to the difference in the inclusion criteria (70% of patients presented with a METAVIR stage at least equal to F2). The heterogeneous recruitment of the Burkinabe study, which included patients already receiving antiviral treatment, could account for the better results.

Conversely, patients selected in our study represent a very homogeneous population of chronic HBV patients, naïve to treatment and newly referred, but the proportion of patients with significant or severe fibrosis (12 with F2, 7 with F3, and none with F4) do not allow any firm statistical conclusion on the correlation between liver histology and non invasive markers.

In our study, we focused on FT and FM, as these biochemical markers are validated and widely implemented for HCV, in France. Low-cost, easier and simpler non-invasive methods of assessing liver fibrosis such as APRI or Hepascore showed similar poor performances with AUROCs at 0.62, CI95%: [0.45–0.79] and 0.63, CI95%: [0.47–0.78] respectively (data not shown).

With regard to the three non-invasive markers performed on the entire population of 225 patients, a large proportion of subjects

Table 3. Values of parameters used to scoring FibroTest® and Fibrometer® in the 7 patients with LSM<7 kPa and FibroTest® METAVIR scoring stages ≥F3.

Age	PT	TB	GGT	Platelets	HA	Urea	A2 M	Hapto	ApoA1	ALT	AST	LSM	FT	FM
19	99	22.2	27	42	25	2.82	3.81	.78	.59	39	31	4.8	F4	F2–F3
25	94	22.2	33	214	19	5.98	2.94	<0.1	1.62	52	37	5.3	F3–F4	F1–F2
30	93	12	30	169	19	4.48	2.89	<0.1	1.2	38	38	5.6	F3–F4	F1–F2
23	76	8.6	21	157	19	2.99	4.6	<0.1	.90	31	35	4.6	F4	F2–F3
24	56	25.7	24	167	22	3.65	3.37	<0.1	1.2	35	53	6.3	F4	F2–F3
26	84	12	45	237	19	1.99	3.29	<0.1	1.11	40	30	6.1	F4	F1–F2
24	80	12	31	196	58	4.32	3.1	<0.1	1.12	31	26	5.3	F4	F1–F2

Normal values: PT (prothrombin time):>70%, TB (total bilirubin): <20 µmol/L, GGT<73 IU/L, Platelets:>150 Giga/L, HA (Hyaluronic acid) <100 µg/L, Urea: 3.3–8.3 mmol/L, A2M (Alpha-2 macroglobulin): 1.3–3 g/L, Hapto (Haptoglobin): 0.64–1.7 g/L, ApoA1 (Apolipoprotein A1): 1.04–2.02 g/L, ALT: 72 IU/L, AST: 59 IU/L.

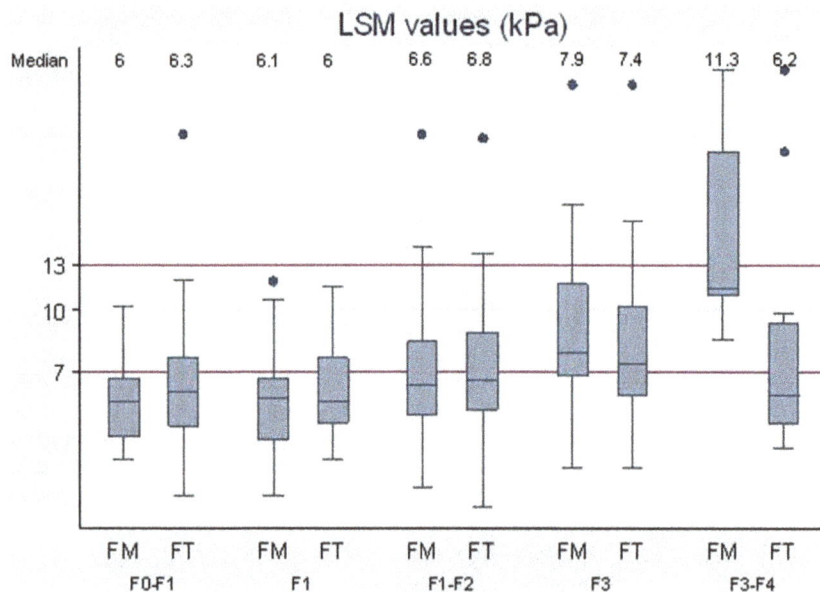

Figure 3. LSM values for each FibroTest® and Fibrometer® stage of fibrosis.

displayed values that fell into the grey zone F1/F2: 36% ranged between 7 and 13 kPa for FibroScan®, 26% for Fibrometer® and up to 51% for FibroTest®.

For subjects with an LSM value of less than 7 kPa and for whom treatment is not in theory indicated, we found 6% of subjects for whom the FT indicated a severe fibrosis; 12% of patients tested with the FT and 8% with FM revealed significant fibrosis. Haptoglobin values could explain the major disparity observed between LSM and FT. Dakar is now malaria-free, but chronic malaria and sickle-cell anaemia which may alter liver function were not examined in this study.

If we apply the cut-off of 7.2 kPa (close to 7) for LSM (defined in Marcellin et al.'s recent study of 200 CHB patients as the threshold for treatment), the rate of discordance among the three markers is high. We reached the same conclusions when we used the optimal cut-off of 7.3 kPa, the identical value found by Bonnard in Burkina Faso to identify patients with significant fibrosis.

For subjects with values between 7 and 13 kPa, results were more consistent, since all stages of fibrosis from F0 to F3 were observed; nonetheless, discordance with LB was significant. In contrast, all 11 subjects except two with a LSM value greater than 13 kPa had at least one of the two serum markers indicating significant or severe fibrosis (9/11); in eight out of 11 cases (73%), both FT and FM were concordant and thus indicated significant or severe fibrosis.

The selection of our population for biopsy based on intermediate values of LSM (7–13) skewed our METAVIR fibrosis staging on F1 and F2, the most difficult stages to differentiate. Furthermore, liver biopsy itself has an intrinsic variability, so that part of the misclassification of serum markers is due to failure of liver biopsy itself to accurately differentiate between fibrosis stages.

Still another reason that these markers have performed less well, especially when they have been used more successfully among HCV patients in western countries and among those with more pronounced fibrosis, may involve the nature of African HBV infection.

Despite the high rate of HCC in Senegal, the evolution of these patients with normal ALT is poorly understood and must be considered for specific monitoring in which the LB remains the cornerstone of fibrosis diagnosis.

Compared to adult HBsAg carriers in the Far East and in Western countries, African patients have a lower rate of HBeAg positivity. The pathogenicity of precore mutants is still incompletely understood but probably generally acquired during long-term persistent infection as escape mutants. Precore and core mutations could be associated with more severe liver fibrosis, with discrepancies between the histological, virological, and biochemical stages. [38].

Nevertheless, considering that only two out of eleven patients with an LSM over 13 kPa had contradictory results on biochemical markers, LSM results over 13 kPa might be a reliable measure for initiating treatment. Conversely, an LSM result under 7 kPa should not rule out significant fibrosis, and LB should therefore be performed. The same rule should be applied to patients with LSM values between 7 and 13 kPa.

As potent antivirals such as Tenofovir become more widely available, the only current means of characterizing CHB remains LB in patients with a viral load greater than 3.2 log/mL and normal ALT. Further investigation of surrogate markers adapted to local epidemiological and virological conditions are critically needed.

Acknowledgments

We would like to thank Dr Françoise Roudot-Thoraval for training Senegalese physicians to FibroScan®, Pr Calès for kindly providing the Fibrometer® formula, Pr Chevalier and Pr Scoazec for interpreting liver biopsies, Dr Elisabeth Delarocque-Astagneau and Dr Tamara Giles-Vernick for reading this manuscript, and the study participants for joining the study.

Author Contributions

Conceived and designed the experiments: MV FS PSM. Performed the experiments: PSM AS J-MS M-LE AB JD AD FF FS. Analyzed the data: MV LC. Contributed reagents/materials/analysis tools: J-MS FS. Wrote the paper: MV FS J-MS LC PSM.

References

1. Lavanchy D (2004) Hepatitis B virus epidemiology, disease burden, treatment, and current and emerging prevention and control measures. J Viral Hepat 11: 97–107.
2. Vray M, Debonne JM, Sire JM, Tran N, Chevalier B, et al. (2006) Molecular epidemiology of hepatitis B virus in Dakar, Senegal. J Med Virol 783: 329–34.
3. McMahon BJ (2008) Natural history of chronic hepatitis B – clinical implications. Medscape 10: 91.
4. EASL Clinical Practice Guidelines: Management of chronic hepatitis B. (2009) J Hepatol 50: 227–42.
5. (2009) AASLD Practice Guidelines: Chronic Hepatitis B: Update 2009 Hepatology 50: 1–36.
6. Castera L, Negre I, Samii K, Buffet C (1999) Pain experienced during percutaneous liver biopsy. Hepatology 30: 1529–30.
7. Cadranel JF, Rufat P, Degos F (2000) Practices of liver biopsy in France: results of a prospective nationwide survey. For the Group of Epidemiology of the French Association for the Study of the Liver (AFEF). Hepatology 32: 477–81.
8. Regev A, Berho M, Jeffers LJ, Milikowski C, Molina EG, et al. (2002) Sampling error and intraobserver variation in liver biopsy in patients with chronic HCV infection. Am J Gastroenterol 97: 2614–8.
9. Bedossa P, Dargère D, Paradis V (2003) Sampling variability of liver fibrosis in chronic hepatitis C. Hepatology 38: 1449–57.
10. Poynard T, Munteanu M, Imbert-Bismut F, Charlotte F, Thabut D, et al. (2004) Prospective analysis of discordant results between biochemical markers and biopsy in patients with chronic hepatitis C. Clin Chem 50: 1344–55.
11. Ziol M, Handra-Luca A, Kettaneh A, Christidis C, Mal F, Kazemi F, et al. (2005) Non invasive assessment of liver fibrosis by measurement of stiffness in patients with chronic hepatitis C. Hepatology 41: 48–54.
12. Imbert-Bismut F, Ratziu V, Pieroni L, Charlotte F, Benhamou Y, et al. (2001) MULTIVIRC Group. Biochemical markers of liver fibrosis in patients with hepatitis C virus infection: a prospective study. Lancet 357: 1069–75.
13. Cales P, Oberti F, Michalak S, Hubert-Fouchard I, Rousselet MC, et al. (2005) A novel panel of blood markers to assess the degree of liver fibrosis. Hepatology 42: 1373–81.
14. Halfon P, Bacq Y, De Muret A, Penaranda G, Bourlière M, et al. (2007) Comparison of test performance for blood tests of liver fibrosis in chronic hepatitis C. J Hepatol 46: 395–402.
15. de Ledinghen V, Poynard T, Wartelle C, Rosenthal E (2008) Non invasive evaluation of liver fibrosis in hepatitis C. Gastroenterol Clin Biol 32: S90–5.
16. Adams LA, Bulsara M, Rossi E, DeBoer B, Speers D, et al. (2005) Hepascore: an accurate validated predictor of liver fibrosis in chronic hepatitis C infection. Clin Chem 51: 1867–73.
17. Leroy V, Hilleret MN, Sturm N, Trocme C, Renversez JC, et al. (2007) Prospective comparison of six non-invasive scores for the diagnosis of liver fibrosis in chronic hepatitis C. J Hepatol 46: 775–82.
18. Boursier J, Vergniol J, Sawadogo A, Dakka T, Michalak S, et al. (2009) The combination of a blood test and Fibroscan improves the non-invasive diagnosis of liver fibrosis. Liver Inter 29: 1507–15.
19. Boursier J, Bacq Y, Halfon P, Leroy V, de Ledinghen V, et al. (2009) Improved diagnostic accuracy of blood tests for severe fibrosis and cirrhosis in chronic hepatitis C. Eur J Gastroenterol Hepatol 21: 28–38.
20. Castera L (2009) Transient elastography and other noninvasive tests to assess hepatic fibrosis in patients with viral hepatitis. J Viral Hepat 16: 300–14.
21. Poynard T, Morra R, Ingiliz P, Imbert-Bismut F, Thabut D, et al. (2008) Biomarkers of liver fibrosis. Adv Clin Chem 46: 131–60.
22. Oliveri F, Coco B, Ciccorossi P, Colombatto P, Romagnoli V, et al. (2008) Liver stiffness in the hepatitis B virus carrier: a non-invasive marker of liver disease influenced by the pattern of transaminases. World J Gastroenterol 14: 6154–62.
23. Marcellin P, Ziol M, Bedossa P, Douvin C, Poupon R, et al. (2009) Non invasive assessment of liver fibrosis by measurement in patients with chronic hepatitis B. Liver Int 29: 242–7.
24. Sebastiani G, Vario A, Guido M, Alberti A (2007) Sequential algorithms combining non-invasive markers and biopsy for the assessment of liver fibrosis in chronic hepatitis B. World J Gastroenterol 13: 525–31.
25. Wu SD, Wang JY, Li L (2010) Staging of liver fibrosis in chronic hepatitis B patients with a composite predictive model: A comparative study. World J Gastroenterol 16: 501–7.
26. Zeng MD, Lu LG, Mao YM, Qiu DK, Li JQ, et al. (2005) Prediction of significant fibrosis in HBeAg-positive patients with chronic hepatitis B by a noninvasive model. Hepatology 42: 1437–45.
27. Fung J, Lai CL, Fong DY, Yuen JC, Wong DK, et al. (2008) Correlation of liver biochemistry with liver stiffness in chronic hepatitis B and development of a predictive model for liver fibrosis. Liver Int 28: 1408–16.
28. Lai CL, Yuen MF (2007) The natural history of chronic hepatitis B. J Viral Hepat 14: 6–10.
29. Bonnard P, Sombie R, Lescure FX, Bougouma A, Guiard-Schmid JB, et al. (2010) Comparison of elastography, serum markers scores, and histology for the assessment of liver fibrosis in hepatitis B virus (HBV) infected patients in Burkina Faso. Am J Trop Med Hyg 82: 454–8.
30. Castera L, Forns X, Alberti A (2008) Non-invasive evaluation of liver fibrosis using transient elastography. J Hepatol 48: 835–47.
31. Nousbaum JB, Cadranel JF, Bonnemaison G, Bourlière M, Chiche L, et al. (2002) Clinical practice guidelines on the use of liver biopsy. Gastroenterol Clin Biol 26: 848–78.
32. Bedossa P, Poynard T (1996) An algorithm for the grading of activity in chronic hepatitis C. The METAVIR Cooperative Study Group. Hepatology 4: 289–93.
33. Landis JR, Koch GG (1977) The measurement of observer agreement for categorical data. Biometrics 3: 159–74.
34. DeLong ER, DeLong DM, Clarke-Pearson DL (1988) Comparing the areas under two or more correlated receiver operating characteristic curves: a nonparametric approach. Biometrics 44: 837–45.
35. Diallo S, Sarr M, Fall Y, Diagne C, Kane MO (2004) Hepatitis B infection in infantile population of Senegal. Dakar Med 49: 136–42.
36. Calès P, de Ledinghen V, Halfon P, Bacq Y, Leroy V, et al. (2008) Evaluating the accuracy and increasing the reliable diagnosis rate of blood tests for liver fibrosis in chronic hepatitis C. Liver Int 28: 1352–62.
37. Sebastiani G, Vario A, Guido M, Alberti A (2008) Performance of noninvasive markers for liver fibrosis is reduced in chronic hepatitis C with normal transaminases. J Viral Hepat 15: 212–8.
38. Ganne-Carrie N, Williams V, Kaddouri H, Trinchet JC, Dziri-Mendil S, et al. (2006) Significance of Hepatitis B virus Genotypes A to E in a cohort of Patients with Chronic Hepatitis B in the Seine Saint Denis District of Paris (France). J Med Virol 78: 335–40.

15

Prospective Validation of ELF Test in Comparison with Fibroscan and FibroTest to Predict Liver Fibrosis in Asian Subjects with Chronic Hepatitis B

Beom Kyung Kim[1,5]**, Hyon Suk Kim**[3]**, Jun Yong Park**[1,2,5]**, Do Young Kim**[1,2,5]**, Sang Hoon Ahn**[1,2,5,6]**,
Chae Yoon Chon**[1,2,5]**, Young Nyun Park**[4]**, Kwang-Hyub Han**[1,2,5,6]**, Seung Up Kim**[1,2,5]*

1 Department of Internal Medicine, Yonsei University College of Medicine, Seoul, Korea, 2 Institute of Gastroenterology, Yonsei University College of Medicine, Seoul, Korea, 3 Department of Laboratory Medicine, Yonsei University College of Medicine, Seoul, Korea, 4 Department of Pathology, Yonsei University College of Medicine, Seoul, Korea, 5 Liver Cirrhosis Clinical Research Center, Yonsei University College of Medicine, Seoul, Korea, 6 Brain Korea 21 Project for Medical Science, Yonsei University College of Medicine, Seoul, Korea

Abstract

Background and Aims: Liver stiffness measurement (LSM) and FibroTest (FT) are frequently used as non-invasive alternatives for fibrosis staging to liver biopsy. However, to date, diagnostic performances of Enhanced Liver Fibrosis (ELF) test, which consists of hyaluronic acid, aminoterminal propeptide of procollagen type-III, and tissue inhibitor of matrix metalloproteinases-1, have not been compared to those of LSM and FT in Asian chronic hepatitis B (CHB) patients.

Methods: Between June 2010 and November 2011, we prospectively enrolled 170 CHB patients who underwent liver biopsies along with LSM, FT, and ELF. The Batts system was used to assess fibrosis stages.

Results: Areas under receiver operating characteristic curves (AUROCs) to predict significant fibrosis (F≥2), advanced fibrosis (F≥3), and cirrhosis (F = 4) were 0.901, 0.860, and 0.862 for ELF, respectively; 0.937, 0.956, and 0.963 for LSM; and 0.896, 0.921, and 0.881 for FT. AUROCs to predict F≥2 were similar between each other, whereas LSM and FT had better AUROCs than ELF for predicting F≥3 (both $p<0.05$), and LSM predicted F4 more accurately than ELF ($p<0.05$). Optimized cutoffs of ELF to maximize sum of sensitivity and specificity were 8.5, 9.4, and 10.1 for F≥2, F≥3, and F = 4, respectively. Using suggested ELF, LSM and FT cutoffs to diagnose F1, F2, F3, and F4, 91 (53.5%), 117 (68.8%), and 110 (64.7%) patients, respectively, were correctly classified according to histological results.

Conclusions: ELF demonstrated considerable diagnostic value in fibrosis staging in Asian CHB patients, especially in predicting F≥2. However, LSM consistently provided better performance for predicting F≥3 and F4.

Editor: Pal Bela Szecsi, Lund University Hospital, Sweden

Funding: This study was supported by the Liver Cirrhosis Clinical Research Center, in part by a grant from the Korea Healthcare technology R & D project, Ministry of Health and Welfare, Republic of Korea (no. A102065), and by the Yonsei Liver Blood Bank (YLBB), in part by a grant from sanofi-aventis Korea. BioPredictive kindly provided the complimentary service for calculation of FT score. The funders had no role in study design, data collection and analysis, decision to publish, or preparation of the manuscript.

Competing Interests: The authors have declared that no competing interests exist.

* E-mail: ksukorea@yuhs.ac

Introduction

Accurate assessment of the severity of liver fibrosis in patients with chronic hepatitis B (CHB) is necessary for not only prediction of the long-term clinical course, but also determination of whether and when to begin antiviral therapy. The most recent guidelines on the management of CHB proposed that the presence of significant fibrosis with detectable serum hepatitis B virus (HBV) DNA indicates antiviral therapy, since viral suppression can reduce liver-related complications in patients with CHB who have significant fibrosis to cirrhosis [1,2]. Conversely, in patients without significant fibrosis and low levels of circulating virus, it is more appropriate to monitor rather than initiate expensive and potentially long-lasting antiviral therapy [1]. Furthermore, since patients with cirrhosis should be entered into the active

surveillance program for early detection of hepatocellular carcinoma (HCC) and other complications associated with hepatic decompensation, including gastroesophageal varices, assessment of fibrosis in patients with CHB has become an important clinical issue for physicians [3].

To-date, liver biopsy has been the gold standard to assess liver fibrosis. It is often limited, however, by its invasiveness, cost, risk of complications, poor acceptance by patients, lack of availability of expert practitioners, and intra/inter-observer variability [4]. These drawbacks have also made sequential liver biopsies unfeasible, especially when repeated examinations are required to monitor the response to antiviral or anti-fibrosis treatment. Consequently, noninvasive approaches combining several biochemical parameters have been introduced, including aspartate aminotransferase (AST)-to-platelet ratio index (APRI) [5], AST-alanine aminotransferase (ALT) ratio [6], Forns test [7], and FibroTest (FT; BioPredictive, Paris, France) [8]. Among them, FT is a commercially available, popular, and non-invasive surrogate, which had been substantially validated in Caucasian patients with chronic hepatitis C (CHC), and thereafter in Asian subjects with CHB [9,10,11,12,13]. Meanwhile, liver stiffness measurement (LSM) using transient elastography (TE; FibroScan®; Echosens, Paris, France), which calculates liver elasticity using a low frequency elastic wave transmitted through the liver, has been introduced recently and proven useful for non-invasive assessment of liver fibrosis among subjects with chronic liver diseases (CLDs) due to various etiologies [14,15,16].

In 2004, the Original European Liver Fibrosis panel of serum markers of liver fibrosis incorporates hyaluronic acid (HA), tissue inhibitor of matrix metalloproteinases-1 (TIMP-1), and aminoterminal propeptide of procollagen type III (P3NP), all of which are involved in the synthesis and degradation of the extracellular matrix. It showed good diagnostic accuracy for the detection of moderate and severe fibrosis in a cohort of patients with mixed etiology CLDs, mainly due to hepatitis C virus (HCV) infection (49%) [17]. Thereafter, it was simplified by removing age while maintaining diagnostic accuracy, to establish the Enhanced Liver Fibrosis Test (ELF, Siemens Diagnostics, NY, USA) [18]. This can accurately predict significant liver fibrosis in independent populations [18,19,20,21]. However, in contrast to other non-invasive surrogate markers available in the current clinical practice, few studies have investigated the diagnostic performance of ELF test in patients with CHB [22]. In particular, no previous study has focused on Asian patients with CHB.

Here, the present study prospectively compared the diagnostic value of ELF test in Asian populations with CHB with that of LSM and FT, two well-known non-invasive alternatives to liver biopsy, and defined optimized thresholds for prediction of liver fibrosis.

Materials and Methods

Patients' eligibility

From the database of the liver cirrhosis clinical research center at Severance Hospital, Yonsei University College of Medicine, Seoul, Korea, consecutive patients with CHB who underwent liver biopsy along with ELF test, LSM and FT on the same day between June 2010 and November 2011, were selected for this study. Liver biopsy was performed to assess the severity of fibrosis and inflammation prior to antiviral therapy.

The exclusion criteria were: previous history of antiviral therapy; the presence of HCC or history of it at the time of liver biopsy; any malignancy other than HCC during the study period; liver biopsy specimen smaller than 20 mm; co-infection with human immunodeficiency virus or HCV; LSM failure or invalid liver stiffness (LS) values with fewer than ten successful acquisitions, a success rate of less than 60%, or interquartile range (IQR)/ median value ratio (IQR/M) greater than 0.3; alcohol ingestion in excess of 40 g/day for more than 5 years; or right-sided heart failure (Figure 1).

This study was performed in accordance with the ethical guidelines of the 1975 Declaration of Helsinki. Written informed consent was obtained from each participant or responsible family member after possible complications of the diagnostic procedures had been explained fully. This study was approved by the institutional review board of Severance Hospital.

Liver biopsy examination

Percutaneous liver biopsy was performed using a 16-g disposable needle immediately following LSM. The liver biopsy specimens were fixed in formalin and embedded in paraffin. Then, sections 4 μm thick were stained with hematoxylin and eosin (H&E) and Masson's trichrome. All liver tissue samples were evaluated by an experienced hepatopathologist who was blinded to the patients' clinical histories. Specimens that were smaller than 20 mm or considered by the pathologists to be unsuitable for fibrosis assessment were excluded from the analysis. Liver histology was evaluated semi-quantitatively according to the Batts and Ludwig scoring system [23]. Fibrosis was staged on a 0–4 scale: F0, no fibrosis; F1, portal fibrosis; F2, periportal fibrosis; F3, septal fibrosis; and F4, cirrhosis. Significant fibrosis was defined as F2 or more and advanced fibrosis as F3 or more.

ELF test

On the same day as LSM and liver biopsy, fasting blood samples were obtained and the serum was stored at −80°C. PIIINP, HA and TIMP-1 were measured using an ADVIA Centaur XP automated immunoanalyzer (Siemens Healthcare Diagnostics, Tarrytown, NY, USA). The ELF score was calculated using the algorithm recommended in the CE-marked assay [ELF = 2.278+0.851 ln(HA)+0.751 ln(PIIINP)+0.394 ln(TIMP-1)].

FT score

On the same day as LSM and liver biopsy, the FT score parameters, including α2-macroglobulin, apolipoprotein A1, haptoglobin, γ-GGT, and total bilirubin, were assessed. The FT score was computed on the BioPredictive website (www. biopredictive.com) as follows: f = 4.467×log[α2-macroglobulin (g/L)]−1.357×log[haptoglobin (g/L)]+1.017×log[γ-GGT (IU/ L)]+0.0281×[age (in years)]+1.737×log[bilirubin (μmol/ L)]−1.184×[apolipoprotein A1 (g/L)]+0.301×sex (female = 0, male = 1)−5.540.

LSM

LSM was performed by one well-trained technician blinded to patients' clinical and laboratory data on the same day as liver biopsy and the laboratory studies, including ELF test and FT. Details of the technique and examination procedure have been published previously [24,25]. The results were expressed in kilopascals (kPa). IQR was defined as an index of intrinsic variability of LS values corresponding to the interval of the LS results containing 50% of the valid measurements between the 25th and 75th percentiles. The median value was considered representative of the elastic modulus of the liver. Only procedures with at least 10 valid measurements, a success rate of at least 60%, and an IQR/M <30% were considered reliable.

Statistical analyses

The major goals of this study were to prospectively validate the diagnostic performance of ELF test to detect histologically confirmed significant fibrosis, advanced fibrosis, and cirrhosis and compared with that of LSM and FT, and to suggest optimal cutoff values of ELF test for Asian patients with CHB. To assess the diagnostic performance of each non-invasive index, receiver operating characteristic (ROC) curves were constructed and the areas under the ROC curves (AUROCs) were calculated. Then, to evaluate the usefulness of the non-invasive method, the sensitivity, specificity, positive predictive value (PPV), and negative predictive value (NPV) were determined from the ROC curves. The Hanley and McNeil test was used to compare the AUROC between two non-invasive models [26]. The most discriminant cutoff values were determined from the ROC curves to maximize the sum of sensitivity and specificity [27].

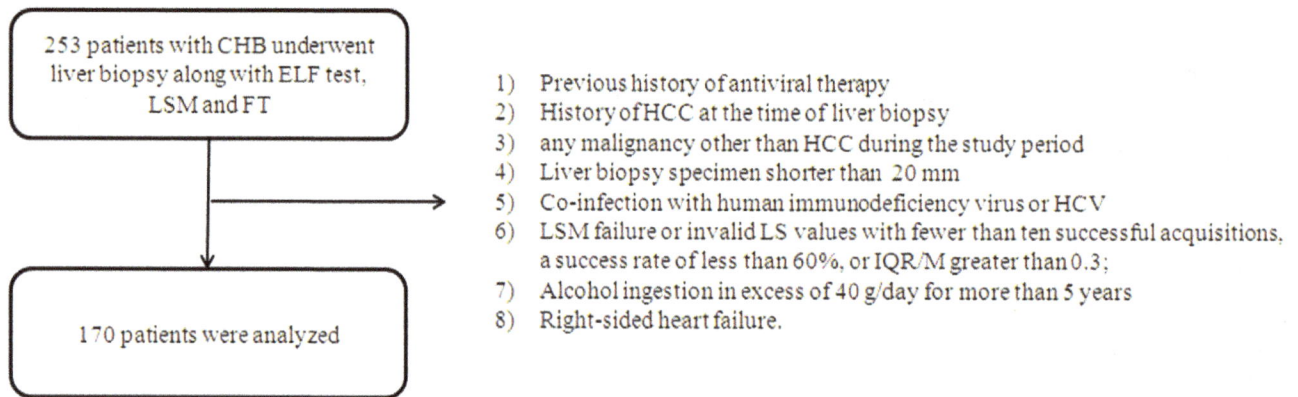

253 patients with CHB underwent liver biopsy along with ELF test, LSM and FT

1) Previous history of antiviral therapy
2) History of HCC at the time of liver biopsy
3) any malignancy other than HCC during the study period
4) Liver biopsy specimen shorter than 20 mm
5) Co-infection with human immunodeficiency virus or HCV
6) LSM failure or invalid LS values with fewer than ten successful acquisitions, a success rate of less than 60%, or IQR/M greater than 0.3;
7) Alcohol ingestion in excess of 40 g/day for more than 5 years
8) Right-sided heart failure.

170 patients were analyzed

Figure 1. Flow chart describing the selection of the study population. Based on the exclusion criteria, 170 subjects were finally recruited for analyses.

Statistical analyses were performed using SAS software, version 9.1.3 (SAS, Cary, NC). In all analyses, $p<0.05$ was considered statistically significant.

Results

Patients' baseline characteristics

A total of 253 consecutive patients were screened for possible inclusion in the study. Based on the exclusion criteria, a total of 170 patients (mean age 45.3 years, 102 male) were included (**Figure 1**).

The patients' characteristics are summarized in **Table 1**. The mean AST level was 45.9 IU/L, while the mean ALT level was 62.9 IU/L. The mean value of the ELF test was 9.56±1.69, while those of the LSM and FT were 12.24±7.76 kPa and 0.55±0.30, respectively. The mean length and the median number of fragments of liver biopsy samples were 21.3 mm and 2, respectively. The fibrosis stages were F0 in 10 (5.9%) patients, F1 in 39 (22.9%), F2 in 36 (21.2%), F3 in 38 (22.4%), and F4 in 47 (27.6%). All patients had adequate liver function.

Diagnostic performances of the ELF test in comparison with LSM and FT

As shown in **Figure 2**, the overall mean values of ELF test increased parallel to the stage of fibrosis (8.01±0.84 in F0-1, 9.24±0.77 in F2, 10.03±1.54 in F3, and 11.10±1.49 in F4, all $p<0.05$ between adjacent fibrosis stages). The Spearman correlation coefficient of ELF test with histological fibrosis stages was 0.724 ($p<0.001$). Similarly, the mean value of the LSM and FT also significantly increased; 5.13±1.54 kPa in F0-1, 7.42±2.53 kPa in F2, 12.18±3.00 kPa in F3, and 23.41±11.66 kPa in F4 for LSM and 0.16±0.08 in F0-1, 0.30±0.16 in F2, 0.61±0.23 in F3, and 0.75±0.20 in F4 for FT (all $p<0.05$ between adjacent fibrosis stages). The Spearman correlation coefficient of LSM and FT with histological fibrosis stages was 0.881 and 0.780, respectively (both $p<0.001$).

With regard to the diagnostic performances of ELF test for prediction of liver fibrosis, the AUROC was 0.901 (95% confidence interval [CI] 0.849–0.953) for significant fibrosis (F≥2) (**Figure 3A**), 0.860 (95% CI 0.805–0.915) for advanced fibrosis (F≥3) (**Figure 3B**), and 0.862 (0.809–0915) for cirrhosis (F = 4) (**Figure 3C**) (**Table 2**). ROC curves and AUROCs of LSM and FT are also shown (**Figure 3** and **Table 2**). The diagnostic performances of each component of ELF (HA, TIMP-1, and P3NP) and FT (α2-macroglobulin, haptoglobin, γ-GGT,

Table 1. Baseline characteristics (n = 170).

Characteristics	Value
Demographic data	
Age (years)	45.3±15.1
Male gender, no. (%)	102 (60.0)
Body mass index (kg/m²)	23.4±2.8
Laboratory data	
Serum albumin (g/dL)	4.2±0.51
Total bilirubin (mg/dL)	1.26±0.90
Aspartate aminotransferase (IU/L)	45.9±21.3
Alanine aminotransferase (IU/L)	62.9±26.1
Prothrombin time (%)	90.2±13.9
Platelet count (10^9/L)	183.9±73.3
Biopsy length (mm)	21.3±0.7
Enhanced liver fibrosis test	9.56±1.69
Liver stiffness (kPa)	12.24±7.76
FibroTest	0.55±0.30
Fibrosis stage, no. (%)	
F0	10 (5.9%)
F1	39 (22.9%)
F2	36 (21.2%)
F3	38 (22.4%)
F4	47 (27.6%)

Values were expressed as mean ± standard deviation, unless indicated otherwise.

bilirubin, and apolipoprotein A1) for prediction of significant fibrosis, advanced fibrosis, and cirrhosis are described in **Table S1**. Overall, the coefficient of variations (CV = standard deviation/mean) of ELF was 17.7%, while those of LSM and FT were 79.7% and 66.1%, respectively.

Among the three non-invasive methods, LSM consistently showed the highest AUROC for prediction of significant fibrosis, advanced fibrosis, and cirrhosis (**Figure 4** and **Table 2**). Although the accuracy of the three markers for prediction of significant fibrosis was statistically equivalent (all $p>0.05$), LSM showed significantly superior diagnostic efficacy over ELF test for

ELF test

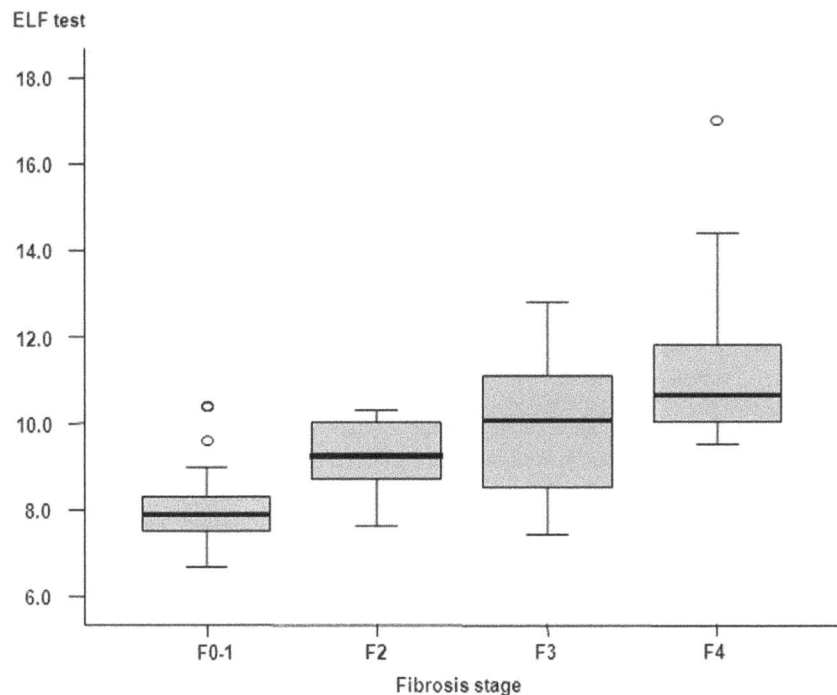

Figure 2. Box plots of ELF test according to fibrosis stage. Boxes and horizontal lines within boxes represent interquartile ranges (IQRs) and median values, respectively. The upper and lower whiskers indicate 75th percentile plus 1.5 IQR and 25th percentile minus 1.5 IQR, respectively. o, mild outlier: a value more than 75th percentile plus 1.5 IQR, but less than 75th percentile plus 3.0 IQR.

predicting advanced fibrosis and cirrhosis (both $p<0.001$), and FT had better AUROCs than ELF test for predicting advanced fibrosis (F≥3) (p = 0.038) (**Figure 4** and **Table 2**).

Determination of the optimal cutoffs for the ELF test

The most discriminant cutoff values for ELF test are indicated in **Table 2**. ELF cutoff values of 8.5, 9.40, and 10.10 generated a sensitivity of 86.0%, specificity of 85.7%, PPV of 93.7% and NPV of 71.2% for F≥2; sensitivity of 83.5%, specificity of 77.7%, PPV of 78.9%, and NPV of 82.5% for F≥3; sensitivity of 70.2%, specificity of 78.9%, PPV of 55.9%, and NPV of 87.4% for F = 4. The corresponding cutoff values of LSM and FT for each

histological stage and their diagnostic indices are shown in detail in **Table 2**.

Agreement between histological results and the ELF test, LSM, or FT

ELF test agreed with liver histology for fibrosis levels of F<2 *vs.* F≥2 in 146 (85.8%) patients, which was higher than LSM (n = 142, 83.5%) and FT (n = 138, 81.2%). However, the ELF predicted the fibrosis stage less accurately (confirmed histologically) for levels F<3 *vs.* F≥3 (n = 135, 79.4%) and F4 (n = 126, 74.1%) than did LSM (n = 158, 92.9% and n = 150, 88.2%,

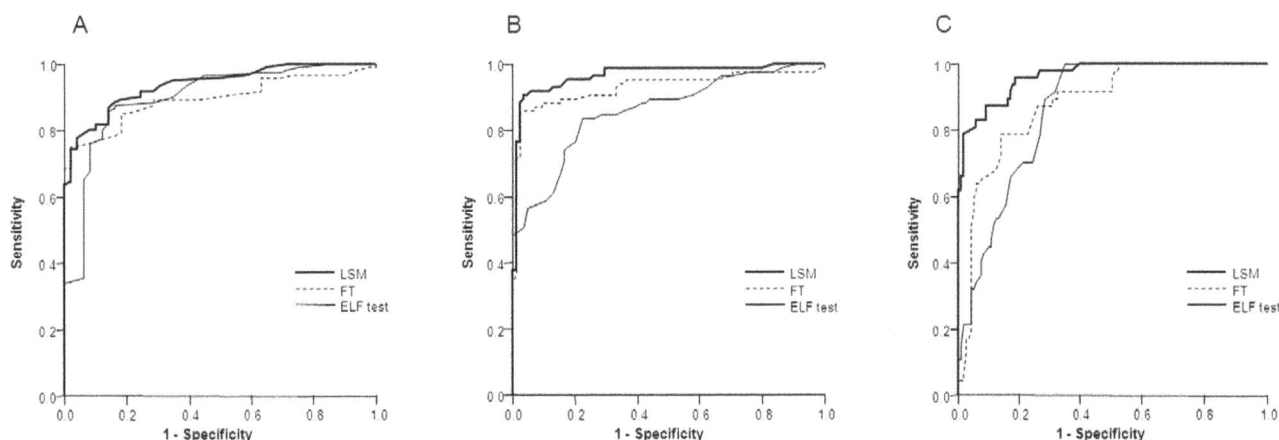

Figure 3. Receiver operating characteristic (ROC) curves for ELF test, LSM and FT in the diagnosis of significant fibrosis (≥F2, A), advanced fibrosis (≥F3, B), and cirrhosis (F = 4, C).

Table 2. Diagnostic performances of LSM, FT and ELF and their suggested optimal cutoff values.

Fibrosis stage	Method	AUROC (95% CI)	Cutoffs	Sensitivity (%)	Specificity (%)	PPV (%)	NPV (%)
	ELF	0.901 (0.849–0.953)	8.50	86.0	85.7	93.7	71.2
F≥2	LSM	0.937 (0.903–0.971)	8.0 kPa	77.7	95.9	97.9	63.5
	FT	0.896 (0.850–0.942)	0.31	75.2	97.9	98.9	61.5
	ELF	0.860 (0.805–0.915)	9.40	83.5	77.7	78.9	82.5
F≥3	LSM*	0.956 (0.929–0.983)	10.1 kPa	90.6	96.5	96.2	91.1
	FT*	0.921 (0.877–0.964)	0.51	85.8	97.7	97.3	87.4
	ELF	0.862 (0.809–0915)	10.10	70.2	78.9	55.9	87.4
F = 4	LSM*	0.963 (0.937–0.989)	14.0 kPa	87.2	91.1	78.8	94.9
	FT	0.881 (0.828–0.935)	0.67	78.7	78.8	68.5	91.4

Abbreviations: ELF, enhanced liver fibrosis; LSM, liver stiffness measurement; FT, FibroTest; AUROC, area under the receiver operating characteristics curve; CI, confidence interval; PPV, positive predictive value; NPV, negative predictive value.
*p<0.05 compared to AUROC of ELF using Hanley and McNeil test.

respectively) or FT (n = 155, 91.2% and n = 141, 82.9%, respectively) (**Table 3**).

In addition, when using the suggested cutoffs of ELF test, LSM, and FT to diagnose each histological fibrosis stage (F1, F2, F3, and F4), 91 (53.5%), 117 (68.8%), and 110 (64.7%) patients (gray-colored area in **Table 3**) were correctly classified according to histological results, meaning that liver biopsy could have been replaced with these non-invasive methods (**Table 3**).

Discordance between histological results and ELF test

Discordant results between fibrosis stages estimated by liver biopsy and ELF test were identified in 79 (46.5%) patients. On multivariate analysis, only the presence of histological cirrhosis was identified as a single significant factor, which was negatively associated with discordance between liver biopsy and ELF test (p<0.001; odds ratio 0.249, 95% CI 0.116–0.533), although, on univariate analysis, the mean ALT level differed significantly between patients with non-disconcordance and discordance (65

$vs.$76 IU/L, p = 0.035), along with the proportion of subjects with histological cirrhosis.

Discussion

Most studies that proposed ELF test as a good non-invasive alternative to liver biopsy have focused primarily on populations with HCV infection or nonalcoholic fatty liver disease [18,28] or those with mixed etiologies including viral hepatitis, primary biliary cirrhosis, $etc.$ [19,22,29]. Since the diagnostic cutoffs of such non-invasive indices based on biochemical parameters can vary, even when the etiology is the same, possibly due to different distribution of fibrosis stages and different baseline biochemical profiles, a new study to generate standardized results in Asian patients with CHB is warranted. To the best of our knowledge, this is the first study to assess the diagnostic value of ELF test and to define new cutoff values for each fibrosis stage optimized for a homogenous Asian population with CHB.

Although the underlying mechanisms of fibrosis progression in chronic viral hepatitis are expected to be similar, differences

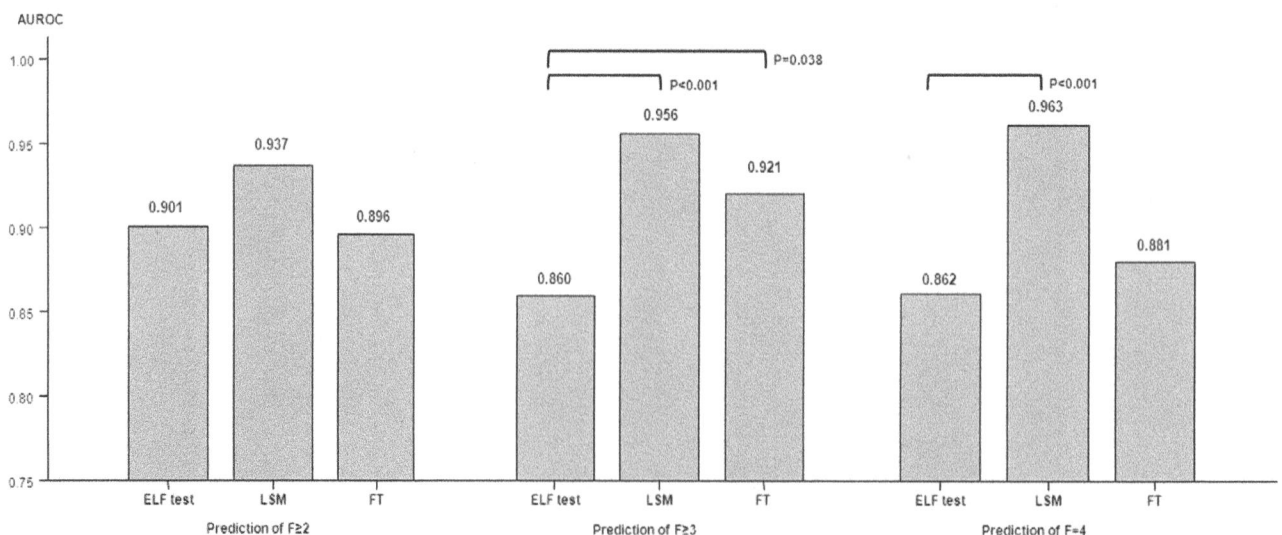

Figure 4. Detailed AUROCs of ELF test, LSM and FT in the diagnosis of significant fibrosis (≥F2), advanced fibrosis (≥F3), and cirrhosis (F = 4).

Table 3. Distribution and agreement of fibrosis stages according to histology and ELF, LSM or FT (n = 170).

Fibrosis stage estimated by histology	Fibrosis stage estimated by ELF			
	F0-1	F2	F3	F4
	ELF<8.5	8.5≤ELF<9.4	9.4≤ELF<10.1	ELF≥10.10
F1	41	4	1	3
F2	7	12	9	8
F3	9	5	5	19
F4	0	0	14	33

Fibrosis stage estimated by histology	Fibrosis stage estimated by LSM			
	F0-1	F2	F3	F4
	LS<8.0 kPa	8.0≤LS<10.1 kPa	10.1≤LS<14.0 kPa	LS≥14.0 kPa
F1	45	3	1	0
F2	20	13	2	1
F3	4	3	18	13
F4	0	1	5	41

Fibrosis stage estimated by histology	Fibrosis stage estimated by FT			
	F0-1	F2	F3	F4
	FT<0.31	0.31≤FT<0.51	0.51≤FT<0.67	FT≥0.67
F1	47	2	0	0
F2	21	12	2	1
F3	5	1	14	18
F4	4	2	4	37

Abbreviations: ELF, Enhanced Liver Fibrosis; LSM, liver stiffness measurement; FT, FibroTest.

according to etiology may affect the diagnostic accuracy of non-invasive tests [30,31]. For example, patients with CHC often have steatosis, which may influence baseline biochemical parameters, and they also tend to have micronodular cirrhosis. In contrast, CHB patients frequently experience a wide range of fluctuations in necroinflammatory activity that can result in overestimation of liver fibrosis but also have macronodular cirrhosis, which can result in underestimation of liver fibrosis [2,31]. These clinico-pathological differences have been suggested to explain the different diagnostic performance and cutoff values of noninvasive markers such as LSM and FT among studies [9,25,32]. Hence, in the present study, we focused primarily on Asian patients with CHB and investigated the accuracy and applicability of ELF test in comparison with LSM and FT, which are the most popular indices used currently in clinical practice.

This study has several advantages. First, we prospectively recruited patients who underwent not only the baseline blood tests and LSM but also FT and ELF test on the same day as liver biopsy, and the diagnostic performance of ELF test was compared to those of LSM and FT, both of which are currently preferred in France over liver biopsy due to their excellent diagnostic values [10], and have also been recently validated in Asian populations with CHB [13,24,33,34]. Furthermore, a relatively large number of subjects from a single center were consecutively enrolled in this study, and the distribution of our population was homogeneous and representative of patients with CHB seen in clinical practice. Therefore, the optimal cutoff values of ELF test derived from our study are expected to ultimately be used as reference values for future studies to elaborate its role in Asian patients with CHB. Last, we considered only biopsy specimens of 20 mm or larger.

Given that intra- and inter-observer variability may exist in histological assessment of fibrosis staging, obtaining specimens of adequate size is of utmost importance to ensure the greatest possible degree of uniformity [4].

In the present study, the diagnostic performance of ELF test was comparable to that of the LSM or FT for predicting significant fibrosis (F≥2); AUROC 0.901 vs. 0.937 or 0.896. This is consistent with several other reports [12,35], suggesting that non-invasive tests have similar accuracy for detection of significant fibrosis each other. However, LSM consistently had significantly better performance than ELF test in predicting both advanced fibrosis (F≥3) (AUROC 0.956 vs. 0.860) and cirrhosis (F = 4) (AUROC 0.963 vs. 0.862). A recent meta-analysis demonstrated a similar finding, that LSM may be much more accurate for cirrhosis than for less severe fibrosis stages [16]. Regarding comparison between ELF test and FT, the diagnostic value of ELF test was significantly lower than that of FT for diagnosis of advanced fibrosis (F≥3) (0.860 vs. 0.921); however, the performance of the ELF test and FT for diagnosing significant fibrosis (F≥2) (0.901 vs. 0.896) and cirrhosis (F4) (0.862 vs. 0.881) was actually equivalent (all $p>0.05$). In contrast, Friedrich-Rust et al. [19] proposed that ELF test (AUROC 0.91) can diagnose cirrhosis with comparable diagnostic accuracy to LSM (AUROC 0.94) and FT (AUROC 0.92). However, this study was limited in that only a small portion of the study cohort underwent both LSM and ELF. On the other hand, another recent study [21] insisted that LSM showed greater accuracy than ELF for detecting significant fibrosis and cirrhosis. Taken together, given these controversial results, the performance of ELF test as a non-invasive alternative compared to LSM or FT should be further validated.

Using the Youden method [27], we suggested ELF cutoff values of 8.5, 9.4, and 10.1 for F≥2, F≥3, and F = 4, respectively. However, Parkes *et al.* [18] reported 10.2 with a maximum sum of sensitivity (70%) and specificity (85%) for diagnosis of F≥3, while Guecho *et al.* [36] suggested 9.00, 9.33, and 9.35 for F≥2, F≥3, and F = 4, respectively. The suggested thresholds and intervals between adjacent stages may vary among studies, and they may be influenced by etiologies, sample size, and the baseline characteristics of populations. Thus, further external investigations with larger sample sizes and a balanced fibrosis stage distribution are needed to validate our data in Asian subjects with CHB.

Regarding discordant results between the histological examination and ELF test, the presence of histological cirrhosis ultimately proved to be a single significant factor with a negative association with the discordant results. Although the lower trend of ALT level in those with non-discordance compared to those with discordance seen on univariate analysis (mean value 65 vs. 76 IU/L, respectively; $p = 0.035$) did not reduce the discordance rate independently on multivariate analysis, it might be inferred that this negative correlation between the presence of histological cirrhosis and discordances can be in part associated with the different level of ALT in patients with and without histological cirrhosis (mean value 46 vs. 85 IU/L, respectively; $p = 0.039$), as observed in several related studies [13,37,38]. Thus, further studies are required to elucidate the possible confounding variables of ELF test.

This study did have some limitations. First, as this was a cross-sectional study, it is not clear whether repeated determination of ELF score may be useful for tracking the progression of fibrosis and related clinical outcomes, such as occurrence of hepatic decompensation and HCC in individual patients. Therefore, the diagnostic value for prediction of the subsequent development of cirrhosis and its various complications with sequential ELF tests during long-term follow-up must be examined further in a longitudinal study. Second, our population included a small portion of patients with F0 fibrosis. This could have resulted in a selection bias and eventually a spectrum bias, since the diagnostic performance of a given noninvasive test may depend on the disease prevalence. Since our institute is a tertiary referral hospital and one of the largest medical centers in South Korea, cases with advanced disease are likely to be referred for close observation. When we further analyzed the performance of ELF to distinguish F≥1 from F0, the AUROC was also high (0.904, CI 0.841–0.967) with an optimal cutoff value of 8.15. However, this result should be applied in real clinical practice cautiously, considering the small proportion (only 5.9%) of patients with F0 among entire population. Taken together, further studies for external validation based upon a community-based cohort should be performed to provide more generalized results for patients with CHB. Third, if we had enrolled more subjects, the diagnostic accuracy of ELF would have been much better. Indeed, when we added the clinical data of 36 patients with CHB who were further recruited for additional 4 months, concordance rate between fibrosis stages based on histology and ELF had become enhanced up to 61.7% (vs. 53.5%; **Table S2**). Thus, a large-scale study should be followed to provide the solid evidences.

In summary, in a prospective study, we first assessed ELF test in Asian patients with CHB, demonstrating its considerable diagnostic value for prediction of histological fibrosis stage, and the optimal suggested cutoff values are expected to be useful in future studies in those populations. However, LSM consistently provided better diagnostic values in the higher fibrosis stages. We hope that other researchers will evaluate the reproducibility of ELF test and its potential role as a method of classifying liver fibrosis in independent populations.

Author Contributions

Conceived and designed the experiments: BKK SUK. Performed the experiments: BKK HSK SUK. Analyzed the data: BKK SUK. Contributed reagents/materials/analysis tools: JYP DYK SHA CYC YNP KHH. Wrote the paper: BKK SUK.

References

1. Degertekin B, Lok AS (2009) Indications for therapy in hepatitis B. Hepatology 49: S129–137.
2. Leroy V, Kim SU (2012) Can transient elastography be used for the management of chronic hepatitis B patients? Liver int 32: 528–530.
3. Lok AS, McMahon BJ (2007) Chronic hepatitis B. Hepatology 45: 507–539.
4. Bedossa P, Dargere D, Paradis V (2003) Sampling variability of liver fibrosis in chronic hepatitis C. Hepatology 38: 1449–1457.
5. Wai CT, Greenson JK, Fontana RJ, Kalbfleisch JD, Marrero JA, et al. (2003) A simple noninvasive index can predict both significant fibrosis and cirrhosis in patients with chronic hepatitis C. Hepatology 38: 518–526.
6. Sheth SG, Flamm SL, Gordon FD, Chopra S (1998) AST/ALT ratio predicts cirrhosis in patients with chronic hepatitis C virus infection. The American journal of gastroenterology 93: 44–48.
7. Forns X, Ampurdanès S, Llovet JM, Aponte J, Quintó L, et al. (2002) Identification of chronic hepatitis C patients without hepatic fibrosis by a simple predictive model. Hepatology 36: 986–992.
8. Imbert-Bismut F, Ratziu V, Pieroni L, Charlotte F, Benhamou Y, et al. (2001) Biochemical markers of liver fibrosis in patients with hepatitis C virus infection: a prospective study. Lancet 357: 1069–1075.
9. Shaheen AA, Wan AF, Myers RP (2007) FibroTest and FibroScan for the prediction of hepatitis C-related fibrosis: a systematic review of diagnostic test accuracy. Am J Gastroenterol 102: 2589–2600.
10. Halfon P, Munteanu M, Poynard T (2008) FibroTest-ActiTest as a non-invasive marker of liver fibrosis. Gastroenterol Clin Biol 32: 22–39.
11. Myers RP, Tainturier MH, Ratziu V, Piton A, Thibault V, et al. (2003) Prediction of liver histological lesions with biochemical markers in patients with chronic hepatitis B. J Hepatol 39: 222–230.
12. Castéra L, Vergniol J, Foucher J, Le Bail B, Chanteloup E, et al. (2005) Prospective comparison of transient elastography, Fibrotest, APRI, and liver biopsy for the assessment of fibrosis in chronic hepatitis C. Gastroenterology 128: 343–350.
13. Kim BK, Kim SU, Kim HS, Park JY, Ahn SH, et al. (2012) Prospective Validation of FibroTest in Comparison with Liver Stiffness for Predicting Liver Fibrosis in Asian Subjects with Chronic Hepatitis B. PLoS One 7: e35825.
14. Cho SW, Cheong JY (2007) [Clinical application of non-invasive diagnosis for hepatic fibrosis]. Korean J Hepatol 13: 129–137.
15. Friedrich-Rust M, Ong MF, Martens S, Sarrazin C, Bojunga J, et al. (2008) Performance of transient elastography for the staging of liver fibrosis: a meta-analysis. Gastroenterology 134: 960–974.
16. Tsochatzis EA, Gurusamy KS, Ntaoula S, Cholongitas E, Davidson BR, et al. (2011) Elastography for the diagnosis of severity of fibrosis in chronic liver disease: a meta-analysis of diagnostic accuracy. J Hepatol 54: 650–659.
17. Rosenberg WM, Voelker M, Thiel R, Becka M, Burt A, et al. (2004) Serum markers detect the presence of liver fibrosis: a cohort study. Gastroenterology 127: 1704–1713.
18. Parkes J, Guha IN, Roderick P, Harris S, Cross R, et al. (2011) Enhanced Liver Fibrosis (ELF) test accurately identifies liver fibrosis in patients with chronic hepatitis C. J Viral Hepat 18: 23–31.
19. Friedrich-Rust M, Rosenberg W, Parkes J, Herrmann E, Zeuzem S, et al. (2010) Comparison of ELF, FibroTest and FibroScan for the non-invasive assessment of liver fibrosis. BMC Gastroenterol 10: 103.
20. Mayo MJ, Parkes J, Adams-Huet B, Combes B, Mills AS, et al. (2008) Prediction of clinical outcomes in primary biliary cirrhosis by serum enhanced liver fibrosis assay. Hepatology 48: 1549–1557.

21. Crespo G, Fernandez-Varo G, Marino Z, Casals G, Miquel R, et al. ARFI, Fibroscan, ELF, and their combinations in the assessment of liver fibrosis: a prospective study. J Hepatol.
22. Lee MH, Cheong JY, Um SH, Seo YS, Kim DJ, et al. (2010) Comparison of surrogate serum markers and transient elastography (Fibroscan) for assessing cirrhosis in patients with chronic viral hepatitis. Dig Dis Sci 55: 3552–3560.
23. Batts KP, Ludwig J (1995) Chronic hepatitis. An update on terminology and reporting. American journal of surgical pathology 19: 1409–1417.
24. Kim SU, Ahn SH, Park JY, Kang W, Kim DY, et al. (2008) Liver Stiffness Measurement in Combination With Noninvasive Markers for the Improved Diagnosis of B-viral Liver Cirrhosis. J Clin Gastroenterol 43: 267–271.
25. Castera L, Forns X, Alberti A (2008) Non-invasive evaluation of liver fibrosis using transient elastography. J Hepatol 48: 835–847.
26. Hanley JA, McNeil BJ (1983) A method of comparing the areas under receiver operating characteristic curves derived from the same cases. Radiology 148: 839–843.
27. Fluss R, Faraggi D, Reiser B (2005) Estimation of the Youden Index and its associated cutoff point. Biom J 47: 458–472.
28. Guha IN, Parkes J, Roderick P, Chattopadhyay D, Cross R, et al. (2008) Noninvasive markers of fibrosis in nonalcoholic fatty liver disease: Validating the European Liver Fibrosis Panel and exploring simple markers. Hepatology 47: 455–460.
29. Parkes J, Roderick P, Harris S, Day C, Mutimer D, et al. (2010) Enhanced liver fibrosis test can predict clinical outcomes in patients with chronic liver disease. Gut 59: 1245–1251.
30. Kim BK, Kim do Y, Park JY, Ahn SH, Chon CY, et al. (2010) Validation of FIB-4 and comparison with other simple noninvasive indices for predicting liver fibrosis and cirrhosis in hepatitis B virus-infected patients. Liver int 30: 546–553.
31. Chang PE, Lui HF, Chau YP, Lim KH, Yap WM, et al. (2008) Prospective evaluation of transient elastography for the diagnosis of hepatic fibrosis in Asians: comparison with liver biopsy and aspartate transaminase platelet ratio index. Alimentary pharmacology & therapeutics 28: 51–61.
32. Castera L, Foucher J, Bertet J, Couzigou P, de Ledinghen V (2006) FibroScan and FibroTest to assess liver fibrosis in HCV with normal aminotransferases. Hepatology 43: 373–374; author reply 375.
33. Kim BK, Han KH, Park JY, Ahn SH, Chon CY, et al. (2010) A novel liver stiffness measurement-based prediction model for cirrhosis in hepatitis B patients. Liver int 30: 1073–1081.
34. Jung KS, Kim SU, Ahn SH, Park YN, Kim do Y, et al. (2011) Risk assessment of hepatitis B virus-related hepatocellular carcinoma development using liver stiffness measurement (FibroScan). Hepatology 53: 885–894.
35. Castera L (2009) Transient elastography and other noninvasive tests to assess hepatic fibrosis in patients with viral hepatitis. J Viral Hepat 16: 300–314.
36. Guechot J, Trocme C, Renversez JC, Sturm N, Zarski JP (2012) Independent validation of the Enhanced Liver Fibrosis (ELF) score in the ANRS HC EP 23 Fibrostar cohort of patients with chronic hepatitis C. Clin Chem Lab Med 50: 693–699.
37. Kim SU, Seo YS, Cheong JY, Kim MY, Kim JK, et al. (2010) Factors that affect the diagnostic accuracy of liver fibrosis measurement by Fibroscan in patients with chronic hepatitis B. Aliment Pharmacol Ther 32: 498–505.
38. Kim SU, Kim JK, Park YN, Han KH (2012) Discordance between liver biopsy and Fibroscan(R) in assessing liver fibrosis in chronic hepatitis b: risk factors and influence of necroinflammation. PLoS One 7: e32233.

16

A New Model using Routinely Available Clinical Parameters to Predict Significant Liver Fibrosis in Chronic Hepatitis B

Wai-Kay Seto[1], Chun-Fan Lee[2,3], Ching-Lung Lai[1], Philip P. C. Ip[4], Daniel Yee-Tak Fong[5], James Fung[1], Danny Ka-Ho Wong[1], Man-Fung Yuen[1]*

1 Department of Medicine, the University of Hong Kong, Queen Mary Hospital, Hong Kong, 2 Department of Biostatistics, Singapore Clinical Research Institute, Singapore, 3 Center for Quantitative Medicine, Duke-NUS Graduate Medical School, Singapore, 4 Department of Pathology, the University of Hong Kong, Queen Mary Hospital, Hong Kong, 5 Department of Nursing Studies, the University of Hong Kong, Queen Mary Hospital, Hong Kong

Abstract

Objective: We developed a predictive model for significant fibrosis in chronic hepatitis B (CHB) based on routinely available clinical parameters.

Methods: 237 treatment-naïve CHB patients [58.4% hepatitis B e antigen (HBeAg)-positive] who had undergone liver biopsy were randomly divided into two cohorts: training group (n = 108) and validation group (n = 129). Liver histology was assessed for fibrosis. All common demographics, viral serology, viral load and liver biochemistry were analyzed.

Results: Based on 12 available clinical parameters (age, sex, HBeAg status, HBV DNA, platelet, albumin, bilirubin, ALT, AST, ALP, GGT and AFP), a model to predict significant liver fibrosis (Ishak fibrosis score $\geq$3) was derived using the five best parameters (age, ALP, AST, AFP and platelet). Using the formula log(index+1) = 0.025+0.0031(age)+0.1483 log(ALP)+0.004 log(AST)+0.0908 log(AFP+1)−0.028 log(platelet), the PAPAS (Platelet/Age/Phosphatase/AFP/AST) index predicts significant fibrosis with an area under the receiving operating characteristics (AUROC) curve of 0.776 [0.797 for patients with ALT <2×upper limit of normal (ULN)] The negative predictive value to exclude significant fibrosis was 88.4%. This predictive power is superior to other non-invasive models using common parameters, including the AST/platelet/GGT/AFP (APGA) index, AST/platelet ratio index (APRI), and the FIB-4 index (AUROC of 0.757, 0.708 and 0.723 respectively). Using the PAPAS index, 67.5% of liver biopsies for patients being considered for treatment with ALT <2×ULN could be avoided.

Conclusion: The PAPAS index can predict and exclude significant fibrosis, and may reduce the need for liver biopsy in CHB patients.

Editor: John E. Tavis, Saint Louis University, United States of America

Funding: These authors have no support or funding to report.

* E-mail: mfyuen@hkucc.hku.hk

Introduction

Up to 40% of patients with chronic hepatitis B (CHB) would develop cirrhotic complications or hepatocellular carcinoma (HCC) during their lifetime [1]. While several clinical parameters, including male gender, older age, higher levels of alanine aminotransferase (ALT) and serum HBV DNA have been identified as risk factors for severe liver disease [2,3,4], the golden standard in assessing disease severity remains to be liver biopsy. Liver biopsy is still recommended for certain CHB patients, especially those with an ALT level of <2×upper limit of normal (ULN) [5,6]. However, up to 2% of patients develop complications from liver biopsy [7,8]. Others problems like intra-observer variation and sampling error are also unavoidable [9,10,11]. There is thus an increasing demand for developing predictive models of fibrosis based on non-invasive markers.

Many predictive models of fibrosis, including the AST/platelet radio index (APRI) and FIB-4 index, were based on patients with chronic hepatitis C [12,13,14,15,16,17]. Using such models to predict liver fibrosis in CHB patients had produced conflicting results [18,19]. Only a minority of models were based on CHB patients [20,21,22,23], and these models were limited by a disproportionate percentage of either hepatitis B e antigen (HBeAg)-positive or −negative patients. Some of these studies also lack patients with normal serum ALT [20,21]. A recently-derived model is the aspartate aminotransferase (AST)/platelet/gamma-glutamyl transpeptidase (GGT)/α-fetoprotein (AFP) (APGA) index, but this is limited by its correlation with transient elastography and not actual liver histology [24]. Another factor limiting the use of other non-invasive models is that markers used in prediction may not be routinely available in non-research laboratories [18,20,25,26].

The aim of this study is to create a predictive model based on routinely-available clinical parameters to accurately predict significant fibrosis in both HBeAg-positive and -negative CHB.

Methods

Patients

The current study included treatment-naïve patients who were enrolled into therapeutic drug trials between 1994 and 2008 in the Department of Medicine, the University of Hong Kong, Queen Mary Hospital. All patients were positive for hepatitis B surface antigen (HBsAg) for at least 6 months, with a HBV DNA level of more than 2,000 IU/mL, and a serum ALT of less than 10 times the ULN prior to recruitment. Patients with decompensated cirrhosis or concomitant liver disease, including chronic hepatitis C or D virus infection, primary biliary cirrhosis, autoimmune hepatitis, Wilson's disease, and significant intake of alcohol (20 grams per day for female, 30 grams per day for male) were excluded. Written consent was obtained prior to liver biopsy, and all trials had been approved by the Institutional Review Board of the University of Hong Kong.

Patient demographics and laboratory parameters (altogether 12 variables) were recorded at the time of liver biopsy. These include age, gender, HBeAg status, HBV DNA levels, albumin, bilirubin, ALT, AST, alkaline phosphatase (ALP), GGT, AFP and platelet count. The ULN of ALT was based on the respective drug trial, ranging from 45 to 53 U/L in men and 31 to 43 U/L in women. Serum HBV DNA levels were measured by three different assays, as follow: a branched DNA assay (Versant HBV DNA 3.0 assay, Bayer Health-Care Diagnostic Division, Tarrytown, NY), with a lower limit of quantification of 400 IU/mL in 33 patients, Cobas Amplicor HBV Monitor Test (Roche Diagnostic, Branchburg, NJ) with a lower limit of quantification of 60 IU/mL in 88 patients, and Cobas Taqman assay (Roche Diagnostic, Branchburg, NJ) with a lower limit of quantification of 12 IU/mL in 116 patients.

Liver Biopsy

An 18G sheathed cutting needle (Temno Evolution, Cardinal Health, McGaw Park, IL) was used for liver biopsy for 33 patients, with a minimum length of 1.5 cm obtained. For the remainder of the cohort, a 17G core aspiration needle (Hepafix, B. Braun Melsungen AG, Germany) was used, with a minimum length of 2 cm obtained. Histologic grading of necroinflammation and staging of liver fibrosis were performed using the Knodell histologic activity index [27] and Ishak fibrosis score [28] respectively, by a single histopathologist blinded to the patients' laboratory data. Significant fibrosis was defined as an Ishak score of 3 or more, meaning the presence of at least bridging fibrosis.

Statistical analysis

The primary endpoint of the present study was to determine whether there were associations between significant fibrosis which were present in 77 patients (32.4%) in the entire cohort, and the 12 routinely-available clinical parameters mentioned above. Data was randomly divided into a training cohort and a validation cohort. Concerning the optimal sample size of this study, with 32.4% of our patient cohort having significant fibrosis and allowing a 10% error for a 95% confidence interval, 84 patients were needed in each cohort for the study to be adequately powered. A training cohort consisting of 108 patients (45.6%) was used to develop the model. The remaining 129 patients (54.4%) formed the validation cohort. All statistical analyses were performed using SPSS version 16.0 (SPSS Inc., Chicago, IL), SAS system version 9.1, R version 2.81 and STATA/SE 9.2.

To create a new predictive model, all variables were subjected to a logarithmic transformation for a better model fit. The sequence of variables in order of their associations with significant liver fibrosis (co-efficient path) was determined by L1 regularized regression. The area under the receiving operating characteristics (AUROC) curve was determined for each number of variables used for the prediction of significant fibrosis. The number of variables used was decided when the addition of extra variables failed to give a relatively better accuracy. A new predictive model was then created with the optimal cut-off value determined as the value with the highest sensitivity and specificity. Using the new regression model, the AUROC, sensitivity, specificity, positive and negative predictive values and likelihood ratios were calculated.

This new predictive model was compared to three pre-existing non-invasive indexes using routinely-available clinical parameters: the APRI, the FIB-4 index and the APGA index. The APRI was calculated using [AST (U/L)/(ULN of AST)/platelet count $(\times 10^9/L)] \times 100$ [12]. The FIB-4 index was calculated using [age (years)$\times$AST (U/L)]/$\{[PLT (10^9/L)] \times (ALT(U/L)]^{1/2}\}$f [13]. The APGA index was calculated using log(index) = 1.44+0.1490 log[GGT (U/L)]+0.3308log [AST (U/L)]−0.5846log [platelet count $(\times 10^9/L)]+0.1148log [AFP (ng/mL)+1] [24].

The Mann-Whitney U test was used for continuous variables with a skewed distribution; the chi-squared test was used for categorical variables. Correlation between different predictive models with significant fibrosis was performed using Spearman correlation co-efficient. A two-sided p value of <0.05 was considered statistically significant.

Results

A total of 237 patients with all 12 clinical parameters available were recruited. The characteristics of all 237 patients at the time of liver biopsy, including a comparison between the training and validation cohorts, are shown in Table 1. The median age was 38.2 years and 98 patients (41.3%) were HBeAg-positive. Twenty-five patients (10.5%) had a normal ALT level. Significant fibrosis and cirrhosis were present in 77 patients (32.4%) and 5 patients (2.1%) respectively. The percentage of patients with significant fibrosis in patients with ALT $\geq$2$\times$ULN and <2$\times$ULN were 39.6% (44 out of 111 patients) and 26.2% (33 out of 126 patients) respectively.

The sequence of variables added at each step under the AUROC curve is shown in Figure 1. The addition of the first 5 variables (AFP, ALP, age, AST, platelet count) achieved a best fit in the regression model. The further addition of variables only increases the complexity of the formula without achieving a marked improvement in prediction accuracy. Using L1 regularized regression, a new predictive model for significant fibrosis, named the PAPAS index (Platelet/Age/Phosphatase/AFP/AST), was derived as follows:

$$\log(\text{Index}+1) = 0.0255 + 0.0031 \times \text{age(years)} +$$
$$0.1483 \times \log[\text{ALP(U/L)}\} + 0.004 \times$$
$$\log[\text{AST(U/L)}] + 0.0908 \times \log[\text{AFP(ng/mL)}+1] -$$
$$0.028 \times \log[\text{platelet count}(10^9/L)].$$

The AUROC for predicting significant fibrosis was 0.701 for the training cohort and 0.776 for the validation cohort (Figure 2). There was no significant difference in the AUCs of both training and validation groups (p = 0.270). The PAPAS index was then

Table 1. Characteristics of 237 patients included in model.

	Total	Training	Validation	*p* value
Number of patients	**237**	**108**	**129**	
Age (years)	38.2 (18–63)	36.4 (18–63)	40.0 (18–61)	0.695
Number of male patients	160 (67.2%)	73 (67.6%)	87 (67.4%)	0.980
Number of HBeAg-positive patients	98 (41.3%)	42 (38.9%)	56 (43.4%)	0.481
Albumin (g/L)	46 (36–54)	46 (37–54)	45 (36–53)	0.156
Bilirubin (umol/L)	12 (3–96)	12 (3–96)	12 (3–31)	0.348
ALP (U/L)	76 (20–242)	73.5 (33–145)	76 (20–242)	0.283
AST (U/L)	54 (16–304)	52 (16–304)	55 (18–304)	0.490
ALT (U/L)	87 (14–507)	80.5 (15–469)	95 (14–507)	0.334
Number of patients with				
• **Normal ALT**	25 (10.5%)	10 (9.3%)	15 (11.6%)	
• **ALT 1–2×ULN**	101 (42.6%)	46 (42.6%)	55 (42.6%)	
• **ALT >2×ULN**	111 (46.8%)	52 (48.1%)	59 (45.7%)	
GGT (U/L)	33 (5–160)	30.5 (6–134)	35 (5–160)	0.999
AFP (ng/mL)	4 (1–178)	4 (1–178)	4 (1–86)	0.420
Platelet (×10⁹/L)	201 (93–334)	206.5 (95–331)	198 (93–334)	0.571
HBV DNA (log IU/mL)	6.77 (2.70–14.0)	6.99 (3.50–11.8)	6.76 (2.70–14.0)	0.148
Number of patients with significant necroinflammation (NI≥7)	120 (50.6%)	47 (43.5%)	73 (56.6%)	0.339
Number of patients with significant fibrosis (F≥3)	77 (32.4%)	30 (27.8%)	47 (36.4%)	0.091
• **F6**	5 (2.1%)	3 (2.8%)	2 (1.6%)	
• **F5**	15 (6.3%)	7 (6.5%)	8 (6.2%)	
• **F4**	25 (10.5%)	13 (12.0%)	12 (9.3%)	
• **F3**	32 (13.5%)	7 (6.5%)	25 (19.4%)	
• **F2**	59 (24.8%)	28 (25.9%)	31 (24.0%)	
• **F1**	71 (29.8%)	32 (29.6%)	39 (30.2%)	
• **F0**	30 (12.6%)	18 (16.7%)	12 (9.3%)	

Continuous variables expressed in median (range) F = Ishak Fibrosis Score.

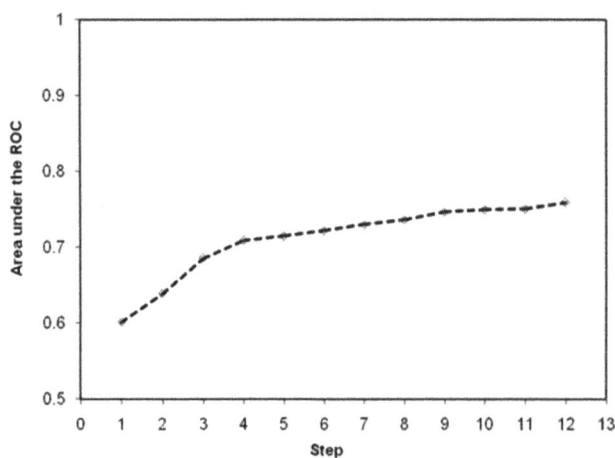

Figure 1. Area under the receiver operating characteristics (AUROC) curve at each step. Steps 1–12 as listed in their order: AFP, ALP, age, AST, platelet count, albumin, HBV DNA, GGT, gender, bilirubin, HBeAg status, ALT.

compared with three previously published non-invasive indices i.e. the APRI, the FIB-4 index and the APGA index. The boxplots of the four indices in predicting significant fibrosis are shown in Figure 3. APRI, the FIB-4 index, the APGA index and the PAPAS index all correlated well with significant fibrosis [$r = 0.337$, 0.338, 0.418 and 0.426 respectively (all p<0.001)]. The AUROC for predicting significant fibrosis in the validation cohort for all four models is shown in Figure 4a. The AUC of the PAPAS index, APGA index, FIB-4 index and APRI were 0.776, 0.758, 0.723 and 0.708 respectively (Table 2). The AUC of the PAPAS index was significantly better than APRI (p = 0.009). There were no significant differences between the AUCs of PAPAS index, APGA index and FIB-4 index. For patients with ALT <2×ULN, the AUROC for all for indices is shown in Figure 4b. The AUC of the PAPAS index improved to 0.797 (Table 3). The accuracy and correlation coefficients of the PAPAS index are the best among the 4 models.

The sensitivity, specificity, predictive values and likelihood ratios of all four indices are shown in Table 4, using the various cut-offs suggested for each model. Using an optimal cut-off of 1.662, the PAPAS index had a sensitivity of 73.3% and a specificity of 78.2% in predicting significant fibrosis. The negative predictive value was 88.4%.

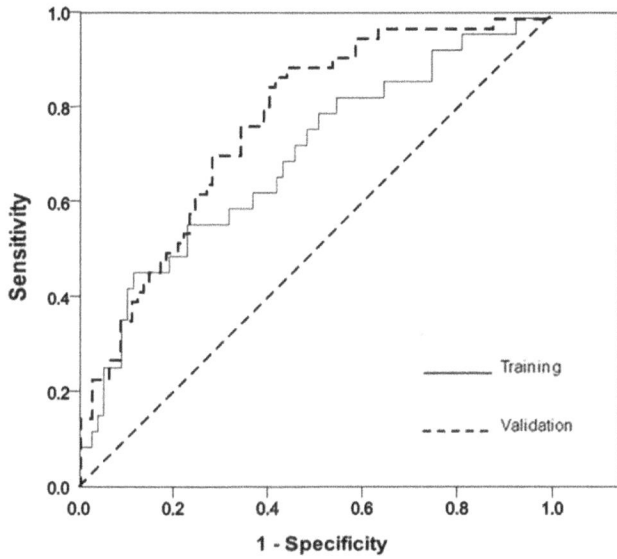

Figure 2. Comparison of receiver operating characteristics (ROC) curves of training and validation cohorts in predicting significant fibrosis for the PAPAS index.

One hundred and twenty-six patients (53.2%) among our total patient cohort had an ALT level of <2×ULN, a patient group in whom liver biopsies are recommended before considering treatment. Among this group, 85 patients (67.5%) had a score less than the optimal cut-off of 1.662, suggesting that these patients do not have significant fibrosis and liver biopsies could be avoided. Seventy-five out of these 85 patients (88.2%) had insignificant fibrosis (Ishak stage 0 to 2) on actual histology. For the remaining 10 patients (11.2%), 5 had stage 3 fibrosis and 5 had stage 4 fibrosis. If the revised ULN of ALT as suggested by Prati et al (30 U/L for men, 19 U/L for women) [29] was used, 39 patients would have an ALT level of <2×ULN, of which 30 patients (76.9%) could avoid liver biopsy by having a score of less than 1.662. Twenty-eight out of these 30 patients (93.3%) had insignificant fibrosis. For the remaining 2 patients (6.7%), one had stage 3 fibrosis and another had stage 4 fibrosis.

Discussion

Given the invasiveness of liver biopsy, the development of non-invasive markers for liver fibrosis has always been an attractive option, especially since non-invasive markers for fibrosis in CHB are not well-established. Liver biopsy itself also has its limitations, thus using the AUROC in evaluating non-invasive markers of fibrosis could never reach the perfect value of 1.0. In fact, it had

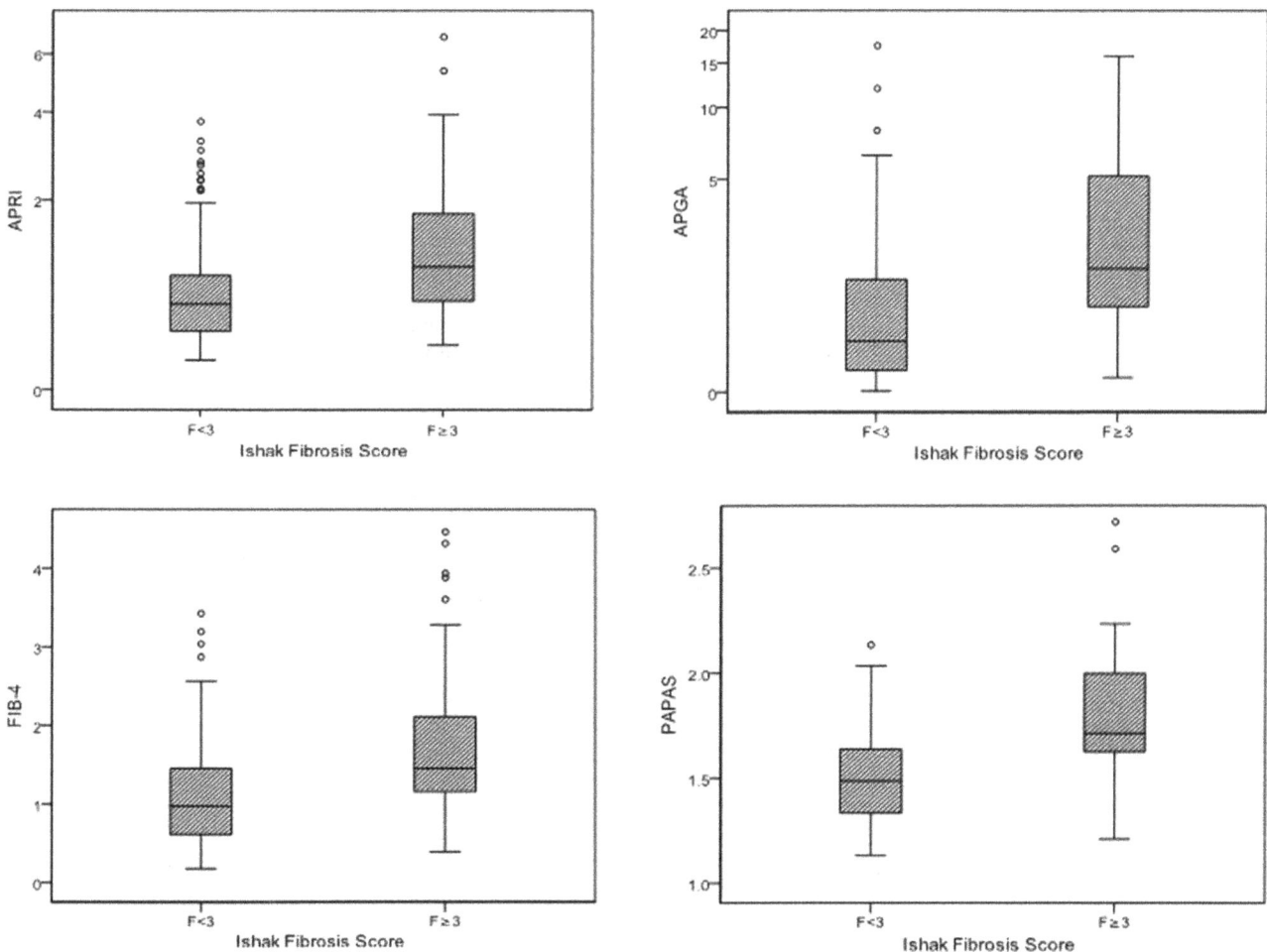

Figure 3. Model values based on Ishak fibrosis score. The top and bottom of each box represents the 25th and 75th percentile interval, the line through the box in the median and the error bars are the 5th and 95th percentile intervals.

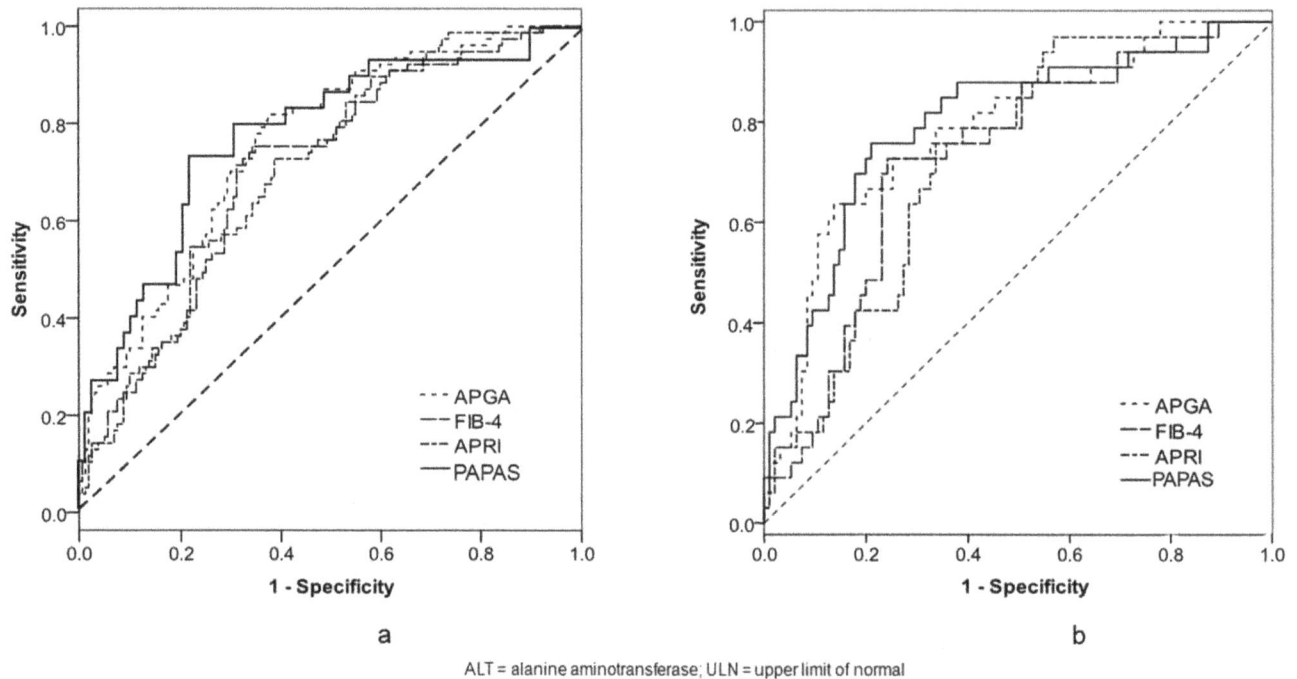

ALT = alanine aminotransferase; ULN = upper limit of normal

Figure 4. Comparison of ROC curves of different predictive models in predicting significant fibrosis for (a) all patients and (b) patients with ALT <×2 ULN.

been shown previously that a perfect marker for significant fibrosis would not even reach an AUROC of 0.90 [30,31], which is the reason for many previous studies can only obtain an AUROC range of 0.76–0.88 [30].

The PAPAS index obtained an AUROC of 0.776 for the prediction of significant fibrosis. The AUROC improves to 0.797 for patients with ALT <2×ULN, the group of patients with liver biopsy recommended before considering treatment. The sensitivity and specificity of our model were both equally high at 73.3% and 78.2% respectively, and a high negative predictive value of 88.4% was achieved at the optimal cut-off value. The AUROC obtained was superior to other models of fibrosis based on commonly-available clinical parameters used in our cohort. Two such models, the FIB-4 index and APRI, were initially created based on patients with chronic hepatitis C, and therefore might not be suitable for CHB patients. According to one study, the AUROC of APRI in 218 CHB patients in predicting fibrosis was only 0.63 [19]. Two other such models based on chronic hepatitis C patients, Fibrotest and Actitest, achieved satisfactory results in CHB patients, but were limited by the requirement of using special and non-routinely

available biomarkers. In addition, the majority of the study population was HBeAg-negative [18]. The disproportionate representation of either HBeAg-positive or HBeAg-negative patients was also seen in other non-invasive models for CHB [20,21,22]. Our study had a good mixture of both HBeAg-positive (41.3%) and -negative patients, making it more representative of the whole spectrum of CHB population. Our study also had patients with different ALT ranges, including a proportion of patients with normal ALT.

A high negative predictive value meant the predictive model would excel in excluding CHB patients with significant fibrosis. For patients with an ALT level of <2×ULN, 67.5% of our cohort would be able to avoid the invasiveness of a liver biopsy. Among this subgroup of patients, 88.2% actually had insignificant fibrosis from histology. While 11.8% (10 out of 85) of patients had a discordance between the predictive model score and actual histology, this figure is lower than other studies validating non-invasive models of liver fibrosis [32,33]. If the revised ULN of ALT as suggested by Prati et al [29] was used, the percentage of patients able to avoid liver biopsy would further increase to 76.9%.

Table 2. Area under curve (AUC) of the validation cohort using the PAPAS index, APGA index, FIB-4 index and APRI for significant fibrosis in all patients.

	AUC for significant fibrosis	95% confidence intervals
PAPAS	0.776	0.694–0.854
APGA	0.757	0.674–0.840
FIB-4	0.723	0.635–0.810
APRI	0.708	0.625–0.800

Table 3. Area under curve (AUC) of the validation cohort using the PAPAS index, APGA index, FIB-4 index and APRI for significant fibrosis in patients with ALT <2×ULN.

	AUC for significant fibrosis	95% confidence intervals
PAPAS	0.797	0.706–0.888
APGA	0.784	0.693–0.875
FIB-4	0.726	0.629–0.823
APRI	0.727	0.636–0.818

Table 4. Sensitivity, specificity, predictive values and likelihood ratios of scores according to different cut-offs for predicting significant fibrosis.

	Optimal cut-off	Sensitivity	Specificity	PPV	NPV	LR+	LR−
PAPAS	1.662	73.3%	78.2%	56.4%	88.4%	3.365	0.341
APGA	6.687	16.9%	98.1%	81.3%	71.0%	9.027	0.847
FIB-4	1.45	51.9%	74.4%	49.4%	76.3%	2.028	0.646
	3.25	9.09%	99.4%	87.5%	69.4%	14.670	0.915
APRI	0.5	89.6%	40.6%	42.1%	89.0%	1.509	0.256
	1.5	29.9%	88.1%	54.8%	72.3%	2.516	0.796

PPV = positive predictive value.
NPV = negative predictive value.
LR+ = positive likelihood ratio.
LR− = negative likelihood ratio.

The PAPAS index was based on five common clinical parameters: age, ALP, AST, AFP and platelet count. All 5 parameters had been shown in previous studies to be associated with significant fibrosis in CHB [20,21,24]. Age is a valuable predictor since progression of fibrosis in CHB is time-dependent [34,35]. Increased fibrosis results in a reduced clearance of AST and hence an elevated serum level [36]. A low platelet count has also been associated with advanced liver fibrosis through the altered production of thrombopoietin [37]. The addition of extra variables other than these five parameters did not further improve the accuracy of the current predictive model. Both ALT and HBV DNA levels, known to fluctuate during the natural history of CHB [38], were not included in the PAPAS index. While previous studies had shown several markers, including hyaluronic acid, α-2 macroglobulin and apolipoprotein A_1, to have a predictive value in CHB, these markers may not be available in the routine evaluation of chronic liver diseases. Using them in predictive models might hinder their widespread use [18,20,25,26].

Many predictive models in previous studies [15,21,22,25] were created using stepwise regression, a prediction method based on identified independent variables to achieve a best-fit model [39]. While commonly used, stepwise regression had been shown to be prone to errors of sampling, measurement and specification [40]. Moreover, a rigid setup in computer programming and a misreading in the order of importance of various predictor variables could result in serious misinterpretation of results [41]. L1 regularized regression adopted in the present study identifies the order in which variables enter or leave the created model, allowing more flexibility in finding a regularized fit with any given number of parameters [42], and has been increasingly used in the design of predictive models in different clinical studies [24,43,44,45].

The current study has certain limitations. Our study only had Chinese CHB patients. Given that 67.6% of patients in our study cohort had limited fibrosis, the study would be biased towards having a high negative predictive value. The PAPAS index was not statistically superior to both the APGA index and FIB-4 index, probably due to the limited number of patients in our present study. Hence, external validation of the PAPAS index with an independent validation cohort would be important before considering widespread use. Body mass index and cholesterol levels were not available in our study, thus we were unable to

compare our model with other predictive indices, including the Forns index [15,21]. Given that the current patient cohort consists of patients with potential to be recruited into drug trials, there would be fewer patients with an inactive disease and low viral load. Our predictive model might not be applicable to this group of patients. However, our cohort included patients with HBV DNA $\geq$2000 IU/mL, which is the threshold level suggested by CHB guidelines in commencing treatment. Due to the small number of patients with histologic cirrhosis, we were unable to create a predictive model for cirrhosis, which would have less measurement and observer error in detection if possible [11]. Similar to previous models based on CHB patients [20,21], the PAPAS index did not achieve a high positive predictive value. Therefore, the PAPAS index will be best applicable in excluding patients with insignificant fibrosis in whom treatment may not be necessary at the time of measurement. For patients with the score above the optimal cut-off level of 1.662, the decision of treatment should be considered in conjunction with other disease parameters or viral markers.

A possible method to improve the diagnostic accuracy of predictive models is to combine the available clinical parameters with imaging or transient elastography. The former had been attempted by including the spleen size on imaging, with a high positive predictive value for cirrhosis obtained [23]. The accuracy of transient elastography in CHB is hindered whenever the ALT levels are elevated [46], but this could be improved by combining transient elastography with a non-invasive predictive model like the Forns index [47]. The sequential use of non-invasive markers is also another option [48], although such studies are lacking in CHB patients.

In conclusion, the PAPAS index, a newly-designed predictive model using routinely-available clinical parameters, can accurately predict significant liver fibrosis in CHB patients, and potentially reduce the need for liver biopsies. Further studies would be needed to validate this model and compare it with other non-invasive models of fibrosis in CHB.

Author Contributions

Conceived and designed the experiments: W-KS M-FY. Performed the experiments: PPCI JF DK-HW. Analyzed the data: C-FL DY-TF. Wrote the paper: W-KS C-FL C-LL M-FY.

References

1. Lai CL, Yuen MF (2007) The natural history and treatment of chronic hepatitis B: a critical evaluation of standard treatment criteria and end points. Ann Intern Med 147: 58–61.

2. Chen CJ, Yang HI, Su J, Jen CL, You SL, et al. (2006) Risk of hepatocellular carcinoma across a biological gradient of serum hepatitis B virus DNA level. JAMA 295: 65–73.

3. Yuen MF, Yuan HJ, Wong DK, Yuen JC, Wong WM, et al. (2005) Prognostic determinants for chronic hepatitis B in Asians: therapeutic implications. Gut 54: 1610–1614.

4. Iloeje UH, Yang HI, Su J, Jen CL, You SL, et al. (2006) Predicting cirrhosis risk based on the level of circulating hepatitis B viral load. Gastroenterology 130: 678–686.

5. Lok AS, McMahon BJ (2009) Chronic hepatitis B: update 2009. Hepatology 50: 661–662.

6. Liaw YF, Leung N, Kao JH, Piratvisuth T, Gane E, et al. (2008) Asian-Pacific consensus statement on the management of chronic hepatitis B: a 2008 update. Hepatol Int 2: 263–283.

7. Piccinino F, Sagnelli E, Pasquale G, Giusti G (1986) Complications following percutaneous liver biopsy. A multicentre retrospective study on 68,276 biopsies. J Hepatol 2: 165–173.

8. Rockey DC, Caldwell SH, Goodman ZD, Nelson RC, Smith AD (2009) Liver biopsy. Hepatology 49: 1017–1044.

9. Abdi W, Millan JC, Mezey E (1979) Sampling variability on percutaneous liver biopsy. Arch Intern Med 139: 667–669.

10. ter Borg F, ten Kate FJ, Cuypers HT, Leentvaar-Kuijpers A, Oosting J, et al. (2000) A survey of liver pathology in needle biopsies from HBsAg and anti-HBe positive individuals. J Clin Pathol 53: 541–548.

11. Regev A, Berho M, Jeffers LJ, Milikowski C, Molina EG, et al. (2002) Sampling error and intraobserver variation in liver biopsy in patients with chronic HCV infection. Am J Gastroenterol 97: 2614–2618.

12. Wai CT, Greenson JK, Fontana RJ, Kalbfleisch JD, Marrero JA, et al. (2003) A simple noninvasive index can predict both significant fibrosis and cirrhosis in patients with chronic hepatitis C. Hepatology 38: 518–526.

13. Sterling RK, Lissen E, Clumeck N, Sola R, Correa MC, et al. (2006) Development of a simple noninvasive index to predict significant fibrosis in patients with HIV/HCV coinfection. Hepatology 43: 1317–1325.

14. Imbert-Bismut F, Ratziu V, Pieroni L, Charlotte F, Benhamou Y, et al. (2001) Biochemical markers of liver fibrosis in patients with hepatitis C virus infection: a prospective study. Lancet 357: 1069–1075.

15. Forns X, Ampurdanes S, Llovet JM, Aponte J, Quinto L, et al. (2002) Identification of chronic hepatitis C patients without hepatic fibrosis by a simple predictive model. Hepatology 36: 986–992.

16. Adams LA, Bulsara M, Rossi E, DeBoer B, Speers D, et al. (2005) Hepascore: an accurate validated predictor of liver fibrosis in chronic hepatitis C infection. Clin Chem 51: 1867–1873.

17. Koda M, Matunaga Y, Kawakami M, Kishimoto Y, Suou T, et al. (2007) FibroIndex, a practical index for predicting significant fibrosis in patients with chronic hepatitis C. Hepatology 45: 297–306.

18. Myers RP, Tainturier MH, Ratziu V, Piton A, Thibault V, et al. (2003) Prediction of liver histological lesions with biochemical markers in patients with chronic hepatitis B. J Hepatol 39: 222–230.

19. Wai CT, Cheng CL, Wee A, Dan YY, Chan E, et al. (2006) Non-invasive models for predicting histology in patients with chronic hepatitis B. Liver Int 26: 666–672.

20. Zeng MD, Lu LG, Mao YM, Qiu DK, Li JQ, et al. (2005) Prediction of significant fibrosis in HBeAg-positive patients with chronic hepatitis B by a noninvasive model. Hepatology 42: 1437–1445.

21. Hui AY, Chan HL, Wong VW, Liew CT, Chim AM, et al. (2005) Identification of chronic hepatitis B patients without significant liver fibrosis by a simple noninvasive predictive model. Am J Gastroenterol 100: 616–623.

22. Mohamadnejad M, Montazeri G, Fazlollahi A, Zamani F, Nasiri J, et al. (2006) Noninvasive markers of liver fibrosis and inflammation in chronic hepatitis B-virus related liver disease. Am J Gastroenterol 101: 2537–2545.

23. Kim BK, Kim SA, Park YN, Cheong JY, Kim HS, et al. (2007) Noninvasive models to predict liver cirrhosis in patients with chronic hepatitis B. Liver Int 27: 969–976.

24. Fung J, Lai CL, Fong DY, Yuen JC, Wong DK, et al. (2008) Correlation of liver biochemistry with liver stiffness in chronic hepatitis B and development of a predictive model for liver fibrosis. Liver Int 28: 1408–1416.

25. Cales P, Oberti F, Michalak S, Hubert-Fouchard I, Rousselet MC, et al. (2005) A novel panel of blood markers to assess the degree of liver fibrosis. Hepatology 42: 1373–1381.

26. Montazeri G, Estakhri A, Mohamadnejad M, Nouri N, Montazeri F, et al. (2005) Serum hyaluronate as a non-invasive marker of hepatic fibrosis and inflammation in HBeAg-negative chronic hepatitis B. BMC Gastroenterol 5: 32.

27. Knodell RG, Ishak KG, Black WC, Chen TS, Craig R, et al. (1981) Formulation and application of a numerical scoring system for assessing histological activity in asymptomatic chronic active hepatitis. Hepatology 1: 431–435.

28. Ishak K, Baptista A, Bianchi L, Callea F, De Groote J, et al. (1995) Histological grading and staging of chronic hepatitis. J Hepatol 22: 696–699.

29. Prati D, Taioli E, Zanella A, Della Torre E, Butelli S, et al. (2002) Updated definitions of healthy ranges for serum alanine aminotransferase levels. Ann Intern Med 137: 1–10.

30. Mehta SH, Lau B, Afdhal NH, Thomas DL (2009) Exceeding the limits of liver histology markers. J Hepatol 50: 36–41.

31. Castera L, Pinzani M (2010) Biopsy and non-invasive methods for the diagnosis of liver fibrosis: does it take two to tango? Gut 59: 861–866.

32. Castera L, Vergniol J, Foucher J, Le Bail B, Chanteloup E, et al. (2005) Prospective comparison of transient elastography, Fibrotest, APRI, and liver biopsy for the assessment of fibrosis in chronic hepatitis C. Gastroenterology 128: 343–350.

33. Castera L, Sebastiani G, Le Bail B, de Ledinghen V, Couzigou P, et al. (2010) Prospective comparison of two algorithms combining non-invasive methods for staging liver fibrosis in chronic hepatitis C. J Hepatol 52: 191–198.

34. Poynard T, Mathurin P, Lai CL, Guyader D, Poupon R, et al. (2003) A comparison of fibrosis progression in chronic liver diseases. J Hepatol 38: 257–265.

35. Fung J, Lai CL, But D, Wong D, Cheung TK, et al. (2008) Prevalence of fibrosis and cirrhosis in chronic hepatitis B: implications for treatment and management. Am J Gastroenterol 103: 1421–1426.

36. Kamimoto Y, Horiuchi S, Tanase S, Morino Y (1985) Plasma clearance of intravenously injected aspartate aminotransferase isozymes: evidence for preferential uptake by sinusoidal liver cells. Hepatology 5: 367–375.

37. Adinolfi LE, Giordano MG, Andreana A, Tripodi MF, Utili R, et al. (2001) Hepatic fibrosis plays a central role in the pathogenesis of thrombocytopenia in patients with chronic viral hepatitis. Br J Haematol 113: 590–595.

38. Chu CJ, Hussain M, Lok AS (2002) Quantitative serum HBV DNA levels during different stages of chronic hepatitis B infection. Hepatology 36: 1408–1415.

39. Freed MN, Ryan JM, Hess RK (1991) Handbook of Statistical Procedures and Their Computer Applications to Education and the Behavioral Sciences. New York: American Council on Education and Macmillan Publishing Company.

40. Edirisooriya G (1995) Stepwise Regression Is a Problem, Not a Solution. Education Resources Information Center (ERIC; http://www.eric.ed.gov): ED393890. 16 p.

41. Welge P (1990) Three Reasons Why Stepwise Regression Methods Should Not Be Used by Researchers. Education Resources Information Center (ERIC; http://www.eric.ed.gov): ED316583. 22 p.

42. Park MY, Hastie T (2007) L1-regularization path algorithm for generalized linear models. Journal of the Royal Statistical Society: Series B (Statistical Methodology) 69: 659–677.

43. Fleisher AS, Sun S, Taylor C, Ward CP, Gamst AC, et al. (2008) Volumetric MRI vs clinical predictors of Alzheimer disease in mild cognitive impairment. Neurology 70: 191–199.

44. Guo W, Lin S (2009) Generalized linear modeling with regularization for detecting common disease rare haplotype association. Genetic Epidemiology 33: 308–316.

45. Parkman HP, Jacobs M, Mishra AK, Kramarczyk J, Gaughan J, et al. (2010) W1392 DNA Microarray SNP Analysis of Domperidone Efficacy in Patients With Gastroparesis. Gastroenterology 138: S-714.

46. Fung J, Lai CL, Cheng C, Wu R, Wong DK, et al. (2011) Mild-to-Moderate Elevation of Alanine Aminotransferase Increases Liver Stiffness Measurement by Transient Elastography in Patients With Chronic Hepatitis B. Am J Gastroenterol 106(3): 492–496.

47. Wong GLH, Wong VWS, Choi PCL, Chan AWH, Chan HLY (2010) Development of a non-invasive algorithm with transient elastography (Fibroscan) and serum test formula for advanced liver fibrosis in chronic hepatitis B. Alimentary Pharmacology & Therapeutics 31: 1095–1103.

48. Sebastiani G, Halfon P, Castera L, Pol S, Thomas DL, et al. (2009) SAFE biopsy: a validated method for large-scale staging of liver fibrosis in chronic hepatitis C. Hepatology 49: 1821–1827.

17

Serum Apoptosis Markers Related to Liver Damage in Chronic Hepatitis C: sFas as a Marker of Advanced Fibrosis in Children and Adults While M30 of Severe Steatosis Only in Children

Pamela Valva[1]*, **Paola Casciato**[2], **Carol Lezama**[3], **Marcela Galoppo**[3], **Adrián Gadano**[2], **Omar Galdame**[2], **María Cristina Galoppo**[3], **Eduardo Mullen**[4], **Elena De Matteo**[1], **María Victoria Preciado**[1]

1 Laboratory of Molecular Biology, Pathology Division, Hospital de Niños Ricardo Gutiérrez, Buenos Aires, Argentina, 2 Liver Unit, Hospital Italiano de Buenos Aires, Buenos Aires, Argentina, 3 Liver Unit of University of Buenos Aires at Hospital de Niños Ricardo Gutiérrez, Buenos Aires, Argentina, 4 Pathology Division, Hospital Italiano de Buenos Aires, Buenos Aires, Argentina

Abstract

Background: Liver biopsy represents the gold standard for evaluating damage and progression in patients with chronic hepatitis C (CHC); however, developing noninvasive tests that can predict liver injury represents a growing medical need. Considering that hepatocyte apoptosis plays a role in CHC pathogenesis; the aim of our study was to evaluate the presence of different apoptosis markers that correlate with liver injury in a cohort of pediatric and adult patients with CHC.

Methods: Liver biopsies and concomitant serum samples from 22 pediatric and 22 adult patients with CHC were analyzed. Histological parameters were evaluated. In serum samples soluble Fas (sFas), caspase activity and caspase-generated neoepitope of the CK-18 proteolytic fragment (M30) were measured.

Results: sFas was associated with fibrosis severity in pediatric (significant fibrosis $p = 0.03$, advanced fibrosis $p = 0.01$) and adult patients (advanced fibrosis $p = 0.02$). M30 levels were elevated in pediatric patients with severe steatosis ($p = 0.01$) while in adults no relation with any histological variable was observed. Caspase activity levels were higher in pediatric samples with significant fibrosis ($p = 0.03$) and they were associated with hepatitis severity ($p = 0.04$) in adult patients. The diagnostic accuracy evaluation demonstrated only a good performance for sFas to evaluate advanced fibrosis both in children (AUROC: 0.812) and adults (AUROC: 0.800) as well as for M30 to determine steatosis severity in children (AUROC: 0.833).

Conclusions: Serum sFas could be considered a possible marker of advanced fibrosis both in pediatric and adult patient with CHC as well as M30 might be a good predictor of steatosis severity in children.

Editor: Ravi Jhaveri, University of North Carolina School of Medicine, United States of America

Funding: This study was funded by grants from the International Society for Infectious Diseases, the National Agency for Scientific and Technology Promotion (PICT 2004 N°25344) National Research Council (CONICET) (PIP2010 1392/11). The funders had no role in study design, data collection and analysis, decision to publish, or preparation of the manuscript. No additional external funding received for this study.

Competing Interests: The authors have declared that no competing interests exist.

* E-mail: valvapamela@yahoo.com

Introduction

Hepatitis related to Hepatitis C virus (HCV) is a progressive disease that may result in chronic active hepatitis, cirrhosis, and hepatocellular carcinoma. It is estimated that over 200 million people are infected worldwide, while 80% develop a chronic form [1]. It represents a global health problem since there is no vaccine available, the response to current standard of care therapy is limited and liver failure related to chronic hepatitis C (CHC) virus infection is one of the most common reasons for liver transplants [2]. Liver disease seems to be milder in children than in adults; however, the natural history of HCV infection acquired in infancy and childhood remains poorly characterized and the long-term outcome of the disease is still a matter of debate [3].

Although liver biopsy represents the gold standard for evaluating presence, type and stage of liver fibrosis and for characterizing necroinflammation; it remains an expensive and invasive procedure with inherent risks. Thus, it cannot be performed frequently to monitor therapeutic outcomes [4,5]. Moreover, in children, biopsy is still perceived to carry a higher risk of complications, so it is less accepted than in adults. Therefore, developing noninvasive tests that can accurately predict initial disease stage and progression over time represents a high priority and growing medical need [6,7].

Several less invasive diagnostic methods are currently being validated as potential tools to determine liver damage, namely serum markers and image methods, but they have not been yet incorporated in clinical practice in most countries [8]. Many authors have proposed multiple indexes based on the combination of biochemical markers with clinical data (i.e. Fib-4, Forms or Fibrotest) or biochemical and clinical markers with fibrosis parameters (i.e. Hepascore, Shasta and Fibrometer) to predict fibrosis stage [9,10,11,12,13,14]. Related to that, we have previously studied, in a cohort of pediatric and adult patients, the presence of a pro-fibrogenic cytokine (TGF-ß1) as well as different matrix deposition markers [hyaluronic acid (HA), type III procollagen amino-terminal peptide (PIIINP) and tissue inhibitor of matrix metalloprotein inhibitor-1 (TIMP-1)] related to liver injury during CHC. The results demonstrated that given the diagnostic accuracy of HA, PIIINP, TGF-ß1, their combination may provide a potential useful tool to assess liver fibrosis in adults. On the other hand, in pediatric patients TIMP-1 could be clinically useful for predicting liver fibrosis in patients with CHC [15].

Considering that 1) apoptosis plays a major role in the tissue development and homeostasis and in pathological processes [16]; 2) it has been demonstrated that hepatocyte apoptosis plays a role in liver pathogenesis of CHC; as well as it may be associated with liver fibrogenesis [17,18,19,20]; the aim of our study was to evaluate the presence of different apoptosis markers which correlate with liver injury in a cohort of pediatric and adult patients with CHC infection.

Methods

Patients and samples

Twenty two pediatric patients with CHC (8 male, 14 female; range of age at biopsy: 1–17 years, median: 8 years) from Hospital de Niños Ricardo Gutierrez (HNRG) and 22 adult patients (13 male, 9 female; range of age at biopsy: 38–74 years, median: 51 years) from Hospital Italiano de Buenos Aires (HIBA) were enrolled in the present study.

Diagnosis was based on the presence of anti-HCV antibodies in serum at or after 18 months of age and HCV RNA in plasma at one or more separate occasions. Patients had no other causes of liver disease, autoimmune or metabolic disorders, hepatocellular carcinoma and coinfection with hepatitis B virus and/or human immunodeficiency virus. In adult cases, patients with a history of habitual alcohol consumption were excluded (>80 g/day for men and >60 g/day for women). Patients were naïve of treatment. This study has the approval of the Institutional Review Board and the Ethics Board of both HNRG and HIBA and is also in accordance with the Helsinki Declaration of 1975, as revised in 1983. A written informed consent was obtained from all the included adult patients and from parents of pediatric patients after the nature of the procedure had been fully explained.

Formalin-fixed paraffin-embedded liver biopsies and serum samples at time of biopsy were used for histological and serological analysis, respectively. Histological sections were evaluated by two independent pathologists in a blind manner. Inflammatory activity and fibrosis were assessed using the modified Knodell scoring system (Histological Activity Index, HAI) and METAVIR [21]. According to HAI, each biopsy specimen was categorized as minimal (≤3), mild (4–6), moderate (7–12) or severe hepatitis (>12). Presence of lymphoid follicles as well as of bile duct lesion and grade of steatosis were also evaluated. Steatosis was graded as follows: minimal (1–33% of hepatocytes affected), moderate, (>33%–66%) or severe (>66%). Serum AST and ALT levels and genotype were obtained from clinical records. As controls, serum samples from pediatric (n = 9) and adult (n = 9) healthy subjects without known systemic or liver disease and with normal biological liver test as well as absence of anti-HCV antibodies, were included.

In adult cases, liver samples were not obtained from patients diagnosed as having liver cirrhosis based on clinical, biochemical and imaging findings. Although, there are no pediatric specific guidelines about the need for and timing of a liver biopsy in children, the probability of a child undergoing liver biopsy in this study reflected the current practice at our centre, which is based mostly on the national experts consensus [22]. In two pediatric cases, more than one sample was available.

Quantitative assessment of apoptosis markers

Soluble Fas (sFas), caspase activity and caspase-generated neoepitope of the CK-18 proteolytic fragment (M30) were measured as apoptosis markers.

Serum sFas and M30 were determined by commercial quantitative sandwich enzyme immunoassay technique (*Quantikine Human soluble Fas kit*, R&D Systems Inc; and *M30-Apoptosense ELISA kit*, PEVIVA; respectively) according to the manufacturer's instructions. Serum concentration for each marker was determined from standard curves. Serum sFas was expressed as pg/mL and M30 as U/L.

Serum Caspase activity was determined using a chemiluminescence assay (*Caspase-Glo Assay*, Promega). Briefly, samples were first diluted 1:1 in a buffer containing 50 mM Tris-HCl, 10 mM KCl, 5% glycerol, pH 7.4 and incubated with 25 µl of samples or controls diluted with an equal volume of caspase substrate for 3 h at room temperature. Then, the samples' luminescence was measured for 20 seconds in the Luminometer Junior LB 9509 (*Berthold Technologies GmbH & Co. KG*). Results are expressed as RLU. An activity negative control (25 µl buffer 50 mM Tris-HCl, 10 mM KCl, 5% glycerol, pH 7.4) and positive control (25 µl Human Recombinant activated Caspase-3 Protein, Millipore, CHEMICON 0.04 U/µl in the same buffer) were included in each assay.

Each serum marker concentration was assessed in duplicate.

Operators who perform the laboratory tests were blinded for patient's clinical and histological data.

Statistical analysis

Statistical analysis was performed using GraphPad InStat software, version 3.05. To compare the means between groups, ANOVA or Student's t test were performed. To determine differences between groups not normally distributed, medians were compared using the Mann-Whitney U test or Kruskal Wallis test. Pearson's correlation coefficient was used to measure the degree of association between continuous, normally distributed variables. The degree of association between non-normally distributed variables was assessed using Spearman's nonparametric correlation. To compare categorical variables Fisher's exact Test was applied. P values<0.05 were considered statistically significant. The results are depicted in box plots. Horizontal lines within boxes indicate medians. Horizontal lines outside the boxes represent the 5 and 95 percentiles. Mean is indicated as +.

To assess the ability of the serum apoptosis markers to differentiate hepatitis grade, fibrosis stages and steatosis grade, we calculated the sensitivity and the specificity for each value of each marker and then constructed receiver operating characteristic (ROC) curves by plotting the sensitivity against the reverse specificity at each value. The diagnostic value of each serum marker was assessed by the area under the ROC (AUROC). AUROC of 1.0 is characteristic of an ideal test, whereas 0.5 indicates a test of no diagnostic value. We determined the cut-off value for the diagnosis, as the maximal value at the sum of the sensitivity (Se) and specificity (Sp). The diagnostic accuracy was calculated by sensitivity, specificity and positive and negative predictive values. Area under the ROC, cut off values, positive predictive values (PPV) and negative predictive values (NPV) were determined using the MedCalc demo statistical software (Mariakerke, Belgium).

Results

Clinical and liver biopsy findings

Clinical, virological, and histological features of patients are described in Table 1 (pediatric patients) and Table 2 (adult patients).

In both groups HCV genotype 1 was predominant, 86% in pediatric cases and 77% in adults. The risk factors for HCV infection in children were 46% vertical transmission, 36% transfusion and 18% unknown. In adults, seven cases (32%) had a history of injecting drug abuse, one case (5%) described an occupational exposure to infected blood, four (18%) a transfusion as a risk factor and 10 (45%) an unknown source for transmission. The aspartate aminotransferase (AST) and alanine aminotransferase (ALT) levels at time of biopsy, considering multiple biopsies from the same patient in 2 pediatric cases, were elevated in 52% and 76% serum samples of pediatric patients, respectively and in 59% and 77% serum samples of adult patients as well.

Eighteen percent of pediatric biopsies showed moderate or severe hepatitis, while concerning fibrosis, bridging fibrosis (stage 2 of METAVIR) was predominant among studied biopsies (44%). In adult cases, moderate or severe hepatitis were present in 73% of biopsies and the fibrosis profile displayed was 32% stage 1, 32% stage 2 and 23% stage 3. Finally, 3 adult patients showed absence of fibrosis. The prevalence of significant fibrosis (F≥2) and advanced fibrosis (F≥3) in the pediatric cohort were 64% and 20%, respectively; meanwhile it was 54% F≥2 and 23% F≥3 in adults. Lymphoid follicles, characteristic of CHC in adults, were present in 40% of pediatric and 82% of adult specimens, whereas bile duct lesions were observed in 83% of pediatric and 95% of adult samples. Hepatocellular fat accumulation, typically a mixture of small and large droplet fat, was present in both series (64% of pediatric and 50% of adult cases). Minimal steatosis was observed in 36%, moderate in 12% and severe in 16% of pediatric biopsies; meanwhile in adults minimal, moderate and severe steatosis were present in 27%, 9% and 14%, respectively. The comparative statistical analysis of all histological parameters between pediatric and adult studied patients did not showed any significant difference except for lymphoid follicles (p = 0.01). However, it should be taken into account that adult cases with liver cirrhosis based on clinical, biochemical and imaging findings were not biopsied.

Finally, aminotransferase values were not associated to any parameter of histological liver damage.

Quantitative assessment of sFas, caspase activity and M30

Apoptosis markers were first compared between patients with CHC and healthy subjects. Then in a further analysis CHC patients apoptosis markers were related to histological parameters of liver injury, particularly fibrosis, hepatitis and steatosis severity.

As it is shown in Figure 1, apoptosis markers were significantly increased in serum samples from both pediatric and adult patients with CHC compared to healthy subjects, except for sFas levels in CHC pediatric patient samples which only showed a trend of association (p = 0.07).

With regard to liver damage, sFas was associated with fibrosis severity in both pediatric and adult CHC patients. It was significantly increased in children with significant fibrosis (p = 0.03) and advanced fibrosis (p = 0.01), and in adults with advanced fibrosis (p = 0.02) (Figure 2a). It is worth mentioning that serum sFas levels of pediatric patients with mild fibrosis stages (F1 and F2) showed no significant differences compared with those levels of pediatric healthy subjects. It is in accordance with most noninvasive makers that offer most reliable results at the extreme fibrosis stages. Finally, sFas was not associated with hepatitis severity or steatosis degree in any of the studied age groups (Figure 2b, c).

The M30 association profile related to the histological parameters was different between children and adults. In pediatric cases, M30 levels were elevated in patients with severe steatosis (p = 0.01) (Figure 2c) while in adults no relation with this histological variable was observed. Concerning fibrosis a trend of association between this marker and advanced fibrosis (p = 0.05) in adults was depicted (Figure 2a). Finally, there were no significant differences in serum M30 levels with respect to hepatitis in none of the studied age groups (Figure 2b).

The caspase activity profile in relation to fibrosis severity was similar to that observed for sFas and M30 in both populations. Caspase activity levels were higher in those cases with significant and advanced fibrosis; however, the difference turned out to be statistically significant only in samples from children with significant fibrosis (p = 0.03). In the adult cohort only a trend of association with significant fibrosis was observed (p = 0.08). In turn, in serum samples from adult patients caspase activity was associated with hepatitis severity (p = 0.04) (Figure 2b). No association between steatosis degree and caspase activity was observed in any of the studied groups (Figure 2c).

Diagnostic performance of apoptosis markers

The evaluation of the diagnostic performance was only assessed for those apoptosis markers which had shown to be associated with histological injury variables. Tables 3, 4 and 5 show the diagnostic accuracy of each marker by means of the sensitivity, specificity, positive and negative predictive values.

When considering a less invasive test as good as a liver biopsy to evaluate liver damage, the AUROC of the marker must be equal to or greater than 0.800 [6]. Therefore, in this study, only those markers which AUROC was greater than this value were taken into account. Thus, sFas quantification demonstrated a limited utility as a less invasive marker of significant fibrosis in pediatric patients (AUROC: 0.719), but it could be considered a possible marker of advanced fibrosis both in children and adults (children AUROC: 0.812, NPV 100%, adults AUROC: 0.800, NPV 100%) (Table 3). On the other hand, M30 showed an AUROC of 0.833 and a high NPV (100%) indicating that it might be a good marker of steatosis severity in pediatric patients (Table 4). Finally, despite the observed association between caspase activity and significant fibrosis stage in pediatric patients as well as moderate/severe hepatitis in adults, this marker would not be useful as a less invasive indicator of liver damage. Although, both specificity and PPV were high, AUROC values were very low (Table 5).

The cut off value for sFas to differentiate advanced fibrosis in pediatric patients was 7416.56 pg/ml (100% Se, 55% Sp), whereas in adults it was 13806.67 pg/ml (100% Se, 70.60% Sp) (Table 3). Serum M30 cut off value for diagnosis of severe steatosis in pediatric patients was 114.53 U/L (100% Se, 57.14% Sp) (Table 4).

Table 1. Clinical, virological and histological features of pediatric CHC patients.

	Clinical and serological characteristics				Transaminases		Histological characteristics				
Pediatric Patients	Sex	Ages (ys)	Risk factor for HCV infection	Genotype	AST (U/L)	ALT (U/L)	Knodell	Fibrosis stages #	Lymphoid Follicle	Bile duct damage	Steatosis
1	M	13	T	1a	47	43	8(5+3)	F2	no	no	absent
2	F	14	T	1b	55	86	11(9+2)	F1	no	no	minimal
3	F	4	V	1a/c	46	34	10(7+3)	F2	yes	yes	absent
4	F	17	T	1a/c	39	43	8(4+4)	F3	no	yes	moderate
5	M	4	V	1a/c	84	97	10(9+1)	F1	yes	yes	severe
6 BxI	F	6	V	1a/c	13	11	7(3+4)	F3	no	no	absent
BxII		13			23	21	8(5+3)	F2	no	yes	minimal
7	F	16	Unknown	1a/c	30	41	12(10+2)	F1	yes	yes	minimal
8 BxI	M	3	V	1a/c	71	91	6(5+1)	F1	yes	yes	minimal
BxII		6			314	364	11(8+3)	F2	no	yes	severe
BxIII		13			225	260	21(16+5)	F3	no	yes	moderate
9	F	6	V	1a/c	35	50	8(7+1)	F1	yes	yes	minimal
10	F	8	Unknown	1a	41	38	9(7+2)	F1	yes	yes	absent
11	M	13	Unknown	ND	56	71	10(7+3)	F2	no	yes	absent
12	F	17	V	1a/c	21	11	6(3+3)	F2	no	yes	minimal
13	F	3	V	1a/c	84	137	6(5+1)	F1	yes	yes	moderate
14	F	3	V	1b	65	75	9(6+3)	F2	no	yes	moderate
15	F	1	V	4	57	33	11(7+4)	F3	yes	yes	absent
16	F	17	T	1a/c	22	16	10(7+3)	F2	yes	yes	minimal
17	M	1	T	1b	159	213	14(11+3)	F2	no	yes	minimal
18	F	8	T	1b	10	12	6(5+1)	F1	yes	no	absent
19	M	15	T	ND	58	76	15(10+5)	F3	no	yes	absent
20	F	6	V	1a/c	56	55	6(5+1)	F1	no	yes	severe
21	M	15	T	1b	20	24	13(10+3)	F2	yes	yes	absent
22	M	12	Unknown	1a/c	83	113	11(8+3)	F2	no	yes	minimal

F: female, M: male. ND: not determined Bx I, Bx II, Bx III denote: multiple liver biopsies. Risk factor for HCV infection: T: transfusion, V: vertical transmission.
ALT: alanine aminotransferase; AST: aspartate aminotransferase. Normal ALT and AST levels were ≤32 and ≤48 IU/L, respectively when test was done at 37°C.
#Fibrosis stages according to METAVIR.

Table 2. Clinical, virological and histological features of adult CHC patients.

Adult Patients	Sex	Ages (ys)	Risk factor for HCV infection	Genotype	Transaminases		Knodell	Fibrosis stages #	Lymphoid Follicle	Bile duct damage	Steatosis
					AST (U/L)	ALT (U/L)					
1	M	38	Unknown	1b	82	89	6(5+1)	F1	yes	yes	absent
2	F	52	T	1b	45	52	8(6+2)	F1	yes	yes	minimal
3	M	42	Unknown	1a	44	56	9(8+1)	F1	yes	yes	absent
4	F	62	T	1a	42	32	11(7+4)	F3	no	yes	moderate
5	M	48	DA	1b	40	63	10(7+3)	F2	no	yes	severe
6	M	40	DA	1a	34	45	10(6+4)	F3	yes	yes	moderate
7	M	47	Unknown	1a	29	54	8(6+2)	F1	yes	yes	minimal
8	M	40	DA	2a	63	79	4(4+0)	F0	yes	no	absent
9	M	41	DA	3a	79	86	7(4+3)	F2	no	yes	absent
10	F	61	Unknown	1a	31	28	17(12+5)	F3	yes	yes	absent
11	F	72	Unknown	1a/c	52	71	9(6+3)	F2	yes	yes	minimal
12	F	74	T	1*	106	85	15(12+3)	F2	yes	yes	absent
13	M	62	Unknown	1b	22	32	10(7+3)	F2	no	yes	absent
14	F	55	Unknown	3b	49	60	8(6+2)	F1	yes	yes	severe
15	F	67	Unknown	2a	28	26	6(6+0)	F0	yes	yes	minimal
16	F	41	Unknown	1a	192	105	6(2+4)	F3	yes	yes	absent
17	M	51	OE	1b	65	74	5(4+0)	F0	yes	yes	absent
18	M	51	DA	1a	73	109	10(7+3)	F2	yes	yes	minimal
19	F	67	T	1b	106	103	13(9+4)	F3	yes	yes	absent
20	M	73	Unknown	1b	31	42	8(6+2)	F1	yes	yes	absent
21	M	41	DA	1a	32	50	10(7+3)	F2	yes	yes	severe
22	M	47	DA	3	38	59	3(2+1)	F1	yes	yes	minimal

F: female, M: male.
*Subtype not determined Risk factor for HCV infection: T: transfusion, DA: drug abuse, OE: occupational exposure.
ALT: alanine aminotransferase; AST: aspartate aminotransferase. Normal ALT and AST levels were ≤40 and ≤42 IU/L, respectively when test was done at 37°C.
#Fibrosis stages according METAVIR.

Discussion

Apoptosis has been implicated in the pathogenesis of a number of hepatic disorders, including viral hepatitis, autoimmune diseases, non-alcoholic steatohepatitis, alcohol-induced injury, cholestasis and hepatocellular cancer [23,24,25,26,27]. There is increasing evidence suggesting that liver cell damage in CHC is mediated by apoptosis induction, which has been proposed in view of pathomorphologic features of infected hepatocytes [17,24,28,29]. Several viral proteins display either apoptotic or antiapoptotic features according to the model under study [18,30]; in turn, both *in vitro* studies or *in vivo* models with whole virus demonstrated its ability to induce apoptosis. Our previous study

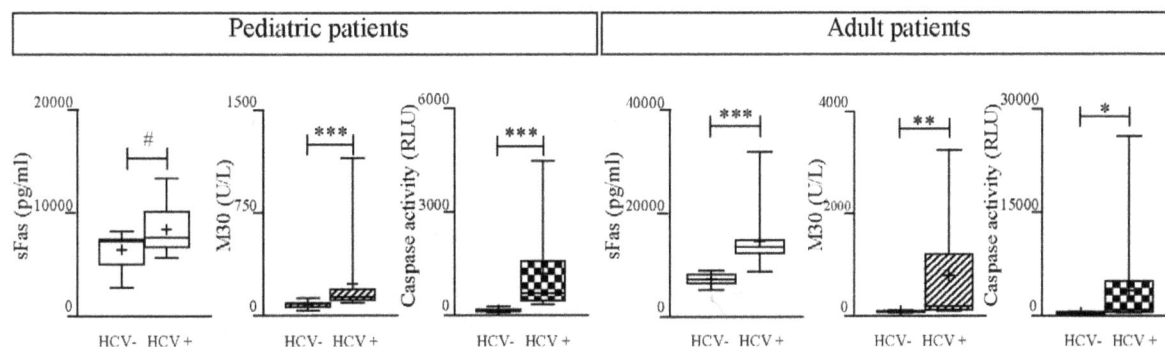

Figure 1. Apoptosis markers in serum samples from CHC patients vs healthy subjects. *$p<0.05$; ** $p<0.001$; ***$p<0.0001$;·# trend of association $p<0.07$.

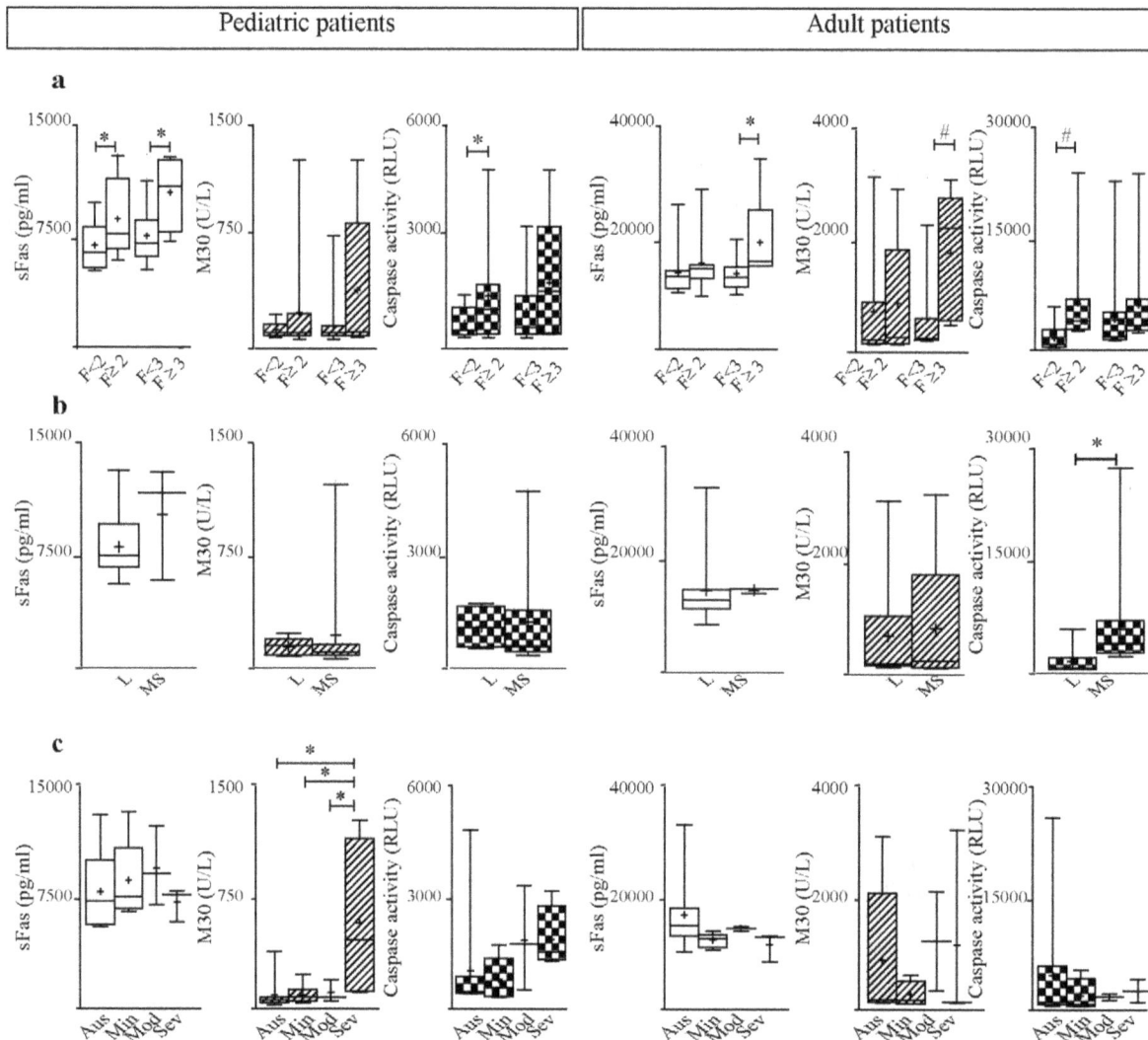

Figure 2. Serum markers related to liver damage in CHC patients. a) fibrosis, b) hepatitis and c) steatosis severity. Fibrosis stages according METAVIR. Significant fibrosis (F≥2) and advanced fibrosis (F≥3). * p<0.05;·# trend of association p<0.08.

demonstrated that apoptosis of hepatocytes is a prominent feature observed in liver biopsies of patients with CHC and that it is related to the pathogenesis of the disease [20]. Here, we evaluated whether the apoptosis markers were a remarkable feature in serum samples of pediatric and adult CHC patients and analyzed their relation to liver damage. According to available data and their importance in the pathogenesis, three components of the apoptosis process were selected for evaluation: **1)** *sFas*, since it has been proposed that apoptosis triggered by Fas/FasL is a major cause of hepatocyte damage together with the observed high Fas/FasL expression levels which correlate with liver injury during CHC [31,32,33,34,35]; **2)** *caspase activity*, since it has been reported that caspases are activated in HCV infected patient hepatocytes and are responsible for most of the morphological changes of the apoptotic cells [36]; and **3)** *M30*, since CK18 is the major intermediate filament of hepatocytes which is, in turn, a caspase substrate whose cleavage contribute to cellular collapse during apoptosis.

According to previously published data, this study showed that serum sFas levels were high in patients with CHC [31,37,38,39,40,41,42]; however, the clinical relevance of circu-

lating sFas is not completely understood. As described above, Fas/FasL interaction is the primary initiator of the extrinsic apoptosis pathway in the liver, hence the elimination of apoptotic bodies in pathological conditions may induce an inflammatory reaction with the consequent activation of stellate cells, which in turn favors the development of liver fibrosis [43]. Several authors postulated that sFas is associated with liver damage severity because significantly increased sFas levels were observed in patients with terminal disease stages such as cirrhosis and HCC [31,44]. In turn, Toyoda et al reported that sFas levels in CHC patients correlated with hepatitis severity [45]. Kakiuchi et al corroborated this result, but on the other hand, reported that this marker is not associated with fibrosis severity [40]. In contrast, the results herein indicated that sFas was not related to hepatitis severity, but instead was associated with fibrosis severity. It is important to note that despite the higher sFas levels detected in CHC children compared to healthy subjects, only a trend of association was observed. A possible explanation for this observation would be that sFas levels in pediatric patients with mild fibrosis stages were similar to those of pediatric healthy subjects; furthermore in our studied series the group of children with severe fibrosis was small since a severe stage

Table 3. Diagnostic accuracy of sFas for significant and advance fibrosis in CHC patients.

SIGNIFICANT FIBROSIS (F≥2)	AUROC	95% CI	Cut off *	Se%	Sp%	PPV	NPV
PEDIATRIC PATIENTS	0.719	0.500–0.881	6815.14	86.67	55.56	76.5	71.4
ADVANCED FIBROSIS (F≥3)	AUROC	95% CI	Cut off *	Se%	Sp%	PPV	NPV
PEDIATRIC PATIENTS	0.812	0.602–0.941	7416.56	100	55	30.8	100
ADULT PATIENTS	0.800	0.577–0.938	13806.67	100	70.60	50	100

*pg/ml.

Table 4. Diagnostic accuracy of M30 for steatosis severity in pediatric CHC patients.

SEVERE STEATOSIS	AUROC	95% CI	Cut off * Se%	Sp%	PPV	NPV
PEDIATRIC PATIENTS	0.833	0.634–0.951	114.53 100	57.14	30.8	100

*U/L.

of fibrosis is not commonly present in CHC patients during infancy and childhood.

With respect to activation of caspases, the current results corroborate that apoptosis is an important event in CHC, as we have previously observed when investigating caspase activity and M30 expression in liver samples from CHC patients [20]. The assessment of caspases activation and M30 showed high values in the two types of samples tested, but in none of the two age groups these markers detected on liver biopsies correlated with their corresponding marker in serum. Since liver and serum are distinct compartments, one possible explanation for the lack of correlation may be that apoptotic cells are rapidly eliminated and therefore, would not be detected in biopsy. Meanwhile, although the exact mechanism of secretion of M30 in the blood has not been determined yet, it is postulated that serum M30 is released as a result of necrosis secondary to apoptosis. In favor of the latter, we observed correlations between M30 and terminal apoptotic cells (TUNEL+ cells) in both pediatric and adult patients (pediatric patients r = 0.533 p = 0.02; adult patients r = 0.535 p = 0.02) (for technical information see Methods S1).

According to that previously described for adult cohorts [28], M30 levels and caspase activity were significantly increased in serum samples from pediatric and adult patients with respect to control subjects. However, their relation to liver damage is still controversial. Bantel et al found that serum M30 quantification is a highly sensitive method to early detect fibrosis severity [28]. They observed that M30 levels were associated with more severe stages of fibrosis only in patients with normal transaminase values, but no association between M30 and either hepatitis or fibrosis severity in general adult CHC patients was found. On the other hand, Seidel et al found that both M30 and caspase activity were elevated in adult patients with severe steatosis [46]. Finally, Papatheodoridis et al found that M30 is associated with global liver damage severity, because its levels correlated with hepatitis severity, fibrosis and steatosis [47]. In contrast, Joka et al describe that M65, another epitope which is present in both caspase-cleaved and uncleaved CK-18, is more sensitive and specific than M30 for the detection of lower fibrosis stages and steatosis severity in many forms of chronic liver disease, including CHC; although M65 and M30 were not individually analyzed in the context of each disease etiology [48]. In our report each marker showed a different association profile related to liver damage in each of the studied cohorts. Higher levels of caspase activity were observed in adult cases with more severe hepatitis as well as in children with significant fibrosis. While M30 showed a trend of association with advanced fibrosis, it did not correlate with steatosis degree in adult patients. Concerning children, this marker was significantly increased in cases with severe steatosis. This last finding is particularly important since M30 is being widely studied as a marker of the steatosis severity both in pediatric and adult patients with Non Alcoholic Steatohepatitis [49,50,51,52,53,54].

Table 5. Diagnostic accuracy of Caspase activity for significant fibrosis and moderate/severe hepatitis in CHC patients.

SIGNIFICANT FIBROSIS (F≥2)							
	AUROC	95% CI	Cut off *	Se%	Sp%	PPV	NPV
PEDIATRIC PATIENTS	0.656	0.436–0.836	1490	37.5	100	100	44.4
MODERATE/SEVERE HEPATITIS							
	AUROC	95% CI	Cut off *	Se%	Sp%	PPV	NPV
ADULT PATIENTS	0.744	0.510–0.907	676	86.67	83.33	92.9	71.4

*RLU.

A major clinical challenge is finding the best means for evaluating liver impairment in the increasing number of CHC infected patients [2,9,55]. Prognosis and treatment of CHC are partly dependent on the assessment of histological activity, namely cell necrosis and inflammation, and on the degree of liver fibrosis. These parameters have so far been provided by liver biopsy, because conventional laboratory tests are unable to precisely evaluate liver lesions. Biopsy, due to its limitations and risks, is no longer considered mandatory as the 1st-line indicator of liver injury in CHC patients [56,57,58,59]. In addition to the risks related to an invasive procedure, liver biopsy has been associated with sampling errors mostly due to suboptimal biopsy size [60,61,62]. To avoid these pitfalls, several markers have been proposed as noninvasive alternatives for predicting liver damage; but few, particularly those which combine clinical and biochemical parameters, have been applied to pediatric patients [63,64]. In this study, the observed relationships between sFas, M30 and caspase activity and liver damage prompted us to assess the diagnostic value of apoptosis markers as potential indicators of liver damage.

Herein, based on AUROC values it was demonstrated that sFas could be a marker of advanced fibrosis both in children and adults and, in turn, M30 could be a good predictor of steatosis severity in children. However, despite the observed association between caspase activity and significant fibrosis in children as well as with hepatitis severity in adult patients, this marker would not be useful as a less invasive indicator of liver damage. Unfortunately, although there are many studies that evaluate these serum apoptosis markers in CHC patients related to liver damage, they do not assess their diagnostic value. This makes it impossible to compare the determined diagnostic accuracy of these markers for the diagnosis of liver injury severity with other reports.

There are several articles that analyze AST-to-platelet ratio (APRI) and AST-to-ALT ratio (AAR) as surrogate indirect serum markers of liver fibrosis. As we previously describe when assessed in our cohorts [15], these approaches did not improve the diagnostic accuracy performance of sFas in pediatric series, since neither APRI nor AAR reached the 0.800 AUROC value proposed to be enough for staging fibrosis. In adults APRI showed a low performance which does not reach the 0.800 AUROC value, while AAR diagnostic value is comparable with the sFas one to predict advanced fibrosis (Table S1).

It should not be ignored that the present study has certain limitations. First, this was in fact a retrospective study, with a quite limited number of cases, so this makes it difficult to validate the utility of serum markers. Second, due to medical management protocols from our institutions, pediatric patients without liver fibrosis (F0) and adults with cirrhosis or hepatic decompensation were not available for this study. Third, since we did not take into account biopsy length and fragmentation, the potential for sampling error and understaging of fibrosis remains possible. Anyway, the molecules here proposed turned out to be easily measurable markers, which can be interpreted in a simple manner. The study of a larger number of cases, perhaps in a multicenter study, will confirm the results obtained in this work and discuss the possibility of adding apoptosis markers to panels that included matrix deposition, clinical and biochemical parameters. Taking into account our previous results on fibrogenesis process direct markers (15) (Table S1), we propose the addition of apoptosis markers, particularly sFas combined with TIMP-1 in pediatric patients and sFas with TGF-ß1, HA, PIIINP in adult patients to more accurately assess liver fibrosis severity.

In conclusion, serum sFas could be considered a possible marker of advanced fibrosis both in pediatric and adult patient with CHC as well as M30 could be a good predictor of steatosis severity in children. Perhaps if these parameters are validated in the near future, they could be easily performed and interpreted and, therefore, could be potentially translatable to the bedside.

Acknowledgments

The authors thank Dr Rey Rodolfo (CEDIE-CONICET, HNRG) for his help with the chemiluminescence assay and Livellara B (Liver Unit, HIBA) for preserving adult serum samples.

Author Contributions

Performed pathological reviews: EDM EM. Assisted in data interpretation and analysis: PC MG CL OG AG MCG. Conceived and designed the experiments: PV MVP. Performed the experiments: PV. Analyzed the data: PV MVP PC. Contributed reagents/materials/analysis tools: EDM EM PC MG CL OG AG MCG. Wrote the paper: PV PC MVP.

References

1. Lavanchy D (2009) The global burden of hepatitis C. Liver Int 29 74–81.
2. Ghany MG, Strader DB, Thomas DL, Seeff LB (2009) Diagnosis, management, and treatment of hepatitis C: an update. Hepatology 49: 1335–1374.
3. Mohan N, Gonzalez-Peralta RP, Fujisawa T, Chang MH, Heller S, et al. (2010) Chronic hepatitis C virus infection in children. J Pediatr Gastroenterol Nutr 50: 123–131.
4. Bravo A, Sheth S, Chopra S (2001) Liver biopsy. N Engl J Med 344: 495–500.
5. Thampanitchawong P, Piratvisuth T (1999) Liver biopsy:complications and risk factors. World J Gastroenterol 5: 301–304.
6. Afdhal N, Nunes D (2004) Evaluation of liver fibrosis: a concise review. Am J Gastroenterol 99: 1160–1174.
7. Martínez SM, Crespo G, Navasa M, X F (2011) Noninvasive assessment of liver fibrosis. Hepatology 53: 325–335.
8. Manning D, Afdhal N (2008) Diagnosis and quantitation of fibrosis. Gastroenterology 134: 1670–1681.
9. Ahmad W, Ijaz B, Gull S, Asad S, Khaliq S, et al. (2011) A brief review on molecular, genetic and imaging techniques for HCV fibrosis evaluation. Virol J 8: 53.
10. Ahmad W, Ijaz B, Javed FT, Gull S, Kausar H, et al. (2011) A comparison of four fibrosis indexes in chronic HCV: development of new fibrosis-cirrhosis index (FCI). BMC Gastroenterol 11: 44.
11. Macías J, Mira J, Gilabert I, Neukam K, Roldán C, et al. (2011) Combined use of aspartate aminotransferase, platelet count and matrix metalloproteinase 2 measurements to predict liver fibrosis in HIV/hepatitis C virus-coinfected patients. HIV Med 12: 12–21.
12. Moreno S, Garcia-Samaniego J, Moreno A, Ortega E, Pineda J, et al. (2009) Noninvasive diagnosis of liver fibrosis in patients with HIV infection and HCV/HBV co-infection. Viral Hepat 16: 249–258.
13. Forns X, Ampurdanès S, Llovet J, Aponte J, Quintó L, et al. (2002) Identification of chronic hepatitis C patients without hepatic fibrosis by a simple predictive model. Hepatology 36: 986–992.
14. Sebastiani G, Castera L, Halfon P, Pol S, Mangia A, et al. (2011) The impact of liver disease aetiology and the stages of hepatic fibrosis on the performance of non-invasive fibrosis biomarkers: an international study of 2411 cases. Aliment Pharmacol Ther 34: 1202–1216.
15. Valva P, Casciato P, Diaz Carrasco JM, Gadano A, Galdame O, et al. (2011) The role of serum biomarkers in predicting fibrosis progression in pediatric and adult hepatitis C virus chronic infection. PLoS One 6: e23218.
16. Wyllie A, Kerr J, Currie A (1980) Cell death: the significance of apoptosis. Int Rev Cytol 68: 251–306.
17. Bantel H, Schulze-Osthoff K (2003) Apoptosis in hepatitis C virus infection. Cell Death Differ 10: S48–58.
18. Fischer R, Baumert T, Blum H (2007) Hepatitis C virus infection and apoptosis. World J Gastroenterol 13: 4865–4872.
19. Rust C, Gores G (2000) Apoptosis and liver disease. Am J Med 108: 567–574.
20. Valva P, De Matteo E, Galoppo MC, Gismondi MI, Preciado MV (2010) Apoptosis markers related to pathogenesis of pediatric chronic hepatitis C virus infection: M30 mirrors the severity of steatosis. J Med Virol 82: 949–957.
21. Theise N, Bordenheimer H, Ferrel L (2007) Acute and chronic viral hepatitis. In: Burt AD, Portmann BC, Ferrel LD, editors. MacSweens Pathology of the liver. London: Churchill-Livingstone. 5° edition cap 8: 418–419.
22. Consenso Argentino de Hepatitis C (2007) Documento final Consenso Argentino Hepatitis C, Asociación Argentina para el Estudio de las Enfermedades del Hígado.
23. Ghavami S, Hashemi M, Kadkhoda K, Alavian S, Bay G, et al. (2005) Apoptosis in liver diseases–detection and therapeutic applications. Med Sci Monit 11: 337–345.
24. Que F, Gores G (1996) Cell death by apoptosis: basic concepts and disease relevance for the gastroenterologist. Gastroenterology 110: 1238–1243.
25. Patel T, Gores G (1995) Apoptosis and hepatobiliary disease. Hepatology 21: 1725–1741.
26. Thompson C (1995) Apoptosis in the pathogenesis and treatment of disease. Science 267: 1456–1462.
27. Zekri AR, Bahnassy AA, Hafez MM, Hassan ZK, Kamel M, et al. (2011) Characterization of chronic HCV infection-induced apoptosis. Comp Hepatol 10: 4.
28. Bantel H, Lügering A, Heidemann J, Volkmann X, Poremba C, et al. (2004) Detection of apoptotic caspase activation in sera from patients with chronic HCV infection is associated with fibrotic liver injury. Hepatology 40: 1078–1087.
29. Kerr J, Cooksley W, Searle J, Halliday J, Halliday W, et al. (1979) The nature of piecemeal necrosis in chronic active hepatitis. Lancet 2: 827–828.
30. Mengshol J, Golden Mason L, Rosen H (2007) Mechanisms of Disease: HCV-induced liver injury. Nat Clin Pract Gastroenterol Hepatol 4: 622–634.
31. El Bassiouny A, El-Bassiouni N, Nosseir M, Zoheiry M, El-Ahwany E, et al. (2008) Circulating and hepatic Fas expression in HCV-induced chronic liver disease and hepatocellular carcinoma. Medscape J Med 10: 130.
32. Bortolami M, Kotsafti A, Cardin R, Farinati F (2008) Fas/FasL system, IL-1beta expression and apoptosis in chronic HBV and HCV liver disease. J Viral Hepat 15: 515–522.
33. El-Bassiouni A, Nosseir M, Zoheiry M, El-Ahwany E, Ghali A, et al. (2006) Immunohistochemical expression of CD95 (Fas), c-myc and epidermal growth factor receptor in hepatitis C virus infection, cirrhotic liver disease and hepatocellular carcinoma. APMIS 114: 420–427.
34. Kanto T, Hayashi N (2006) Immunopathogenesis of hepatitis C virus infection: multifaceted strategies subverting innate and adaptive immunity. Intern Med 45: 183–191.
35. Kiyici M, Gurel S, Budak F, Dolar E, Gulten M, et al. (2003) Fas antigen (CD95) expression and apoptosis in hepatocytes of patients with chronic viral hepatitis. Eur J Gastroenterol Hepatol 15: 1079–1084.
36. Bantel H, Lugering A, Poremba C, Lugering N, Held J, et al. (2001) Caspase activation correlates with the degree of inflammatory liver injury in chronic hepatitis C virus infection. Hepatology 34: 758–767.
37. Panasiuk A, Parfieniuk A, Zak J, Flisiak R (2010) Association among Fas expression in leucocytes, serum Fas and Fas-ligand concentrations and hepatic inflammation and fibrosis in chronic hepatitis C. Liver Int 30: 472–478.
38. Zaki Mel S, Auf FA, Ghawalby NA, Saddal NM (2008) Clinical significance of serum soluble Fas, Fas ligand and fas in intrahepatic lymphocytes in chronic hepatitis C. Immunol Invest 37: 163–170.
39. Raghuraman S, Abraham P, Daniel HD, Ramakrishna BS, Sridharan G (2005) Characterization of soluble FAS, FAS ligand and tumour necrosis factor-alpha in patients with chronic HCV infection. J Clin Virol 34: 63–70.
40. Kakiuchi Y, Yuki N, Iyoda K, Sugiyasu Y, Kaneko A, et al. (2004) Circulating soluble Fas levels in patients with hepatitis C virus infection and interferon therapy. J Gastroenterol 39: 1189–1195.
41. Lapinski TW, Kowalczuk O, Prokopowicz D, Chyczewski L (2004) Serum concentration of sFas and sFasL in healthy HBsAg carriers, chronic viral hepatitis B and C patients. World J Gastroenterol 10: 3650–3653.
42. Ozaslan E, Kilicarslan A, Simsek H, Tatar G, Kirazli S (2003) Elevated serum soluble Fas levels in the various stages of hepatitis C virus-induced liver disease. J Int Med Res 31: 384–391.
43. Canbay A, Friedman S, Gores G (2004) Apoptosis: the nexus of liver injury and fibrosis. Hepatology 39: 273–278.
44. Zekri AR, Alam El-Din HM, Bahnassy AA, Zayed NA, Mohamed WS, et al. (2010) Serum levels of soluble Fas, soluble tumor necrosis factor-receptor II, interleukin-2 receptor and interleukin-8 as early predictors of hepatocellular carcinoma in Egyptian patients with hepatitis C virus genotype-4. Comp Hepatol 9: 1.
45. Toyoda M, Kakizaki S, Horiguchi N, Sato K, Takayama H, et al. (2000) Role of serum soluble Fas/soluble Fas ligand and TNF-alpha on response to interferon-alpha therapy in chronic hepatitis C. Liver 20: 305–311.
46. Seidel N, Volkmann X, Langer F, Flemming P, Manns M, et al. (2005) The extent of liver steatosis in chronic hepatitis C virus infection is mirrored by caspase activity in serum. Hepatology 42: 113–120.
47. Papatheodoridis GV, Hadziyannis E, Tsochatzis E, Georgiou A, Kafiri G, et al. (2010) Serum apoptotic caspase activity in chronic hepatitis C and nonalcoholic Fatty liver disease. J Clin Gastroenterol 44: e87–95.
48. Joka D, Wahl K, Moeller S, Schlue J, Vaske B, et al. (2012) Prospective biopsy-controlled evaluation of cell death biomarkers for prediction of liver fibrosis and nonalcoholic steatohepatitis. Hepatology 55: 455–464.

49. Lebensztejn DM, Wierzbicka A, Socha P, Pronicki M, Skiba E, et al. (2011) Cytokeratin-18 and hyaluronic acid levels predict liver fibrosis in children with non-alcoholic fatty liver disease. Acta Biochim Pol 58: 563–566.

50. Tamimi TI, Elgouhari HM, Alkhouri N, Yerian LM, Berk MP, et al. (2011) An apoptosis panel for nonalcoholic steatohepatitis diagnosis. J Hepatol 54: 1224–1229.

51. Feldstein AE, Wieckowska A, Lopez AR, Liu YC, Zein NN, et al. (2009) Cytokeratin-18 fragment levels as noninvasive biomarkers for nonalcoholic steatohepatitis: a multicenter validation study. Hepatology 50: 1072–1078.

52. Yilmaz Y, Dolar E, Ulukaya E, Akgoz S, Keskin M, et al. (2007) Soluble forms of extracellular cytokeratin 18 may differentiate simple steatosis from nonalcoholic steatohepatitis. World J Gastroenterol 13: 837–844.

53. Fitzpatrick E, Mitry RR, Quaglia A, Hussain MJ, DeBruyne R, et al. (2010) Serum levels of CK18 M30 and leptin are useful predictors of steatohepatitis and fibrosis in paediatric NAFLD. J Pediatr Gastroenterol Nutr 51: 500–506.

54. Wieckowska A, Zein N, Yerian L, Lopez A, McCullough A, et al. (2006) In vivo assessment of liver cell apoptosis as a novel biomarker of disease severity in nonalcoholic fatty liver disease. Hepatology 44: 27–33.

55. Kershenobich D, Razavi HA, Sanchez-Avila JF, Bessone F, Coelho HS, et al. (2011) Trends and projections of hepatitis C virus epidemiology in Latin America. Liver Int 31 Suppl 2: 18–29.

56. Castera L, Pinzani M (2010) Biopsy and non-invasive methods for the diagnosis of liver fibrosis: does it take two to tango? Gut 59: 861–866 2010.

57. Gebo KA, Herlong HF, Torbenson MS, Jenckes MW, Chander G, et al. (2002) Role of liver biopsy in management of chronic hepatitis C: a systematic review. Hepatology 36: S161–172.

58. Poynard T, Ratziu V, Benhamou Y, Thabut D, Moussalli J (2005) Biomarkers as a first-line estimate of injury in chronic liver diseases: time for a moratorium on liver biopsy?. Gastroenterology 128: 1146–1148

59. Sebastiani G, Alberti A (2006) Non invasive fibrosis biomarkers reduce but not substitute the need for liver biopsy. World J Gastroenterol 12: 3682–3694.

60. Poynard T, Halfon P, Castera L, Charlotte F, Le Bail B, et al. (2007) Variability of the area under the receiver operating characteristic curves in the diagnostic evaluation of liver fibrosis markers: impact of biopsy length and fragmentation. Aliment Pharmacol Ther 25: 733–739.

61. Colloredo G, Guido M, Sonzogni A, G L (2003) Impact of liver biopsy size on histological evaluation of chronic viral hepatitis: the smaller the sample, the milder the disease. J Hepatol 39: 239–244.

62. Regev A, Berho M, Jeffers LJ, Milikowski C, Molina EG, et al. (2002) Sampling error and intraobserver variation in liver biopsy in patients with chronic HCV infection. Am J Gastroenterol 97: 2614–2618.

63. Hermeziu B, Messous D, Fabre M, Munteanu M, Baussan C, et al. (2010) Evaluation of FibroTest-ActiTest in children with chronic hepatitis C virus infection. Gastroenterol Clin Biol 34: 16–22.

64. El-Shabrawi MH, Mohsen NA, Sherif MM, El-Karaksy HM, Abou-Yosef H, et al. (2010) Noninvasive assessment of hepatic fibrosis and necroinflammatory activity in Egyptian children with chronic hepatitis C virus infection using FibroTest and ActiTest. Eur J Gastroenterol Hepatol 22: 946–951.

18

Eligibility and Safety of Triple Therapy for Hepatitis C: Lessons Learned from the First Experience in a Real World Setting

Benjamin Maasoumy, Kerstin Port, Antoaneta Angelova Markova, Beatriz Calle Serrano, Magdalena Rogalska-Taranta, Lisa Sollik, Carola Mix, Janina Kirschner, Michael P. Manns, Heiner Wedemeyer, Markus Cornberg*

Department of Gastroenterology, Hepatology and Endocrinology, Hannover Medical School, Hannover, Germany

Abstract

Background: HCV protease inhibitors (PIs) boceprevir and telaprevir in combination with PEG-Interferon alfa and Ribavirin (P/R) is the new standard of care in the treatment of chronic HCV genotype 1 (GT1) infection. However, not every HCV GT1 infected patient is eligible for P/R/PI therapy. Furthermore phase III studies did not necessarily reflect real world as patients with advanced liver disease or comorbidities were underrepresented. The aim of our study was to analyze the eligibility and safety of P/R/PI treatment in a real world setting of a tertiary referral center.

Methods: All consecutive HCV GT1 infected patients who were referred to our hepatitis treatment unit between June and November 2011 were included. Patients were evaluated for P/R/PI according to their individual risk/benefit ratio based on 4 factors: Treatment-associated safety concerns, chance for SVR, treatment urgency and nonmedical patient related reasons. On treatment data were analyzed until week 12.

Results: 208 patients were included (F3/F4 64%, mean platelet count 169/nl, 40% treatment-naïve). Treatment was not initiated in 103 patients most frequently due to safety concerns. 19 patients were treated in phase II/III trials or by local centers and a triple therapy concept was initiated at our unit in 86 patients. Hospitalization was required in 16 patients; one patient died due to a gastrointestinal infection possibly related to treatment. A platelet count of <110/nl was associated with hospitalization as well as treatment failure. Overall, 128 patients were either not eligible for therapy or experienced a treatment failure at week 12.

Conclusions: P/R/PI therapies are complex, time-consuming and sometimes dangerous in a real world setting, especially in patients with advanced liver disease. A careful patient selection plays a crucial role to improve safety of PI based therapies. A significant number of patients are not eligible for P/R/PI, emphasizing the need for alternative therapeutic options.

Editor: John E. Tavis, Saint Louis University, United States of America

Funding: BM was supported by the Integrated Research and Treatment Center Transplantation (IFB-Tx) funded by the German Federal Ministry of Education and Research (Bundesministerium für Bildung und Forschung; BMBF). Publication costs were covered by the DFG (Deutsche Forschungsgemeinschaft)-Project "Open Access Publizieren". The funders had no role in study design, data collection and analysis, decision to publish, or preparation of the manuscript.

Competing Interests: The authors have read the journal's policy and declare the following conflicts concerning Peg-Interferon alpha-2a (Roche), Peg-Interferon alpha-2b (Merck), Ribavirin (Roche, Merck), Boceprevir (Merck), Telaprevir (Janssen-Cilag): BM received travel grants from Merck and Janssen-Cilag, KP received lecture fees from Roche and Janssen-Cilag, AM declares no conflict, BCS received lecture fees from Merck, MRT declares no conflict, LS declares no conflict, JK declares no conflict, CM declares no conflict, MPM received grants, lectural fees and/or consult fees from Roche, Merck and Janssen-Cilag, HW received grants, lectural fees and/or consult fees from Roche, Merck and Janssen-Cilag.

* E-mail: Cornberg.Markus@mh-hannover.de

Introduction

Hepatitis C virus (HCV) infection remains a global health burden with approximately 160 million chronically infected individuals worldwide [1] including 8–11 million patients in Europe [2]. Chronic HCV infection is a major cause of liver cirrhosis and hepatocellular carcinoma [3,4]. An effective antiviral treatment with sustained virological response (SVR) is associated with a significant improvement of the overall clinical outcome in particular at more advanced stages of the disease with severe liver fibrosis [5].

Combination therapy of pegylated interferon alfa and ribavirin (P/R) has been the standard of care since more than 10 years [6]. Recently the approval of the protease inhibitors (PI) boceprevir (BOC) and telaprevir (TLV) as first generation of new direct acting antivirals (DAA) has been a milestone in the therapy of chronic HCV genotype 1 infection. In phase III studies 67–75% of the therapy-naïve patients achieved SVR after a triple therapy consisting of P/R and PI [7,8]. Even higher SVR rates of up to 80% were observed in those, who experienced a relapse after a previous therapy with P/R [9,10]. In addition, the overall safety profile appeared to be moderate in these trials [7–10]. Despite these encouraging results there still remain some challenges ahead. SVR rates with PI-based triple therapies were much lower in patients with a previous null-response to P/R, especially in those individuals who also had advanced liver fibrosis and cirrhosis [11]. Furthermore, phase III trials do not necessarily reflect real world setting since the study population was highly selective. For example, patients with liver cirrhosis were underrepresented in these studies and those with advanced cirrhosis, low platelets or with additional risk factors like higher age or comorbidities were entirely excluded. Preliminary week 16 results of the French early access program (CUPIC) investigating the new triple therapy only in those with advanced liver fibrosis revealed a totally different safety profile with alarming rates of severe adverse effects (SAE) of up to 49% and a mortality rate of up to 2% [12]. In addition, it has to be considered that a certain part of the infected population is not eligible for the new therapies at the first place. Since current therapy concepts are still based on interferon alfa, several contraindications may prevent antiviral therapy. Various DAAs are currently in preclinical and clinical development and encouraging results have been published recently suggesting the introduction of interferon-free regimens in the near future [13]. Thus, it might well be a preferable alternative to wait for more efficient and safer treatment options in patients with only mild liver disease. In addition, limited resources may prevent treatment of all eligible patients.

The aim of our study was to analyze the eligibility and safety of new triple therapy concepts for the treatment of chronic HCV genotype 1 infection in a real world setting of a German tertiary referral center.

Patients and Methods

Patient Selection

All consecutive patients with chronic HCV genotype 1 infection who were referred to our hepatitis outpatient clinic between June 1st and November 30th 2011 were included. Excluded were patients with antiviral treatment at the time of their initial presentation during this time period. All patients were evaluated for a triple therapy concept. Figure 1 gives a schematic overview of the selection algorithm of our study. We recorded all reasons that influenced whether treatment was initiated or not until May 31st 2012. Patient data were analyzed anonymously.

This study has been conducted according to the principles expressed in the Declaration of Helsinki. The ethical committee of Hannover Medical School approved this research project and waived the need for written informed consent because of the anonymous evaluation of patient data from patient records. For routinely assessment of IL28B genotype written informed consent was obtained.

Assessment of Baseline Parameters

Routine laboratory parameters like hemoglobin level, platelet counts, ALT, AST and INR were measured by standard procedures. HCV RNA levels were detected using Roche COBAS TaqMan, Version 1. Extraction of the RNA was done automatically by COBAS AmpliPrep (Roche) according to the manufactures instructions. In those patients who gave written informed consent, assessment of the IL28B genotype (rs12979860) was performed as described previously using the Light Mix Kit rs12979860 TIB MOLBIOL [14]. The stage of liver fibrosis is described according to the METAVIR-Score. The majority of patients were classified using transient elastography/Fibroscan (84%). For classification the following cut off values were used: F0/

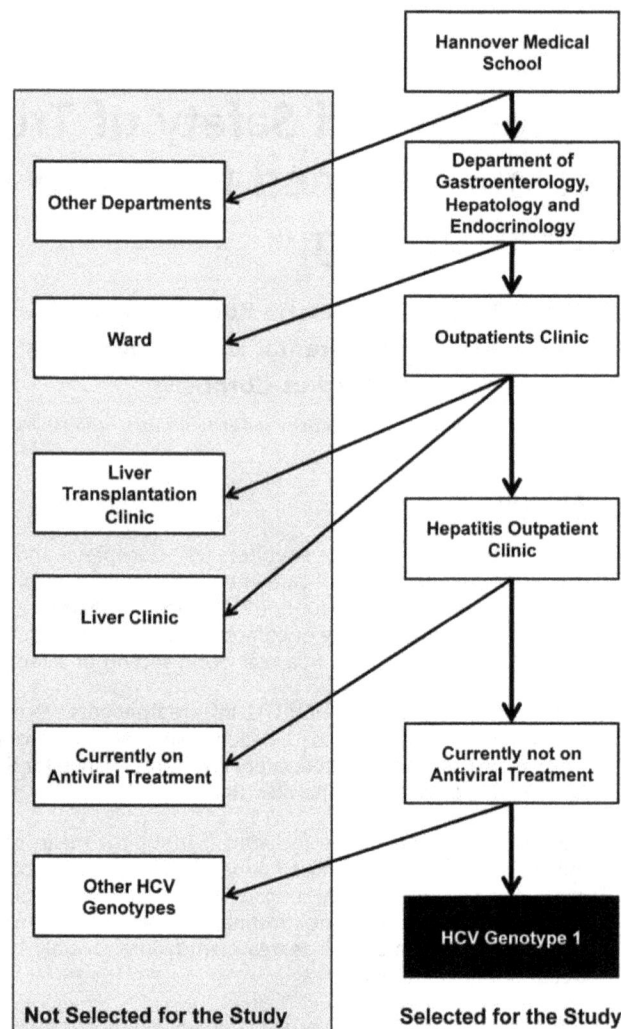

Figure 1. Selection of the study cohort.

F1:<7.1 kPa; F1/F2: $\geq$ 7.1 kPa; F2 $\geq$ 8.7 kPa; F3: $\geq$ 9.5 kPa; F3/F4: $\geq$ 12.5 kPa; Definite cirrhosis: $\geq$ 14.5 kPa [15,16]. In the remaining cases the stage of fibrosis was determined based on a liver biopsy or obvious clinical parameters indicating liver cirrhosis.

Triple Therapy Concepts

Different triple therapy concepts were considered. Some patients were treated with an individualized lead-in phase followed by the treatment protocol according to the approved label. These individualized concepts were planned for cases of uncertain treatment tolerability or low chances for SVR. In a few patients individualized lead-in phases included episodes with RBV mono-therapy prior to the standard BOC or TLV treatment protocol i.e. in cases of uncertain RBV tolerance or in some patients with thrombocytopenia with the purpose to increase or stabilize platelet count. Davis et al. have shown that IFN-induced decrease of platelet count was less pronounced if RBV is co-administered [17]. In addition we also used a P/R lead-in prior to the TLV label regimen with or without previous RBV mono-therapy. For patients who were started on a triple therapy concept at our hepatitis outpatient clinic until May 31st 2012 safety and efficacy data were analyzed until treatment week 12 of the standard treatment regimen according to label. In those patients treated with an individualized lead-in concept week 0 of therapy was defined as the start of the approved standard treatment (4 weeks P/R, 24–44 weeks P/R/BOC or 12 weeks P/R/TLV).

Definition of Treatment Failure

Treatment failure was defined as either virological failure or a permanent discontinuation of all antiviral medication due treatment intolerance i.e. in cases of AEs. Virological failure was defined along with the futility rules according to the respective labels: A) HCV RNA level ≥ 1,000 IU/ml at week 4 and/or week 12 of triple therapy including TLV. B) HCV RNA ≥100 IU/ml at treatment week 12 of a BOC protocol. C) Virological breakthrough was defined as an increase of HCV RNA level of>1 log.

In addition, patients with liver cirrhosis and previous null-response to P/R were also classified as virological failure, if they achieved<1 log decline of HCV RNA after a four-week lead-in phase with P/R. According to previously published studies chances for SVR have to be estimated as very low in these cases [18]. Thus we decided not to continue treatment due to an inadequate risk/benefit ratio.

Statistical Analysis

All data are either presented as absolute numbers or as mean ± SD unless otherwise stated. Continuous data we analyzed with t-test and categorical data with χ2 tests.

Results

Patients and Evaluation Process

Baseline characteristics of the study cohort are shown in Table 1. 55% of the patients were male. Mean age was 52.9 years. The majority of patients were infected with HCV genotype 1b (62%) and the predominant IL28B genotype was CT (44%), whereas IL28B CC was present in only 18% of the individuals. Only 40% of the patients were treatment-naïve. Platelet counts below 150/nl were detected in 84 (40%) patients and 35 patients (17%) had platelets of<90/nl. The mean hemoglobin concentration was 14.3 g/dl including 21 individuals with hemoglobin levels<13 g/dl (men) or 12 g/dl (women). Baseline serum ALT levels were elevated in the majority of patients but only 15 patients had ALT levels of more than five times the upper limit of normal (ULN). Advanced liver fibrosis (F3/F4 according to METAVIR) was present in 133 (64%) individuals including 88 (42%) patients with definite cirrhosis. Only nine patients (4.3%) had a Child-Pugh Score of B indicating pre-selection of patients referred for antiviral therapy to our hepatitis treatment unit. Patients with decompensated cirrhosis are being referred to our liver transplant outpatient clinic.

Of the 208 patients, eleven were included into clinical phase II or III trials and were therefore not further considered for this analysis. Treatment was not initiated in 103 patients. The remaining 94 patients were considered for a triple therapy concept, of which eight preferred treatment at other centers. Thus, treatment was started in 86 patients at our hepatitis outpatient clinic. Patients who received antiviral therapy at our center were more likely to be male, to be infected with HCV genotype 1b, to have higher ALT levels and to show a more advanced stage of liver fibrosis than patients who were not treated. Treated patients were more often patients with previous treatment failure, which explains the lower prevalence of IL28B CC in the treated population (Table 1).

Factors that Influenced the Decision not to Start P/R/PI

Four key factors were considered to calculate the risk/benefit ratio during evaluation process: (i) Therapy-associated safety concerns, (ii) chances for SVR, (iii) treatment urgency and (iv) nonmedical patient related reasons. Sometimes one of these factors completely dominated final decision i.e. in some patients with obvious interferon intolerance. Still, in many patients two or more of these factors significantly influenced the final decision indicating the complexity of the evaluation process.

(i) In 66 (64%) patients risk of SAEs during P/R/PI treatment was considerable. This was majorly related to comorbidities affecting 48 (47%) patients, most frequently the risk of exacerbation of an autoimmune reaction during treatment with interferon alfa since 18 patients were either recipients of organ transplants or had a history of an autoimmune disease. Severe psychological instability and disorders like severe depression i.e. with a history of a suicidal attempt or psychosis were relevant in 15 cases. Cardiovascular diseases i.e. a history of heart attacks, bypass or present congestive heart failure were important in eight and a low level of hemoglobin in seven individuals. Other comorbidities as impaired renal function, thyroidal dysfunction or severe diabetes were only relevant in a few patients. Besides comorbidities liver related morbidity played an essential role as well. Overall, in 10 patients with an advanced stage of liver disease risk of hepatic decompensation during antiviral treatment was estimated as to high. Thrombocytopenia had a significant impact on the negative evaluation in 12 subjects. In addition, advanced age (> 70 years) linked to a limited physical capacity was a reason that prevented treatment in eight patients. Six individuals reported poor tolerability of the previous treatment. Two patients were pregnant at the time of presentation.(ii) In seven (6.8%) patients mainly with advanced fibrosis, a history of treatment failures and further negative predictors, the chance to achieve SVR was considered to be too low to reach an acceptable risk/benefit ratio.

(iii) Thirty-one (30%) patients were considered to have no urgent treatment indication in our view, as the stage of liver fibrosis was not advanced limiting the benefit of an immediate treatment.

(iv) Finally, nonmedical patient related reasons played an important role in thirty-two patients (31%). All patients were widely informed about their liver related prognosis, risks, benefits and conditions of current triple therapy concepts as well as the chances for alternative treatment options that may be accessible in the future. Eighteen patients decided to wait for future treatment options. Twelve patients were either completely lost to follow up or missed appointments and were considered as incompliant. In seven cases a triple therapy concept was not possible due to social or work related reasons i.e. two subjects were professional drivers. In Table 2 we have listed the factors that influenced treatment decision.

Safety and Effort of Triple Therapy

Overall, 406 visits during 1022 treatment weeks (one visit every 2.5 weeks) were documented. During the investigated time period several cases of cytopenia occurred that required dose modifications of the antiviral therapy. Thirty-two patients (37%) experienced at least one episode of significant anemia (Hb<10 g/dl). In 12 (14%) of these patients, hemoglobin level dropped to a

Table 1. Baseline characteristics of the study cohort.

		All Patients (A)	Patients selected for Antiviral Treatment (B)	Patients Treated with a Triple Therapy Concept (C)	Not Treated (D)	p-value C vs. D
Patient number		208	105	86	103	
Scheduled for						
	TLV			61 (71%)		
	BOC			25 (29%)		
Mean Age ± SD (years)		52.9 ± 12	52.6 ± 10.1	53.5 ± 10.4	53.1 ± 13.7	0.41
Gender						
	Male (m)	115 (55%)	65 (62%)	55 (64%)	50 (49%)	0.16
	Female (f)	93 (45%)	40 (38%)	31 (36%)	53 (51%)	0.11
HCV genotype						
	1a	75 (36%)	34 (32%)	26 (30%)	41 (40%)	0.27
	1b	128 (62%)	69 (66%)	58 (67%)	59 (57%)	0.38
	Mixed/n.d.	5 (2.4%)	2 (1.9%)	2 (2.3%)	3 (3%)	0.80
IL28B genotype						
	CC	38 (18%)	12 (11%)	10 (12%)	26 (25%)	< 0.01
	CT	92 (44%)	55 (52%)	52 (60%)	37 (36%)	0.11
	TT	29 (14%)	17 (16%)	13 (15%)	12 (12%)	0.84
	N/A	49 (24%)	21 (20%)	11 (13%)	28 (27%)	
Treatment experienced						
	Yes	124 (60%)	70 (67%)	63 (73%)	54 (52%)	< 0.05
	No	84 (40%)	35 (33%)	23 (27%)	49 (48%)	0.07
Platelet counts (/nl)						
	Mean ± SD	169 ± 77.6	166 ± 69	158 ± 68.7	172 ± 85.4	0.11
	> 149	121 (58%)	60 (57%)	46 (53%)	61 (59%)	0.61
	90–149	49 (24%)	29 (28%)	25 (29%)	20 (19%)	0.17
	< 90	35 (17%)	14 (13%)	14 (16%)	21 (20%)	0.52
	N/A	3 (1.4%)	2 (1.9%)	1 (1.2%)	1 (1%)	
Hemoglobin (g/dl)						
	Mean ± SD	14.3 ± 1.77	14.5 ± 1.64	14.6 ± 1.61	14.2 ± 1.87	0.05
	<13 (m), <12 (f)	21 (10%)	6 (5.7%)	5 (5.8%)	15 (15%)	0.07
ALT						
	Mean ± SD	95.5 ± 81.6	102 ± 82.2	102 ± 76.4	88.9 ± 80.4	0.13
	< ULN	46 (22%)	16 (15%)	13 (15%)	30 (29%)	< 0.05
	1–2×ULN	82 (39%)	45 (43%)	36 (42%)	37 (36%)	0.51
	2–5×ULN	64 (31%)	35 (33%)	31 (36%)	29 (28%)	0.34
	> 5×ULN	15 (7.2%)	8 (7.6%)	6 (7%)	7 (6.8%)	0.96
	N/A	1 (0.5%)	1 (1%)	0 (0%)	0 (0%)	
Fibrosis Stage						
	F0–F2	72 (35%)	22 (21%)	11 (13%)	50 (49%)	< 0.0001
	F3/F4	133 (64%)	82 (78%)	74 (86%)	51 (50%)	< 0.01
	N/A	3 (1.4%)	1 (1%)	1 (1.2%)	2 (1.9%)	
De Ritis ratio						
	≤ 1	131 (63%)	69 (66%)	58 (67%)	62 (60%)	0.53
	> 1	76 (37%)	35 (33%)	28 (33%)	41 (40%)	0.41
	N/A	1 (0.5%)	1 (1%)	0 (0%)	0 (0%)	
Child-Pugh Score						
	5	167 (80%)	83 (79%)	67 (78%)	84 (82%)	0.78
	6	18 (8.7%)	10 (9.5%)	9 (10%)	8 (7.8%)	0.54
	> 6	9 (4.3%)	3 (2.9%)	2 (2.3%)	6 (5.8%)	0.24

Table 1. Cont.

		Patients selected for Antiviral Treatment (B)	Patients Treated with a Triple Therapy Concept (C)	Not Treated (D)	p-value C vs. D
	All Patients (A)				
N/A	14 (6.7%)	9 (8.6%)	8 (9.3%)	5 (4.9%)	

TLV: telaprevir; BOC: boceprevir; N/A: not available; n.d.: not differentiated; SD: standard deviation.

concentration of less than 8.5 g/dl. In 12 patients anemia was countered by blood transfusions. Less commonly thrombocytopenia (20%) and neutropenia (12%) reached a stage where dose modifications are recommended. Ribavirin dose reduction was required in 31 patients (36%) predominantly due to anemia. In 11 patients (13%) a temporary discontinuation became necessary. The dosage of pegylated interferon alfa was reduced in 20 (23%) patients and six (7%) required a temporary discontinuation.

Twenty-one hospitalizations related to antiviral therapy have been documented in 16 patients (19%). Most frequent reason was a severe or symptomatic anemia (62%), followed by infections (14%) and hepatic decompensations (14%). Overall, the rate of treatment-associated hospitalization was estimated as 0.99/patient treatment year. The 16 patients who were referred to hospital were at a similar age as the remaining patients (53.9 vs. 53.4 years) but more likely to have a more advanced liver disease at baseline indicated by a significantly higher MELD-Score (9.6 vs. 7.3) and a lower platelet count (107.5/nl vs. 169.9/nl). Platelets<110/nl (48% hospitalized patients) and>five points in the Child-Pugh Score (45% hospitalized patients) were associated with a high risk

of hospitalization. In contrast, only four out of 60 patients (6.7%) who had none of the above-mentioned risk factors required hospitalization (Table 3).

Treatment Failure at Week 12

Of the 86 patients that were started on a triple therapy concept 20 (23%) dropped out before week 12 of the approved treatment regimen. In 10 of these patients treatment was stopped due to a virological failure, while seven had to discontinue because of AEs and one patient died after a gastrointestinal infection. In two patients, both poor tolerability as well as poor virological response contributed equally. Of those, who maintained on therapy, four patients had to stop at week 12 because they met futility criteria. In addition, one patient experienced a SAE at week 12 of therapy that resulted in a permanent discontinuation. As a result, 25 out of 86 patients (29%) had to be classified as a treatment failure at week 12 (Figure 2).

Patients that discontinued had a significantly lower platelet count at baseline (123/nl vs. 172/nl, p<0.001). More than half of the patients with a baseline platelet count of less than 110/nl had

Table 2. Factors that influenced the decision not to treat with P/R/PI.

Factor			Frequency n (% of 86 patients)
Treatment associated safety concerns			**66 (64%)***
	Comorbidities		48 (47%)
		Autoimmune exacerbation	18 (17%)
		Neuro-psychiatric diseases	15 (15%)
		Cardiovascular diseases	8 (7.8%)
		Anemia	7 (6.8%)
		Other comorbidities	9 (8.7%)
	Risk of hepatic decompensation		10 (9.7%)
	Thrombocytopenia¶		12 (12%)
	Age		8 (7.8%)
	Intolerance to previous P/R treatment		6 (5.8%)
	Need for other urgent procedures		6 (5.8%)
	Pregnancy		2 (1.9%)
Poor chance for SVR			**7 (6.8%)***
Treatment urgency§			**31 (30%)***
Nonmedical patient related reasons			**32 (31%)***
	Patient wish		18 (17%)
	Poor compliance/LTFU		12 (12%)
	Social reasons (i.e. bus driver)		7 (6.8%)

*More than factor could have influenced treatment decision.
¶Eleven patients with platelets <60/nl; one patient with a platelet count of 89/nl and several other risk factors.
§Based on individual risk for disease progression and current stage of liver fibrosis (majority F0/F1:71%; remaining patients with Fibroscan result <9 kPa and one patient with F2 in liver biopsy)

Table 3. Baseline characteristics of patients who were hospitalized until week 12.

		No hospitalization until week 12	Hospitalization until week 12	p-value
Number of patients		70 (81%)	16 (19%)	
Treatment Regimen				
	P/R/TLV	43 (61%)*	12 (75%)	0.51
	P/R/BOC	19 (27%)*	2 (13%)	0.29
	P/R Lead-In¶	9 (13%)	2 (13%)	0.99
Mean Age ± SD (years)		53.4 ± 10.2	53.9 ± 11.4	0.45
Gender				
	Male (m)	49 (70%)	6 (38%)	0.14
	Female (f)	21 (30%)	10 (63%)	0.05
Treatment experienced				
	Yes	51 (73%)	12 (75%)	0.93
	No	19 (27%)	4 (25%)	0.88
Platelet Count (/nl)				
	Mean ± SD	170 ± 65.7	108 ± 57.3	< 0.01
	< 110	11 (16%)	10 (63%)	< 0.001
	N/A	1 (1.4%)	0 (0%)	
Hemoglobin (g/dl)				
	Mean ± SD	14.8 ± 1.56	13.5 ± 1.40	< 0.01
	< 13 (m),<12 (f)	3 (4.3%)	2 (13%)	0.23
ALT				
	Mean ± SD	100 ± 71.4	108 ± 94.7	0.39
	< ULN	9 (13%)	4 (25%)	0.26
	1–2×ULN	32 (46%)	4 (25%)	0.25
	2–5×ULN	25 (36%)	6 (38%)	0.91
	> 5×ULN	4 (5.7%)	2 (13%)	0.36
Fibrosis stage				
	F0–F2	10 (14%)	1 (6.3%)	0.41
	F3/F4	59 (84%)	15 (94%)	0.75
	N/A	1 (1.4%)	0 (0%)	
De Ritis ratio				
	≤ 1	50 (71%)	8 (50%)	0.35
	> 1	20 (29%)	8 (50%)	0.18
Child-Pugh Score				
	5	58 (83%)	9 (56%)	0.34
	> 5	6 (8.6%)	5 (31%)	< 0.05
	N/A	6 (8.6%)	2 (13%)	
MELD				
	Mean ± SD	7.33 ± 2.24	9.60 ± 2.89	< 0.01
	≤ 8	56 (80%)	8 (50%)	0.19
	> 8	8 (11%)	7 (44%)	< 0.01
	> 10	2 (2.9%)	5 (31%)	< 0.001
	N/A	6 (8.6%)	1 (6.3%)	

P: pegylated interferon alfa; R: ribavirin; TLV: telaprevir; BOC: boceprevir; N/A: not available; n.d.: not differentiated; SD: standard deviation
*One patient switched from TLV to BOC after week 2 of therapy
¶Patients that discontinued treatment during/after the lead-in phase and never received a PI

to be classified as a treatment failure at week 12 of therapy. Patients infected with HCV genotype 1a were more likely to experience a treatment failure (p<0.05). IL28B CC genotype was associated with a superior treatment outcome. None of the 10 patients with the IL28B CC genotype that started a triple therapy experienced a virological failure until week 12 of treatment.

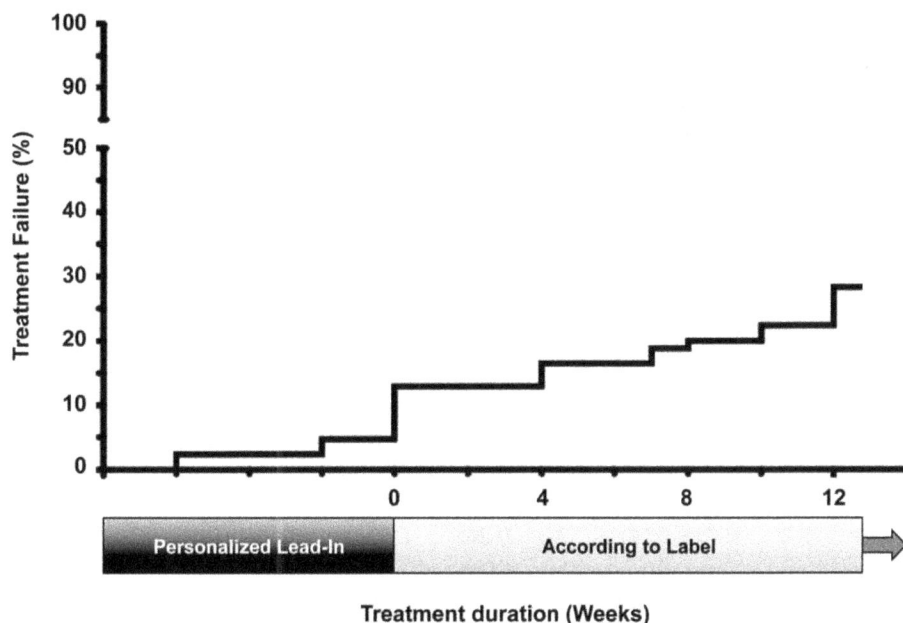

Figure 2. Treatment failures during the observed time period.

However, one patient experienced a lethal AE. No significant difference could be observed between TLV and BOC in those receiving at least one dose of PI (p = 0.73) (Table 4).

Overall, 128 patients (65%) were either not eligible or experienced a treatment failure at week 12 (Figure 3).

Discussion

Pivotal phase III trials investigating the efficacy and safety of triple therapy including boceprevir or telaprevir showed excellent response rates with a reasonable safety profile. However, considerable concerns have been raised to what extend the new treatment concepts can be translated into clinical practice as only highly selected patients qualified for registration trials [11]. At this stage it remains unclear what proportion of the total HCV genotype 1-infected population is eligible for treatment and which patients will subsequently benefit from the novel therapeutic options. Here we describe our initial experience in selecting patients for and treating with PI-based antiviral treatment regimens. Selection of patients for treatment was based on four main factors, which were treatment-associated safety concerns, chance for SVR, treatment urgency and nonmedical patient related reasons. It has to be considered that the here studied patient population has already been preselected by the referral approach. Patients with decompensated cirrhosis and other obvious contraindications for therapy are managed by other clinics at our center, i.e. by the liver transplant unit (Figure 1). Still, so-called difficult-to-treat patients including those with advanced liver disease, previous treatment failures and individuals with comorbidities were overrepresented in this cohort. Subsequently, safety concerns for P/R/PI played a major role for not selecting patients for therapy. On the other side, mild liver disease and patient's wish were also frequent reasons for not initiating therapy at this stage with more convenient interferon free regimens on the horizon (11, 13). Interestingly, poor chance to achieve SVR played a minor role not to start therapy mainly due to high expectations in efficacy and the opportunity of the lead-in phase. In the end, treatment was not initiated in half of the patients, including several

patients with the most urgent medical need as well as individuals likely being the easiest to treat. Considering the referral approach to our hepatitis treatment unit, we suggest that the proportion of HCV-infected patients not qualifying for current treatment options can be estimated to be even higher than 50% if the here used evaluation criteria are applied.

Management of adverse events was an enormous effort in this cohort. Patients were seen almost every two weeks at our outpatient clinic and the overall frequency of consultations was certainly considerably higher since we did not assess visits at the general practitioner, local hospitals and telephone calls. Although we only analyzed the first treatment period, hospitalization became already necessary in nearly one out of five patients. Anemia was the most prevalent side effect requiring frequent hemoglobin monitoring and blood transfusions.

Infections represent the most serious complication of interferon alfa-based treatment of hepatitis C. Death of one patient during the first 12-week treatment period and an additional death of a patient at week 14 was related to gastrointestinal infection with sepsis.

In contrast to the registration trials a much larger proportion of patients had to stop therapy early during therapy. Both virological treatment failure and adverse events accounted for these early treatment discontinuations. An obvious explanation for virological failure might be the large number of patients with F3/F4 fibrosis and previous treatment failure [19]. In addition, advanced liver fibrosis has been shown to be linked to a higher incidence of adverse events [12]. In our cohort HCV genotype 1a infection and low platelet counts were associated with early treatment failure. The impact of platelet counts suggests that the negative predictive value of liver cirrhosis increases with more advanced stages of cirrhosis.

Platelet counts also predicted the need for hospitalizations during therapy further highlighting the value of this specific marker in the context of new antiviral therapies. Of note only six out of 14 patients with platelet counts of less than 90/nl, which is the recommended cut-off level for treatment eligibility with P/R [20], managed to pass week 12 futility rules. Our data indicate that

Table 4. Baseline characteristics of patients with and without treatment failure until week 12.

		Continued treatment after week 12	Treatment failure until week 12	p-value
Number of patients		61 (71%)	25 (29%)	
Mean Age ± SD (years)		52.8 ± 11.2	55.4 ± 7.81	0.12
Gender				
	Male (m)	38 (62%)	17 (68%)	0.76
	Female (f)	23 (38%)	8 (32%)	0.69
HCV genotype				
	1a	13 (21%)	13 (52%)	< 0.05
	1b	47 (77%)	11 (44%)	0.13
	Mixed/n.d.	1 (1.6%)	1 (4%)	0.49
IL28B				
	CC	9 (15%)	1 (4%)	0.16
	Non-CC	43 (70%)	22 (88%)	0.06
	N/A	9 (15%)	2 (8%)	
Treatment experienced				
	Yes	47 (77%)	16 (64%)	0.52
	No	14 (23%)	9 (36%)	0.29
Platelet count (/nl)				
	Mean ± SD	172 ± 69.3	123 ± 52.5	< 0.001
	<110	10 (16%)	11 (44%)	< 0.05
Hemoglobin (g/dl)				
	Mean ± SD	14.7 ± 1.66	14.4 ± 1.47	0.24
	< 13 (m),<12 (f)	3 (4.9%)	2 (8%)	0.56
ALT				
	Mean ± SD	96.3 ± 70.4	115 ± 87.8	0.17
	< ULN	11 (18%)	2 (8%)	0.28
	1–2×ULN	24 (39%)	12 (48%)	0.57
	2–5×ULN	22 (36%)	9 (36%)	1
	> 5×ULN	4 (6.6%)	2 (8%)	0.82
Fibrosis stage				
	F0–F2	8 (13%)	3 (12%)	0.88
	F3/F4	52 (85%)	22 (88%)	0.95
	N/A	1 (1.6%)	0 (0%)	
De Ritis ratio				
	≤ 1	42 (69%)	16 (64%)	0.80
	> 1	19 (31%)	9 (36%)	0.29
Child-Pugh Score				
	5	48 (79%)	19 (76%)	0.67
	> 5	6 (9.8%)	5 (20%)	0.29
	N/A	7 (11%)	1 (4%)	

N/A: not available; n.d.: not differentiated; SD: standard deviation.

even higher platelet levels have to be considered as a predictive marker for poor treatment outcome since six out of seven patients with a baseline platelet count between 90 and 110/nl either needed to be referred to hospital and/or experienced a virological failure. Platelets<110/nl were also significantly associated with treatment failure at week 12. By further follow-up, 70% of patients with platelets<110/nl required hospitalization at some point and 2 of these patients died (data not shown). We therefore suggest that low platelet count of<110/nl is a marker for advanced liver disease with a high risk for serious adverse events during P/R/PI treatment. In addition, more than 5 points in the Child-Pugh score was another valuable predictive marker for adverse events and hospitalization.

Our study was not designed to directly compare the two available PIs. Many of the observed adverse events are certainly related to P/R since some patients discontinued treatment even before taking a single dose of a PI. It was not the aim of this study to attribute treatment-associated risk and effort to a single

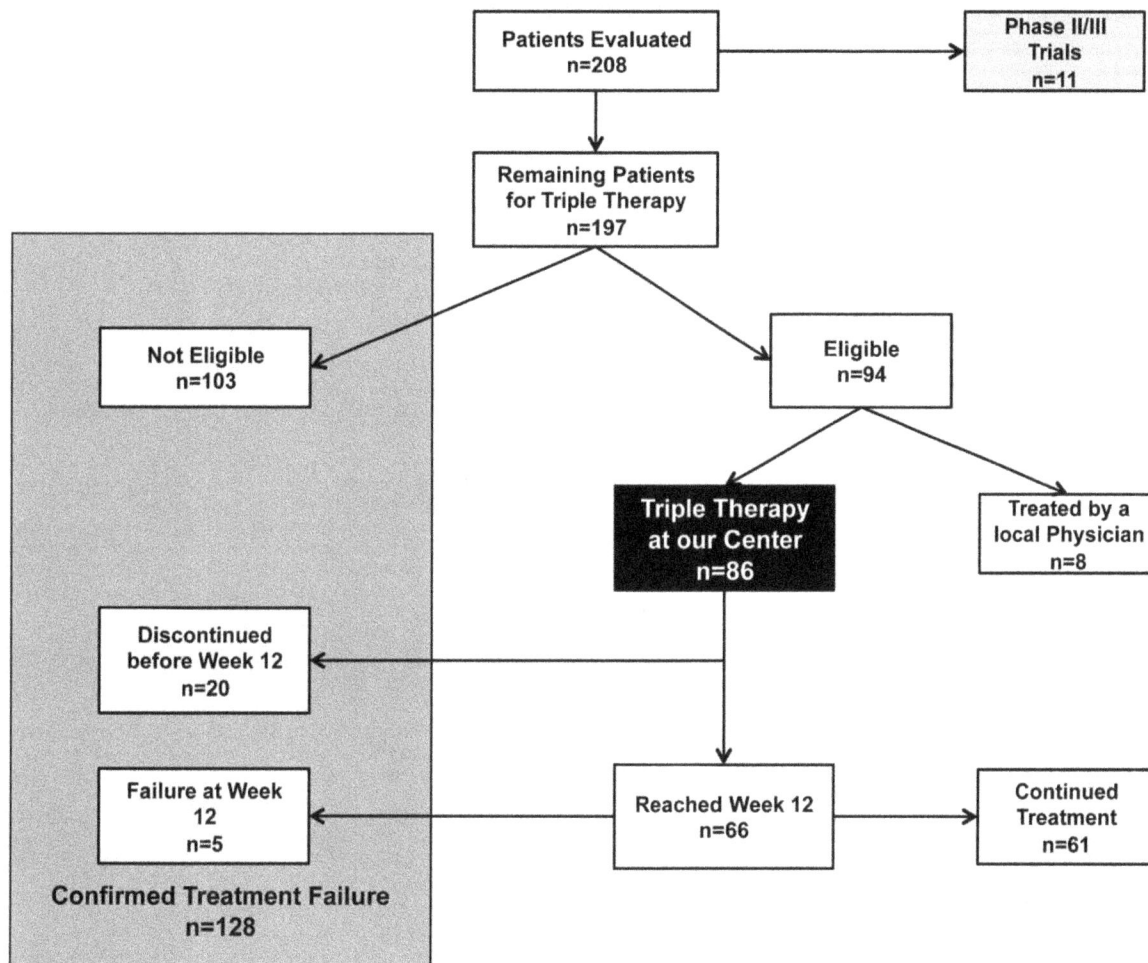

Figure 3. Overall outcome of the evaluation process and treatment period.

component of the antiviral therapy regimen. We could already demonstrate that, in contrast to pivotal registration trials, safety and efficacy of currently available antiviral regimens are limited in a real world cohort. In addition treatment required enormous recourses both in terms of time and monitoring visits as well as by the management of side effects. On the other side HCV RNA became undetectable in most of the patients who reached week 12 of therapy. Thus it is crucial to identify reliable markers for the prediction of both safety and efficacy. In our opinion a lead-in phase regardless of the later used PI can be a valuable tool in patients with uncertain treatment tolerability and offer additional information on chances for SVR. Early discontinuation may prevent SAEs and even some lethal complications. According to our data platelet count and Child-Pugh Score, markers for advanced liver disease, seem to be valuable tools to identify patients with a high therapy associated risk and a poor treatment outcome. However, specific cut-offs to determine ineligibility for triple therapy (i.e. platelet count <110/nl, Child-Pugh Score >5) warrants further validation in larger cohorts. Still, the risk/benefit ratio should be well calculated in patients with advanced cirrhosis indicated by such risk factors. If treatment will be initiated in such patients a very close monitoring and early management of adverse events is essential.

We here presented our first experiences with new triple therapies, rising considerable safety concerns at least in certain

populations. However, overall safety of these new treatments will certainly improve with more "real world" data and more experience gained regarding the optimal management of adverse events in particular anemia. According to recently published data RBV dose reduction as first line strategy is done much more rapidly in our center, which seemed to decrease the number of hospitalizations in following cohorts [21]. More effective strategies to meet severe infections need to be developed. High efficacy of PI-based therapies raises high ambitions to treat a huge amount of patients. This may lead to an underestimation of risk factors. Our data suggest, that patients need to be selected very carefully since a sensible patient selection is the first and may be the most important step to ensure a reasonable safety profile and a high efficacy. From a retrospective point of view we might slightly shift our patient selection to a cohort with less advanced liver disease. In our opinion ideal candidates for current PI based therapies are those with middle stage fibrosis (F2–F3) and well-compensated cirrhosis as well as prevalence of some positive predictors for SVR. Including some more easier-to-treat patients would certainly reduce the huge effort that is required for therapy management. A more balanced patient cohort may also permit to treat a higher number of HCV-infected individuals even more cost-effectively. Conclusions of our study are supported by a recently published, huge epidemiologic study comparing different approaches to the initiation of antiviral treatment. Here it has been demonstrated that starting treatment as soon as liver fibrosis has reached F2 might be a more effective strategy than delaying treatment until higher stages of fibrosis have been established [22]. We here identified valuable pretreatment markers to predict both safety and efficacy, which may help to select the appropriate patients in the future. However, further studies will certainly be necessary to develop a valuable scoring system for this selection process. According to the poor outcome of patients with advanced disease and the small benefit for those at very early stages of the disease, it has to be concluded that despite the improvements that have been achieved during the last year safer and more efficient treatment options are still urgently needed.

Acknowledgments

The authors thank Janet Cornberg for her help with the data assessment.

Author Contributions

Assesment of data: BM KP AM BCS MRT LS CM JK. Conceived and designed the experiments: BM MPM HW MC. Analyzed the data: BM HW MC. Wrote the paper: BM MPM HW MC.

References

1. Lavanchy D (2011) Evolving epidemiology of hepatitis C virus. Clin Microbiol Infect 17: 107–115.
2. Cornberg M, Razavi HA, Alberti A, Bernasconi E, Buti M, et al. (2011) A systematic review of hepatitis C virus epidemiology in Europe, Canada and Israel. Liver Int 31 Suppl 2: 30–60.
3. (2011) EASL Clinical Practice Guidelines: management of hepatitis C virus infection. J Hepatol 55: 245–264.
4. Sarrazin C, Berg T, Ross RS, Schirmacher P, Wedemeyer H, et al. (2010) [Prophylaxis, diagnosis and therapy of hepatitis C virus (HCV) infection: the German guidelines on the management of HCV infection]. Z Gastroenterol 48: 289–351.
5. Veldt BJ, Heathcote EJ, Wedemeyer H, Reichen J, Hofmann WP, et al. (2007) Sustained virologic response and clinical outcomes in patients with chronic hepatitis C and advanced fibrosis. Ann Intern Med 147: 677–684.
6. Manns MP, Wedemeyer H, Cornberg M (2006) Treating viral hepatitis C: efficacy, side effects, and complications. Gut 55: 1350–1359.
7. Jacobson IM, McHutchison JG, Dusheiko G, Di Bisceglie AM, Reddy KR, et al. (2011) Telaprevir for previously untreated chronic hepatitis C virus infection. N Engl J Med 364: 2405–2416.
8. Poordad F, McCone JJ, Bacon BR, Bruno S, Manns MP, et al. (2011) Boceprevir for untreated chronic HCV genotype 1 infection. N Engl J Med 364: 1195–1206.
9. Bacon BR, Gordon SC, Lawitz E, Marcellin P, Vierling JM, et al. (2011) Boceprevir for previously treated chronic HCV genotype 1 infection. N Engl J Med 364: 1207–1217.
10. Zeuzem S, Andreone P, Pol S, Lawitz E, Diago M, et al. (2011) Telaprevir for retreatment of HCV infection. N Engl J Med 364: 2417–2428.
11. Dusheiko G, Wedemeyer H (2012) New protease inhibitors and direct-acting antivirals for hepatitis C: interferon's long goodbye. Gut.
12. Hezode C, Dorival C, Zoulim F, Poynard T, Mathurin P, et al. (2012) Safety of telaprevir or boceprevir in combination with peginterferon alfa/ribavirin, in cirrhotic non responders. First results of the french early access program (anrs co20-cupic). Journal of Hepatology 56 Suppl 2: S4.
13. Lok AS, Gardiner DF, Lawitz E, Martorell C, Everson GT, et al. (2012) Preliminary study of two antiviral agents for hepatitis C genotype 1. N Engl J Med 366: 216–224.
14. Sarrazin C, Susser S, Doehring A, Lange CM, Muller T, et al. (2011) Importance of IL28B gene polymorphisms in hepatitis C virus genotype 2 and 3 infected patients. J Hepatol 54: 415–421.
15. Ziol M, Handra-Luca A, Kettaneh A, Christidis C, Mal F, et al. (2005) Noninvasive assessment of liver fibrosis by measurement of stiffness in patients with chronic hepatitis C. Hepatology 41: 48–54.
16. de Ledinghen V, Vergniol J (2008) Transient elastography (FibroScan). Gastroenterol Clin Biol 32: 58–67.
17. Davis GL, Esteban-Mur R, Rustgi V, Hoefs J, Gordon SC, et al. (1998) Interferon alfa-2b alone or in combination with ribavirin for the treatment of relapse of chronic hepatitis C. International Hepatitis Interventional Therapy Group. N Engl J Med 339: 1493–1499.
18. Foster GR, Zeuzem S, Andreone P, Pol S, Lawitz EJ, et al. (2011) Subanalyses of the telaprevir lead-in arm in the realize study: response at week 4 is not a substitute for prior null response categorization. Journal of Hepatology 54 Suppl 1: S3–S4.
19. Poordad F, Bronowicki JP, Gordon SC, Zeuzem S, Jacobson IM, et al. (2012) Factors That Predict Response of Patients With Hepatitis C Virus Infection to Boceprevir. Gastroenterology.
20. Pegasys Label information.
21. Poordad F, Lawitz E, Reddy KR, Afdhal NH, Hezode C, et al. (2012) A randomized trial comparing ribavirin dose reduction versus erythropoietin for anemia management in previously untreated patients with chronic hepatitis c receiving boceprevir plus peginterferon/ribavirin. Journal of Hepatology 56: S559–S559.
22. Deuffic-Burban S, Deltenre P, Buti M, Stroffolini T, Parkes J, et al. (2012) Predicted effects of treatment for HCV infection vary among European countries. Gastroenterology 143: 974–985.e14.

19

Activation of TGF-β1 Promoter by Hepatitis C Virus-Induced AP-1 and Sp1: Role of TGF-β1 in Hepatic Stellate Cell Activation and Invasion

Lance D. Presser, Steven McRae, Gulam Waris*

Department of Microbiology and Immunology, H.M. Bligh Cancer Research Laboratories, Rosalind Franklin University of Medicine and Science, Chicago Medical School, Chicago, Illinois, United States of America

Abstract

Our previous studies have shown the induction and maturation of transforming growth factor-beta 1 (TGF-β1) in HCV-infected human hepatoma cells. In this study, we have investigated the molecular mechanism of TGF-β1 gene expression in response to HCV infection. We demonstrate that HCV-induced transcription factors AP-1, Sp1, NF-κB and STAT-3 are involved in TGF-β1 gene expression. Using chromatin immunoprecipitation (ChIP) assay, we further show that AP-1 and Sp1 interact with TGF-b1 promoter in vivo in HCV-infected cells. In addition, we demonstrate that HCV-induced TGF-β1 gene expression is mediated by the activation of cellular kinases such as p38 MAPK, Src, JNK, and MEK1/2. Next, we determined the role of secreted bioactive TGF-β1 in human hepatic stellate cells (HSCs) activation and invasion. Using siRNA approach, we show that HCV-induced bioactive TGF-β1 is critical for the induction of alpha smooth muscle actin (α-SMA) and type 1 collagen, the markers of HSCs activation and proliferation. We further demonstrate the potential role of HCV-induced bioactive TGF-β1 in HSCs invasion/cell migration using a transwell Boyden chamber. Our results also suggest the role of HCV-induced TGF-β1 in HCV replication and release. Collectively, these observations provide insight into the mechanism of TGF-β1 promoter activation, as well as HSCs activation and invasion, which likely manifests in liver fibrosis associated with HCV infection.

Editor: Ching-Ping Tseng, Chang Gung University, Taiwan

Funding: This work was supported in part by the American Cancer Society, Illinois Division, Inc., 09-14, National Institutes of Health/National Institute of Allergy and Infectious Diseases grant R21:A1078532, and by the Rosalind Franklin University of Medicine and Science-H.M. Bligh Cancer Research Fund to G.W. The funders had no role in study design, data collection and analysis, decision to publish, or preparation of the manuscript.

* E-mail: gulam.waris@rosalindfranklin.edu

Introduction

HCV infection causes chronic hepatitis in a significant number of infected individuals, which may gradually progress to liver fibrosis, cirrhosis and subsequently to hepatocellular carcinoma (HCC) [1]. HCV is an enveloped, single-stranded, positive-sense RNA virus which is approximately 9.6 kb in length, contains both 5′ and 3′ untranslated regions (UTRs), and encodes a single polyprotein of about 3000 amino acids [2]. The 5′ UTR contains the internal ribosome entry site (IRES) which is required for cap-independent translation of the polyprotein. The polyprotein is cleaved by host and viral proteases into structural proteins (core, E1, and E2) and nonstructural proteins (p7, NS2, NS3, NS4A, NS4B, NS5A, and NS5B) [2,3]. Until 2005, the studies of molecular mechanisms of HCV replication and pathogenesis had been hampered by the lack of an efficient cell culture system or a suitable small-animal model. The development of a productive HCV (genotype 2a) infection system provided a major breakthrough which allows the production of infectious virions in cell culture [4,5,6].

The molecular mechanisms underlying liver injury and fibrosis in chronic HCV remain unclear. TGF-β1 is the major profibrogenic cytokine which regulates the production and deposition of the major extracellular matrix molecules (ECM) [7]. It has been reported that HCV infection is associated with a significant increase in TGF-β1 expression and secretion in liver and serum respectively [8,9]. Previously, we and others have demonstrated an increased secretion of bioactive TGF-β1 from HCV-infected cells [10,11,12,13,14]. In addition, several other viruses have been shown to activate TGF-β1, and in some cases, TGF-β1 has a positive effect on the replication of the virus [15]. For instance it has been previously reported that TGF-β1 enhances replication of respiratory syncytial virus in lung epithelial cells [16]. Human cytomegalovirus induces TGF-β1 activation in renal tubular epithelial cells after epithelial-to-mesenchymal transition [13]. TGF-β1 has also been shown to play an important role in HIV/HCV co-infection as HIV increases HCV replication in a TGF-β1 dependent manner [11].

TGF-β1 has been shown to be regulated by transcription factors such as AP-1, Sp1, NF-κB, EGR-1, USF, ZF9/core promoter binding protein, and STAT-3 in various experimental systems [10,17,18,19,20,21,22,23,24,25,26,27]. It has been well documented that cellular kinases play key roles in HCV-mediated pathogenesis by activating downstream transcription factors. We and others have shown the activation of various cellular kinases in response to HCV-infection such as JNK, p38 MAPK, ERK, Src,

PI3K and JAK, and these kinases induce transcription factors Nrf2, NF-κB, AP-1, Sp1, HIF-1α, ATF6, SREBPs, and STAT-3 [10,12,17,26,28,29,30,31,32,33,34,35].

Human hepatic stellate cells (HSCs) comprise approximately 15% of all liver cells and are the major cell type involved in liver fibrogenesis [36,37,38]. HSCs are normally in a "quiescent" or quiet state but can become activated by the binding of bioactive TGF-β1 to TGF-β1 receptors on HSCs [37,39]. Upon activation, HSCs up regulate the production of ECM proteins and become invasive [37,39].

In the present study, we first demonstrate the mechanisms of TGF-β1 promoter activation and then the effect of secreted bioactive TGF-β1 on HSC activation and invasion. We show that transcription factors AP-1, Sp1, NF-κB, and STAT-3 play critical role in TGF-β1 gene expression. Furthermore, we demonstrate increased HSCs activation and invasion when HSCs were incubated with conditioned medium (CM) from HCV-infected cells which contain bioactive TGF-β1. We also determined the role of TGF-β1 in HCV production and release. These data collectively demonstrate the mechanisms for TGF-β1 gene expression by HCV infection, and the role of TGF-β1 on HSC activation and invasion which leads to liver fibrosis.

Materials and Methods

Cell Lines

The human hepatoma cell line, Huh-7.5, was obtained from Dr. C. Rice (Rockefeller University, NY) (Blight et al., 2002). Huh-7.5 cells were cultured at 37°C in a humidified atmosphere containing 5% CO_2 with Dulbecco's modified Eagle's medium (DMEM) supplemented with 10% fetal calf serum, 100 U of penicillin/ml, and 100 μg of streptomycin sulfate/ml. The human hepatic stellate cell (HSC) line, LX-2 was obtained from Dr. S. Friedman (Mount Sinai Hospital, NY) [40]. LX-2 cells were cultured in DMEM as described above. For HSCs activation experiments LX-2 cells were serum starved in serum free DMEM for 48 h before use.

Plasmids, Reagents and Antibodies

The infectious J6/JFH-1 cDNA (HCV genotype 2a) was obtained from Dr. C. Rice (Rockefeller University, NY). The TGF-β1 promoter luciferase-reporter plasmids (phTG1 −1362/+11, phTG5 −453/+11, phTG6 −323/+11, phTG7 −175/+11, phTG7-4 −60/+11) were provided by Dr. S. J. Kim (National Cancer Institute, MD) [19,41]. The HCV nonstructural (NS) protein NS3 expression plasmids pFlag-NS3, pFlag-NS3/4A, were provided by Dr. M. Gale (University of Washington, WA) [41]. The wild-type HCV NS5A expression vector was obtained from Dr. A. Siddiqui (University of California San Diego, CA). The dominant negative c-Jun plasmid (pcDNA3.1/His-TAM67) as well as (AP-1)₄-luciferase-reporter construct was obtained from Dr. Nancy Colburn (National Cancer Institute, MD). The dominant negative mutants of STAT-3 (pSG5hSTAT3-β; a mutation at Tyr 705 of STAT-3, and STAT3-S727A, a mutation at Ser 727 of STAT-3), and the STAT-3 reporter plasmid pLucTKS3 (driven by the thymidine kinase promoter with seven copies of upstream STAT-3 binding sites from the human C-reactive protein gene) was obtained from Dr. Richard Jove (Moffitt Cancer Center, FL). The plasmid bearing the IκBα S32A/S36A (Ser to Ala) mutated gene under control of the CMV promoter was obtained from Dr. Robert Scheinman (University of Colorado Health Sciences Center, CO). The plasmid p3x-κB-Luc (luciferase reporter driven by the minimal fos promoter with three upstream NF-κB binding sites from MHC class I) was a generous gift from Dr. J. Martin (University of Colorado at Boulder, CO). All the primary antibodies were used according to the manufacturer's protocol: HCV NS3 (Virogen, MA), α-SMA (Abcam, MA), GAPDH, STAT-3, IκBα, c-jun, c-fos, Sp1 and TGF-β1 (Cell Signaling, MA), furin and TSP-1 (Santa Cruz Biotechnology, CA).

HCV Cell Culture Infection System

The plasmid pFL-J6/JFH1 encoding the HCV J6/JFH-1 genome was linearized with XbaI for in vitro transcription using the Ampliscribe T₇ transcription kit (Epicentre Technologies, WI). Fifteen micrograms of J6/JFH-1 RNA was delivered into Huh-7.5 cells by electroporation as described previously [6,29]. Cells were passaged every 3–5 days; the presence of HCV in these cells and the corresponding supernatants were determined as described

Table 1. Oligonucleotides used in PCR, site-directed mutagenesis, and ChIP assays.

Target genes	Sense Primers	Antisense Primers
*AP-1	5'-TTGTTTCCCAGCCTGACTCTC-3'	5'-TGTGGGTCACCAGAGAAAGAG -3'
*Sp1	5'-AGGAGGCAGCACCCTGTTT-3'	5'-ACCGTCCTCATCTCGCGT-3'
HCV	5'-CGGGAGAGCCATAGTGG-3'	5'-AGTACCACAAGGCCTTTCG-3'
TGFβ-1	5'-CAACAATTCCTGGCGATACC-3'	5'-GAACCCGTTGATGTCCACTT-3'
Col1A1	5'-GGCGGCCAGGGCTCCGAC-3'	5'-AATTCCTGGTCTGGGCACC-3'
Furin	5'-GAGATTGAAAACACCAGCGAA-3'	5'-GCGGTGCCATAGAGTACGAG-3'
TSP-1	5'-GTGTTTGACATCTTTGAACTC-3'	5'-CCAAAGACAAACCTCACATTC-3'
α-SMA	5'-CAGCACCGCCTGGATAGCC-3'	5'-AGGCACCCCTGAACCCGAA-3'
18S rRNA	5'-ACATCCAAGGAA GGCAGCAG-3'	5'-TCGTCACTACCTCCCCGG-3'
HCV Taqman probe	5'-6FAM-CTGCGGAACCGGTGAGTACAC-TAMRA-3'	
Site directed mutagenesis primers: Mutated bases are italicized.		
AP-1	5'-TGTTTCCCAGCCTGG*TT*CTCCTTCCGTTCTGG-3'	5'-AAGGGTCGGACCAAGAGGAAGGCAAGACCCAG-3'
Sp1	5'-AGCCGGGGGAGCC*TA*CCCCCTTTCCCCCAGGG-3'	5'-GCCCCTCGGATGGGGGAAAGGGGGTCCCGAC-3'

*Primers used in ChIP assay.

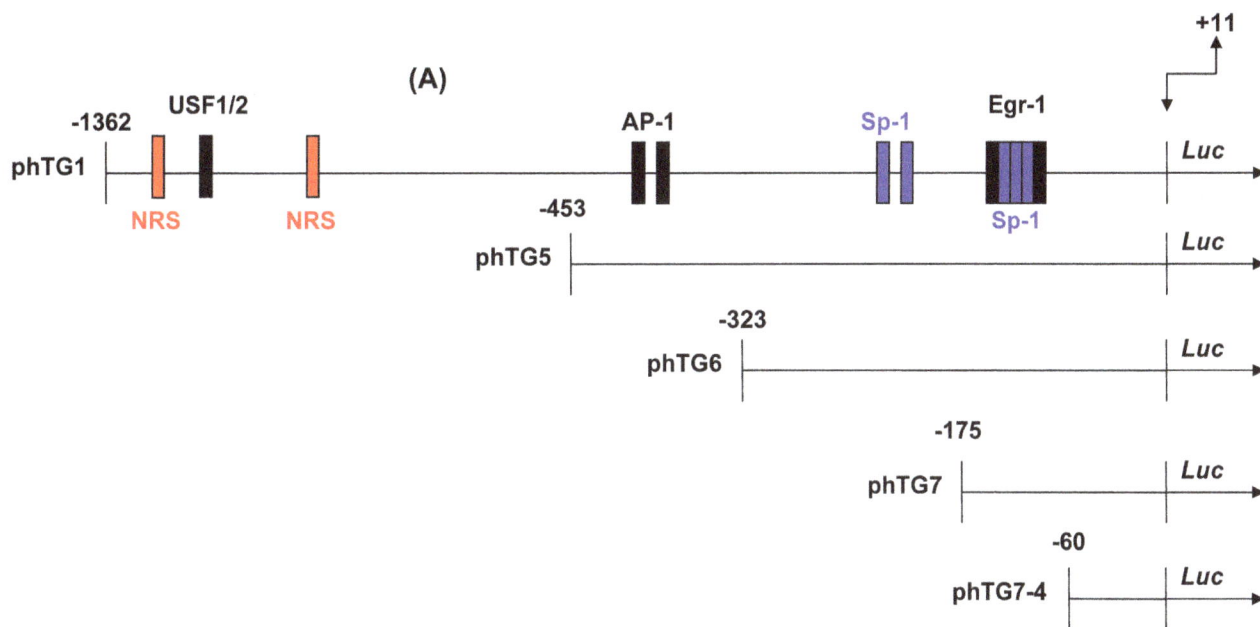

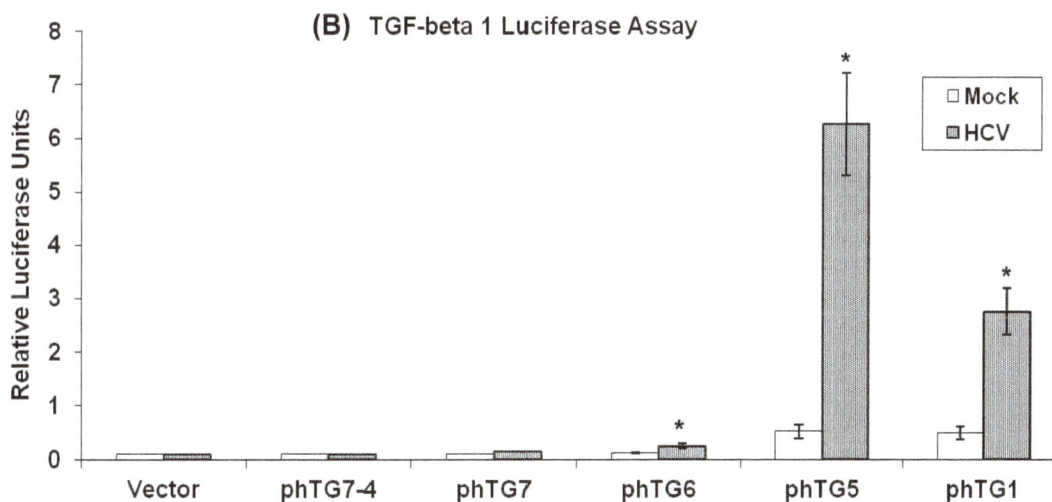

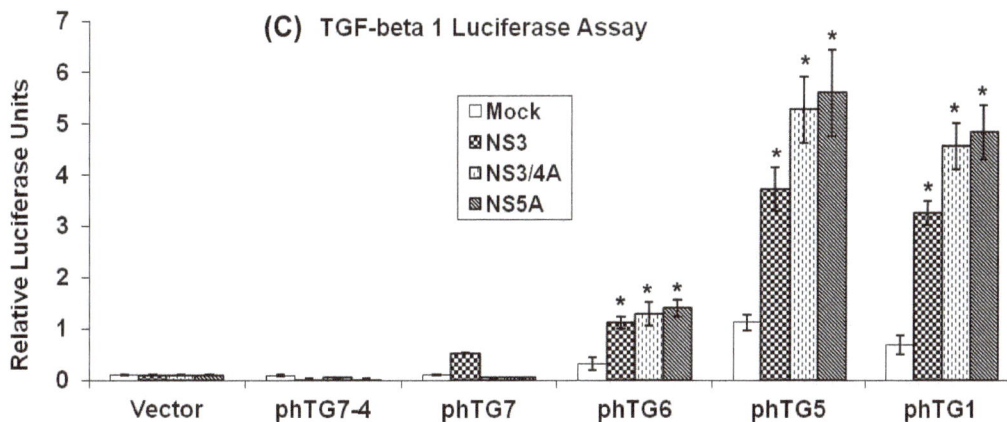

Figure 1. HCV activates TGF-β1 promoter. A) Wild-type TGF-β1 promoter luciferase reporter (phTG1) and various deletion constructs (phTG5, phTG6, phTG7, and phTG7-4) are shown. Two negative regulatory sequences (NRS) are shown in the region between −453 and −1362 as well as an USF1/2 binding region. Two AP-1 binding sites are located between −453 and −323. Two Sp1 binding sites are located between −323 and −175. Three Sp1 sites and two Egr-1 sites are located between −175 and −60. B) Mock- and HCV-infected cells were transfected with TGF-β1 promoter-luciferase reporter constructs (phTG1, TG5, TG6, TG7, TG7-4) or vector control (500 ng) using Lipofectamine 2000 according to the manufacturer's instructions (Invitrogen, CA). At 36 h post transfection cellular lysates were subjected to dual-luciferase reporter assay. The values represent the means standard deviations of three independent experiments performed in triplicate. * denotes p<0.05 compared to mock cells. C) Mock cells were transfected with TGF-β1 promoter-luciferase reporter constructs (phTG1, TG5, TG6, TG7, TG7-4) or vector control (500 ng) along with plasmids expressing HCV NS3, NS3/4A, or NS5A (500 ng), as described above. At 36 h post transfection cellular lysates were subjected to dual-luciferase reporter assay. The values represent the mean standard deviations of three independent experiments performed in triplicate. * denotes p<0.05 compared to mock cells. The data represent luciferase activity relative to mock cells.

previously [6,29]. The cell-free virus was propagated in Huh-7.5 cell cultures, as described previously [4]. The expression of HCV protein in HCV-infected cells was analyzed using western blot assays. The viral titer in cell culture supernatant was expressed as focus forming unit (ffu) ml^{-1}, which was determined by the average number of HCV-NS5A-postitive foci detected at the highest dilutions as described previously [6]. The HCV positive cell culture supernatant was used to infect naive Huh-7.5 cells at appropriate dilutions (moi of 1) for 5–6 h at 37°C and 5% CO_2 [12,29]. Cells were then plated in complete DMEM for 5–7 days. In most of the experiments, HCV-infected cells at day 6–7 were used. The cell culture supernatant collected from Huh-7.5 cells expressing JFH-1/GND (replication defective virus) was used as a negative control.

Western Blotting

Cells were harvested and cellular lysates were prepared by incubating in radioimmune precipitation (RIPA) buffer (50 mM Tris-HCl, pH 7.5, 150 mM NaCl, 1% NP-40, 0.5% sodium deoxycholate, 0.1% SDS, 1 mM sodium orthovanadate, 1 mM sodium formate, and 10 μl/ml protease inhibitor cocktail (Thermo Scientific, IL) for 30 min on ice. Cellular lysates were subjected to SDS-PAGE. Gels were electroblotted on to nitrocellulose membrane (Thermo Scientific, IL) in 25 mM Tris, 192 mM glycine and 20% methanol. Membranes were incubated for 1 h in blocking buffer [20 mM Tris-HCl, pH 7.5, 150 mM NaCl, 0.5% Tween-20, 5% dry milk], probed with primary antibody for 1 h at room temperature (RT) and washed twice for 10 min with blocking buffer without milk followed by incubation with secondary antibody for 1 h at RT. After an additional washing step with blocking buffer, immunoblots were visualized using the Odyssey Infrared Imaging System (LI-COR Biosciences, NE).

Preparation of Nuclear Lysates

Mock and HCV-infected cells were washed with ice-cold PBS and lysed in hypotonic buffer (20 mM HEPES, pH 7.9, 10 mM KCl, 0.1 mM Na$_3$VO$_4$, 1 mM EDTA, 10% glycerol, 1 mM PMSF, 3 mg/ml aprotinin, 1 mg/ml pepstatin, 20 mM NaF and 1 mM DTT with 0.2% NP-40) on ice for 15 min followed by centrifugation at 4°C for 1 min. The nuclear pellet was washed one time with ice-cold PBS and resuspended in high salt buffer (hypotonic buffer with 20% glycerol and 420 mM NaCl) at 4°C by rocking for 30 min. After centrifugation for 5 min the clarified nuclear lysates were used for electrophoretic mobility shift assay.

Electrophoretic Mobility Shift Assay (EMSA)

EMSA were performed using the Odyssey infrared EMSA kit according to the manufacturer's protocols (LI-COR Biosciences). The duplex oligonucleotides containing the putative AP-1 and Sp1 binding sites on human TGF-β1 promoter (AP-1; 5′-CTTGTTTCCCAGCC*TGACTCT*CCTTCCGTTCT-3′; Sp1; 5′-AGCCGGGGAGC*CCGCCCCC*TTTCCCCCAGGG-3′ the

AP-1 and Sp1 binding sites are italicized) were labeled at 5′-end with IRDye 700 infrared dye (Integrated DNA Technologies). For mobility shift assay, equal amounts of nuclear lysates (10 μg) were incubated with 50 nM of IRDye 700 labeled probes. The competition reactions were performed with a 200-fold molar excess of unlabeled consensus probe prior to addition of labeled probe. The supershift was performed by incubation of nuclear lysate and probe complex with antibody for 20 min. The DNA-protein complexes were resolved by 5% polyacrylamide gel electrophoresis in 0.5 X TBE buffer. The gels were visualized using a LI-COR Odyssey imaging system.

Chromatin Immunoprecipitation (ChIP) Assay

The ChIP assay was performed using SimpleChIP Enzymatic Chromatin IP Kit (Cell Signaling, Cat#9003). Briefly, mock- and HCV-infected cells (5×10^7 cells) were fixed in 1% formaldehyde for 10 min to crosslink the DNA and the DNA-associated-proteins. The reaction was quenched using 125 nM glycine for 5 min. The cell pellet was washed two times with ice-cold PBS and suspended in ice-cold buffer A containing DTT, PMSF and protease inhibitor cocktail. The nuclei were pelleted by centrifugation at 3,000 rpm for 5 min at 4°C. The supernants were removed and the pellet was suspended in ice-cold buffer B+ DTT. The lysate was incubated with 5 μl micrococcal nuclease for 20 min at 37°C to digest DNA to length approximately to 150–900 bp. The samples were suspended in 1X ChIP buffer and sonicated for 30 seconds using Qsonica Q700. The sonicated lysate was centrifuged at 10,000 rpm for 10 min at 4°C to remove debris. The supernatant (cross-linked chromatin preparation) were incubated with anti-c-Jun (1:50), c-Fos (1:50) and Sp1 (1:100) antibody or a normal rabbit IgG followed by an isolation procedure using Protein G magnetic beads. The DNA-protein interaction was reversed by heating to 65°C for 12 h. The AP-1 and Sp1 binding sites on the immunoprecipitated DNA was determined by quantitative RT-PCR using SYBR green dye and AP-1 and Sp1 primers (Table 1). The PCR products were visualized on 1% agarose gel stained with 0.5 μg/ml ethidium bromide.

Lipid Droplet Staining

Mock- and HCV-infected cells on glass cover slips were fixed with 4% paraformaldehyde and permeabilized as described above. The cells were incubated with a fluorescent dye; BODIPY 493/503 (4,4-difluoro-3a,4a-diaza-s-indacene) (Invitrogen, CA) for lipid droplet staining. After washing with PBS, cells were mounted with antifade reagent containing DAPI (4, 6-diamidino-2 phenylindole) (Invitrogen, CA) and observed under a laser scanning confocal microscope (Zeiss LSM 510).

RNA Interference

Mock- and HCV-infected cells were transfected with TGF-β1 siRNA (siTGF-β1), sifurin, siTSP-1 and siGFP according to the

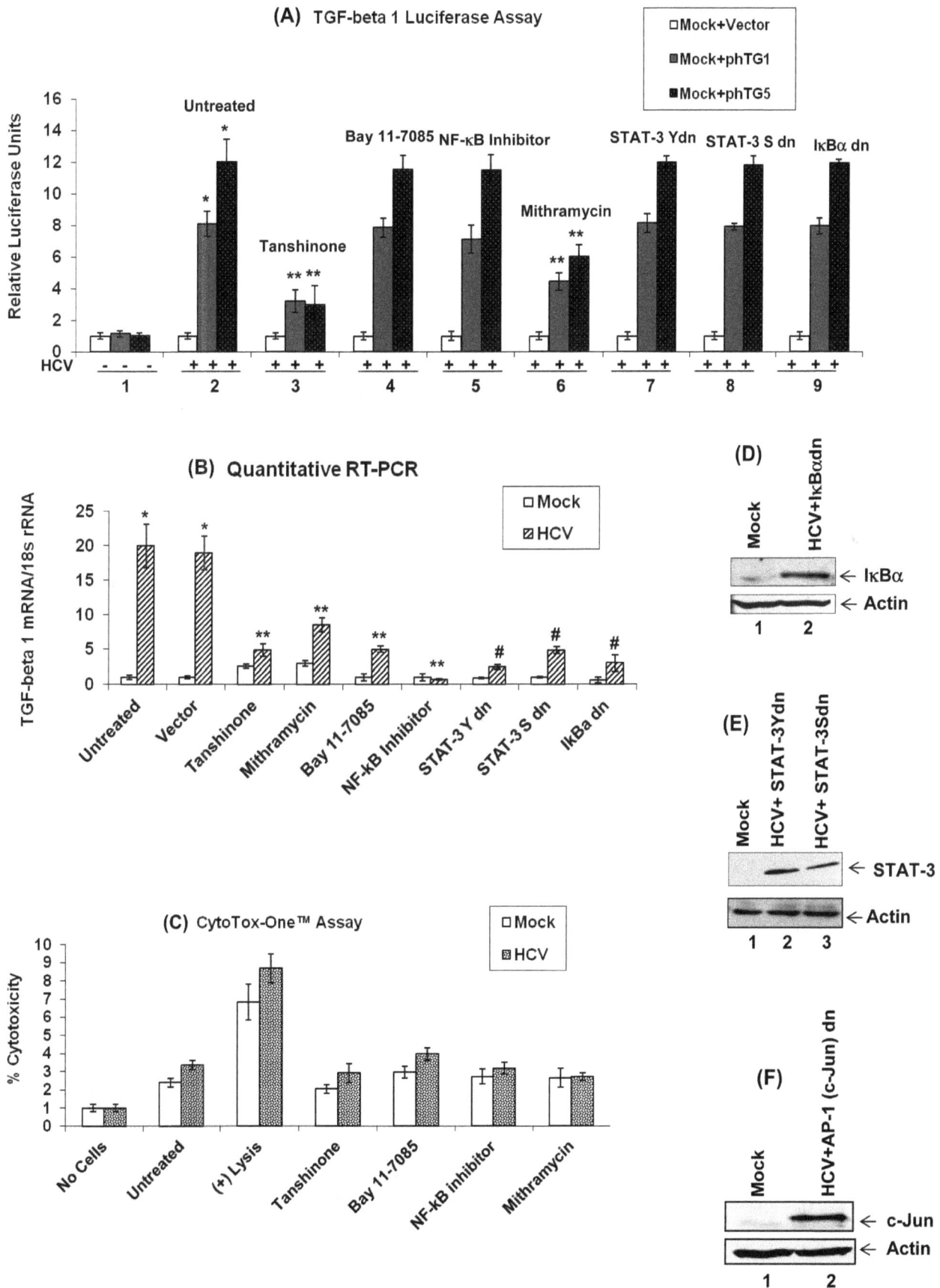

(A) TGF-beta 1 Luciferase Assay

□Mock+Vector
■Mock+phTG1
■Mock+phTG5

(B) Quantitative RT-PCR

□Mock
▨HCV

(C) CytoTox-One™ Assay

□Mock
▨HCV

(D)

(E)

(F)

Figure 2. Role of HCV-induced transcription factors on TGF-β1 promoter activation. A) Mock- and HCV-infected cells were transfected with 500 ng of wild-type (phTG1 −1362/+11), deletion mutant (phTG5 −453/+11) TGF-β1 promoter-luciferase reporter constructs and vector control. At 36 h posttransfection, cells were incubated with inhibitors of AP-1 (Bar#1; Tanshinone IIA, 80 μM), IkB kinase (Bar#4 and 5; Bay 11-7085, 80 μM and NF-κB activation inhibitor 80 μM), and Sp1 (Bar# 6; Mithramycin A, 100 μM) as described in Materials and Methods. Mock- and HCV-infected cells were also transfected with 500 ng of TGF-β1 promoter-luciferase reporter and 500 ng of the dominant negative mutants of STAT-3 (Bar#7; pSG5hSTAT3-β; mutation of STAT-3 tyrosine phosphorylation site 705 into phenylalanine; Bar#8; STAT3-S727A; mutation of STAT-3 serine phosphorylation site 727 into alanine) and the inhibitory subunit of NF-κB (Bar#9; IkBα S32A/S36A; mutation of IkBα serine 32,36 into alanine). Cellular lysates were subjected to dual-luciferase reporter assay. The values represent the means standard deviations of three independent experiments performed in triplicate. * denotes $p<0.05$ compared to mock cells. ** denotes $p<0.05$ compared to untreated promoter. B) Mock- and HCV-infected cells were treated with the inhibitors and dn mutants as described above. Total cellular RNA was extracted and TGF-β1 mRNA was analyzed using TGF-β1 specific primers and SYBR green probe. The values represent the means standard deviations of three independent experiments performed in triplicate. * denotes $p<0.05$ compared to mock cells. ** denotes $p<0.05$ compared to untreated promoter. # denotes $p<0.05$ compared to vector control. C) Mock- and HCV-infected cells were treated with inhibitors or transfected with dominant negative mutants as described above. Samples were tested for cytotoxicity using CytoToxONE homogenous membrane integrity assay as described in Materials and Methods. The data represent luciferase activity relative to mock cells. D, E, and F) HCV-infected cells were transfected with vectors expressing dominant negative proteins of IkBα (IkBα S32A/S36A), STAT-3 (pSG5hSTAT3-β and STAT3-S727A), and AP-1 (pcDNA3.1/His-TAM67). At 48 h posttransfection, cellular lysates were prepared and subjected to western blot analysis using anti-IkBα, STAT-3, and c-Jun antibodies. Actin was used as a protein loading control.

manufacturer's protocol (Santa Cruz Biotechnology, CA). Each siRNA consists of pools of three to five target-specific 19–25 nt siRNA designed to knockdown the target gene expression. For each transfection, two solutions were prepared. Solution A: 60 pmol of siRNA duplex was mixed with 100 μl siRNA transfection medium. Solution B: 6 μl of transfection reagent was added to 100 μl siRNA transfection medium. Solutions A and B were allowed to incubate at RT for 20 min. Solutions A and B were combined, and allowed to incubate another 20 min at RT. The combined solutions were then added to the cells in six well plates, and then incubated for 5 h at 37°C and 5% CO_2, and the transfection solution was replaced with complete DMEM growth media.

Luciferase Assay

Mock- and HCV-infected Huh-7.5 cells were transfected with wild-type and mutant TGF-β1 promoter-luciferase constructs. At 36 h post transfection, cells were serum starved for 4–5 h. Cells were harvested and cellular lysates were analyzed for luciferase activity using the dual-luciferase reporter assay kit (Promega, WI). All transfections included a renilla expression vector to serve as an internal control. In all the experiments the data represent luciferase activity relative to mock cells.

Inhibitor Treatments

The cells were serum starved for 4 h and treated with inhibitors against p38 MAPK (SB203580, 10 μM), JNK (SP600125, 30 μM), PI3K (LY294002, 50 μM), Src (SU6656, 10 μM), JAK 2/3 (AG490, 100 μM), and MEK1/2 (UO126, 20 μM) (Calbiochem, MA) at indicated concentrations for 12 h. The cells were also treated with inhibitors against transcription factors AP-1 (Tanshinone IIA, 80 μM) (Enzo, NY), phosphorylation of IkBα/NF-κB pathway (Bay 11-7085, 80 μM) (Calbiochem, MA), NF-κB (80 μM) (Cat# 481406; Calbiochem, MA) and SP1 (Mithramycin A, 100 μM) (Sigma, MO).

TGF-β1 ELISA

The cell culture supernatant from mock- and HCV-infected cells were harvested, and centrifuged at 1000 rpm for 10 min to remove cell debris. After centrifugation, the conditioned medium (CM) were collected. The secreted TGF-β1 protein in CM was determined by ELISA according to the manufacturer's protocol (Promega, WI). A standard curve was constructed by serial dilutions of human recombinant TGF-β1. TGF-β1 levels were measured in triplicate determinations.

Detection of Bioactive TGF-β1 Using Mink Lung Epithelial Cell Luciferase Assay

Mink lung epithelial cells (MLECs) containing bioactive TGF-β1 sensitive plasminogen activator inhibitor promoter-luciferase construct (PAI/L) was a kind gift from Dr. D. B. Rifkin and were assayed as previously described [12,42,43]. The assay is based on the ability of bioactive TGF-β1 to bind to MLEC receptors. This results in a dose-dependent increase in luciferase activity. Briefly, MLEC were plated in 96 well plates at a concentration of 2.5×10^5 cells per well in regular DMEM and incubated for 24 h at 37°C. Next, cells were incubated with CM from HCV-infected cells for 24–48 h. Cells were then washed twice with PBS, and lysed with 50 μl of reporter lysis buffer (Promega, WI). Twenty microliter of cell extract and 90 μl of luciferase assay reagent were added to 96 well white opaque flat bottom plate and light emission is measured for 10 s in a Bio-TEK Synergy HT Multi-Detection microplate reader. TGF-β1 standards were prepared by adding 2 μl human recombinant TGF-β1 to 500 μl of 0.2% FBS DMEM into a polypropylene tube. The standard stock solution is then serially diluted to obtain standards from 1000–125 pg/ml.

Quantitative Real-time RT-PCR

Total RNA was extracted from mock- and HCV-infected cells using TRIzol (Invitrogen, CA). HCV RNA was quantified by real-time RT-PCR using an ABI PRISM 7500 Sequence Detector (Applied Biosystems, CA). Amplifications were conducted in triplicate using HCV specific primers and 6-carboxyfluorescein (6FAM)- and tetrachloro-6-carboxyfluorescein (TAMRA)-labeled probes (Applied Biosystems, CA). The sequences for the primers and probes were designed using Primer Express software (Applied Biosystems, CA) (Table 1). Amplification reactions were performed in a 25 μl mix using RT-PCR core reagents kit and the template RNA. Reactions were performed in a 96-well spectrofluorometric thermal cycler under the following conditions: 2 min at 50°C, 30 min at 60°C, 10 min at 95°C, 44 cycles of 20 s at 95°C and 1 min at 62°C. Fluorescence was monitored during every PCR cycle at the annealing step. At the termination of each PCR run, the data was analyzed by the automated system and amplification plots were generated. To determine the HCV RNA copy number, standards ranging from 10^1 to 10^8 copies/μg were used for comparison.

SYBR Green RT-PCR

The expression of cellular genes in mock- and HCV-infected cells were quantified by real-time RT-PCR using their respective primers (Table 1). Total cellular RNA was extracted using TRIzol

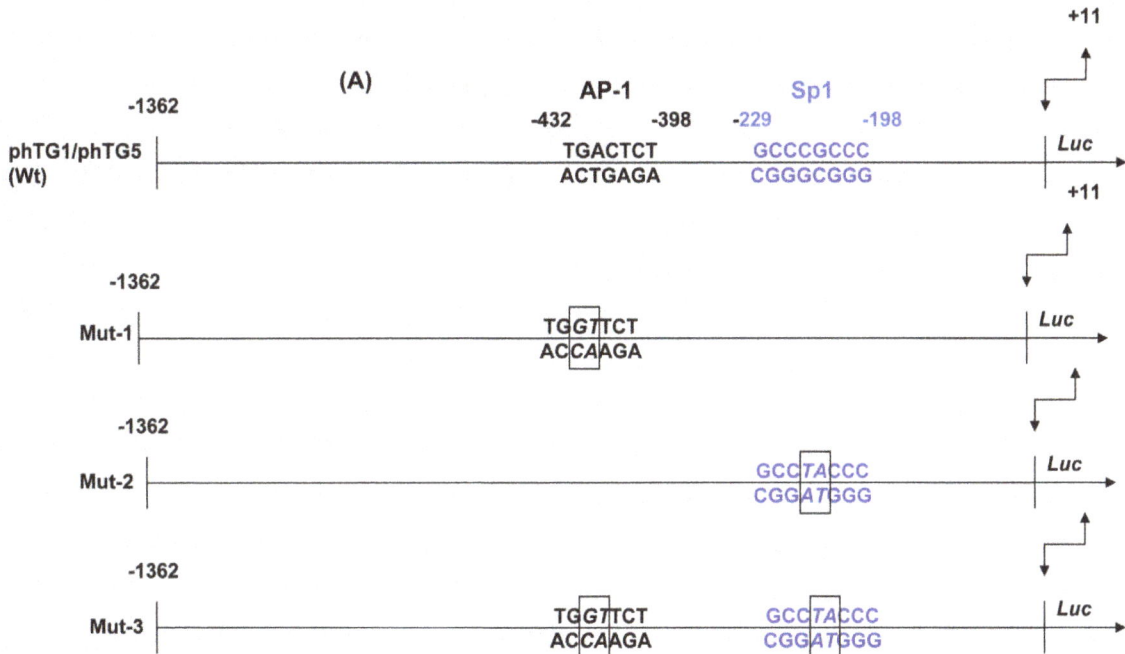

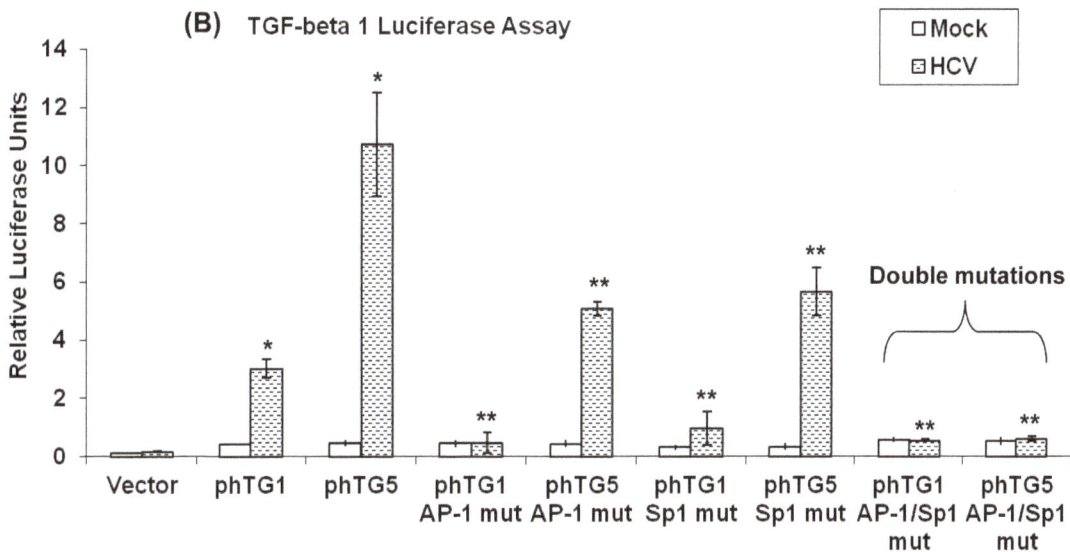

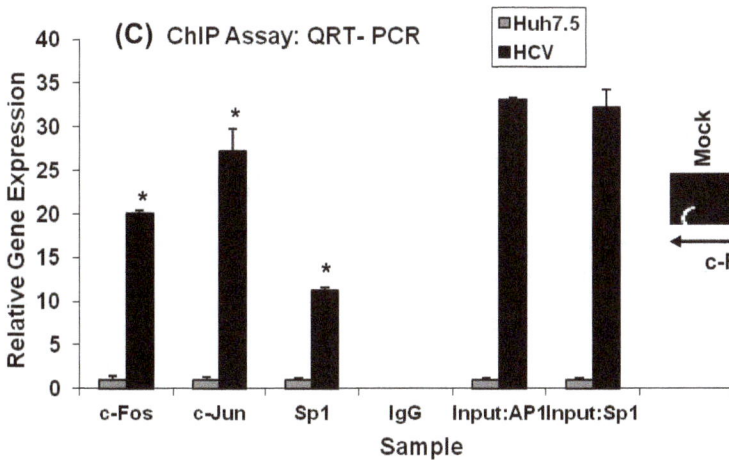

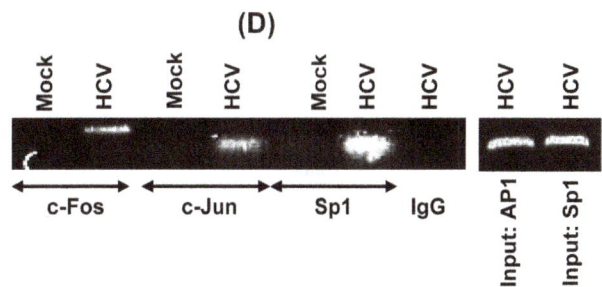

Figure 3. Mutational analysis of AP-1 and Sp1 binding sites on TGF-β1 promoter-luciferase reporter. A) AP-1 and Sp1 binding sites on TGF-β1 promoter sequences were deduced from sequence data as described previously [19]. The pGL3 vector includes the wild-type TGF-β1 fragment −1362/+11 fused to the luciferase gene and was used as a template for the site-directed mutagenesis as described in Materials and Methods. The AP-1 and Sp1 binding site were mutated by a change of two bases in the consensus sequence as indicated. Substituted bases are italicized and highlighted with a box. The wild-type and mutated plasmids used for the transfection experiments are shown. B) Mock- and HCV-infected cells were transfected with 500 ng of the wild-type phTG1 and phTG5 and mutant TGF-β1 luciferase constructs (Mut-1, Mut-2, Mut-3). At 36 h posttransfection cellular lysates were harvested and subjected to dual-luciferase reporter assay. The values represent the means standard deviations of three independent experiments performed in triplicate. * denotes p<0.05 compared to mock cells. ** denotes p<0.05 compared to wild type phTG1 and phTG5 constructs. C) Cross-linked chromatin preparation from mock and HCV-infected cells were immunoprecipitated with anti-c-Jun, c-Fos and Sp1 antibody or a normal rabbit IgG. The AP-1 and Sp1 binding sites on the immunoprecipitated DNA was determined by quantitative RT-PCR using the primers and SYBR green probe. Amplification of input chromatin (input) prior to immunoprecipitation were served as positive controls for chromatin extraction and PCR amplification. Chromatin immunoprecipitation using a non-specific antibody (normal human IgG) served as negative controls. The data represent luciferase activity relative to mock cells. The values represent the means standard deviations of three independent experiments performed in triplicate. * denotes p<0.05 compared to mock cells. D) Five microliters of the PCR products were visualized on 1% agarose gel stained with 0.5 μg/ml ethidium bromide.

and treated with DNase using RQ1 RNase-free DNase prior to cDNA production. The cDNA was reverse-transcribed from 1 μg of total RNA using oligo(dT) primers according to the manufacturer's protocol (Applied Biosystems, CA). Quantitative RT-PCR was carried out using SYBR green master mix and specific primer sets. Amplification reactions were performed under the following conditions: 2 min at 50°C, 10 min at 95°C, 40 cycles for 15 s at 95°C, and 1 min at 60°C. Relative transcript levels were calculated using ΔΔCt method as specified by the manufacturer.

Site-directed Mutagenesis

The base substitution mutations of AP-1 and Sp1 binding sites on TGF-β1 promoter-luciferase reporter constructs were carried out by oligonucleotide-mediated mutagenesis as described previously [44]. Site-directed mutagenesis was performed using AP-1 and Sp1 primers (Table 1). The PCR reactions were performed with wild-type TGF-β1 promoter-luciferase construct and AP-1 and Sp1 mutagenesis primers according to the manufacturer's protocol (Stratagene, CA). Briefly, reaction buffer (5 μL), dsDNA template (30 ng), oligonucleotide primers (125 ng each), dNTP mix (1 μL), 1 μL PfuTurbo DNA polymerase (2.5 U/μL), and 35 μL ddH2O were added to a final volume of 50 μL. PCR amplification reactions were performed under the following conditions: Segment 1, 1 cycle at 95°C for 30 s; Segment 2, 16 cycles at 95°C for 30 s; 55°C for 1 minute, 68°C for 8 min. At the end of reaction, samples were digested with DpnI and transformed into DH5α competent cells (Invitrogen, CA). Clones were tested by restriction digestion and the base substitution mutations were confirmed by DNA sequencing.

CytoTox-ONE™ Homogeneous Membrane Integrity Assay

Mock- and HCV-infected cells in 96-well plates were treated with various inhibitors. The assay plate was equilibrated to RT for 20–30 min. CytoTox-ONE reagent (Promega, WI) was added into the wells and incubated at RT while shaking for 30 seconds. Plate was next incubated at RT for 10 min without shaking. 50 μl stop solution was added to each well in the same order as CytoTox-ONE reagent. Plate was again incubated at RT while shaking for 10 seconds. Fluorescence was recorded with an excitation wavelength of 560 nm and emission wavelength of 590 nm. Cytotoxicity was calculated by subtracting the average fluorescence values of the culture medium background from all fluorescence values of the experimental wells. The average fluorescence values from kinase inhibitor treated cells were used to calculate the percent cytotoxicity for a given experimental treatment. Percent cytotoxicity = 100 × (experimental - culture

medium background)/(maximum LDH release – culture medium background). The cytotoxicity levels were measured in triplicate.

CytoSelect™ 24-well Cell Invasion Assay

Conditioned medium from mock- and HCV-infected cells transfected with siTGF-β1, and siGFP were collected. LX-2 cells were plated at a concentration of 1×10^6 cells/ml in serum free DMEM for 48 h in the upper chamber. Five hundred micro liters CM from mock- and HCV-infected cells transfected with siTGF-β1, and siGFP were placed into the lower chamber to stimulate cell invasion. Following incubation for 48 h at 37°C in 5% CO2 atmosphere, media was carefully aspirated from the insert. Cotton-tipped swabs were used to gently swab the interior of the inserts to remove non-invasive cells. Next, inserts were transferred to a clean well containing 400 μL of cell stain solution and incubated for 10 min at RT. Inserts were then washed several times in ddH2O and allowed to dry. Next, inserts were transferred to an empty well and 200 μL of extraction solution was added to the lower chamber of each well and incubated at RT for 10 min on an orbital shaker. One hundred micro-molar of each sample was transferred to a 96-well microtiter plate and the absorbance was recorded at 560 nm.

Statistical Analysis

Error bars show the standard deviations of the means of data from three individual trials. Two-tailed unpaired t-tests were used to compare experimental conditions to those of the respective controls. The significance level was set at p value of 0.05.

Results

HCV Activates TGF-β1 Promoter

In our previous studies we have shown the induction and maturation of TGF-β1 by HCV infection [12]. In this study, we sought to investigate the molecular mechanism(s) of TGF-β1 promoter activation leading to the secretion of bioactive TGF-β1, activation and invasion of human HSCs. To initiate this study, we have incubated human hepatoma cell line Huh-7.5 cells with HCV cell culture supernatant as described previously [12,28,29]. Mock- and HCV-infected cells were transiently-transfected with wild-type (phTG1 −1362/+11) and various deletion mutants of TGF-β1 promoter-luciferase reporter constructs (phTG5 −453/+11, phTG6 −323/+11, phTG7 −175/+11, phTG7-4 −60/+11) (Fig. 1A). We observed approximately 6 fold and 3 fold increase in luciferase activity by phTG5 and phTG1 respectively in HCV-infected cells compared to mock-infected cells (Fig. 1B). However, we did not observe TGF-β1 promoter-luciferase activation in cells transfected with deletion mutants (phTG7, and phTG7-4). These results suggest that the region between −1362 to −323 is

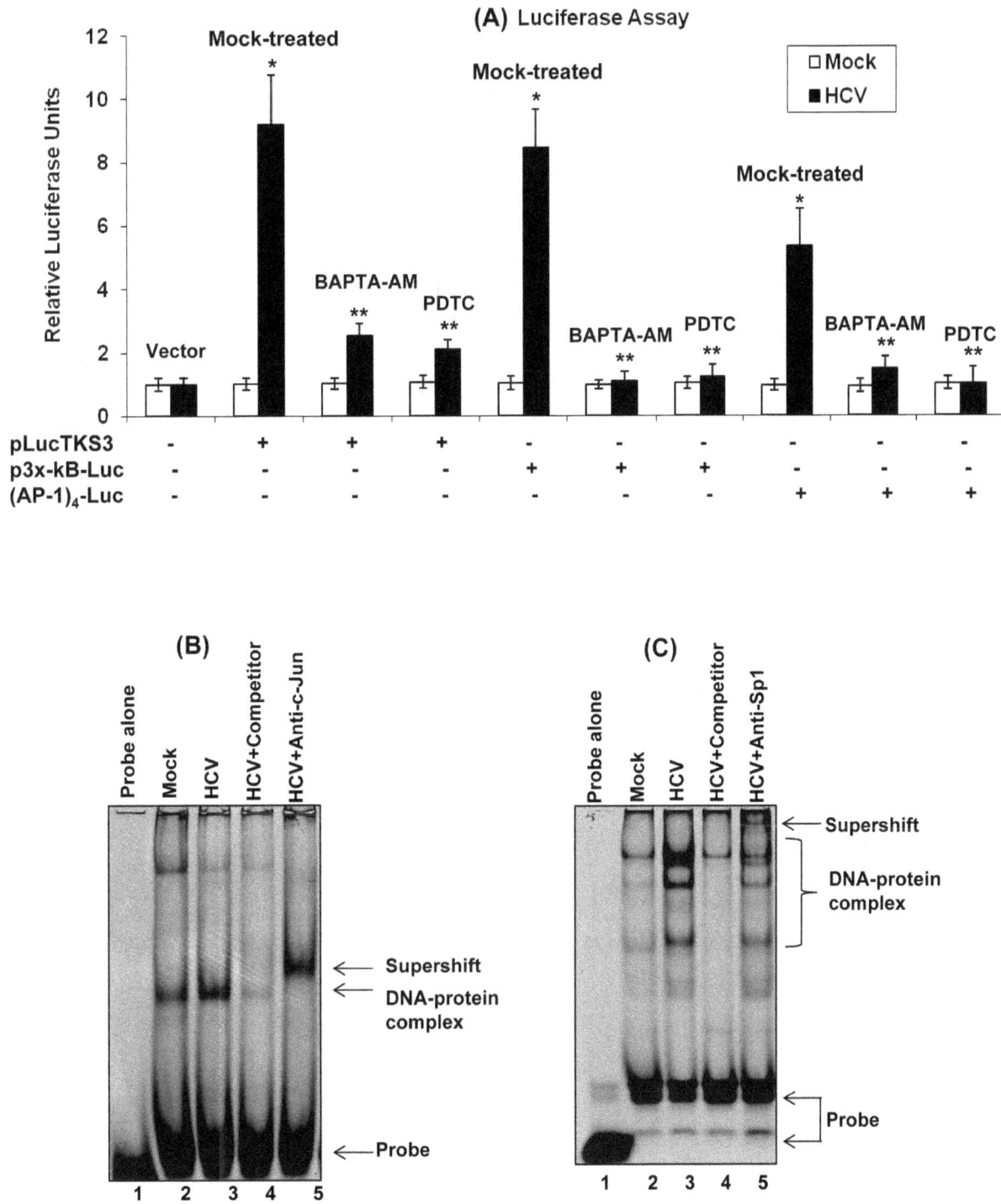

Figure 4. Effect of HCV-induced signaling pathways on transcription factor activation. A) Mock- and HCV-infected cells were transfected with 500 ng of pLucTKS3, p3x-κB-Luc, or (AP-1)₄-Luc reporter constructs. At 36 h posttransfection cells were treated with intracellular calcium chelator (BAPTA-AM, 50 μM) or antioxidant (PDTC, 100 μM). Cellular lysates were harvested and subjected to dual-luciferase reporter assay. The values represent the means standard deviations of three independent experiments performed in triplicate. *denotes p<0.05 compared to mock cells. **denotes p<0.05 compared to HCV-infected mock-treated with inhibitors. The data represent luciferase activity relative to mock cells. B and C) EMSA was carried out in the presence of IRDye 700-labeled oligonucleotides derived from TGF-β1 promoter (contains AP-1 and Sp1 binding sites) and nuclear lysates from mock (Huh7.5) and HCV-infected cells. Lane 1, probe alone; lanes 2 and 3, equal amounts of nuclear lysates from mock and HCV-infected cells; lane 4, same as lane 3 but incubated with 200-fold excess of unlabeled oligonucleotides; lane 5, DNA-protein complex incubated with anti-c-Jun or anti-Sp1 for 20 min at RT.

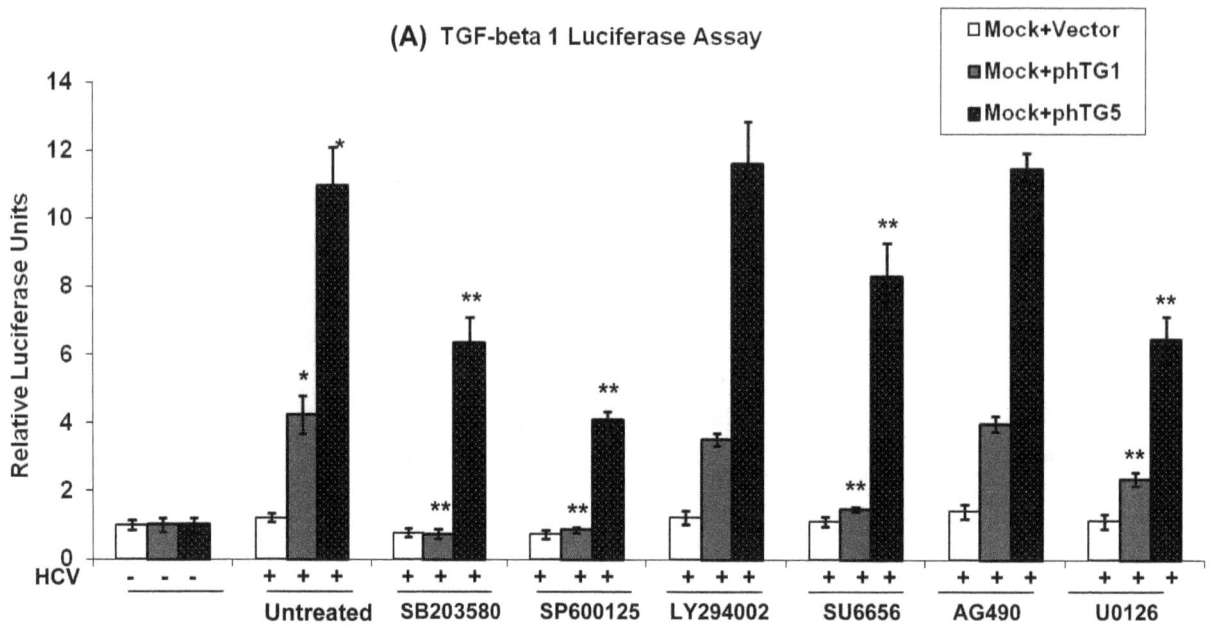

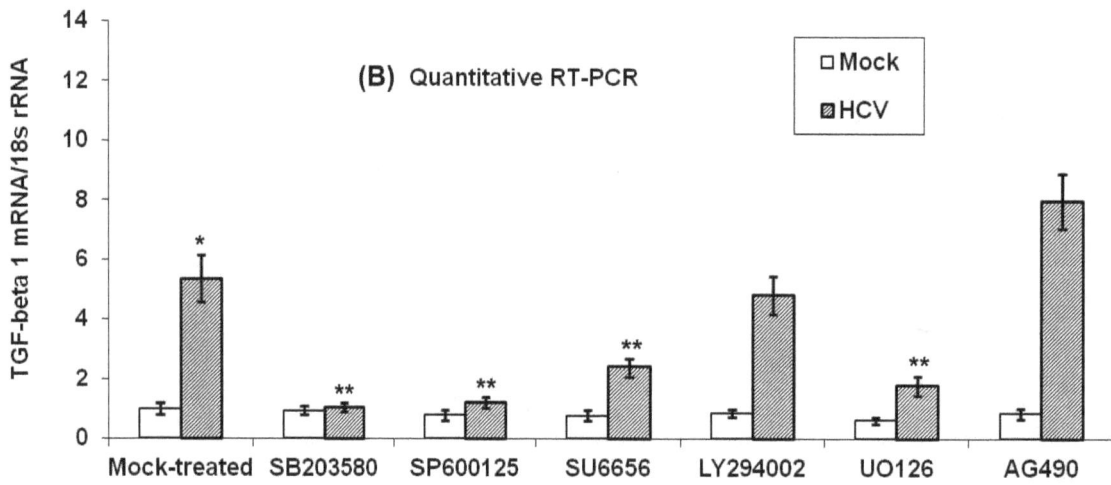

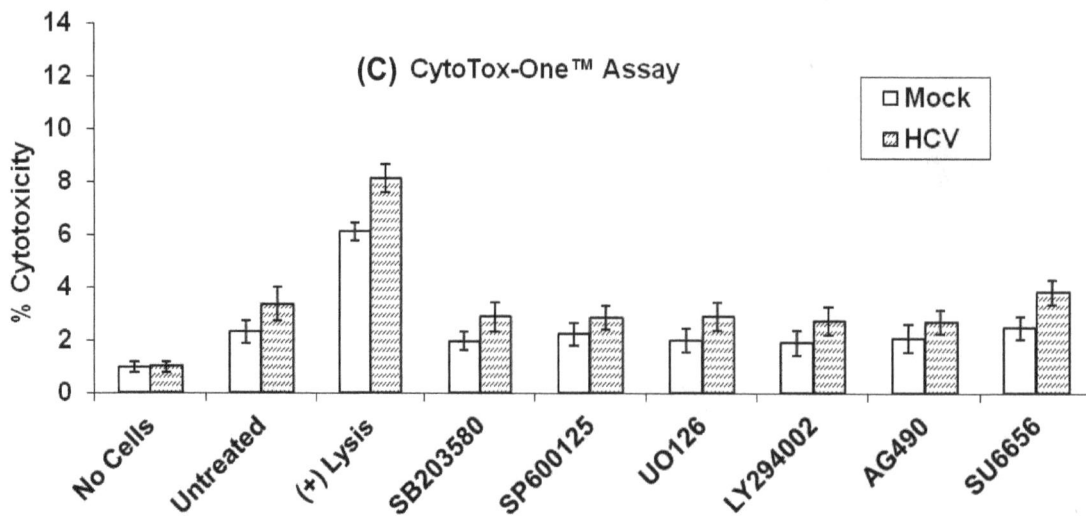

Figure 5. Role of HCV-induced cellular kinases on TGF-β1 promoter activation. A) Mock- and HCV-infected cells were transfected with 500 ng of phTG1 and phTG5 TGF-β1 promoter-luciferase reporter. At 36 h posttransfection cells were serum starved for 4 h and treated with inhibitors against p38 MAPK (SB203580, 10 μM), JNK (SP600125, 30 μM), PI3K (LY294002, 50 μM), Src (SU6656, 10 μM), JAK 2/3 (AG490, 100 μM), and MEK1/2 (UO126, 20 μM) for 12 h. Cellular lysates were subjected to dual-luciferase reporter assay. The values represent the means standard deviations of three independent experiments performed in triplicate. *denotes p<0.05 compared to mock cells. **denotes p<0.05 compared to HCV-infected mock-treated cells. B) Mock- and HCV-infected cells were treated with kinase inhibitors as described in Materials and Methods. Total cellular RNA was extracted and TGF-β1 mRNA was analyzed using TGF-β1 specific primers and SYBR green fluorescent dye. The values represent the means standard deviations of three independent experiments performed in triplicate. *denotes p<0.05 compared to mock cells. **denotes p<0.05 compared to HCV-infected mock-treated cells. C) Mock- and HCV-infected cells were treated with kinase inhibitors as described in Materials and Methods. Cells were subjected to growth inhibition assay using CytoToxONE homogenous membrane integrity assay as described in Materials and Methods.

responsible for the TGF-β1 promoter-luciferase activation in HCV-infected cells.

Previously, we have shown that HCV nonstructural (NS) proteins (NS3, NS3/4A, and NS5A) were able to induce TGF-β1 activation and secretion [12]. To demonstrate the effect of HCV NS3, NS3/4A, and NS5A on TGF-β1 promoter activation, Huh-7.5 cells were cotransfected with TGF-β1 promoter-luciferase reporter constructs along with HCV NS3, NS3/4A, and NS5A expression vectors. The results show increased luciferase activity of phTG5 and phTG1 by NS3, NS3/4A, and NS5A (Fig. 1C).

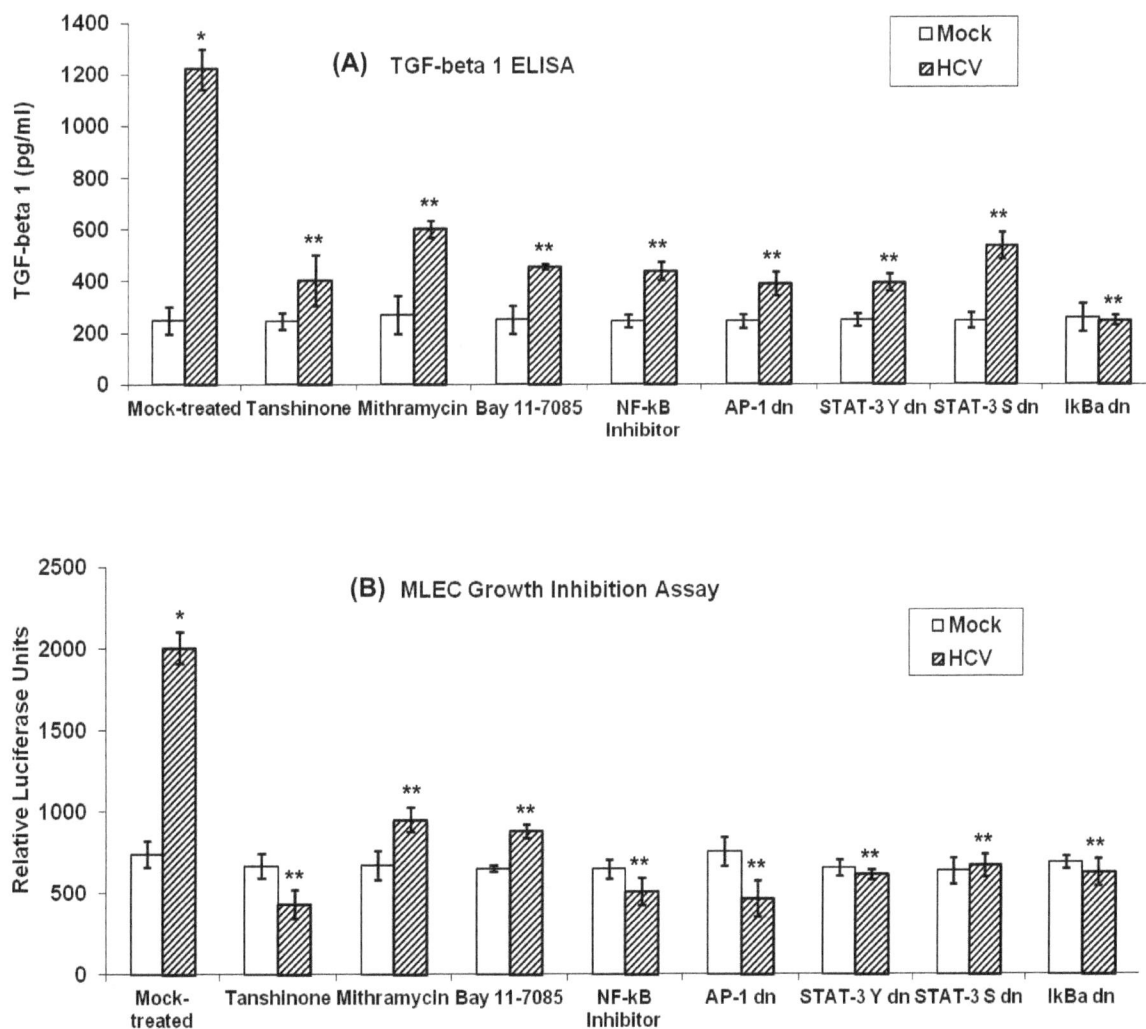

Figure 6. Effect of HCV-induced transcription factors on TGF-β1 secretion. A) Mock- and HCV-infected cells were treated with inhibitors of AP-1, Sp1, IkB kinase or transfected with dn mutants of AP-1, STAT-3, or IkBα. At 36 h posttransfection, total secreted TGF-β1 in CM were determined by TGF-β1 specific ELISA. The values represent the means standard deviations of three independent experiments performed in triplicate. *denotes p<0.05 compared to mock cells. **denotes p<0.05 compared to HCV-infected mock-treated cells. B) CM as described above, were subjected to growth inhibition assay using mink lung epithelial cells as described in Materials and Methods. The data shown here represent the means standard deviations of three independent experiments performed in triplicate. *denotes p<0.05 compared to mock cells. **denotes p<0.05 compared to HCV-infected mock-treated cells.

(A) Quantitative RT-PCR

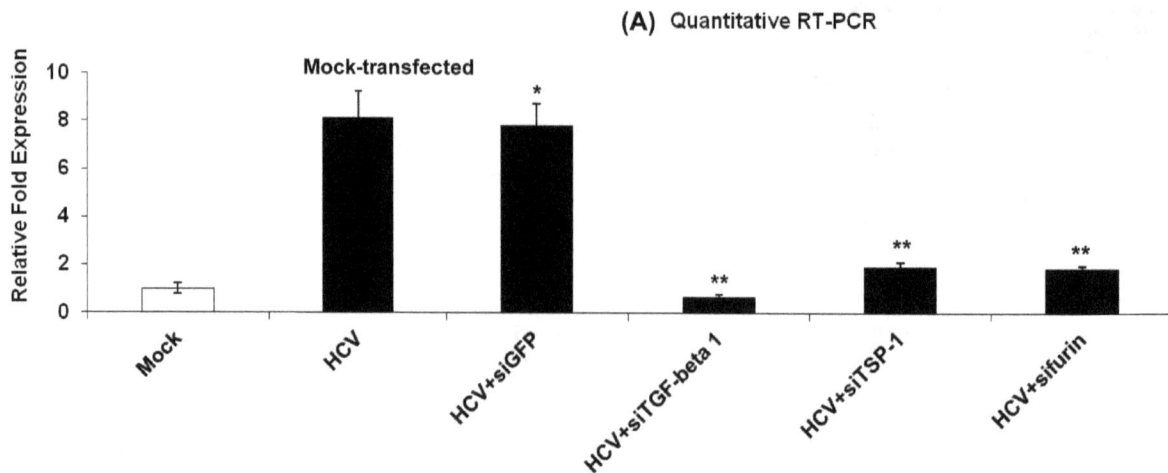

(B)

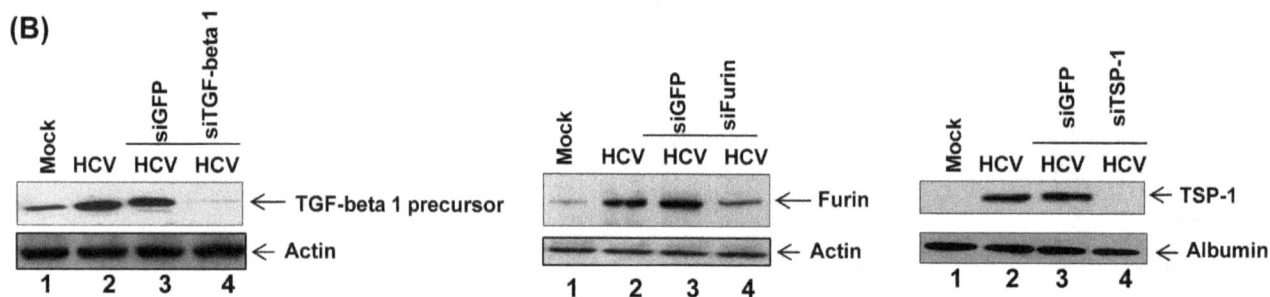

(C) Quantitative RT-PCR

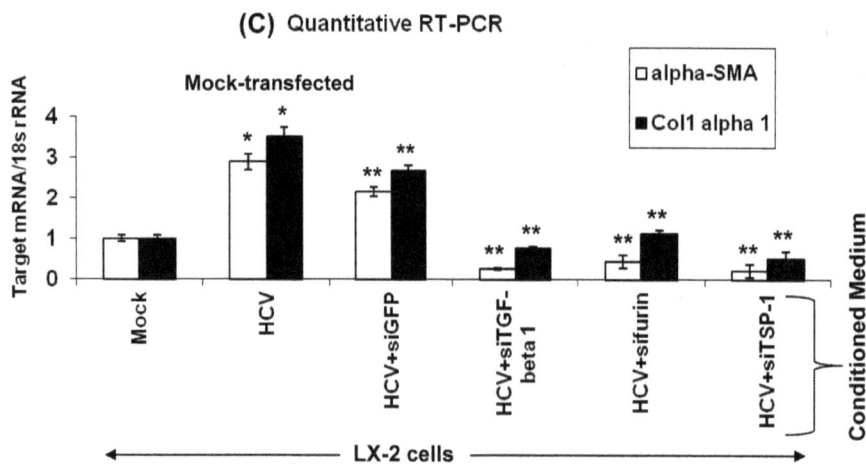

(D)

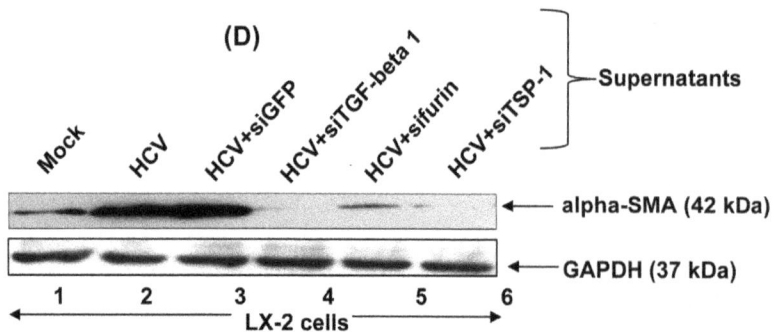

Figure 7. Effect of HCV-induced TGF-β1, furin, and TSP-1 on hepatic stellate cells activation. A) Mock- and HCV-infected cells were transfected with siGFP, siTGF-β1, sifurin, and siTSP-1 as described in Materials and Methods. To determine the levels of silencing, total cellular RNA was extracted, and subjected to quantitative RT-PCR using furin, TSP-1, and TGF-β1 specific primers. The data shown here represent the means standard deviations of three independent experiments performed in triplicate. *denotes p<0.05 compared to mock cells. **denotes p<0.05 compared to HCV-infected mock-transfected cells. B) Equal amounts of cellular lysates from above siRNA transfected cells were subjected to western blot analysis using anti-TGF-β1, furin, and TSP-1 antibodies. Lane 1, Lysates from mock (Huh7.5) cells; lane 2, HCV-infected cells; lanes 3 and 4, HCV-infected cells transfected with siGFP or siTGF-β1, sifurin and siTSP-1. Actin and albumin were used as protein loading controls. C) HSC line, LX-2 was grown and serum starved for 48 h prior to incubation with conditioned medium (CM) collected from HCV-infected Huh-7.5 cells transfected with siGFP, siTGF-β1, sifurin, or siTSP-1 for 24 h. Total cellular RNA was extracted from LX-2 cells and the levels of α-SMA and Col 1 alpha 1 mRNA were determined by quantitative RT-PCR. The data shown here represent the means standard deviations of three independent experiments performed in triplicate. *denotes p<0.05 compared to LX-2 cells incubated with CM from mock cells. **denotes p<0.05 compared to LX-2 cells incubated with CM from HCV-infected cells. D) Cellular lysates from cells as described above were subjected to immunoblot analysis using antibodies against α-SMA and GAPDH. Lanes 1 and 2, lysates from LX-2 cells incubated with CM from mock- and HCV-infected cells; Lanes 3–6, lysates from LX-2 cells incubated with CM from HCV-infected cells transfected with siGFP, siTGF-β1, sifurin, and siTSP-1. Bottom panel shows the protein loading control immunoblotted with anti-GAPDH primary antibody.

However, deletion mutant phTG6 showed modest activity. In contrast, deletion mutants, phTG7 and phTG7-4 did not show any activity by HCV NS proteins (Fig. 1C).

Role of HCV-induced Transcription Factors on TGF-β1 Promoter Activation

Previously, several transcription factors such as EGR-1, USF, ZF9/core promoter biding protein, AP-1, Sp1, NF-kB, and STAT-3 have been shown to bind to TGF-β1 promoter [10,17,18,20,21,22,23,25,27]. Since we observed increased luciferase activity of wild-type (phTG1) and deletion mutant (phTG5) in HCV-infected cells, we have used these luciferase constructs in our further studies. To determine if HCV-induced transcription factors activate TGF-β1 promoter, mock- and HCV-infected cells were transfected with phTG1 and phTG5 promoter-luciferase reporters followed by treatment with the inhibitors of AP-1 (Tanshinone IIA), Sp1 (Mithramycin), IkBα phosphorylation (Bay 11-7085), NF-κB, and cotransfected with the dominant negative (dn) mutants of NF-kB and STAT-3. The results show increased luciferase activity of phTG1 and phTG5, which was reduced upon treatment with AP-1 and Sp1 inhibitors (Fig. 2A). In contrast, we did not observe any effect of the inhibitors of IkBα and NF-kB as well as dn mutants of IkBα and STAT-3 (Fig. 2A). This is not unexpected as phTG1 and phTG5 do not contain the binding sites for NF-kB and STAT-3 (Fig. 1A).

To examine if HCV-induced NF-kB and STAT-3 have any effects on endogenous TGF-β1 promoter activation, mock- and HCV-infected cells were incubated with the inhibitors and dn mutants as described in figure 2A. Total cellular RNA was harvested and subjected to quantitative RT-PCR. We observed a 20 fold increased TGF-β1 mRNA expression, which was reduced in cells treated with the inhibitors of AP-1, Sp1, IkBα, NF-κB, and dn mutants of IkBα and STAT-3 (Fig. 2B). These results suggest that endogenous TGF-β1 promoter is regulated by HCV-induced AP-1, Sp1, NF-kB, and STAT-3. The cellular toxicity assay was performed by CytoTox-One cytotoxicity assay. Untreated cells showed approximately 2.5–3.5% cytotoxicity, whereas the positive lysis control cells showed approximately 7–9% cytotoxicity (Fig. 2C). Mock- or HCV-infected cells treated with the inhibitors did not cause significant cytotoxicity (Fig. 2C). The expression of IkBα, STAT-3 and AP-1 dominant negative proteins in HCV-infected cells are shown by western blot assay (Fig. 2D–2F).

Role of AP-1 and Sp1 Binding Sites on HCV-induced TGF-β1 Promoter Activation

To demonstrate the role of AP-1 binding site (−432/−398) and Sp1 binding site (−229/−198) on HCV-induced TGF-β1 promoter activation, we mutated the binding sites of AP-1 and

Sp1 in phTG1 and phTG5 using site-directed mutagenesis (Fig. 3A). The mutations were confirmed by DNA sequence analysis from the Genomics Core Facility at Northwestern University, IL. Mock- and HCV-infected cells were transfected with wild-type and mutated reporter constructs. The results showed increased luciferase activity of wild-type phTG1 and phTG5, however, a mutation in AP-1 and Sp1 binding sites individually resulted in a decrease in HCV-mediated TGF-β1 promoter-luciferase activity (Fig. 3B). To determine if these effects were synergistic, we introduced double mutations in TGF-β1 promoter constructs. Our results showed a significant decrease in TGF-β1 promoter activity in HCV infected cells that were transfected with TGF-β1 promoter-luciferase constructs containing mutations in AP-1 and Sp1 binding sites (Fig. 3B), suggesting the synergistic effect of AP-1 and Sp1 on TGF-β1 promoter-luciferase reprter.

To determine whether AP-1 and Sp1 interact with the TGF-β1 promoter *in vivo* in HCV-infected cells, ChIP assay was performed using c-Jun, c-Fos, and Sp1 antibody. The DNA qRT-PCR analysis showed that c-Jun, c-Fos and Sp1 specific antibodies immunoprecipitated chromatin from HCV-infected cells (Fig. 3C). However, immunoprecipitation with non-specific antibody (normal human IgG) did not amplify the DNA fragments. The PCR amplification of input chromatin before immunoprecipitation was served as positive control. The amplified DNA fragments were further confirmed by agarose gel electrophoresis (Fig. 3D). These results indicate that AP-1 and Sp1 form a protein-DNA transcriptional regulatory complex by binding to the TGF-β1 promoter in HCV-infected cells.

Effect of HCV-induced Signaling Pathways on Transcription Factor Activation

To determine the role of HCV-induced Ca^{2+} signaling and induction of reactive oxygen species (ROS) on the activation of HCV-induced transcription factors, mock- and HCV-infected cells were transfected with STAT-3, NF-κB, and AP-1 responsive luciferase reporter plasmids. Our data show increased activity of STAT-3, NF-κB, and AP-1 responsive luciferase reporters which were decreased when treated with intracellular Ca^{2+} chelator (BAPTA-AM) or antioxidant (PDTC; pyrrolidine dithiocarbamate) (Fig. 4A).

To determine the binding of HCV-induced AP-1 and Sp1 with oligonucleotide derived from TGF-β1 promoter, we performed the EMSA of c-Jun and Sp1 with labeled probe. Our results showed the increased DNA-protein complex formation in HCV-infected nuclear lysates (Fig. 4B and 4C). The specificity of DNA-protein complexes were confirmed by competition with 200-fold molar excess of unlabeled consensus probe and a supershift of

(A)

LX-2 cells are placed in upper chamber

48 hrs

Invasive LX-2s pass through basement membrane layer and cling to the bottom of the insert membrane

Invasive cells are stained and quantified

Conditioned Media
Serum Free DMEM
•LX-2s
Staining Solution
Basement Membrane Layer

(B)

LX-2 cells + CM from Mock cells

LX-2 cells + CM from HCV-infected cells

LX-2 cells + CM from HCV-infected cells +siGFP

LX-2 cells + CM from HCV-infected cells +siTGF-beta 1

(C) CytoSelect Invasion Assay

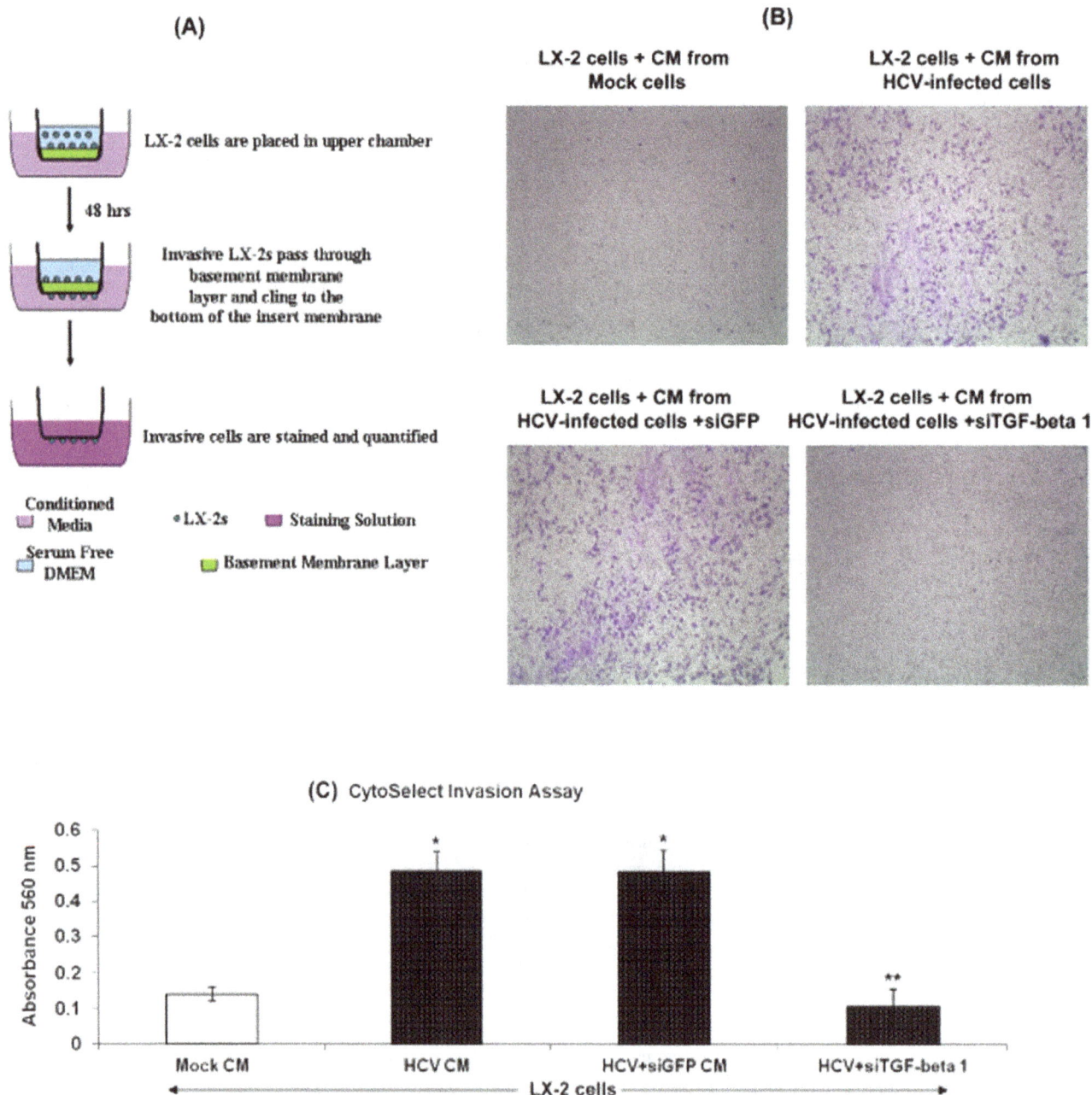

Figure 8. Effect of HCV-induced TGF-β1 on hepatic stellate cell invasion. A) Schematic of invasion assay. B) LX-2 cells were plated in upper chamber in serum free DMEM. CM from mock- and HCV-infected cells as well as HCV-infected cells transfected with siTGF-β1, and siGFP were used in the lower chamber. Boyden chamber was incubated at 37°C for 48 h to examine HSCs invasion. Invasion was assessed by counting migrated cells in multiple microscopic fields per well at 35× magnification. C) The HSC invasion was also quantified using extraction solution and absorbance was recorded at 560 nm according to manufacturer's protocol (Cell Biolabs, Inc., CA). The data shown here represent the means standard deviations of two independent experiments performed in duplicate. *denotes p<0.05 compared to LX-2s treated with CM from mock cells. **denotes p<0.05 compared to LX-2s treated with CM from HCV-infected cells.

DNA-protein complex in the presence of anti-c-Jun and anti-Sp1 antibodies.

Role of HCV-induced Cellular Kinases on TGF-β1 Promoter Activation

Previously, we and others have shown that the activation of transcription factors are regulated by cellular kinases in HCV expressing cells [10,29,31,45]. To demonstrate the role of HCV-

induced cellular kinases in TGF-β1 promoter activation, mock- and HCV-infected cells were transiently-transfected with phTG1 and phTG5 promoter-luciferase reporters followed by treatment with the inhibitors of p38 MAPK (SB203580), JNK (SP600125), Src (SU6656), PI3K (LY294002), JAK (AG490), and MEK1/2 (U0126). The results show increased activity of phTG1 and phTG5 in HCV-infected cells, which was abrogated in HCV-infected cells treated with inhibitors of p38 MAPK, JNK, Src, and MEK1/2, but not with PI3K and JAK (Fig. 5A).

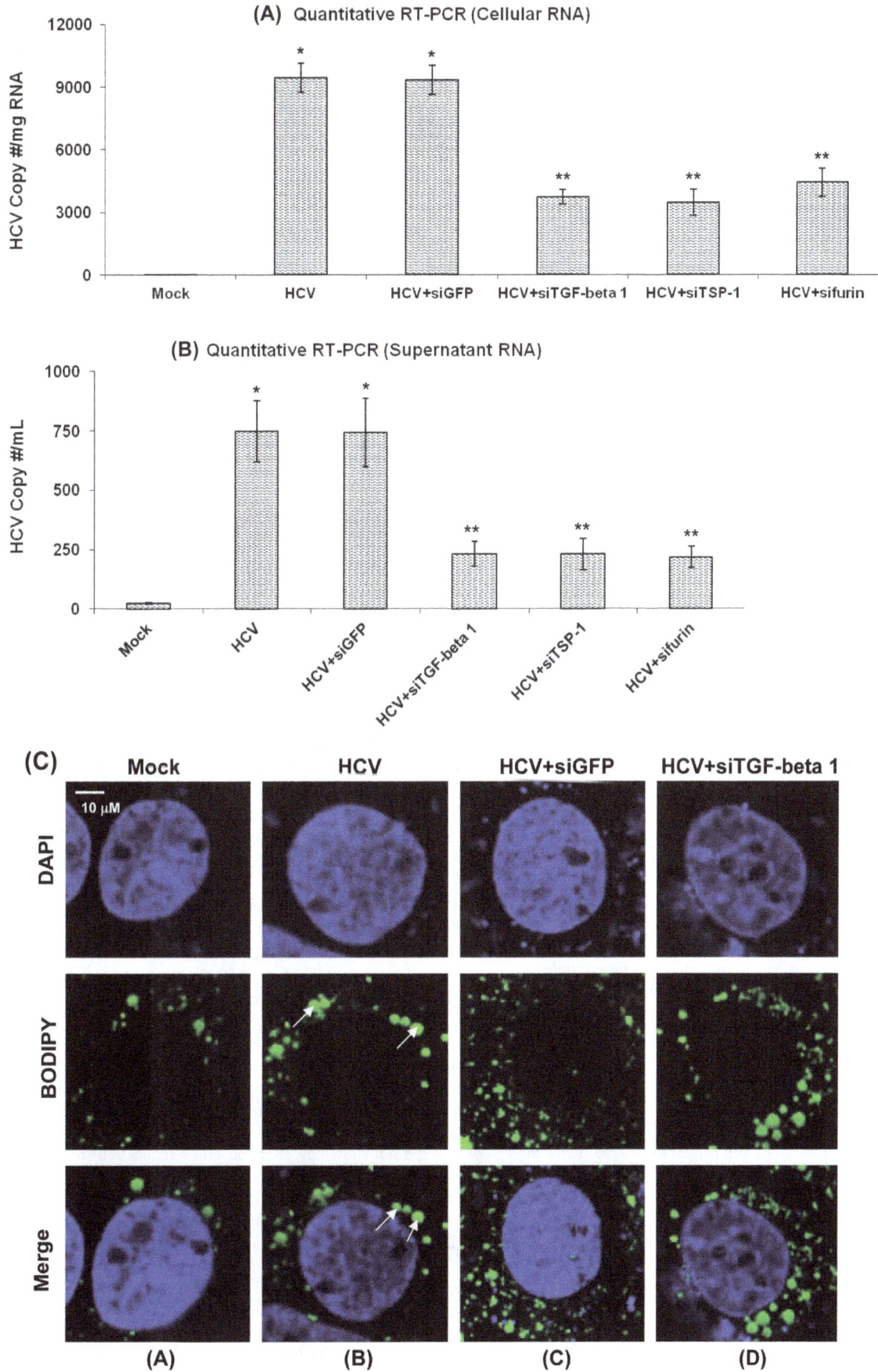

(A) Quantitative RT-PCR (Cellular RNA)

(B) Quantitative RT-PCR (Supernatant RNA)

(C)

Figure 9. Effect of TGF-β1, furin, and TSP-1 on HCV replication and release. A) Total cellular RNA was collected at day 4 from mock, HCV-infected cells, and those transfected with siRNA, and the level of HCV RNA was determined by quantitative RT-PCR. The data shown here represent the means standard deviations of three independent experiments performed in triplicate. *denotes $p < 0.05$ compared to mock cells. **denotes $p < 0.05$ compared to HCV-infected mock-transfected cells. B) Two milliliters of CM were collected from above cells at day 7, and the level of HCV release was determined by quantitative RT-PCR as described in Materials and Methods. The data shown here represent the means standard deviations of three independent experiments performed in triplicate. *denotes $p < 0.05$ compared to mock cells. **denotes $p < 0.05$ compared to HCV-infected, mock-transfected cells. C) Mock, HCV-infected cells, as well as HCV-infected cells transfected with siTGF-β1, and siGFP were prepared for confocal laser-scanning microscopy as described in Materials and Methods. Briefly, cells were incubated with BODIPY for 1 h at RT, and washed with PBS. DAPI was used as a nuclear stain. Arrows indicate lipid droplets. Bar, 10 μM.

To demonstrate the effect of these kinases on endogenous TGF-β1 gene expression, mock- and HCV-infected cells were incubated the kinase inhibitors as described above. Total cellular RNA was subjected to quantitative RT-PCR. We observed increased expression of TGF-β1 mRNA in HCV-infected cells, which was abrogated in the presence of the inhibitors of p38 MAPK, JNK, Src, and MEK1/2 (Fig. 5B). To determine the level of toxicity caused by the kinase inhibitors in the HCV-infected cells, CytoTox-One cytotoxicity assay was performed. We did not observe any cytotoxicity in cells treated with above kinase inhibitors (Fig. 5C).

Effect of HCV-induced Transcription Factors on TGF-β1 Secretion

To determine the role of HCV-induced AP-1, Sp1, NF-κB, and STAT-3 on TGF-β1 secretion, mock- and HCV-infected cells were incubated with the inhibitors of AP-1 (Tanshinone IIA), Sp1 (Mithramycin), IκBα (Bay 11-7085), and NF-κB, or transfected with the dn mutants of AP-1 (TAM67), STAT-3 (STAT-3β, STAT-3 S727A), and IkBα (IkBα S32, 36 to alanine 32, 36) as described in figure 2. Conditioned media (CM) were collected from these cells and subjected to TGF-β1 ELISA. We observed approximately 1250 pg/ml of TGF-β1 in CM collected from HCV-infected cells, which was significantly reduced by treatment with above inhibitors or transfected with dn mutants (Fig. 6A).

The bioactive TGF-β1 in CM was quantified by a standard growth inhibition assay using mink lung epithelial cells (MLEC) as described previously [12,42,43]. In this assay, MLEC stably transfected with the PAI/L demonstrate a dose-dependent increase in luciferase activity which indirectly corresponds to growth inhibition. MLEC were incubated with CM from mock- and HCV-infected cells treated with above inhibitors or transfected with above dn mutants. MLEC cells were then lysed, and subsequent luciferase assay was performed. HCV-infected cells secreted approximately 2.6 fold more bioactive TGF-β1 compared to mock-infected cells. Increased secretion of bioactive TGF-β1 by HCV-infection was significantly reduced by treatment with above inhibitors or dn mutants (Fig. 6B).

Effect of HCV-induced TGF-β1, Furin, and TSP-1 on Hepatic Stellate Cells Activation

Hepatic stellate cells (HSCs) are the primary cell type involved in liver fibrosis [7]. To demonstrate the effect of secreted TGF-β1 from HCV-infected cells on HSCs, LX-2 cells were incubated with CM from mock- and HCV-infected cells as well as HCV-infected cells transfected with siGFP, siTGF-β1, siTSP-1, and sifurin. In our previous studies we have shown that furin and TSP-1 are involved in the proteolytic processing (maturation) of TGF-β1 [12]. To determine the knock down of TGF-β1, TSP-1, and furin by their siRNA, quantitative RT-PCR and western blot assay were performed. We observed reduced expression of TGF-β1, TSP-1, and furin mRNA and protein at 72 h posttransfection (Fig. 7A and 7B).

LX-2 cells were incubated with CM from HCV-infected cells. The results showed increased expression of LX-2 cells activation markers, α-smooth muscle actin (α-SMA) and collagen type 1 α 1 (Col1A1) mRNA, which was reduced in LX-2 cells incubated with CM collected from HCV-infected cells transfected with siTGF-β1, siTSP-1, or sifurin (Fig. 7C). To further demonstrate the activation of LX-2, western blot analysis of α-SMA was performed. The results show a significant increase in α-SMA expression following incubation with conditioned media from HCV-infected cells (Fig. 7D), which was reduced in LX-2 cells incubated with conditioned media from HCV-infected cells transfected with siTGF-β1, siTSP-1, or sifurin (Fig. 7D).

Effect of HCV-induced TGF-β1 on HSC Invasion

To evaluate the effect of TGF-β1 from HCV-infected cells on HSCs, LX-2 cells in serum-free DMEM were plated in the upper chamber of the CytoSelect Cell Invasion Assay. CM from HCV-infected cells transfected with siTGF-β1 or siGFP was used in the lower chamber to stimulate cell invasion (Fig. 8A). The results showed increased invasion of LX-2 cells when incubated with CM from HCV-infected cells, which was reduced in LX-2 cells incubated with CM collected from HCV-infected cells transfected with siTGF-β1 but not with siGFP (Fig. 8B). Using extraction solution, we also quantified the invading cells by recording the absorbance of the samples at 560 nm. The results show an increased invasion of LX-2 cells when incubated with CM from HCV-infected cells, which was reduced in LX-2 cells incubated with CM from HCV-infected cells transfected with siTGF-β1 but not with siGFP (Fig. 8C).

Effect of TGF-β1, Furin, and TSP-1 on HCV Replication and Release

To evaluate the effect of TGF-β1, furin, and TSP-1 on HCV replication, and release, we used RNA interference approach as described in figure 7A. Total cellular RNA was extracted from cells as well as supernatant from mock and HCV-infected cells and subjected to quantitative RT-PCR analysis using HCV-specific primers and Taqman probe. We observed an increase in HCV replication in HCV-infected cells (Fig. 9A), which was significantly reduced in HCV-infected cells transfected with siTGF-β1, siTSP-1 or sifurin (Fig. 9A). However, transfection of siGFP (negative control) did not show any effect on HCV replication (Fig. 9A).

Similarly, we observed an increase in HCV RNA in the supernatant of HCV-infected cells, which was significantly reduced in HCV-infected cells transfected with siTGF-β1, siTSP-1, or sifurin (Fig. 9B) but not with siGFP (negative control) (Fig. 9B). These results suggest the role of HCV-induced TGF-β1, furin, and TSP-1 in HCV replication and release.

Previously, lipid droplets have been shown to play a critical role in HCV assembly and secretion [46,47,48,49]. To demonstrate the effect of HCV-induced TGF-β1 on lipid droplet formation, cells were subjected to lipid droplet staining as described in

Materials and Methods. The results showed no change in lipid droplet formation (Fig. 9C).

Discussion

Chronic HCV infection can lead to liver fibrosis, cirrhosis, and eventually hepatocellular carcinoma by various mechanisms. Although induction of profibrogenic molecules such as TGF-β1 has been shown to play an important role in the pathogenesis of HCV, little is understood about the mechanism of HCV-mediated liver fibrosis [10,12].

Liver fibrosis is defined as the excessive accumulation of ECM proteins including multiple types of collagens, fibronectin, laminin, and other molecules that are associated with chronic liver diseases [50]. Accumulation of ECM proteins distorts the hepatic architecture by forming scar tissue and the subsequent development of nodules of regenerating hepatocytes defines the progression of fibrosis to cirrhosis [51]. HSCs are the primary source of ECM and activation of HSCs by various stimuli often leads to fibrosis [52]. The initial activation of HSCs is likely to be a result of stimuli produced by neighboring cells e.g. hepatocytes, or Kupffer cells, these stimuli include ROS, lipid peroxides, growth factors, and inflammatory cytokines [52].

TGF-β1 is the most potent fibrogenic stimulus to HSCs and elevated TGF-β1 expression has been implicated in the pathogenesis of various diseases including liver fibrosis, and HCC [53]. Previous studies related to HCV-mediated liver fibrosis have been conducted in HSCs. In the absence of inflammation, TGF-β1 is secreted from HSC and Kupffer cells, but not from hepatocytes. However, during liver injury and inflammation, hepatocytes can become a major source of TGF-β1 [10,12,54,55,56,57]. Secreted bioactive TGF-β1 from hepatocytes can activate HSCs leading to the secretion of ECM proteins [43].

In the present study, we investigated the molecular mechanisms of TGF β1 promoter activation in response to HCV, as well as the effect of secreted TGF-β1 on human HSCs activation and invasion. Using a series of TGF-β1 promoter-luciferase constructs, we demonstrate that the region between −323 and −453 is responsible for TGF-β1 promoter activation in response to HCV-infection (Fig. 1B). Previous studies have demonstrated two AP-1 binding sites between −323 and −453 [44]. In addition, our results show modest level of activity by phTG6 which contains known Sp1 binding sites. phTG1 showed decreased activity compared phTG5 because phTG1 is known to contain negative regulatory regions [19].

One of the effects of HCV translation/replication activities in the ER is the activation of cellular transcription factors [35]. Previously, HCV proteins (core, NS3, and NS5A) have been shown to induce various transcription factors (STAT-3, Sp1, NF-κB, and AP-1) through multiple signaling pathways [30,31,43,50]. Our results showed a significant decrease in TGF-β1 promoter activation in HCV-infected cells treated with inhibitors of AP-1 and Sp1. However, we did not observe a reduction of TGF-β1 promoter activation when cells were treated with inhibitors of NF-κB, or transfected with dominant negative forms of NF-κB or STAT-3, as the TGF-β1 promoter phTG1 (−1362/+11) does not contain binding sites for NF-κB and STAT-3.

However, endogenous TGF-β1 gene expression was significantly reduced by NF-κB inhibitors and dominant negative forms of NF-κB and STAT-3 as well as inhibitors of AP-1 and Sp1. Previous studies have demonstrated a far upstream TGF-β1 promoter region at positions −3155 and −2515 upstream of the transcription initiation site [21]. This region contains STAT-3 binding site which is far upstream from TGF-β1 promoter-

luciferase and would explain the discrepancy between TGF-β1 promoter-luciferase and endogenous TGF-β1 mRNA results. Similarly, NF-κB has been shown to be activated by HCV-infection and plays an important role in TGF-β1 promoter activation; however TGF-β1 promoter region −1362 to +11 does not contain any NF-κB binding sites. Therefore, it could be possible that NF-κB is either binding directly to a secondary promoter region upstream, or is indirectly regulating the TGF-β1 promoter region via interactions with other cellular proteins [10,11,45].

Previously, AP-1 and Sp1 transcription factors have been shown to play an important role in the induction of TGF-β1 in various systems [19,22,44,58]. Transcriptional regulation of TGF-β1 by v-src gene products has been shown to be mediated through the AP-1 complex [58]. AP-1 proteins have been shown to mediate hyperglycemia-induced activation of TGF-β1 promoter in mesangial cells [44]. Sp1 is known to play an important role in HPV E6- and E7-mediated activation of the TGF-β1 promoter [22]. Our results are consistent with these previous studies.

AP-1, STAT-3, Sp1, and NF-κB are activated by upstream cellular kinases and belong to a category of rapid acting transcription factors. AP-1 and NF-κB are both complexes that have been shown to be phosphorylated and activated in response to HCV gene expression [31,45]. STAT-3, although not a complex like AP-1 and NF-κB, has also been shown to be activated by HCV gene expression [30]. Sp1 has been shown to be activated by p38 MAPK but the mechanism has not been defined [59]. We and others have shown the activation of cellular kinases JNK, p38 MAPK, JAK2, ERK1/2, Src and PI3K/Akt signaling in HCV-infected cells [10,29,31,34,45,60]. In this study, we observed that the activation of TGF-β1 promoter is mediated through the activation of cellular kinases such as JNK, p38 MAPK, Src, and ERK.

Human hepatic stellate cells are the primary cell type responsible for liver fibrosis following their activation into fibrogenic myofibroblast-like cells [7,37]. In this study, the fibrogenic effect of TGF-β1 secreted from HCV-infected Huh-7.5 cells was studied by examining the status of the well known markers of HSCs activation, α-SMA and ColIA1. Our results showed a significant decrease of α-SMA and ColIAI mRNA expression and α-SMA protein expression in HSCs incubated with CM from HCV-infected cells transfected with siTGF-β1, siFurin, or siTSP-1. These data suggest that secreted bioactive TGF-β1 is regulated by host proteins furin and TSP-1, and bioactive TGF-β1 plays an important role in the activation of HSCs. Our data is in agreement with previously published work on TGF-β1 stimulation of HSCs and elucidates the role of secreted TGF-β1 from HCV-infected cells [61,62,63,64]. Another hallmark of HSC activation is an invasive phenotype [64]. We observed an increase in LX-2 invasion when incubated with CM from HCV-infected cells, and a significant decrease of invasive phenotype with CM from HCV-infected cells transfected with siTGF-β1. This data suggests that TGF-β1 secreted from HCV-infected cells plays a critical role in invasive potential of HSCs.

Previous studies have shown that TGF-β1 increased replication of respiratory syncytial virus and JC virus [15,65]. Our previous studies have demonstrated that siTGF-β1 decreased replication of HCV [12]. However, the underlying mechanism by which TGF-β1 enhances HCV replication is unknown. Previously, the stimulation as well as suppression of HCV replication by exogenous addition of TGF-β1 has been demonstrated in HCV replicon system [11,66]. Endogenous TGF-β1 has been shown to induce intracellular signaling pathways including activation of hypoxia inducible factor-1 (HIF-1) and direct interaction of TGF-β1 with STAT-5 leading to liver fibrosis [17,67].

Lipid droplets (LDs) are mainly involved in lipid storage but can also be involved in vesicular transport and cellular signaling [68]. Several clinical studies have demonstrated that chronic HCV infection is associated with enhanced accumulation of LDs in the liver [69,70,71]. Previous studies have shown that LDs have a critical role in the production of infectious HCV particles [46,47,48,49]. Our data suggests that TGF-β1 is required for the release of infectious HCV particles without affecting LD biogenesis (Fig. 9C), suggesting that TGF-β1 may be regulating HCV release through LD-independent mechanisms.

In summary, we show TGF-β1 promoter activation by HCV-infection is dependent on transcription factors AP-1, Sp1, STAT-3, and NF-κB. Our results also show the activation of these transcription factors is dependent on the activation of cellular kinases. These studies provide greater insight into the molecular mechanisms of TGF-β1 promoter activation by HCV infection. Our results also demonstrate the role of secreted TGF-β1 from HCV-infected cells in the activation and invasion of HSCs suggesting invasive potential of activated HSCs. In addition, our results demonstrate the role of TGF-β1 in HCV replication and release. The results of these studies provide ideas for new concepts and a framework to develop novel strategies of treatment of chronic HCV infection associated with liver fibrosis.

Acknowledgments

We thank Dr. Takaji Wakita (NIID, Tokyo, Japan), and Dr. Charles Rice (Rockefeller University, NY) for the generous gift of HCV genotype 2a (JFH-1) and J6/JFH-1 infectious cDNA and Huh-7.5 cell line; Dr. S.J. Kim (NIH/HCI, MD); for TGF-β1 reporter constructs' Dr. Daniel Rifkin (NYU, NY) for the mink lung epithelial cell line (Mv1Lu TGF-β1 sensitive PAI-1/L); Dr. Scott Friedman (Mount Sinai Hospital, NY) for the LX-2 cell line; Dr. Nancy Colburn (NCI, MD) for the dominant negative c-Jun plasmid (pcDNA3.1/His-TAM67) as well as (AP-1)₄-luciferase-reporter construct.

Author Contributions

Conceived and designed the experiments: LP SM GW. Performed the experiments: LP SM. Analyzed the data: LP SM GW. Contributed reagents/materials/analysis tools: LP SM GW. Wrote the paper: LP GW.

References

1. Alter MJ (2007) Epidemiology of hepatitis C virus infection. World J Gastroenterol 13: 2436–2441.
2. Bartenschlager R, Lohmann V (2000) Replication of the hepatitis C virus. Baillieres Best Pract Res Clin Gastroenterol 14: 241–254.
3. Blight KJ, Kolykhalov AA, Rice CM (2000) Efficient initiation of HCV RNA replication in cell culture. Science 290: 1972–1974.
4. Lindenbach BD, Evans MJ, Syder AJ, Wolk B, Tellinghuisen TL, et al. (2005) Complete replication of hepatitis C virus in cell culture. Science 309: 623–626.
5. Wakita T, Pietschmann T, Kato T, Date T, Miyamoto M, et al. (2005) Production of infectious hepatitis C virus in tissue culture from a cloned viral genome. Nat Med 11: 791–796.
6. Zhong J, Gastaminza P, Cheng G, Kapadia S, Kato T, et al. (2005) Robust hepatitis C virus infection in vitro. Proc Natl Acad Sci U S A 102: 9294–9299.
7. Schuppan D, Krebs A, Bauer M, Hahn EG (2003) Hepatitis C and liver fibrosis. Cell Death Differ 10 Suppl 1: S59–67.
8. Grungreiff K, Reinhold D, Ansorge S (1999) Serum concentrations of sIL-2R, IL-6, TGF-beta1, neopterin, and zinc in chronic hepatitis C patients treated with interferon-alpha. Cytokine 11: 1076–1080.
9. Wilson LE, Torbenson M, Astemborski J, Faruki H, Spoler C, et al. (2006) Progression of liver fibrosis among injection drug users with chronic hepatitis C. Hepatology 43: 788–795.
10. Lin W, Tsai WL, Shao RX, Wu G, Peng LF, et al. (2010) Hepatitis C virus regulates transforming growth factor beta1 production through the generation of reactive oxygen species in a nuclear factor kappaB-dependent manner. Gastroenterology 138: 2509–2518, 2518 e2501.
11. Lin W, Weinberg EM, Tai AW, Peng LF, Brockman MA, et al. (2008) HIV increases HCV replication in a TGF-beta1-dependent manner. Gastroenterology 134: 803–811.
12. Presser LD, Haskett A, Waris G (2011) Hepatitis C virus-induced furin and thrombospondin-1 activate TGF-beta1: role of TGF-beta1 in HCV replication. Virology 412: 284–296.
13. Shin JY, Hur W, Wang JS, Jang JW, Kim CW, et al. (2005) HCV core protein promotes liver fibrogenesis via up-regulation of CTGF with TGF-beta1. Exp Mol Med 37: 138–145.
14. Taniguchi H, Kato N, Otsuka M, Goto T, Yoshida H, et al. (2004) Hepatitis C virus core protein upregulates transforming growth factor-beta 1 transcription. J Med Virol 72: 52–59.
15. McCann KL, Imani F (2007) Transforming growth factor beta enhances respiratory syncytial virus replication and tumor necrosis factor alpha induction in human epithelial cells. J Virol 81: 2880–2886.
16. Gibbs JD, Ornoff DM, Igo HA, Zeng JY, Imani F (2009) Cell cycle arrest by transforming growth factor beta1 enhances replication of respiratory syncytial virus in lung epithelial cells. J Virol 83: 12424–12431.
17. Hosui A, Kimura A, Yamaji D, Zhu BM, Na R, et al. (2009) Loss of STAT5 causes liver fibrosis and cancer development through increased TGF-{beta} and STAT3 activation. J Exp Med 206: 819–831.
18. Kim KS, Jung HS, Chung YJ, Jung TS, Jang HW, et al. (2008) Overexpression of USF increases TGF-beta1 protein levels, but G1 phase arrest was not induced in FRTL-5 cells. J Korean Med Sci 23: 870–876.
19. Kim SJ, Glick A, Sporn MB, Roberts AB (1989) Characterization of the promoter region of the human transforming growth factor-beta 1 gene. J Biol Chem 264: 402–408.
20. Kim Y, Ratziu V, Choi SG, Lalazar A, Theiss G, et al. (1998) Transcriptional activation of transforming growth factor beta1 and its receptors by the Kruppel-like factor Zf9/core promoter-binding protein and Sp1. Potential mechanisms for autocrine fibrogenesis in response to injury. J Biol Chem 273: 33750–33758.
21. Ogata H, Chinen T, Yoshida T, Kinjyo I, Takaesu G, et al. (2006) Loss of SOCS3 in the liver promotes fibrosis by enhancing STAT3-mediated TGF-beta1 production. Oncogene 25: 2520–2530.
22. Peralta-Zaragoza O, Bermudez-Morales V, Gutierrez-Xicotencatl L, Alcocer-Gonzalez J, Recillas-Targa F, et al. (2006) E6 and E7 oncoproteins from human papillomavirus type 16 induce activation of human transforming growth factor beta1 promoter throughout Sp1 recognition sequence. Viral Immunol 19: 468–480.
23. Qi W, Gao S, Wang Z (2008) Transcriptional regulation of the TGF-beta1 promoter by androgen receptor. Biochem J 416: 453–462.
24. Weigert C, Brodbeck K, Klopfer K, Haring HU, Schleicher ED (2002) Angiotensin II induces human TGF-beta 1 promoter activation: similarity to hyperglycaemia. Diabetologia 45: 890–898.
25. Weigert C, Brodbeck K, Sawadogo M, Haring HU, Schleicher ED (2004) Upstream stimulatory factor (USF) proteins induce human TGF-beta1 gene activation via the glucose-response element-1013/−1002 in mesangial cells: up-regulation of USF activity by the hexosamine biosynthetic pathway. J Biol Chem 279: 15908–15915.
26. Xiang Z, Qiao L, Zhou Y, Babiuk LA, Liu Q (2010) Hepatitis C virus nonstructural protein-5A activates sterol regulatory element-binding protein-1c through transcription factor Sp1. Biochem Biophys Res Commun 402: 549–553.
27. Yoo YD, Chiou CJ, Choi KS, Yi Y, Michelson S, et al. (1996) The IE2 regulatory protein of human cytomegalovirus induces expression of the human transforming growth factor beta1 gene through an Egr-1 binding site. J Virol 70: 7062–7070.
28. Burdette D, Haskett A, Presser L, McRae S, Iqbal J, et al. (2012) Hepatitis C virus activates interleukin-1beta via caspase-1-inflammasome complex. J Gen Virol 93: 235–246.
29. Burdette D, Olivarez M, Waris G (2010) Activation of transcription factor Nrf2 by hepatitis C virus induces the cell-survival pathway. J Gen Virol 91: 681–690.
30. Gong G, Waris G, Tanveer R, Siddiqui A (2001) Human hepatitis C virus NS5A protein alters intracellular calcium levels, induces oxidative stress, and activates STAT-3 and NF-kappa B. Proc Natl Acad Sci U S A 98: 9599–9604.
31. Qadri I, Iwahashi M, Capasso JM, Hopken MW, Flores S, et al. (2004) Induced oxidative stress and activated expression of manganese superoxide dismutase during hepatitis C virus replication: role of JNK, p38 MAPK and AP-1. Biochem J 378: 919–928.
32. Tardif KD, Mori K, Siddiqui A (2002) Hepatitis C virus subgenomic replicons induce endoplasmic reticulum stress activating an intracellular signaling pathway. J Virol 76: 7453–7459.
33. Tardif KD, Waris G, Siddiqui A (2005) Hepatitis C virus, ER stress, and oxidative stress. Trends Microbiol 13: 159–163.
34. Waris G, Felmlee DJ, Negro F, Siddiqui A (2007) Hepatitis C virus induces proteolytic cleavage of sterol regulatory element binding proteins and stimulates their phosphorylation via oxidative stress. J Virol 81: 8122–8130.
35. Waris G, Tardif KD, Siddiqui A (2002) Endoplasmic reticulum (ER) stress: hepatitis C virus induces an ER-nucleus signal transduction pathway and activates NF-kappaB and STAT-3. Biochem Pharmacol 64: 1425–1430.

36. Bauer M, Schuppan D (2001) TGFbeta1 in liver fibrosis: time to change paradigms? FEBS Lett 502: 1–3.
37. Friedman SL (2000) Molecular regulation of hepatic fibrosis, an integrated cellular response to tissue injury. J Biol Chem 275: 2247–2250.
38. Rockey DC (2001) Hepatic blood flow regulation by stellate cells in normal and injured liver. Semin Liver Dis 21: 337–349.
39. Ikeda K, Wakahara T, Wang YQ, Kadoya H, Kawada N, et al. (1999) In vitro migratory potential of rat quiescent hepatic stellate cells and its augmentation by cell activation. Hepatology 29: 1760–1767.
40. Xu L, Hui AY, Albanis E, Arthur MJ, O'Byrne SM, et al. (2005) Human hepatic stellate cell lines, LX-1 and LX-2: new tools for analysis of hepatic fibrosis. Gut 54: 142–151.
41. Johnson CL, Owen DM, Gale M Jr (2007) Functional and therapeutic analysis of hepatitis C virus NS3.4A protease control of antiviral immune defense. J Biol Chem 282: 10792–10803.
42. Abe M, Harpel JG, Metz CN, Nunes I, Loskutoff DJ, et al. (1994) An assay for transforming growth factor-beta using cells transfected with a plasminogen activator inhibitor-1 promoter-luciferase construct. Anal Biochem 216: 276–284.
43. Schulze-Krebs A, Preimel D, Popov Y, Bartenschlager R, Lohmann V, et al. (2005) Hepatitis C virus-replicating hepatocytes induce fibrogenic activation of hepatic stellate cells. Gastroenterology 129: 246–258.
44. Weigert C, Sauer U, Brodbeck K, Pfeiffer A, Haring HU, et al. (2000) AP-1 proteins mediate hyperglycemia-induced activation of the human TGF-beta1 promoter in mesangial cells. J Am Soc Nephrol 11: 2007–2016.
45. Waris G, Livolsi A, Imbert V, Peyron JF, Siddiqui A (2003) Hepatitis C virus NS5A and subgenomic replicon activate NF-kappaB via tyrosine phosphorylation of IkappaBalpha and its degradation by calpain protease. J Biol Chem 278: 40778–40787.
46. Aizaki H, Morikawa K, Fukasawa M, Hara H, Inoue Y, et al. (2008) Critical role of virion-associated cholesterol and sphingolipid in hepatitis C virus infection. J Virol 82: 5715–5724.
47. Barba G, Harper F, Harada T, Kohara M, Goulinet S, et al. (1997) Hepatitis C virus core protein shows a cytoplasmic localization and associates to cellular lipid storage droplets. Proc Natl Acad Sci U S A 94: 1200–1205.
48. Perlemuter G, Sabile A, Letteron P, Vona G, Topilco A, et al. (2002) Hepatitis C virus core protein inhibits microsomal triglyceride transfer protein activity and very low density lipoprotein secretion: a model of viral-related steatosis. Faseb J 16: 185–194.
49. Shi ST, Polyak SJ, Tu H, Taylor DR, Gretch DR, et al. (2002) Hepatitis C virus NS5A colocalizes with the core protein on lipid droplets and interacts with apolipoproteins. Virology 292: 198–210.
50. Bataller R, Brenner DA (2005) Liver fibrosis. J Clin Invest 115: 209–218.
51. Bataller R, Gines P (2002) [New therapeutic strategies in liver fibrosis: pathogenic basis]. Med Clin (Barc) 118: 339–346.
52. Hui AY, Friedman SL (2003) Molecular basis of hepatic fibrosis. Expert Rev Mol Med 5: 1–23.
53. Rossmanith W, Schulte-Hermann R (2001) Biology of transforming growth factor beta in hepatocarcinogenesis. Microsc Res Tech 52: 430–436.
54. Canbay A, Friedman S, Gores GJ (2004) Apoptosis: the nexus of liver injury and fibrosis. Hepatology 39: 273–278.
55. Gao C, Gressner G, Zoremba M, Gressner AM (1996) Transforming growth factor beta (TGF-beta) expression in isolated and cultured rat hepatocytes. J Cell Physiol 167: 394–405.
56. Jeong WI, Do SH, Yun HS, Song BJ, Kim SJ, et al. (2004) Hypoxia potentiates transforming growth factor-beta expression of hepatocyte during the cirrhotic condition in rat liver. Liver Int 24: 658–668.
57. Takehara T, Tatsumi T, Suzuki T, Rucker EB 3rd, Hennighausen L, et al. (2004) Hepatocyte-specific disruption of Bcl-xL leads to continuous hepatocyte apoptosis and liver fibrotic responses. Gastroenterology 127: 1189–1197.
58. Birchenall-Roberts MC, Ruscetti FW, Kasper J, Lee HD, Friedman R, et al. (1990) Transcriptional regulation of the transforming growth factor beta 1 promoter by v-src gene products is mediated through the AP-1 complex. Mol Cell Biol 10: 4978–4983.
59. D'Addario M, Arora PD, McCulloch CA (2006) Role of p38 in stress activation of Sp1. Gene 379: 51–61.
60. Mannova P, Beretta L (2005) Activation of the N-Ras-PI3K-Akt-mTOR pathway by hepatitis C virus: control of cell survival and viral replication. J Virol 79: 8742–8749.
61. Shi YF, Zhang Q, Cheung PY, Shi L, Fong CC, et al. (2006) Effects of rhDecorin on TGF-beta1 induced human hepatic stellate cells LX-2 activation. Biochim Biophys Acta 1760: 1587–1595.
62. Yang C, Zeisberg M, Mosterman B, Sudhakar A, Yerramalla U, et al. (2003) Liver fibrosis: insights into migration of hepatic stellate cells in response to extracellular matrix and growth factors. Gastroenterology 124: 147–159.
63. Lin YL, Hsu YC, Chiu YT, Huang YT (2008) Antifibrotic effects of a herbal combination regimen on hepatic fibrotic rats. Phytother Res 22: 69–76.
64. Sancho-Bru P, Juez E, Moreno M, Khurdayan V, Morales-Ruiz M, et al. (2010) Hepatocarcinoma cells stimulate the growth, migration and expression of pro-angiogenic genes in human hepatic stellate cells. Liver Int 30: 31–41.
65. Ravichandran V, Jensen PN, Major EO (2007) MEK1/2 inhibitors block basal and transforming growth 1beta1-stimulated JC virus multiplication. J Virol 81: 6412–6418.
66. Murata T, Ohshima T, Yamaji M, Hosaka M, Miyanari Y, et al. (2005) Suppression of hepatitis C virus replicon by TGF-beta. Virology 331: 407–417.
67. McMahon S, Charbonneau M, Grandmont S, Richard DE, Dubois CM (2006) Transforming growth factor beta1 induces hypoxia-inducible factor-1 stabilization through selective inhibition of PHD2 expression. J Biol Chem 281: 24171–24181.
68. Martin S, Parton RG (2006) Lipid droplets: a unified view of a dynamic organelle. Nat Rev Mol Cell Biol 7: 373–378.
69. Piodi A, Chouteau P, Lerat H, Hezode C, Pawlotsky JM (2008) Morphological changes in intracellular lipid droplets induced by different hepatitis C virus genotype core sequences and relationship with steatosis. Hepatology 48: 16–27.
70. Sato S, Fukasawa M, Yamakawa Y, Natsume T, Suzuki T, et al. (2006) Proteomic profiling of lipid droplet proteins in hepatoma cell lines expressing hepatitis C virus core protein. J Biochem 139: 921–930.
71. Siagris D, Christofidou M, Theocharis GJ, Pagoni N, Papadimitriou C, et al. (2006) Serum lipid pattern in chronic hepatitis C: histological and virological correlations. J Viral Hepat 13: 56–61.

20

Contribution of the ELFG Test in Algorithms of Non-Invasive Markers towards the Diagnosis of Significant Fibrosis in Chronic Hepatitis C

Jean-Pierre Zarski[1,2]*, Nathalie Sturm[2,3], Jérôme Guechot[4], Elie-Serge Zafrani[5], Michel Vaubourdolle[4], Sophie Thoret[6], Jennifer Margier[6], Sandra David-Tchouda[7], Jean-Luc Bosson[6]

1 Hepato-Gastroenterology Clinic, DIGIDUNE Pole, Grenoble University Hospital, Grenoble, France, 2 INSERM/UJF U823 IAPC unit, Institut Albert Bonniot, Grenoble, France, 3 Department of Pathological Anatomy and Cytology, Biology Pole, Grenoble University Hospital, Grenoble, France, 4 Biochemistry A Laboratory, Saint Antoine Hospital, Assistance Publique-Hôpitaux de Paris, Paris, France, 5 Pathology Department, Henri Mondor Hospital Center, Assistance Publique-Hôpitaux de Paris, Paris Est Creteil University, Créteil, France, 6 UJF-Grenoble 1/CNRS/Clinical Research Centre-Inserm CIC03/TIMC-IMAG UMR 5525/Themas, Grenoble University Hospital, Grenoble, France, 7 Medical-Economics unit, Clinical Research Administration, Grenoble University Hospital, Grenoble, France

Abstract

Background and Aims: We aimed to determine the best algorithms for the diagnosis of significant fibrosis in chronic hepatitis C (CHC) patients using all available parameters and tests.

Patients and Methods: We used the database from our study of 507 patients with histologically proven CHC in which fibrosis was evaluated by liver biopsy (Metavir) and tests: Fibrometer®, Fibrotest®, Hepascore®, Apri, ELFG, MP3, Forn's, hyaluronic acid, tissue inhibitor of metalloproteinase-1 (TIMP1), MMP1, collagen IV and when possible Fibroscan™. For the first test we used 90% negative predictive value to exclude patients with F≤1, next an induction algorithm was applied giving the best tests with at least 80% positive predictive value for the diagnosis of F≥2. The algorithms were computed using the R Software C4.5 program to select the best tests and cut-offs. The algorithm was automatically induced without premises on the part of the investigators. We also examined the inter-observer variations after independent review of liver biopsies by two pathologists. A medico-economic analysis compared the screening strategies with liver biopsy.

Results: In "intention to diagnose" the best algorithms for F≥2 were Fibrometer ®, Fibrotest®, or Hepascore® in first intention with the ELFG score in second intention for indeterminate cases. The percentage of avoided biopsies varied between 50% (Fibrotest® or Fibrometer®+ELFG) and 51% (Hepascore®+ELFG). In "per-analysis" Fibroscan™+ELFG avoided liver biopsy in 55% of cases. The diagnostic performance of these screening strategies was statistically superior to the usual combinations (Fibrometer® or Fibrotest®+Fibroscan™) and was cost effective. We note that the consensual review of liver biopsies between the two pathologists was mainly in favor of F1 (64–69%).

Conclusion: The ELFG test could replace Fibroscan in most currently used algorithms for the diagnosis of significant fibrosis including for those patients for whom Fibroscan™ is unusable.

Editor: Joerg F. Schlaak, University Hospital of Essen, Germany

Funding: The ANRS (French Agency for Research on AIDS and Viral Hepatitis) funded the main study (HCEP 23) (http://www.anrs.fr/). The funders had no role in study design, data collection and analysis, decision to publish, or preparation of the manuscript.

Competing Interests: The authors have declared that no competing interests exist.

* E-mail: JPZarski@chu-grenoble.fr

Introduction

Blood tests and transient elastography (Fibroscan™) have been developed with the objective of replacing liver biopsy for the diagnosis of liver fibrosis in chronic hepatitis C (CHC). Retrospective and recent independent prospective studies have shown that the four most validated non-invasive methods, Fibrotest®, Fibrometer®, Hepascore® and Fibroscan™ have similar performances for the diagnosis of significant fibrosis (METAVIR F≥2) in CHC [1–5]. These methods have been recently approved after an independent systematic review by the French National Authority for Health for the first line assessment of fibrosis in naïve patients with CHC [6]. Other blood tests have also been

proposed for the diagnosis of liver fibrosis in CHC: FIB-4 [7], Forns' score [8], MP3 [9], Apri [10], ELFG [11], and Hyaluronic acid [12]. However, in our recent study their diagnostic performance seemed to be lower than that of the four most validated tests [13].

The performance of these non-invasive methods for the diagnosis of significant fibrosis or cirrhosis may be improved when they are combined, as suggested by recently proposed algorithms. These use either two blood tests sequentially, such as the Sequential Algorithm for Fibrosis Evaluation (SAFE) [14,15] or are based on agreement between a blood test and Fibroscan™ results, as for the Bordeaux Algorithm (BA) [16]. To date the most used and validated algorithm has been Fibrotest®+Fibroscan™. However, this strategy has some limitations requiring an expensive Fibroscan™ machine that is not always available; it cannot be used in about 10% of cases, often because of obesity, and gives uninterpretable results in another 10% of cases [17]. For this combination the positive predictive value (PPV) and/or negative predictive value (PPV) have not always been determined and number of avoided biopsies was only 30–50% for the diagnosis of significant fibrosis [2,16]. Moreover, in constructing these algorithms, all the available blood tests had not been introduced in the statistical analysis model. Furthermore the relative cost of the different screening strategies has not been thoroughly analysed.

Using data from the FIBROSTAR study [13] we aim here to determine simple screening strategy algorithms that can be used in routine clinical practice by most physicians with the best accuracy for the diagnosis of significant fibrosis in CHC. We also consider the relative costs of the screening strategies in comparison with liver biopsy in this indication.

Patients and Methods

Ethics Statement

The main 'FIBROSTAR' study protocol was approved by the regional ethics committee "Comité de Protection des Personnes (CPP) Sud-Est 5" France. All patients gave written informed consent.

Patients

Our patient population, along with the study inclusion and exclusion criteria, has been previously described [13]. Briefly, treatment naïve consecutive adult patients with histologically proven hepatitis C were prospectively included. Patients with compensated cirrhosis could be included, but those with co-existing liver disease were excluded. Liver biopsies were performed as part of normal clinical care for staging and grading of the liver disease before antiviral treatment.

Biological Scores of Liver Fibrosis

Blood sampling and handling were previously reported in detail [13] and methods are summarized in Text S1. We emphasize here that cholesterol, platelet count and prothrombin time were immediately measured in each centre; all other biochemical parameters, aspartate aminotransferase (ASAT), alanine amino-transferase (ALAT), gamma glutamyl transpeptidase (GGT), Bilirubin, Urea, Apolipoprotein A1, Alfa-2 macroglobulin, Haptoglobin) were measured in a centralized laboratory. All the tests were performed blind of clinical and histological data.

Each biochemical parameter was firstly evaluated alone then the following blood tests were introduced in the analysis: Fibrotest®, Fibrometer®, Forns score, Apri, MP3, ELFG, Hepascore®, FIB-4, hyaluronic acid and collagen IV [18]. Blood test scores were calculated according to the published formulae, the patent for Fibrotest® or by courtesy of the manufacturer (BioLivescale) for Fibrometer®. The list of variables included in each test and the measurement techniques were previously described [13].

Liver stiffness measurement by transient elastography (Fibroscan™)

Measurements were made as previously described [13] by the operator who performed the liver biopsy. Liver stiffness measurement (LSM) failure was defined as zero valid shots (after at least 10 attempts) and "unreliable examinations" were defined as fewer than 10 valid shots or an interquartile range (IQR)/LSM greater than 30% or a success rate less than 60% [19].

Liver biopsy

Liver biopsies and fibrosis scoring according to the METAVIR scale were performed as described by two senior liver pathologists (NS and ESZ) with an inter-observer κ agreement of 0.48 and a weighted κ agreement of 0.75 [13]. Biopsies were examined for steatosis, prevalence of non-alcoholic steatohepatitis and iron deposits. To be considered for scoring, biopsies less than 20 mm had to measure at least 15 mm and/or contain at least 11 portal tracts.

Statistical Analysis and Automated Algorithm

In first intention we used one of the four tests that have been shown to perform best according to the published studies [13] and that have been validated by the French health authorities (HAS) (Fibrotest® or Fibrometer® or Hepascore® or Fibroscan™) [6] to identify patients with no or mild fibrosis (METAVIR F≤1) using cut-offs given by a 90% negative predictive value (NPV). Then, we constructed C4.5 algorithms using an automated program to determine the most effective second test, with a positive predictive value (PPV) of 80%, to identify patients with significant fibrosis (METAVIR F≥2). For each algorithm we calculated the number of biopsies avoided. The algorithm gave the cut-offs to be used when making clinical decisions and these are consistent with several publications in the field [20].

The C4.5 algorithm was performed on R software (version 2.9.1). It is a decision tree algorithm (statistical classifier) that uses Shannon's entropy measure. At each node, the program chooses the variable that best separates the populations (the difference in entropies must be maximal).The process is then repeated on the subgroups obtained. The algorithm is automatically induced without premises [21].

In a *post hoc* analysis we performed a principal component analysis (PCA) of the main tests: Fibrotest®, Fibrometer®, ELFG, Hepascore®, ELFG and Fibroscan™.

Medico-economic analysis

To meet current requirements for optimization of health spending, a *post hoc* cost analysis of different screening strategies was conducted. A hospital perspective was chosen and only medical costs were included. As complications related to liver biopsy are heterogeneous and rare (3 per 1,000), they were not included in this analysis. Costs of blood tests were based on reimbursement rates by French Health Insurance (FHI), to which we added the cost of the scoring algorithm where appropriate. For each screening strategy, the described cost included the non-invasive tests plus liver biopsy cost if needed.

Regarding the cost of screening by transient elastography (Fibroscan™) and the cost of the liver biopsy, the cost of reimbursement by FHI was considerably lower than the real cost of performing the procedures by the hospital. Thus we calculated the cost for the hospital then performed a sensitivity analysis. This sensitivity analysis permitted us to vary the costs for liver biopsy and to allow for cost recovery of the medical device (Fibroscan™). Lastly, to take into account the very high variability of the cost of the biopsy and to allow greater transposability of costs from one hospital to another, we set three levels of liver biopsy cost based on published data and the cost in our hospital: 800 Euros, 1,000 Euros and 1,200 Euros. Further details of the economic analysis are provided in Text S2.

Results

Patients' characteristics

Figure 1 shows the flow chart for the 512 patients included in the main study between November 2006 and July 2008. Their main demographic, laboratory and histological features have been previously described (13) and are presented here as Table S1. Table 1 presents the results of different blood tests, selected pertinent parameters and Fibroscan™ in both the intention to diagnose and per-protocol populations. No statistical difference was observed between the two groups regarding these parameters.

Proposed algorithms

The results of different algorithms are presented in Figure 2 with cut-offs for the blood tests and Fibroscan™ and the number of avoided liver biopsies. First we selected and entered the four most validated tests into the model (Fibrotest®, Fibrometer®, Hepascore® and Fibroscan™). The cut-off was determined with a 90% NPV that excluded patients with no or mild fibrosis F≤1. Second, when the value was superior to the cut-off, the computer automatically introduced another test in the model and calculated the PPV, thus giving the number of patients with moderate or severe fibrosis (F≥2). With this method, the ELFG was always chosen by the computer whatever the first test introduced in the model. In the intermediate zone ("impossible to conclude") we considered that liver biopsy was mandatory. This procedure gave the number of liver biopsies avoided.

We explored the interest of introducing a third test in the model. However we did not observe any significant increase in the number of biopsies avoided when we compared the diagnostic performance of algorithms with 2 or 3 tests (data not shown). Nevertheless, the third test selected by the software was always Fibroscan™.

We also compared the diagnostic performance of our algorithms with the usual combinations published in the literature (Table 2 and Figure S1). The number of avoided liver biopsies was significantly lower with the SAFE algorithm (16%) and higher with

the "Bordeaux" algorithm (68%). However the predictive values were lower with this latter combination (NPV: 80% and PPV: 84%)

Finally we considered the inter-observer variations after independent histological analysis of liver biopsies by two pathologists, especially for F1/F2, but also for other lesions considered in the histological examination.

No significant difference was observed for the different algorithms concerning all the histological lesions, especially the

Table 1. Scores from the different tests and selected parameters for the 507 CHC patients having all the blood tests (intention to diagnose population) and the 396 CHC patients with all the blood tests and reliable Fibroscan™ (per protocol population).

Non-Invasive Test	n = 507	n = 396
Hepascore®	0.5±0.3	0.5±0.3
Fibroscan™	9.7±7.3	9.7±7.3
Fibrotest®	0.5±0.3	0.5±0.3
Fibrometer®	0.6±0.3	0.6±0.3
Apri	0.3±0.4	0.3±0.4
ELFG	−0.8±0.9	−0.8±0.9
MP3	0.3±0.1	0.3±0.1
Hyaluronic acid (µg/L)	69.7±101.5	67.4±99.2
TIMP1* (µg/L)	173.8±69.0	170.5±67.6
MM1**(µg/L)	4.4±3.4	4.2±3.3
PIIINP***(µg/L)	5.4±4.1	5.3±4.4
Collagen-IV (µg/L)	170.5±85.0	170.3±86.9

*TIMP1: tissue inhibitor of metalloproteinase-1; **MM1: matrix metalloproteinase-1;
***PIIINP: N-terminal peptide of type III procollagen.

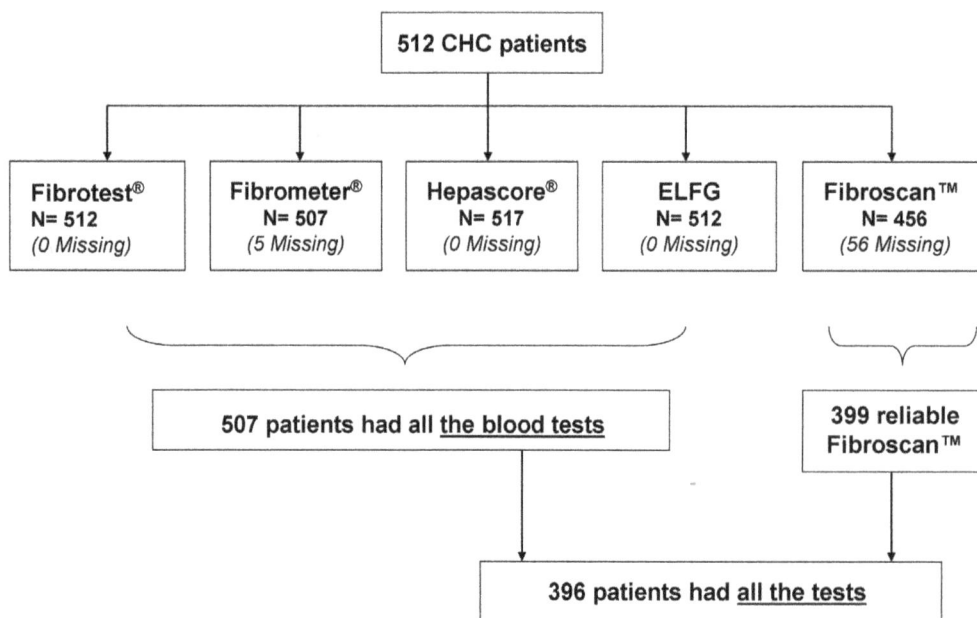

Figure 1. Study Flow Chart. N: number of chronic hepatitis C patients with test results; and the number of patients without the test or with missing test data are shown in parentheses.

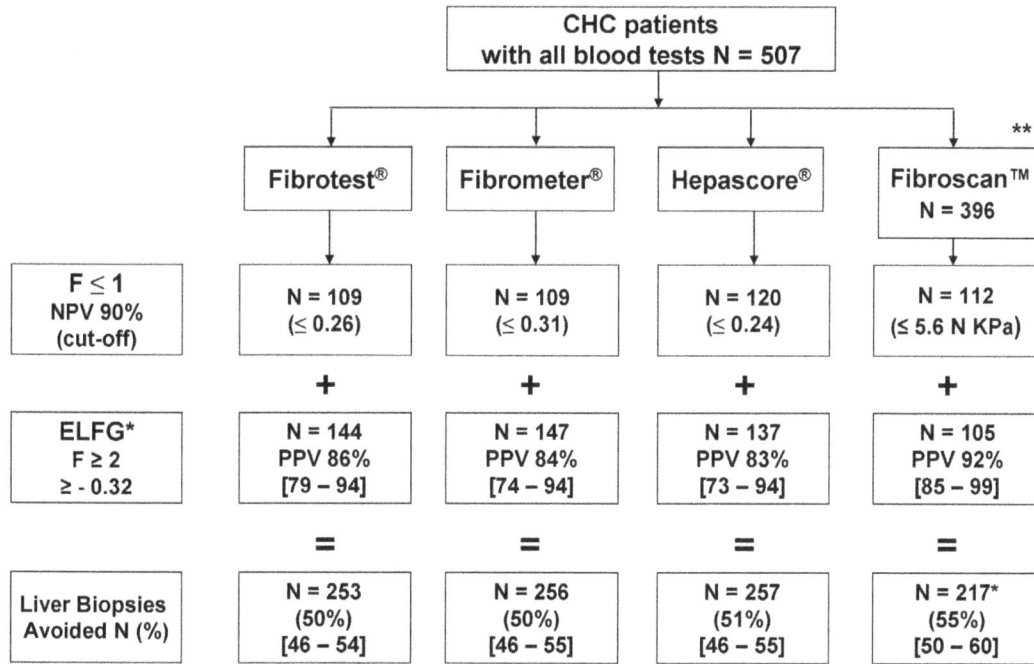

Figure 2. Proposed algorithm: automatically determined by the C4.5 program with the number of avoided liver biopsies. The bottom line gives the total number of liver biopsies avoided following one of the three most validated blood tests or Fibroscan followed by the ELFG test for those patients for whom the first test was not conclusive. N: number of patients; F: Metavir liver biopsy Fibrosis score; NPV: Negative Predictive Value with the cut-off in parentheses; PPV: Positive Predictive Value with the cut-off range in brackets. * = cut-off = >−0.32; ** = per protocol analysis.

number of discordances for F1/F2 staging, between the pathologists (Table 3). Moreover, the quality of the liver biopsy (length, number of portal-tracts, number of septa/length of biopsy), the METAVIR activity index, the rate of steatosis and the presence of steatohepatitis or iron deposits were not statistically different between patients with discordances and those without discordances. The consensual review of liver biopsies by the two pathologists was mainly in favor of F1 (64–69%).

Principal Component Analysis

ELFG was located differently in the PCA space with respect to Fibrotest®, Fibrometer® and Hepascore®, which were grouped close together and also not so close to Fibroscan™ (Figure S2).

Medico-economic analysis

When one test alone was inconclusive, the less expensive strategies were "Bordeaux" and Hepascore+ELFG. However the "Bordeaux" screening strategy includes Fibroscan™ and the cost of Fibroscan™ depends on the extent to which the instrument is used i.e. on the number of procedures per year (Figure 3). Most

strategies that included the ELFG blood test were cheaper, except ELFG+Fibroscan™ when the Fibroscan™ device is infrequently used (less than 10 procedures per month).

Discussion

Several algorithms have been proposed to improve the performance of the four validated tests (Fibrometer®, Fibrotest®, Hepascore® and Fibroscan™) for the staging of significant fibrosis in CHC patients. The most used is Fibrotest®+Fibroscan™. However, these algorithms have been constructed a priori without necessarily using all the tests available.

Here, we used an original methodology in which the algorithms were generated using an automated computerized induction method, which selected the appropriate tests and cut-offs from the full range of available tests. The cut-off for the first test was determined with a 90% NPV, and then the automated C4.5 induction program alone identified the best second test with a minimum of 80% PPV for the diagnosis of significant fibrosis (F≥2) without any intervention on the part of the investigators.

Table 2. Comparison between proposed algorithm, with ELFG, and published algorithms (that include Fibroscan™) in terms of number of patients with avoided liver biopsies.

	Fibrometer®	Fibrotest®	Hepascore®	Fibroscan™
	(N = 507)	(N = 507)	(N = 507)	(N = 396)
ELFG (cut-off:≤ −0.32)	256 (50%)	253 (50%)	257 (51%)	217 (55%)
Fibroscan™ (cut-off: 5.6 KPa)	109 (21%)	109 (21%)	120 (24%)	–

Table 3. Characteristics of liver biopsy for each algorithm, when liver biopsy is required, and in the overall population.

	Fibrometer®	Fibrotest®	Hepascore®	Fibroscan™	4 algorithms	Overall
	+ELFG	+ELFG	+ELFG	+ELFG		population
	N = 271	N = 271	N = 259	N = 192	N = 119	N = 507
Length of biopsy (mm)	25.3±8.4	25.1±8.6	25.5±8.6	25.2±8.5	23.9±8.2	25.4±8.5
Number of portal tracts	21.0±8.3	20.7±8.7	21.1±8.7	20.9±8.4	20.3±8.6	20.6±8.4
Discordances between the 2 pathologists for fibrosis staging	N = 78 (29%)	N = 83 (31%)	N = 82 (32%)	N = 59 (31%)	N = 37 (31%)	N = 154 (30.5%)
Number (%) of discordances F1/F2	N = 46 (59%)	N = 47 (57%)	N = 45 (55%)	N = 29 (49%)	N = 20 (54%)	N = 72 (47%)
Consensual review of	30 F1 (65%)	30 F1 (64%)	29 F1 (64%)	20 F1 (69%)	13 F1 (65%)	48 F1 (67%)
	16 F2 (35%)	17 F2 (36%)	16 F2 (36%)	9 F2 (31%)	7 F2 (35%)	24 F2 (33%)

As shown in Figure 2, the better screening strategies for the diagnosis of significant fibrosis in "intention to diagnose" were Fibrometer®, Fibrotest® or Hepascore® in combination with the ELFG score. In "per-protocol analysis" the performance of the combination Fibroscan™+ELFG was similar to those combining two blood tests. The number of avoided liver biopsies varied between 50% and 55%. The diagnostic performance was better in terms of avoided liver biopsies compared to the usual combinations (Fibrometer®, Fibrotest® or Hepascore® plus Fibroscan™). When we added a third test diagnostic performance was not

improved, contrary to previously published results [22]. Our study clearly shows a better diagnostic performance than the SAFE algorithm [15] in terms of the number of avoided liver biopsies. In the "Bordeaux" algorithm [16] the NPV and PPV were lower than with the ELFG algorithm.

The cut-off for ELFG was the same whatever the first test used (−0.32). Several components of ELFG are direct markers of fibrosis and could explain the renewed interest in this test. Indeed, our "Principal Component Analysis" (Figure S2) describing the characteristics of different tests on two dimensions showed that

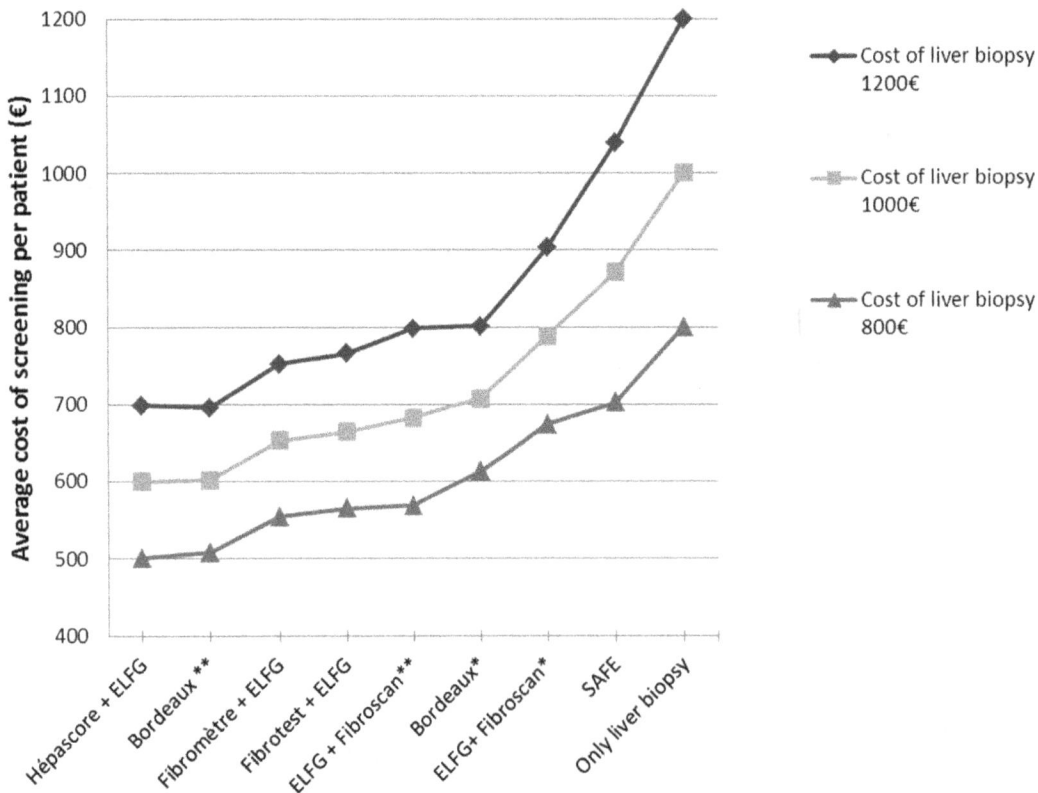

Figure 3. Economic analysis. Average cost of screening per patient (in euros) of the various combinations of tests, taking 3 levels of liver biopsy cost based on published data and the cost in our hospital: 800 Euros, 1,000 Euros and 1,200 Euros. *Cost of Fibroscan, for use equivalent to 10 acts per month. * *Cost of Fibroscan, for use equivalent to 32 acts per month.

ELFG provides different and complementary information to the other blood tests, closer to that of LSM.

In our main study the performance of Fibroscan™ was markedly reduced as results were unavailable or unreliable in more than 20% of cases, whereas the advantage of combining two blood tests for the diagnosis of significant fibrosis was highlighted.

In cases of discordant results, the choice of whether to perform a liver biopsy must be discussed because it is not a perfect "gold standard" [23,24]. Any disagreements between the two pathologists in fibrosis staging were similar for all the combinations and occurred throughout the study population (Table 3). The quality of liver biopsy, the number of septa in the biopsy and the associated histological lesions could not explain these discrepancies. However the consensual review of the biopsy by both pathologists showed that the majority of patients (64–69%) had mild fibrosis (F1) when the discrepancy for staging was F1 or F2.

We also performed a cost-benefit analysis and compared the different strategies. To our knowledge, only one medico-economic study has been published in this field [20]. In that study the cost of liver biopsy was estimated 700 euros and the cost of Fibrotest® was 100 euros in absence of reimbursement by the social security. However the cost of Fibroscan™ was not taken into account and the cost of the Bordeaux algorithm not analyzed. The SAFE strategy was cheaper than other algorithms. In the present study, that includes all blood tests and Fibroscan™, we find the lowest cost strategies include ELFG. This result reinforces the interest of this test, as it is complementary to the others, as seen in the principal component analysis. From an economic perspective, the strategies that include Fibroscan™ seem to be particularly interesting only when the rate of use of Fibroscan™ is high. In other words, a hospital that doesn't have a Fibroscan™ instrument should invest only if the frequency of use will be sufficient to offset the capital outlay.

In conclusion the use of the ELFG score following one of the three validated blood tests shows promise for improving the diagnosis of significant fibrosis in chronic hepatitis C and is cost-economic. Our algorithm using one of the validated blood tests (Fibrotest®, Fibrometer®, Hepascore®) is relatively cheap and ELFG could clearly replace Fibroscan™ allowing liver fibrosis to be staged in all CHC patients, including those who are overweight.

Supporting Information

Figure S1   Other previously published algorithms applied to Fibrostar database.

Figure S2   Principal Component Analysis of the five main tests.

Table S1   Demographic, laboratory, and histological characteristics of the 507 CHC patients having all the blood tests and the 396 CHC patients with all the tests and reliable Fibroscan™.

Text S1   Details of laboratory tests with formulae for the calculation of the scores.

Text S2   Details of calculation of costs for the economic analysis.

Text S3   The ANRS HCEP-23 FIBROSTAR study group.

Acknowledgments

We thank Dr Alison Foote (Grenoble Clinical Research Centre, Inserm CIC03) for critically reading and editing the manuscript with particular attention to English usage. We also thank the members of the ANRS HCEP-23 FIBROSTAR study group, listed in Text S3, for their participation in the main study.

Author Contributions

Conceived and designed the experiments: JPZ NS. Performed the experiments: NS ESZ JG MV. Analyzed the data: ST SDT JM JLB. Contributed reagents/materials/analysis tools: JLB. Wrote the paper: JPZ JG ST JM SDT.

References

1. Adams L, Bulsara M, Rossi E, DeBoer B, Speers D, et al. (2005) Hepascore: an accurate validated predictor of liver fibrosis in chronic hepatitis C infection. Clin Chem 51: 1867–1873.
2. Cales P, Oberti F, Michalak S, Hubert-Fouchard I, Rousselet M-C, et al. (2005) A novel panel of blood markers to assess the degree of liver fibrosis. Hepatology 42: 1373–1381.
3. Imbert-Bismut F, Ratziu V, Pieroni L, Charlotte F, Benhamou Y, et al. (2001) Biochemical markers of liver fibrosis in patients with hepatitis C virus infection: a prospective study. Lancet 357: 1069–1075.
4. Ziol M, Handra-Luca A, Kettaneh A, Christidis C, Mal F, et al. (2005) Noninvasive assessment of liver fibrosis by measurement of stiffness in patients with chronic hepatitis C. Hepatology 41: 48–54.
5. Degos F, Perez P, Roche B, Mahmoudi A, Asselineau J, et al. (2005) Diagnostic accuracy of FibroScan and comparison to liver fibrosis biomarkers in chronic viral hepatitis: A multicenter prospective study (the FIBROSTIC study). J Hepatol 53: 1013–1021.
6. Haute Autorité de Santé (HAS) France (2006) Methods of Assessment of Hepatic Fibrosis during chronic liver disease [Méthodes d'évaluation de la fibrose hépatique au cours des hépatopathies chroniques] Available: http://www.hassante.fr/portail/upload/docs/application/pdf/rapport_fibrose.pdf.
7. Vallet-Pichard A, Mallet V, Nalpas B, Verkarre V, Nalpas A, et al. (2007) FIB-4: an inexpensive and accurate marker of fibrosis in HCV infection, comparison with liver biopsy and fibrotest. Hepatology 46: 32–36.
8. Forns X, Ampurdanes S, Llovet J, Aponte J, Quintó L, et al. (2002) Identification of chronic hepatitis C patients without hepatic fibrosis by a simple predictive model. Hepatology 36: 986–992.
9. Leroy V, Monier F, Bottari S, Trocme C, Sturm N, et al. (2005) Circulating matrix metalloproteinases 1, 2, 9 and their inhibitors TIMP-1 and TIMP-2 as serum markers of liver fibrosis in patients with chronic hepatitis C: comparison with PIIINP and hyaluronic acid. Am J Gastroenterol 99: 271–279.
10. Wai CT, Greenson J, Fontana RJ, Kalbfleisch JD, Marrero JA, et al. (2005) A simple noninvasive index can predict both significant fibrosis and cirrhosis in patients with chronic hepatitis C. Hepatology 38: 518–526.
11. Rosenberg W, Voelker M, Thiel R, Burt A, Schuppan D, et al. (2004) Serum markers detect the presence of liver fibrosis: a cohort study. Gastroenterology 127: 1704–1713.
12. Guechot J, Laudat A, Loria A, Serfaty L, Poupon R, et al. (1996) Diagnostic accuracy of hyaluronan and type III procollagen amino-terminal peptide serum assays as markers of liver fibrosis in chronic viral hepatitis C evaluated by ROC curve analysis. Clin Chem 42: 558–563.
13. Zarski JP, Sturm N, Guechot J, Paris A, Zafrani ES, et al. (2012) Comparison of 9 blood tests and transient elastography for liver fibrosis in chronic hepatitis C: the ANRS HCEP-23 study. J Hepatol 56: 55–62.
14. Sebastiani G, Vario A, Guido M, Noventa F, Plebani M, et al. (2006) Stepwise combination algorithms of non-invasive markers to diagnose significant fibrosis in chronic hepatitis C. J Hepatol 44: 686–693.
15. Sebastiani G (2009) Non-invasive assessment of liver fibrosis in chronic liver diseases: implementation in clinical practice and decisional algorithms. World J Gastroenterol 15: 2190–203.
16. Castera L, Vergniol J, Foucher J, Le Bail B, Chanteloup E, et al. (2005) Prospective comparison of transient elastography, Fibrotest, APRI, and liver biopsy for the assessment of fibrosis in chronic hepatitis C. Gastroenterology 128: 343–350.
17. Castera L, Foucher J, Bernard PH, Carvalho F, Allaix D, et al. (2010) Pitfalls of liver stiffness measurement: a 5-year prospective study of 13,369 examinations. Hepatology 51: 828–835.
18. Tsutsumi M, Takase S, Urashima S, Ueshima Y, Kawahara H, et al. (1996) Serum markers for hepatic fibrosis in alcoholic liver disease: which is the best marker, type III procollagen, type IV collagen, laminin, tissue inhibitor of metalloproteinase, or prolyl hydroxylase? Alcoholism: Clinical and Experimental Research. 20: 1512–1517.

19. Lucidarme D, Foucher J, Le Bail B, Vergniol J, Castera L, et al. (2009) Factors of accuracy of transient elastography (fibroscan) for the diagnosis of liver fibrosis in chronic hepatitis C. Hepatology 49: 1083–1089.

20. Sebastiani G, Halfon P, Castera L, Mangia A, Di Marco D, et al. (2012) Comparison of three algorithms of non-invasive markers of fibrosis in chronic hepatitis C. Aliment Pharmacol Ther 35: 92–104.

21. Quinlan JR (1993) C4.5: Programs for machine learning, Morgan Kaufmann, San Mateo, CA.

22. Bourliere M, Penaranda G, Renou C, Botta-Fridlund D, Tran A, et al. (2006) Validation and comparison of indexes for fibrosis and cirrhosis prediction in chronic hepatitis C patients: proposal for a pragmatic approach classification without liver biopsies. J Viral Hepat 13: 659–670.

23. Bedossa P, Dargere D, Paradis V (2003) Sampling variability of liver fibrosis in chronic hepatitis C, Hepatology 38: 1449–1457.

24. Poynard T, Ingiliz P, Elkrief L, Munteanu M, Lebray P, et al. (2008) Concordance in a world without a gold standard: a new non-invasive methodology for improving accuracy of fibrosis markers. PLoS One 8: 1–8.

Permissions

All chapters in this book were first published in PLOS ONE, by The Public Library of Science; hereby published with permission under the Creative Commons Attribution License or equivalent. Every chapter published in this book has been scrutinized by our experts. Their significance has been extensively debated. The topics covered herein carry significant findings which will fuel the growth of the discipline. They may even be implemented as practical applications or may be referred to as a beginning point for another development.

The contributors of this book come from diverse backgrounds, making this book a truly international effort. This book will bring forth new frontiers with its revolutionizing research information and detailed analysis of the nascent developments around the world.

We would like to thank all the contributing authors for lending their expertise to make the book truly unique. They have played a crucial role in the development of this book. Without their invaluable contributions this book wouldn't have been possible. They have made vital efforts to compile up to date information on the varied aspects of this subject to make this book a valuable addition to the collection of many professionals and students.

This book was conceptualized with the vision of imparting up-to-date information and advanced data in this field. To ensure the same, a matchless editorial board was set up. Every individual on the board went through rigorous rounds of assessment to prove their worth. After which they invested a large part of their time researching and compiling the most relevant data for our readers.

The editorial board has been involved in producing this book since its inception. They have spent rigorous hours researching and exploring the diverse topics which have resulted in the successful publishing of this book. They have passed on their knowledge of decades through this book. To expedite this challenging task, the publisher supported the team at every step. A small team of assistant editors was also appointed to further simplify the editing procedure and attain best results for the readers.

Apart from the editorial board, the designing team has also invested a significant amount of their time in understanding the subject and creating the most relevant covers. They scrutinized every image to scout for the most suitable representation of the subject and create an appropriate cover for the book.

The publishing team has been an ardent support to the editorial, designing and production team. Their endless efforts to recruit the best for this project, has resulted in the accomplishment of this book. They are a veteran in the field of academics and their pool of knowledge is as vast as their experience in printing. Their expertise and guidance has proved useful at every step. Their uncompromising quality standards have made this book an exceptional effort. Their encouragement from time to time has been an inspiration for everyone.

The publisher and the editorial board hope that this book will prove to be a valuable piece of knowledge for researchers, students, practitioners and scholars across the globe.

List of Contributors

David van der Poorten, Mahsa Shahidi, Enoch Tay, Jayshree Sesha, Vikki Ho, Lionel W. Hebbard and Jacob George
Storr Liver Unit, Westmead Millennium Institute, University of Sydney at Westmead Hospital, Sydney, Australia

Mark W. Douglas
Storr Liver Unit, Westmead Millennium Institute, University of Sydney at Westmead Hospital, Sydney, Australia
Centre for Infectious Diseases and Microbiology, Westmead Hospital, Sydney, Australia

Kayla Tran, Duncan McLeod and Jane S. Milliken
Department of Anatomical Pathology, Institute of Clinical Pathology and Medical Research (ICPMR), Westmead Hospital, Sydney, Australia

Morten Ruhwald
Clinical Research Centre, Copenhagen University Hospital, Hvidovre, Copenhagen, Denmark,

Ellen Sloth Andersen
Department of Infectious Diseases, Copenhagen University Hospital, Hvidovre, Copenhagen, Denmark
Department of Infectious Diseases, Copenhagen University Hospital, Rigshospitalet, Copenhagen, Denmark

Nina Weis
Department of Infectious Diseases, Copenhagen University Hospital, Hvidovre, Copenhagen, Denmark
Faculty of Health Sciences, Copenhagen University, Copenhagen, Denmark

Peer Brehm Christensen and Belinda Klemmensen Moessner
Department of Infectious Diseases, Odense University Hospital, Odense, Denmark

Pamela Valva, Juan M. Diaz Carrasco, Elena De Matteo and María Victoria Preciado
Laboratory of Molecular Biology, Pathology Division, Ricardo Gutiérrez Children's Hospital, Buenos Aires, Argentina

Paola Casciato, Adrian Gadano and Omar Galdame
Liver Unit, Hospital Italiano de Buenos Aires, Buenos Aires, Argentina

María Cristina Galoppo
Liver Unit of University of Buenos Aires at Ricardo Gutiérrez Children's Hospital, Buenos Aires, Argentina

Eduardo Mullen
Pathology Division, Hospital Italiano de Buenos Aires, Buenos Aires, Argentina

Verena Bihrer, Oliver Waidmann, Mireen Friedrich-Rust, Nicole Forestier, Simone Susser, Jörg Haupenthal, Martin Welker, Ying Shi, Jan Peveling-Oberhag, Andreas Polta, Michael von Wagner, Christoph Sarrazin, Jörg Trojan, Stefan Zeuzem, Bernd Kronenberger and Albrecht Piiper
Department of Medicine I, University of Frankfurt/M., Frankfurt, Germany

Heinfried H. Radeke
Institute of Pharmacology/ZAFES, University of Frankfurt/M., Frankfurt, Germany

Bevin Gangadharan, Manisha Bapat, Jan Rossa, Robin Antrobus, David Chittenden, Bettina Kampa, Raymond A. Dwek and Nicole Zitzmann
Oxford Antiviral Drug Discovery Unit, Oxford Glycobiology Institute, Department of Biochemistry, University of Oxford, Oxford, United Kingdom

Paul Klenerman
Nuffield Department of Clinical Medicine, University of Oxford, Oxford, United Kingdom

Eleanor Barnes
Nuffield Department of Clinical Medicine, University of Oxford, Oxford, United Kingdom
Oxford NIHR Biomedical Research Centre, The John Radcliffe Hospital, Headington, Oxford, United Kingdom

Peter Bacchetti and Ross Boylan
Department of Epidemiology and Biostatistics, University of California San Francisco, San Francisco, California, United States of America

David L. Thomas
Department of Medicine, Johns Hopkins University, Baltimore, Maryland, United States of America

Jacquie Astemborski
Department of Medicine, Johns Hopkins University, Baltimore, Maryland, United States of America
Department of Epidemiology, Johns Hopkins Bloomberg School of Public Health, Baltimore, Maryland, United States of America

Shruti H. Mehta
Department of Epidemiology, Johns Hopkins Bloomberg School of Public Health, Baltimore, Maryland, United States of America

Hui Shen and Alexander Monto
Department of Medicine, University of California San Francisco, San Francisco, California, United States of America
Division of Gastroenterology, San Francisco Veterans Affairs Medical Center, San Francisco, California, United States of America

Norah A. Terrault
Department of Medicine, University of California San Francisco, San Francisco, California, United States of America
Department of Surgery, University of California San Francisco, San Francisco, California, United States of America

Trevor G. Bell, Euphodia Makondo and Anna Kramvis
Hepatitis Virus Diversity Research Programme, Department of Internal Medicine, University of the Witwatersrand, Johannesburg, South Africa

Neil A. Martinson
Perinatal HIV Research Unit, University of the Witwatersrand, Johannesburg, South Africa
Johns Hopkins University School of Medicine, Baltmore, Maryland, United States of America

Wai-Kay Seto, James Fung, Danny Ka-Ho Wong, John Chi-Hang Yuen and Ivan Fan-Ngai Hung
Department of Medicine, The University of Hong Kong, Queen Mary Hospital, Hong Kong

Ching-Lung Lai and Man-Fung Yuen
Department of Medicine, The University of Hong Kong, Queen Mary Hospital, Hong Kong
State Key Laboratory for Liver Research, The University of Hong Kong, Queen Mary Hospital, Hong Kong

Philip P. C. Ip
Department of Pathology, The University of Hong Kong, Queen Mary Hospital, Hong Kong

Tirumuru Nagaraja, Appakkudal R. Anand and Ramesh K. Ganju
Department of Pathology, Ohio State University Wexner Medical Center, Columbus, Ohio, United States of America

Li Chen and David R. Brigstock
Center for Clinical and Translational Research, The Research Institute at Nationwide Children's Hospital, Columbus, Ohio, United States of America

Anuradha Balasubramanian and Jerome E. Groopman
Division of Experimental Medicine, Beth Israel Deaconess Medical Center, Harvard Medical School, Boston, Massachusetts, United States of America

Kalpana Ghoshal and Samson T. Jacob
Department of Molecular and Cellular Biochemistry, The Ohio State University, Columbus, Ohio, United States of America

Andrew Leask
Schulich School of Medicine and Dentistry, University of Western Ontario, London, Ontario, Canada

Silvia Cermelli and Laura Beretta
Public Health Sciences Division, Fred Hutchinson Cancer Research Center, Seattle, Washington, United States of America

Anna Ruggieri
Public Health Sciences Division, Fred Hutchinson Cancer Research Center, Seattle, Washington, United States of America
Department of Infectious, Parasitic and Immune-Mediated Disease, Istituto Superiore di Sanita`, Roma, Italy

Jorge A. Marrero
Division of Gastroenterology, Department of Internal Medicine, University of Michigan, Ann Arbor, Michigan, United States of America

George N. Ioannou
Division of Gastroenterology, Department of Medicine, Veterans Affairs Puget Sound Health Care System and University of Washington, Seattle, Washington, United States of America

Milan E. Folkers and Cassie A. Nelson
Department of Medicine, University of Utah, Salt Lake City, Utah, United States of America

Don A. Delker and Christopher I. Maxwell
Department of Medicine, University of Utah, Salt Lake City, Utah, United States of America
Huntsman Cancer Institute, University of Utah, Salt Lake City, Utah, United States of America

Curt H. Hagedorn
Department of Medicine, University of Utah, Salt Lake City, Utah, United States of America
Huntsman Cancer Institute, University of Utah, Salt Lake City, Utah, United States of America
Department of Experimental Pathology, University of Utah, Salt Lake City, Utah, United States of America

David A. Nix
Huntsman Cancer Institute, University of Utah, Salt Lake City, Utah, United States of America

Jason J. Schwartz
Department of Surgery, University of Utah, Salt Lake City, Utah, United States of America

Stella M. Martinez
Liver Unit, Hospital Clinic, IDIBAPS and CIBERehd, Barcelona, Spain

Juliette Foucher
Centre d'Investigation de la Fibrose hépatique, Hôpital Haut-Lévêque, CHU Bordeaux, Pessac, France

Jean-Marc Combis
Clinique Ambroise Paré, Toulouse, France

Dominique Capron
Department of Hepato-Gastroenterology, Amiens University Hospital, Amiens, France

Marc Bourlière
Service d'hépato-gastroentérologie, Hôpital Saint-Joseph, Marseille, France

Damien Lucidarme
Service de Pathologie Digestive, Université Nord de France, Groupe Hospitalier de l'Institut Catholique Lillois/Faculté Libre de Médecine Lille, Lille, France

Shan Liu
Department of Management Science and Engineering, Stanford University, Stanford, California, United States of America

Michaël Schwarzinger
Equipe ATIP-AVENIR/UMR-S 738 INSERM, Paris Diderot University, Paris, France

Fabrice Carrat
UMR-S 707 INSERM, Pierre et Marie Curie University, Paris, France

Jeremy D. Goldhaber-Fiebert
Department of Medicine, Center for Health Policy and Center for Primary Care and Outcomes Research, Stanford University, Stanford, California, United States of America

Papa Saliou Mbaye, Adama Ba and Fatou Fall
Department of Hepatology and Gastroenterology, Principal Hospital, Dakar, Senegal

Anna Sarr and Marie-Louise Evra
Department of Hepatology and Gastroenterology, Abass Ndao Hospital, Dakar, Senegal

François Simon
INSERM U941, University of Medicine Paris-Diderot, Saint-Louis Hospital, Paris, France

Jean-Marie Sire
INSERM U941, University of Medicine Paris-Diderot, Saint-Louis Hospital, Paris, France
Medical Laboratory, Pasteur Institute, Dakar, Senegal

Jean Daveiga
Department of Hepatology and Gastroenterology, Saint-Jean de Dieu Hospital, Thies, Senegal

Aboubakry Diallo
Department of Hepatology and Gastroenterology, Grand-Yoff Hospital, Dakar, Senegal

Loic Chartier and Muriel Vray
Epidemiology Unit of Infectious Diseases, Pasteur Institute, INSERM, Paris, France

Beom Kyung Kim
Department of Internal Medicine, Yonsei University College of Medicine, Seoul, Korea
Liver Cirrhosis Clinical Research Center, Yonsei University College of Medicine, Seoul, Korea

Jun Yong Park, Do Young Kim, Chae Yoon Chon and Seung Up Kim
Department of Internal Medicine, Yonsei University College of Medicine, Seoul, Korea,
Institute of Gastroenterology, Yonsei University College of Medicine, Seoul, Korea
Liver Cirrhosis Clinical Research Center, Yonsei University College of Medicine, Seoul, Korea

Kwang-Hyub Han and Sang Hoon Ahn
Department of Internal Medicine, Yonsei University College of Medicine, Seoul, Korea,
Institute of Gastroenterology, Yonsei University College of Medicine, Seoul, Korea
Liver Cirrhosis Clinical Research Center, Yonsei University College of Medicine, Seoul, Korea
Brain Korea 21 Project for Medical Science, Yonsei University College of Medicine, Seoul, Korea

Hyon Suk Kim
Department of Laboratory Medicine, Yonsei University College of Medicine, Seoul, Korea

Young Nyun Park
Department of Pathology, Yonsei University College of Medicine, Seoul, Korea

Wai-Kay Seto, Ching-Lung Lai, James Fung, Danny Ka-Ho Wong and Man-Fung Yuen
Department of Medicine, the University of Hong Kong, Queen Mary Hospital, Hong Kong,

Chun-Fan Lee
Department of Biostatistics, Singapore Clinical Research Institute, Singapore
Center for Quantitative Medicine, Duke-NUS Graduate Medical School, Singapore

Philip P. C. Ip
Department of Pathology, the University of Hong Kong, Queen Mary Hospital, Hong Kong

Daniel Yee-Tak Fong
Department of Nursing Studies, the University of Hong Kong, Queen Mary Hospital, Hong Kong

Benjamin Maasoumy, Kerstin Port, Antoaneta Angelova Markova, Beatriz Calle Serrano,Magdalena Rogalska-Taranta, Lisa Sollik, Carola Mix, Janina Kirschner, Michael P. Manns, Heiner Wedemeyer and Markus Cornberg
Department of Gastroenterology, Hepatology and Endocrinology, Hannover Medical School, Hannover, Germany

Lance D. Presser, Steven McRae and Gulam Waris
Department of Microbiology and Immunology, H.M. Bligh Cancer Research Laboratories, Rosalind Franklin University of Medicine and Science, Chicago Medical School, Chicago, Illinois, United States of America

Jean-Pierre Zarski
Hepato-Gastroenterology Clinic, DIGIDUNE Pole, Grenoble University Hospital, Grenoble, France
INSERM/UJF U823 IAPC unit, Institut Albert Bonniot, Grenoble, France

Nathalie Sturm
INSERM/UJF U823 IAPC unit, Institut Albert Bonniot, Grenoble, France
Department of Pathological Anatomy and Cytology, Biology Pole, Grenoble University Hospital, Grenoble, France

Jérôme Guechot and Michel Vaubourdolle
Biochemistry A Laboratory, Saint Antoine Hospital, Assistance Publique-Hôpitaux de Paris, Paris, France

Elie-Serge Zafrani
Pathology Department, Henri Mondor Hospital Center, Assistance Publique-Hôpitaux de Paris, Paris Est Creteil University, Créteil, France

Sophie Thoret, Jennifer Margier and Jean-Luc Bosson
UJF-Grenoble 1/CNRS/Clinical Research Centre-Inserm CIC03/TIMC-IMAG UMR 5525/Themas, Grenoble University Hospital, Grenoble, France

Sandra David-Tchouda
Medical-Economics unit, Clinical Research Administration, Grenoble University Hospital, Grenoble, France

Index

www.ingramcontent.com/pod-product-compliance
Lightning Source LLC
Chambersburg PA
CBHW080255230326
41458CB00097B/5007